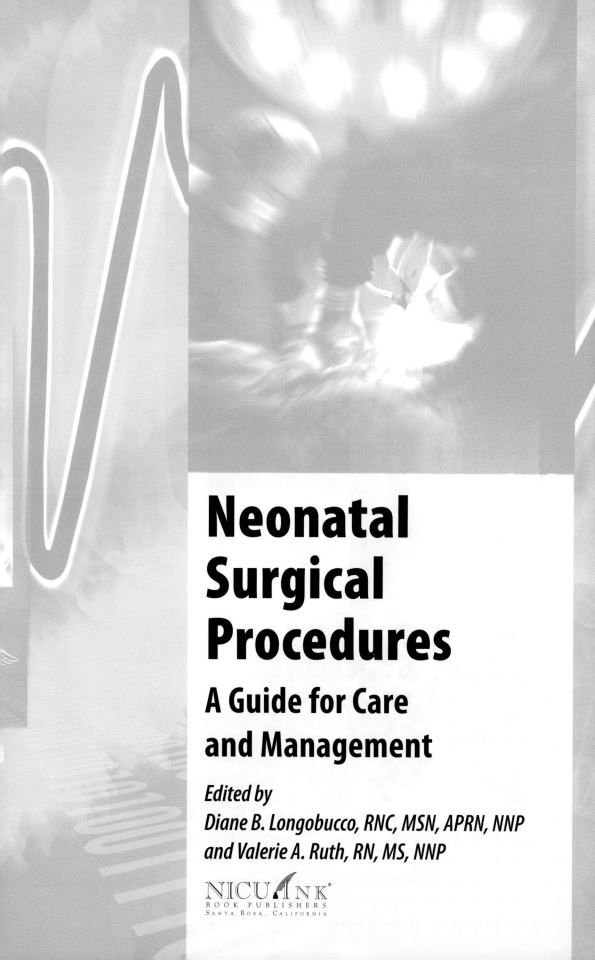

Neonatal Surgical Procedures

A Guide for Care and Management

Edited by
Diane B. Longobucco, RNC, MSN, APRN, NNP
and Valerie A. Ruth, RN, MS, NNP

NICU Ink®
BOOK PUBLISHERS
SANTA ROSA, CALIFORNIA

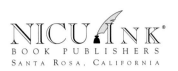

BOOK PUBLISHERS
SANTA ROSA, CALIFORNIA

Copyright © 2007 by NICU Ink®

Editor-in-Chief: Charles Rait, RN, MSEd, PNC

Managing Editor: Suzanne G. Rait, RN

Editorial Coordinator: Tabitha Parker

Editors: Beverley DeWitt, BA
Debbie Fraser Askin, RNC, MN
Sylvia Stein Wright, BA

Reviewers: Linda Helene Genen, MD, MPH, FAAP
Jeanne M. Giebe, RNC, MSN, NNP
Carol M. Greene, RN, MSN, CRNP

Continuing Education Course Content: Debbie Fraser Askin, RNC, MN

Continuing Education Course Reviewers: Angela Burd, RNC, MSN, CCNS
Lori Jackson, RNC, ND, CCRN, NNP
Maria A. Lofgren, MSN, ARNP, APN
Jeanne M. Perino, RN, BSN, NNP
Ruth Snyder, RNC, BSN
Laurel Vessey, RN, BSN

Proofreader: Joanne Gosnell, BA

Indexer: Gerry Lynn Shipe, BSN, MBA

Medical Illustrators: Elizabeth Weadon Massari, MSMI, CMI
Briar Lee Mitchell, MA

Book Design and Composition: Marsha Godfrey Graphics

LIBRARY OF CONGRESS CATALOGING-IN-PUBLICATION DATA

Neonatal surgical procedures : a guide for care and management /
[edited by] Diane B. Longobucco, Valerie A. Ruth.
   p. ; cm.
  Includes bibliographical references and index.
  ISBN-13: 978-1-887571-16-6 (pbk.)
  ISBN-10: 1-887571-16-7 (pbk.)
  1. Newborn infants--Surgery. 2. Pediatric nursing. I.
Longobucco, Diane B., 1962- II. Ruth, Valerie A., 1963-
  [DNLM: 1. Infant, Newborn, Diseases--surgery. 2. Surgical
Procedures, Operative--nursing. 3. Infant, Newborn. 4. Neonatal
Nursing--methods. 5. Perioperative Nursing--methods. WY 161 N4386 2007]
  RD137.5.N46 2007
  617.9'8--dc22   2006039636

Table of Contents

Contributors vii

Acknowledgments ix

Foreword xi

Introduction xiii

Section 1

1 Neonatal Surgical Disorders of the Head, Ears, Eyes, Nose and Throat **1**

Embryology 1

Arteriovenous Malformation 8

Cystic Hygroma 11

Retinopathy of Prematurity 16

Pharyngeal (Branchial) Arch Anomalies 25

Choanal Atresia 28

Cleft Lip and Palate 31

Robin Sequence 37

Laryngomalacia 39

Laryngeal Web 42

Vocal Cord Paralysis 45

Tracheomalacia 47

Craniosynostosis 49

2 Neonatal Pulmonary Disorders **59**

Embryology 59

Congenital Lobar Emphysema 64

Bronchogenic Cyst 68

Congenital Cystic Adenomatoid Malformation 70

Bronchopulmonary Sequestration 76

Pulmonary Lymphangiectasia 84

Congenital Diaphragmatic Hernia 87

Eventration of the Diaphragm 94

Chylothorax 97

Pneumothorax, Pulmonary Intersitial Emphysema, Pneumomediastinum, and Pneumopericardium 101

Nursing Considerations for Neonatal Pulmonary Disorders 106

3 Neonatal Cardiovascular Surgical Conditions **113**

Embryology 114

Prenatal Diagnosis of Congenital Heart Disease 117

Neonatal Diagnosis of Congenital Heart Disease 117

Patent Ductus Arteriosus 121

Tetralogy of Fallot 124

D-Transposition of the Great Arteries 128

Hypoplastic Left Heart Syndrome...131

Total Anomalous Pulmonary Venous Connection............................134

Postoperative Nursing Care...136

4 Neonatal Gastrointestinal Surgical Conditions 141

Embryology...141

Esophageal Atresia and Tracheoesophageal Fistula 146

Gastroesophageal Reflux..151

Gastroschisis...155

Omphalocele 158

Pyloric Stenosis..160

Intestinal Atresia and Stenosis 162

Meconium Ileus..164

Malrotation/Volvulus...166

Hirschsprung's Disease 169

Necrotizing Enterocolitis 171

Anorectal Malformations...175

Inguinal Hernia 181

5 Surgical Conditions of the Liver, Gallbladder, and Biliary Apparatus 189

Embryology...190

Biliary Atresia 190

Neuroblastoma 203

6 Genitourinary Surgical Conditions 217

Embryology...217

Physiology..227

Posterior Urethral Valves..240

Torsion of the Testicle..252

Patent Urachus (of Any Degree) 255

Bladder Exstrophy (Classic)...260

Cloacal Exstrophy...271

Megaureter 279

Prune Belly Syndrome 287

Ureteropelvic Junction Obstruction 294

Ovarian Cysts 303

Newborn Circumcision 309

7 Neurosurgical Conditions 321

Embryology...321

Neurologic Physiology..325

Hydrocephalus and Posthemorrhagic Hydrocephalus.....................326

Myelomeningocele (Spina Bifida) 335

Tethered Cord 340

Spinal Dimples and Sinuses 342

Encephalocele 345

Skull Fracture 348

Extra- and Intracranial Hemorrhage 351

Traumatic Spinal Cord Injury 356

Ethical Considerations 360

8 Surgical Repair of Defects and Injuries of the Extremities in the Neonatal Period 363

Embryology 363

Intrinsic and Extrinsic Limb Reduction Defects 368

Amniotic Band Syndrome 373

Absent Radius 378

Talipes Equinovarus (Clubfoot) 382

Developmental Dysplasia of the Hip 391

Brachial Plexus Injuries 400

Section 2

9 Fluid, Electrolyte, and Nutritional Management of the Postsurgical Neonate 413

General Principles 413

Fluid and Electrolyte Disturbances in Infants with Specific Conditions 426

Fluid and Electrolyte Management 428

Nutritional Management 434

10 Assessment and Management of Postoperative Pain 441

Incidence of Pain in the NICU 441

The Clinical Significance of Pain Management 441

Standards of Practice 442

Assessment of Pain 443

Nonpharmacologic Approaches to Pain Management 445

Pharmacologic Approaches to Pain Management 446

Pain Management for Procedures 454

Parent Education 454

11 Skin Care After Surgical Intervention 457

Anatomy and Embryology 457

Healing of the Skin 461

General Management 462

Treatment of Injured Skin 466

Care of Surgical Wounds Healing by Primary Closure 468

Care of Open Surgical Wounds Healing by Secondary Intention 469

Ostomy Care in the Newborn 469

12 Transport of the Surgical Infant 479

Transport Team Composition and Operation 479

Physiologic Stresses of Transport 484

Dispatch of the Transport Team 489

Care of the Neonate During Transport. 489

Additional Transport Team Responsibilities 498

Transport Equipment and Medications 501

Transport Team Communication. 504

Transport Safety 504

Quality Assurance for Transport. 506

13 Support for the Family of the Surgical Infant. 509

Implementing Culturally Competent, Family-Centered Care 509

Understanding Grief and Loss in the Perinatal/Neonatal Period 516

Section 3

14 Fetal Surgery. 523

Patient Selection for Fetal Intervention 523

Fetal Congenital Diaphragmatic Hernia 525

Congenital Cystic Adenomatoid Malformation 528

Sacrococcygeal Teratoma 530

Myelomeningocele 533

Giant Neck Masses 535

Obstructive Uropathy. 537

Maternal and Fetal Management 540

The Fetal Diagnosis and Treatment Center 541

Future Directions 542

Appendices

A Tracheostomy 547

B Extracorporeal Membrane Oxygenation. 553

C Broviac Insertion 561

D Gastrostomy Tube Placement 563

E Infant Pain Scales 571

F Glossary. 575

G Table of Abbreviations. 587

Index. 591

Continuing Education Course Instructions 664

Contributing Authors

Barbara Bratton, RNC, MS, PNP
University of California Children's Hospital, San Francisco, California

Donna L. Buchanan, APRN, MS, NNP
University of Connecticut Health Center
John Dempsey Hospital, Farmington, Connecticut

Annette Carley, RN, MS, PNP, NNP
University of California, San Francisco, San Francisco, California

Cheryl A. Carlson, RNC, MS, NNP
Children's Hospital
Medical University of South Carolina, Charleston, South Carolina

Alison Kirse Coit, MN, ARNP
Pediatrix Medical Group
Swedish Medical Center, Seattle, Washington

Terese M. Donovan, RNC, MS
University of Connecticut Health Center, Farmington, Connecticut

Kim Friddle, RNC, BSN, BC
Primary Children's Medical Center, Salt Lake City, Utah

Lori J. Howell, RN, MS
The Children's Hospital of Philadelphia, Philadelphia, Pennsylvania

Carol M. Johnson, RN, MSN, CNNP
South Western Arizona Neonatology, Yuma, Arizona

Katherine M. Jorgensen, RNC, MSN/MBA, HonD
Medical University of South Carolina, Charleston, South Carolina
Neonatal Nurse Consultant, KMJ Consulting, Inc., Daniel Island, South Carolina

Tracy Karp, RNC, MS, NNP
Intermountain Healthcare
Primary Children's Medical Center, LDS Hospital, Salt Lake City, Utah

Diane B. Longobucco, RNC, MSN, APRN, NNP
St. Francis Hospital and Medical Center, Hartford, Connecticut

Brenda Lykins, RNC, BSN
Neonatal Nurse Consultant, DuPont, Washington

Nan Nicholes, RNC, MS
Primary Children's Medical Center, Salt Lake City, Utah

Paula Peterson, MS, CPNP
Primary Children's Medical Center, Salt Lake City, Utah

Valerie A. Ruth, RN, MS, NNP
Lucile Packard Children's Hospital
Stanford University Medical Center, Palo Alto, California

Julieanne Schiefelbein, RNC, MAppSc, MA(Ed), RNM, CPNP, CCRN, NNP
Primary Children's Medical Center, Salt Lake City, Utah

Nancy Shaw, MS, NNP
Primary Children's Medical Center, Salt Lake City, Utah

Erica Siddell, PhD, RN
Formerly with Manchester Memorial Hospital, Manchester, Connecticut

Ellen Tappero, RNC, MN, NNP
Neonatology Associates, Ltd., Phoenix, Arizona

Laura Udy, RNC, BSN
Primary Children's Medical Center, Salt Lake City, Utah

Marlene Walden, PhD, RNC, CCNS, NNP
Texas Children's Hospital, Houston, Texas

Judith West, RN, MN, DNS
University of California, San Francisco, San Francisco, California

Tracy M. Widmer, CRNP, MS
Children's Hospital of Philadelphia, Philadelphia, Pennsylvania

Catherine Witt, RNC, MS, NNP
Presbyterian/St. Luke's Medical Center, Denver, Colorado

Sandra Young, RNC, MN, NNP
Calgary Health Region, Alberta, Canada

Jeanette Zaichkin, RNC, MN
Neonatal Nursing Consultant, Olympia, Washington

Acknowledgments

The authors are indebted to the following persons who have contributed to the making of this book in their own unique and invaluable ways.

To my husband, Mario, children, Alyssa and Brett, and parents, Renee and William Blanchette. You have given me never-ending support and encouragement in my career as it has evolved. Thanks for believing in me. I love you "to the moon and back." To my Sitto, who made me feel like the best nurse on earth...I love you and miss you.

To Valerie Ruth. Thank you for pursuing me as an author and coeditor and for allowing me to be part of your "baby." It has been an experience I will never forget.

Thank you also to Joseph Pallis, Susan Arcata, and Catherine Posteraro for your assistance in finding me references, books, manuscripts, and whatever else I needed in a most timely way. I could not have done this easily without your help.

In special memory of Sara Oblon, Tina Wieselberg, Betsy Christenson, and Peter Kurtis. Your years of dedication to neonatal medicine and to our unit is sadly missed, but never forgotten.

Diane

This book would never have been completed without the persistence of Diane Longobucco. You really came through for all of us. Thank you.

I am grateful to the many people who have supported me in my work and development. My father, Joseph, has given me many strengths, especially his instinct for survival. My dear friend, Wes, has shown me that it is possible to live what you speak and give from the heart. And most importantly, my children, Jordan and Will, have kept life wild, wonderful, and fun, even in the midst of hard work. You are always in my heart.

In loving memory of my mother, Joan, and my sister, Debbie, who continue to influence me from within.

Valerie

*T*hank you to all of the authors for your hard work and continued dedication to the project over these years. You are all invaluable to the specialty of neonatal nursing and have so much professional expertise to offer. We are honored you chose to share it with us.

Thanks to Tabitha Parker, whose help, guidance, and organization with editing and putting it all together will never be forgotten. You are truly the most organized person we know.

Debbie Fraser Askin, thank you for all the work you have done behind the scenes, helping to organize the content of the chapters and making sure each topic was covered thoroughly. Your help came along when we needed it most!

A special thanks to Suzanne Rait, "the editor to the editor," for your mentoring and support. Without your encouragement, this project would never have reached fruition. Words cannot express the gratitude for all that you have done both personally and professionally. What started out as a project has ended as a friendship, and we thank you.

And last, but not least, special thanks to Chuck Rait, who believed in and supported this project from the beginning. Your kind heart and easy manner helped to mentor us in the process of developing, writing and publishing this book as new editors. Thank you for giving us this opportunity and for continuing to contribute to neonatal nursing through your conferences, organizations, and publications. You are truly a role model for all.

This book is dedicated to our colleagues at the many institutions that supported our professional development and this work: Saint Francis Hospital and Medical Center, Hartford, Connecticut; University of California San Francisco, San Francisco, California; Encino-Tarzana Regional Medical Center, Encino, California; Good Samaritan Hospital and Medical Center, San Jose, California; and Lucile Packard Children's Hospital at Stanford University Medical Center, Stanford, California.

It is our hope that the knowledge you acquire through reading and using this book will be passed on to the next generation of neonatal nurses and improve the care of the tiny miracles entrusted to us.

Diane and Valerie

Foreword

Although surgeons have treated neonates successfully for decades, only recently has significant progress been made in the improvement in outcome of these fragile infants. Certainly, the discovery and utilization of antimicrobical agents beginning in the late 1930s benefited these patients; but I believe that five important advances have been responsible for the overall improvement in the successful management of surgical neonates.

The first was the development and refinement of supportive ventilation for infants with respiratory failure. It was initially utilized for infants with primary lung disease, but its use with surgically correctable lesions followed immediately. Adding end positive pressure to intermittent positive or negative pressure ventilation further enhanced the use of ventilation in infants requiring surgery. As newer and more sophisticated machines and applications, such as high frequency ventilation, were developed, their use in neonates with surgical disorders improved.

The second advance was the development and progressive improvement of neonatal intravenous nutrition. Although this approach was attempted in the late 1930s, not until the late 1960s and early 1970s had pediatric surgeons demonstrated the feasibility of infusing 20 percent dextrose solutions combined with protein hydrolysates into major blood vessels, thereby providing adequate caloric and protein intake to ensure the growth of these infants. Refinements in the type of amino acids and the development of intravenous fat preparations and careful monitoring techniques further improved the patient's nutritional balance.

The third was the dramatic advancement of imaging techniques that enabled physicians to rapidly recognize and accurately identify various pathologic conditions and to respond more readily by providing appropriate therapeutic measures.

The fourth was the development of techniques to measure chemistries and blood gases in microquantity amounts of blood and serum.

The last was the development of intensive care nurseries, which supplanted the "premature infant care centers." This arena allowed infants with various disorders to be cared for in a "state of the art" environment that presented an opportunity for investigators to carry out innovative clinical studies as well. Simultaneously, there was the emergence of a cadre of nurses who were dedicated to the care of critically ill infants and who were able to recognize and respond to their needs. The interaction that occurred with nurses working in close contact with physicians allowed each to educate the other and, by doing so, decrease the mortality and morbidity rates of infants significantly. This camaraderie was unique, has continued to thrive, and is the basis of successful intensive care units.

The editors and contributors of this text have exemplified and encompassed the major aspects of neonatal surgical care. Each of the chapters discussing the various organ systems begins with the embryology of that system, enhancing the understanding of the developmental abnormalities that occur. Various forms of therapy and their alternatives are clearly presented as well. The chapters on skin care; assessment and management of pain; fluid, electrolyte, and nutritional management; and family-oriented care also enhance the quality of the text.

This text is a wonderful example of the very best in nursing thought and nursing care. Every nurse who cares for infants in an intensive care environment should have this text as part of his or her armamentarium.

Philip Sunshine, MD
Professor of Pediatrics
Division of Neonatal and Developmental Medicine
Stanford University School of Medicine
Palo Alto, California

Introduction

$\mathcal{T}$he impetus for writing this book, which began many years ago, was the need for a concise resource on neonatal surgical procedures that emphasized the care and management as well as the clinical presentation of surgical conditions. Thus, the idea was to create a bedside reference that would not only augment the surgical team's expertise, but also be a place from which the bedside clinician could prepare the staff, infant, and family for what the surgical procedure entailed.

This book is the culmination of the efforts of many people. Author selection was based on representation of geographical regions as well as professional expertise in order to provide the very best and least biased information on the broad scope of surgical procedures addressed. Nurse authors represent a variety of neonatal clinical specialties and geographical regions with the hope that this would limit any geographical bias.

The book was written with the goal of providing a comprehensive overview of neonatal surgical procedures. It is our hope that it is organized in a way that provides the bedside clinician with valuable information in a manner that is easy to locate and read. It is written in outline format to provide the information in a concise manner for easy reference. It is intended to provide a general knowledge base from which surgical correction and medical and nursing management can be understood. The limitations of the book include the rapid advancement of medical practice and surgical technology as well as the nuances of individual practice. The text addresses surgical conditions as they pertain to each body system. This information will provide a basis for the embryology, pathophysiology, diagnosis, surgical management, and nursing management of each condition. Although each chapter is separately authored, all are organized in a similar format. Section 1 begins with a discussion of the many surgical conditions by systems, in a head-to-toe approach. Specific management of fluids, pain control, skin care, transport of the surgical infant, and family support are discussed in Section 2. Section 3 discusses fetal surgery. The text concludes with appendices that provide resource information on tracheostomy, ECMO, broviac insertion, gastrostomy tube, and infant pain scales. A glossary of important terms, a detailed cross-referenced index, and a continuing education test conclude the book. Photographs, illustrations, and figures are included throughout the text to enhance understanding of embryology, pathophysiology, and surgical management.

Although we understand that this book will not eliminate the need for those trips to the library, Internet, or office to sift through those hefty surgical textbooks or for those up-to-the-minute articles in this rapidly evolving medical arena, we hope that it will provide a foundation for management of the surgical neonate.

Diane B. Longobucco, RNC, MSN, APRN, NNP

Valerie A. Ruth, RN, MS, NNP

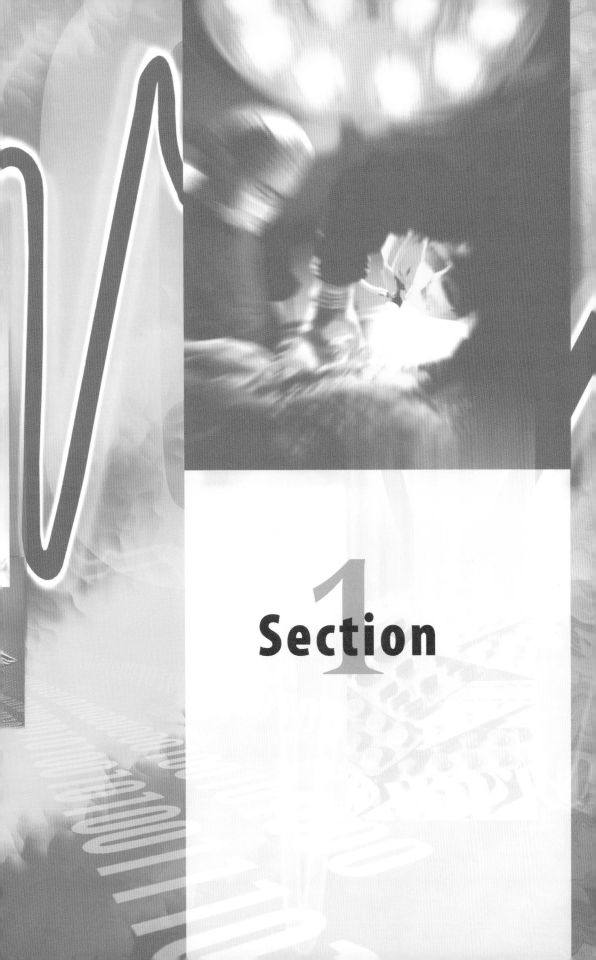

Section 1

Neonatal Surgical Disorders of the Head, Ears, Eyes, Nose, and Throat

Valerie A. Ruth, RN, MS, NNP

There are many anomalies of the head and neck region that may require surgical intervention or repair in the neonatal period. These are discussed in this chapter. Anomalies range from congenital malformations to acquired defects either because of birth trauma or as a complication of prematurity. Diagnosis, the most commonly described and current surgical procedure for repair, postoperative complications, and nursing interventions are discussed. A better understanding of these defects and their surgical repair can aid the clinician in preoperative and postoperative management, as well as in anticipating potential complications.

Embryology

OVERVIEW

A. The human embryo develops rapidly in the first weeks following conception.
   1. The embryonic disc, which develops in the second week of gestation, consists of three layers of cells:
      a. The outer ectoderm
      b. The mesoderm
      c. The inner endoderm
   2. These layers of cells give rise to the tissues and structures that will form the fetus.
B. The structural components of the head and neck develop between the third and eighth week after conception.
C. This section briefly reviews the development of the major structures of the head and neck.

TABLE 1-1 ■ Structures Derived From Pharyngeal Arch Components

Arch	Nerve	Muscles	Skeletal Structures	Ligaments
First (mandibular)	Trigeminal* (CN V)	Muscles of mastication† Mylohyoid and anterior belly of digastric Tensor tympani Tensor veli palatini	Malleus Incus	Anterior ligament of malleus Sphenomandibular ligament
Second (hyoid)	Facial (CN VII)	Muscles of facial expression‡ Stapedius Stylohyoid Posterior belly of digastric	Stapes Styloid process Lesser cornu of hyoid Upper part of body of hyoid bone	Stylohyoid ligament
Third	Glossopharyngeal (CN IX)	Stylopharyngeus	Greater cornu of hyoid Lower part of body of hyoid bone	
Fourth and sixth§	Superior laryngeal branch of vagus (CN X) Recurrent laryngeal branch of vagus (CN X)	Cricothyroid Levator veli palatini Constrictors of pharynx Intrinsic muscles of larynx Striated muscles of esophagus	Thyroid cartilage Cricoid cartilage Arytenoid cartilage Corniculate cartilage Cuneiform cartilage	

CN = cranial nerve

*The ophthalmic division CN V does not supply any pharyngeal arch components.

†Temporalis, masseter, medial, and lateral pterygoids.

‡Buccinator, auricularis, frontalis, platysma, orbicularis oris, and orbicularis oculi.

§The fifth pharyngeal arch is often absent. When present, it is rudimentary and usually has no recognizable cartilage bar. The cartilaginous components of the fourth and sixth arches fuse to form the cartilages of the larynx.

From: Moore KL, and Persaud TVN. 2003. *The Developing Human: Clinically Oriented Embryology*, 7th ed. Philadelphia: Saunders, 207. Reprinted by permission.

WEEK 3[1-5]

A. The central nervous system and rudimentary heart are among the first recognizable structures to develop.
   1. The nervous system arises from a thickening of the ectoderm known as the neural plate.
   2. Elevations of ectodermal tissue, the neural folds, develop along a central groove in the neural plate.
   3. The folds fuse at the junction of the future brain and spinal cord, creating the neural tube and the major divisions of the brain:
      a. Forebrain
      b. Midbrain
      c. Hindbrain
B. Ectodermal cells next to the neural fold form the neural crest cells, which migrate throughout the embryo.
   1. Most connective and skeletal tissue is derived from neural crest cells.
   2. Neural crest cells migrate to the area of the future head and neck.

WEEK 4[1-5]

A. The pharyngeal (branchial) arches form on either side of the foregut.
   1. Neural crest cells migrate into the developing arches, causing the arches to enlarge. The arches:
      a. Consist of a core of mesenchyme tissue

      b. Are covered on the outside by ectoderm

      c. Are covered inside by a layer of endodermal tissue

  2. These arches give rise to structures of the head and neck.

      a. The structures appear as rounded ridges on each side of the head and neck that are separated by pharyngeal grooves.[3,5]

         1) They develop into deep clefts (pharyngeal clefts)[4]

         2) Pharyngeal pouches or outpocketings develop at the same time.[4]

  3. Each arch is composed of:[1]

      a. An aortic arch—a blood vessel arising from the primordial heart

      b. A cartilaginous rod that forms the skeletal structures of the arch

      c. A muscle component

      d. A nerve

  4. Initially, four pairs of pharyngeal arches are visible.

      a. Table 1-1 provides a listing of structures derived from these arches.

  5. The arches are separated from each other by fissures known as pharyngeal grooves.

      a. Four pharyngeal grooves form on each side of the head and neck area from 4–5 weeks.[3,4]

      b. The first groove becomes the external auditory meatus.

      c. The other grooves are eventually obliterated.

  6. Pharyngeal pouches, balloon-like diverticuli, are also found between each arch.

      a. There are four well-developed pairs of pouches; the fifth is undeveloped.

      b. A portion of the first pharyngeal pouch forms:

         1) Tympanic membrane

         2) Middle ear cavity

         3) Eustachian tube

      c. The second pharyngeal pouch forms:

         1) Tonsillar sinus

         2) Palatine tonsil

         3) Tonsillar crypts

         4) Lymphatic nodules

      d. The third pharyngeal pouch forms:[3–5]

         1) Inferior parathyroid gland

         2) Thymus

      e. The fourth pharyngeal pouch includes the fifth pharyngeal pouch and forms:[3,4]

         1) Superior parathyroid gland

         2) Ultimobranchial body[4]

         3) Parafollicular cells (C cells) that produce calcitonin

  7. Many congenital anomalies in these regions are the result of the failure of these apparatus to transform into the adult derivatives. Examples of these anomalies include:[3,5]

      a. Robin sequence

      b. DiGeorge syndrome

      c. Treacher Collins syndrome

B. The face starts to form.

  1. Facial development begins early in the fourth week when five primordia appear around the stomodeum, arising mainly from mesenchyme of the first pharyngeal arch.[4,5]

FIGURE 1-1 ■ Cervical sinus to branchial cyst.

A. Lateral view of the head, neck, and thoracic regions of a 5-week embryo, showing the cervical sinus that is normally present at this stage. **B.** Horizontal section of the embryo, at the level shown in A, illustrating the relationship of the cervical sinus to the pharyngeal arches and pouches. **C.** Diagrammatic sketch of the adult pharyngeal and neck regions, indicating the former sites of openings of the cervical sinus and pharyngeal pouches. The *broken lines* indicate possible courses of branchial fistulas. **D.** Similar sketch showing the embryologic basis of various types of branchial sinus. **E.** Drawing of a branchial fistula resulting from persistence of parts of the second pharyngeal groove and second pharyngeal pouch. **F.** Sketch showing possible sites of branchial cysts and openings of branchial sinuses and fistulas. A branchial vestige is also illustrated.

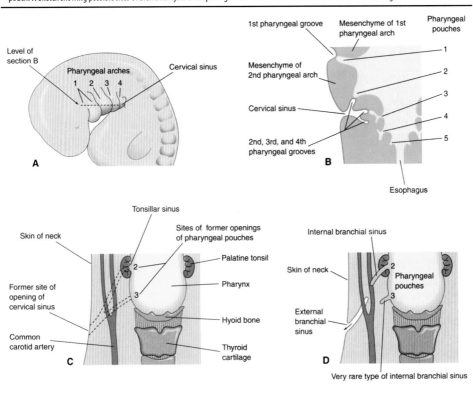

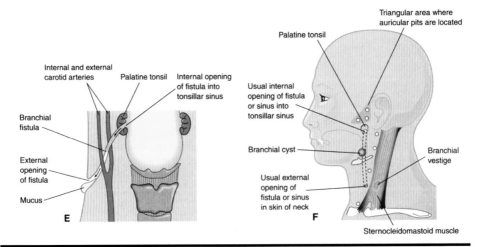

From: Moore KL, and Persaud TVN. 2003. *The Developing Human: Clinically Oriented Embryology,* 7th ed. Philadelphia: Saunders, 213. Reprinted by permission.

      a. Frontonasal prominence, which forms:[3]
        1) Optic vesicles that form the eyes
        2) Forehead
        3) Dorsum and apex of the nose
        4) Nasal septum
        5) Primordial mouth and nose
      b. Paired maxillary prominences, which form:
        1) Upper cheek
        2) Most of upper lip
      c. Paired mandibular prominences, which form:[3]
        1) Chin
        2) Mandible
        3) Lower lip
        4) Lower cheek

  2. The beginning of the lenses, termed the *lens placodes,* are seen on the sides of the head in the area of the optic disc.
  3. Nasal placodes deepen to form the olfactory groove and the nasal pits (which will become the anterior nares).
  4. Development of the tongue begins with a medial swelling and two lateral lingual swellings.[3-5]
  5. Distal tongue buds develop on each side, increase in size, merge, overgrow the median tongue bud, and form the oral part of the tongue.[3-5]
  6. Differentiation of structures is dependent on epithelial mesenchymal interactions.

C. The first endocrine gland to develop, the thyroid gland, appears during the fourth week as the thyroid primordium.[3,5]
  1. As the embryo grows, the thyroid gland descends in the neck.[4]
  2. The thyroglossal duct develops as the thyroid gland descends in the neck.
  3. This is a connection to the tongue, but the connection later disappears.[3-5]

WEEK 5[1-5]

A. Muscles of mastication develop from the first pharyngeal arch.

B. The second pharyngeal arch enlarges.
  1. It overgrows the third and fourth arches and forms a depression known as the cervical sinus (Figure 1-1A).
  2. It gives rise to the muscles of facial expression.

C. The lens placodes fold inward and close within the optic discs.
  1. The optic stalk begins to form the optic nerve.
  2. The retina begins to form in the optic cup.

D. The maxillary prominences begin to fuse with the caudal end of the medial nasal prominences.
  1. Deepening nasal pits become nasal sacs.[3-5]
  2. The oronasal membrane initially separates the nasal sacs from the oral cavity (primitive choanae) until this membrane ruptures, allowing communication between the nasal and oral cavities (definitive choanae).[5]
  3. Elevations on lateral walls of the nasal cavity form the superior, middle, and inferior conchae.[3,5]
  4. Ectoderm epithelium in the roof of each nasal cavity form olfactory receptor cells.
     a. Axons of these cells form olfactory nerves and olfactory bulbs.[3,5]

5. Paranasal sinuses form as outgrowths of the lateral nasal wall.
   a. These become air-filled extensions of the nasal cavities that develop after birth.
   b. These sinuses define the size and shape of the face and add resonance to the voice.[5]
E. Development of the cranium begins as the mesenchyme surrounding the primitive brain forms a capsule (Figure 1-2).

WEEK 6[1-5]

A. The nasal processes begin to fuse, forming the tip of the nose, frenulum, and palate.
   1. These structures shift to a more ventral position.
   2. The maxillary process and the medial nasal fold fuse to form the nostril.
B. Palatogenesis begins toward the end of the fifth week and is complete by the twelfth week, with weeks 6–9 being the critical point in development.[3,5]
   1. The primary palate arises early in week 6, as a mass of mesoderm between the maxillary prominences.[3,5]
   2. The secondary palate develops from the lateral palatine processes that project from the maxillary prominences.
      a. These structures gradually grow toward each other and fuse.
      b. They also fuse with the primary palate and nasal septum beginning in week 6 and ending in week 12 (failure to fuse results in cleft palate).[3-5]
C. Neural crest cells on the edge of the lens differentiate to form the sclera and cornea, and the beginnings of the eyelids appear.
D. Several swellings, the auricular hillocks, form around the pharyngeal groove and give rise to the structures of the external ear.
   1. The ears first form low on the side of the neck and gradually move up with further development of the face.
E. The third pharyngeal pouch differentiates, forming the inferior parathyroid gland and the thymus gland.
F. The superior parathyroid gland is derived from a portion of the fourth pharyngeal pouch.

WEEK 7[1-5]

A. The second, third, and fourth pharyngeal grooves and the cervical sinus have disappeared, giving the neck a smooth appearance.
B. The tip of the nose and the external ear are recognizable.
C. The eyelids become prominent.

WEEK 8[1-5]

A. The facial fissures have now closed, giving the embryo a more human-like facial appearance.
B. The upper and lower jaws have now formed.
C. The eyes are beginning to move medially as the skull shape changes.
   1. Eyelid development continues with fusion of the upper and lower lids beginning.
   2. The conjunctival sac and lacrimal ducts develop.
D. The nasal area and upper lip become better defined.
   1. Nasal cartilage appears above the nose.
   2. Ossification centers appear in the premaxillary and maxillary regions.

FIGURE 1-2 ■ Diagrams illustrating stages in the development of the cranium.

Views of the base of the developing cranium, viewed superiorly (A to C), and laterally (D), are illustrated. **A.** Six weeks, showing the various cartilages that will fuse to form the chondrocranium. **B.** Seven weeks, after fusion of some of the paired cartilages. **C.** Twelve weeks, showing the cartilaginous base of the cranium or chondrocranium formed by the fusion of various cartilages. **D.** Twenty weeks, indicating the derivation of the bones of the fetal cranium.

☐ Cartilaginous neurocranium   ☐ Membranous neurocranium   ☐ Cartilaginous viscerocranium   ■ Membranous viscerocranium

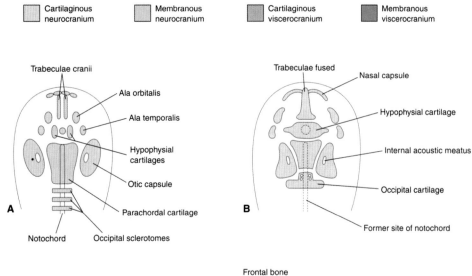

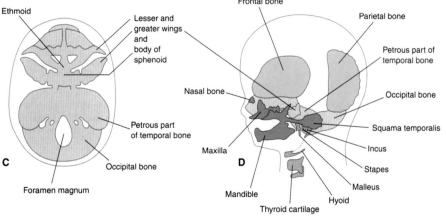

From: Moore KL, and Persaud TVN. 2003. *Before We Are Born: Essentials of Embryology and Birth Defects,* 6th ed. Philadelphia. Saunders, 314. Reprinted by permission.

E. Ossification of the skull is ongoing during this week.
   1. Membranous ossification takes place within the mesenchyme, forming the frontal and parietal bones as well as the bones of the calvarial vault.
   2. Ossification of the sphenoid, temporal, and occipital bones occurs through a process of endochondral ossification.
   3. Parts of the skull remain in a cartilaginous state to:
      a. Allow further forward growth of the cranial base
      b. Facilitate inward rotation of the eye complex

FINAL DEVELOPMENT[1-5]

A. From the end of the embryonic period until gestation is complete, facial appearance changes, mainly as a result of the growth of the underlying brain.
   1. As the brain enlarges, the forehead becomes more prominent, moving the eyes more medially.
   2. The mandible and nose, initially flat, also assume their final appearance over the remaining weeks of gestation.

Arteriovenous Malformation (AVM)

DEFINITION

Malformation of the developing vascular system resulting in the abnormal connections of arteries, arterioles, and capillaries to the venous system, creating a large arteriovenous shunt

PATHOPHYSIOLOGY

A. An AVM develops when there is aberrant arterial drainage of one or more of the cerebral arteries into a midline deep venous structure.[6]
B. AVMs occur most commonly in the parietal, followed by the occipital, lobes.[7]
C. The aneurysmally dilated venous structure contains areas of abnormal and thin-walled blood vessels that lack intervening capillaries to provide venous drainage.
   1. There is a distinct absence of capillaries in the lesion when examined pathologically.[7]
D. The AVM can be so large as to require an increase of as much as 50 percent of the infant's normal blood volume.

ETIOLOGY

A. Although frequently referred to as the vein of Galen malformation, it is now believed that the most common venous structure for drainage of the shunt is the median prosencephalic vein, more commonly known as the vein of Markowski, the embryologic precursor to the vein of Galen. This is the aneurysmally dilated vessel.[6,8,9]
B. The vein of Markowski is normally replaced by the internal cerebral veins, including the vein of Galen, around the eleventh week of gestation.[9,10]
C. The malformation occurs between the sixth and eleventh week of gestation.[9]

INCIDENCE

A. AVMs are the most common neurovascular lesion seen in the neonate.
   1. They represent 30 percent of vascular malformations in the pediatric population.[6,11,12]

CLINICAL PRESENTATION[9,11,13,14]

A. Forty to 60 percent of AVMs present in the newborn period.
   1. Morbidity and mortality are significantly increased when there is clinical presentation in the neonatal period.
B. Congestive heart failure (CHF) is the presenting symptom in >90 percent of neonates.
C. Hydrocephalus or subarachnoid or intraventricular hemorrhage presents in 5–10 percent of neonates.
D. Clinical bruit is most frequently localized over the posterior cranium.
E. Bounding carotid pulses exist.

ASSOCIATIONS

A. There is a high risk for intracranial hemorrhage secondary to backflow and subsequent engorgement of vessels proximal to the lesion.

B. Ischemic brain injury can occur as a secondary effect caused by dilated vessels compressing normal brain tissue.[12]

C. CHF is secondary to:[9,12]
   1. Decreased cerebral vascular resistance caused by a relatively nonresistant void created by the arteriovenous malformation
   2. Increased venous return secondary to increased blood volume

D. There is ischemic heart injury secondary to inadequate perfusion of the coronary arteries that normally occurs during diastole; perfusion is decreased because of low diastolic filling (inadequate pressure and volume).

DIFFERENTIAL DIAGNOSIS

A. Ebstein anomaly

B. Congenital CHF

DIAGNOSIS

A. Chest x-ray demonstrates:
   1. Massively enlarged cardiac silhouette
   2. Possible pulmonary infiltrates secondary to congestive heart failure

B. Cranial ultrasound reveals:
   1. A large echogenic area in the region of the vein of Galen on gray-scale images
   2. Mass effect and mixed echogenicity in the region of the lesion with color-flow Doppler in symptomatic patients[7,13]

C. Doppler study of flow velocity accomplishes the following:
   1. Is diagnostic
   2. Can provide information regarding anatomy and hemodynamics that is useful when employing interventional techniques[9]
   3. Is useful in demonstrating decreased flow following embolization[13]
   4. Provides a useful baseline for follow-up[11]

D. Computed tomography (CT) is useful in evaluating the extent of parenchymal ischemic injury or intracranial hemorrhage.[9]

E. Magnetic resonance imaging (MRI) is most useful for delineating the major arterial feeding vessels.[9,15]

F. Angiography accomplishes the following:[11,13,16]
   1. Defines anatomic details of the aberrant vessel
   2. Delineates the primary arterial feeders
   3. Shows the size and location of the dilated vein

TREATMENT OPTIONS AND NURSING CARE

A. Indication for treatment is intractable, high-output, cardiac failure refractory to medical management such as fluid restriction and inotropic medication.[9,13]

B. Arteriovenous malformation can be treated by:
   1. Surgical excision
   2. Arterial embolization
   3. Venous embolization
   4. Radiosurgery

C. Surgical risk to the neonate is significant because ischemic, myocardial injury has already occurred secondary to high-output failure and can be exacerbated by intra- or postoperative hypotension.[9]

SURGICAL MANAGEMENT

A. Surgical intervention by way of direct craniotomy to repair AVMs has proven unsuccessful in the newborn.[9,13,17] Seventy to 100 percent mortality has been described in several centers.[9,17] Other centers report 70–80 percent survival with 40–50 percent neurologic impairment when surgical intervention is employed in the neonatal period.[13]

B. Staged embolization with cyanoacrylates, metal microcoils, or detachable balloons to reduce blood flow through the malformation is preferred over direct surgical intervention.[6,7,13] The goal of embolization is to mitigate CHF and reduce vascular steal through the malformation, thereby redirecting blood flow to the normal neurovascular system.[6,7]

   1. Staged embolization technique can be done with a liquid adhesive.
      a. The procedure is performed under general anesthesia.[11]
      b. Under direct angiography, catheter sheaths are inserted for the femoral or umbilical arterial approach.[9]
      c. The transtorcular approach involves passing the embolizing catheter from the torcular herophili through the straight sinus of the brain directly into the dilated vessel (Figure 1-3).[9,18]
      d. The sheath tip is positioned, as much as possible, directly into the aberrant vein or feeder arteries.
      e. Transarterial embolization using a liquid adhesive agent composed of a polymerizing compound is attempted initially.[16]
      f. The liquid adhesive agent is injected until a prolongation in blood transit time through the malformation is noted on real-time angiography.[9,13,16]
         1) The amount of liquid adhesive injected is patient dependent and differs depending on the specific lesion.
         2) The limiting factor is blood flow through the lesion.
      g. The patient is then monitored for signs of improvement in CHF.
         1) If CHF does not improve, or worsens after initial improvement, subsequent attempts at embolization are made.
         2) Numerous attempts at embolization are often required.[12]

   2. If staged embolization with a liquid adhesive fails, microcoils transvenously inserted via sheaths from the femoral vein may be used as a secondary approach.[12,18]
      a. This transvenous technique is similar to injection of a liquid adhesive in that catheter sheaths are inserted via the femoral vein.[18]
      b. General anesthesia is used.
      c. The patient is heparinized to maintain patency of the sheaths, which can remain in place for up to 24 hours.[11]
      d. The catheter tip is advanced into the vein of Galen via the transverse sinus.[18]
      e. Small metal coils are used for transvenous embolization. Small metal coils are inserted through the catheter into the AVM to block blood flow to the anomalous structure in an effort to reduce steal from the systemic circulation.
         1) Hundreds of coils, as well as numerous attempts, may be necessary to affect blood flow.[9,13,18]
      f. The threshold for stopping the procedure is hemodynamic instability.[11]
      g. Further attempts at embolization can be made after hemodynamic and metabolic stability are regained.[11]

COMPLICATIONS

A. Complications range from mild to fatal.[6]
  1. Cerebral infarction and ischemic neurologic deficits
  2. Cerebral hemorrhage secondary to venous hemorrhage or perforation of the venous sac during endovascular intervention
  3. Developmental delay secondary to either of the above

POSTOPERATIVE NURSING CARE

A. Monitor:
  1. Vital signs frequently
  2. Hemodynamic status closely for:
    a. Tachycardia
    b. Hypotension
  3. Pulmonary status:
    a. For signs and symptoms of pulmonary edema, which indicates worsening or refractory CHF
    b. For respiratory distress in the event of inadvertent pulmonary embolization (secondary to high flow across the intracranial shunt)[6]
  4. Neurologic status for acute changes secondary to the risk of:
    a. Ischemic injury
    b. Intracranial hemorrhage
B. Observe for signs and symptoms of coagulopathy.
C. Maintain integrity of venous catheters and sheaths because they may be left in place for future embolization procedures.
D. Provide parental support.
  1. Explain the need for close monitoring.
  2. Discuss the importance of minimal stimulation of the infant postoperatively.

OUTCOMES

A. Past prognosis for AVMs presenting in the neonatal period was grim; recent follow-up demonstrates more favorable prognoses for infants treated with embolization.[9,11,12,19,20] However, neonatal morbidity and mortality remain high.[13]
  1. Mortality: 23–75 percent
  2. Morbidity: 21–88 percent
  3. Mortality with endovascular management: 8–33 percent compared with 84 percent a decade ago[12]
B. In cases of severe cardiac failure, the prognosis for CHF itself is poor enough that the outcome is guarded.[11]

Cystic Hygroma

DEFINITION

A. The name means "watery tumor."
B. It is a network of fluid-filled, dilated, lymphatic cysts.

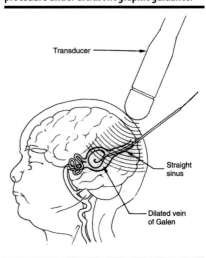

FIGURE 1-3 ■ Transtorcular embolization procedure under ultrasonographic guidance.

From: Abbitt PL, et al. 1990. The role of ultrasound in the management of vein of Galen aneurysms in infancy. *Neuroradiology* 32(2): 86. With kind permission of Springer Science and Business Media.

PATHOPHYSIOLOGY

A. This congenital anomaly of the lymphatic system arises from anomalous embryologic development of the lymphatic system.[3,21]

B. It is a benign, multilobular, multinodular, cystic mass.[22]

C. This cystic structure is lined with endothelial cells and continues to produce lymphatic fluid.[23]

ETIOLOGY

A. The disruption of the normal development of the lymphatic system *in utero* is believed to be the result of maldevelopment of the lymphatic jugular sacs with failure of the structures to connect or drain into the venous system.[3,24]

B. It is primarily congenital. A small percentage are acquired, but present much later and usually develop after some type of trauma, such as surgical intervention, infection, or bleeding into the cystic space.[24]

INCIDENCE

A. Cystic hygromas comprise <5 percent of congenital neck masses, with a worldwide incidence of 1/12,000.[25,26]

B. Forty percent of cystic hygromas appear in the newborn period, and 80–90 percent appear by 2 years of age. The remaining 10–20 percent are usually acquired and appear after age 20.[21,23]

CLINICAL PRESENTATION

A. On physical exam, cystic hygroma is noted as:[23]
1. A nontender, soft, cystic mass
2. Ranging in size from a few millimeters to several centimeters

B. The mass usually grows in proportion to the neonate; however, sudden enlargement can occur following:[3,23]
1. An upper respiratory infection
2. Trauma
3. Spontaneous hemorrhage thought to be caused by excessive lymphatic filtration

C. The infant may present with respiratory obstruction: this is the most serious complication.

D. Large hygromas may involve the oropharynx and trachea, and 3–5 percent of these extend into the mediastinum.[23]

E. Hemorrhage into the cyst can cause nerve compression, resulting in paresthesias and pain.[21,24]

F. Ninety percent of cystic hygromas:
1. Occur in the cervical region
2. Tend to grow along fascial planes and around neurovascular structures
3. Are seen on the left side more often than the right side (2 to 1 predilection)
    a. This is probably secondary to the thoracic duct entering the subclavian vein on the left.[22]

G. The most common location in the neck is the posterior triangle region; neck hygromas may communicate beneath the clavicle with other axillary or mediastinal hygromas.[21,23] This may lead to airway obstruction at birth.

H. Twenty percent occur in the axillae and 5 percent in the mediastinum, retroperitoneum, or pelvis and groin areas.[22,23]

I. Rarely, hygromas undergo spontaneous partial or complete regression.[23]

ASSOCIATIONS

A. Cystic hygromas diagnosed by fetal ultrasound before 30 weeks gestation are most likely associated with a chromosomal abnormality:[27–29]
   1. Turner syndrome
   2. Karyotype abnormalities
   3. Malformation syndromes
B. Development of fetal hydrops adds greatly to the complexity of management.
   1. Generalized effusions (especially in pleural cavities, the pericardium, and the abdomen)
   2. Obstruction of cardiac venous return
   3. CHF
   4. Hypoproteinuria

DIFFERENTIAL DIAGNOSIS

A. Neoplastic tumor[30]

DIAGNOSIS

A. Prenatally:
   1. Ultrasound has identified the anomaly as early as 10 weeks gestation.[31]
   2. Diagnosis made after 30 weeks gestational age is almost always an isolated anomaly.[21]
B. Postnatally, evaluation in the neonatal period includes:[30]
   1. Ultrasonography of the heart and kidneys
   2. Karyotypic analysis
   3. Transillumination can help to distinguish a fluid-filled mass from a more solid lesion.
   4. X-ray is of limited use because:
      a. CT scan and MRI are widely available and can be used for diagnostics as well as preoperatively to determine the extent of the cyst and the underlying structures involved.
   5. CT scan demonstrates multiloculated cystic masses (usually >1 cm) with smooth septations; these appear as a thin-walled mass with homogeneous density, but can be single- or multicystic.
   6. MRI is superior to CT in delineation of soft-tissue structures and is therefore better able to show the extent of the lesion. MRI provides a three-dimensional evaluation of the mass and assists in preoperative surgical planning.[21,30]
   7. Ultrasound may be useful in confirming the diagnosis.

TREATMENT OPTIONS AND NURSING CARE

A. Treatment depends on:
   1. The clinical presentation
   2. The size of the lesion
   3. The anatomic location of the lesion
   4. The complications

B. Acute management is directed toward relief of airway obstruction or dysphagia.[21]

   1. When prenatal diagnosis has been made, a team skilled in addressing airway obstruction issues must be present at the delivery of an infant with a large cystic hygroma of the head and/or neck.

   a. Antenatal use of MRI to define the likelihood of airway obstruction may be helpful.

   b. Needle aspiration is an effective temporizing measure for emergency decompression:[21]

   1) Fluid accumulation in the chest and abdomen often interferes with adequate respiration.

   2) Drain with an 18-gauge over-the-needle catheter that can be left in place after the needle is removed.[22] Allow fluid to drain until there is no further compromise.

C. Expectant management is preferred for the first 18–24 months of life unless there is significant or life-threatening progression of the mass.

D. When cystic hygromas continue to show progressive enlargement with associated symptoms, treatment should not be delayed.

   1. Surgical intervention

   2. Sclerosing therapy

E. Alternatives to surgical excision have been tried with variable success.

   1. Aspiration is not effective for long-term management because of the multiloculated spaces and the rapid reaccumulation of fluid. However, aspiration may be useful with:

   a. The need for emergency decompression **(see B., Acute management, above)**

   b. A large unilocular cyst

   2. Incision and drainage are not indicated except in cases of infection.

   3. Radiotherapy is controversial because of its limited success and the potential for complications.[32]

   a. Radiation should not be used unless other modes of treatment have failed or are contraindicated.

   b. Complications of radiation therapy are dependent on the radiation dose and treatment field; some reported complications include:

   1) Thyroid damage

   2) Bony damage, such as scoliosis, hypoplasia, and benign osteochondromas that can result in symptoms ranging from sensory dissociation to flaccid paresis[33]

   4. Use of sclerosing agents as an alternative to surgical excision has been met with some skepticism.[21,24,34,35]

   a. Sclerosing agents currently in use are:

   1) Bleomycin

   a) Contraindications to use:

   • In infants less than six months of age

   • For lesions with mediastinal involvement

   2) OK-432

   3) Doxycycline

   b. Sclerosing agents are mixed with radiopaque dye and injected via a pigtail catheter placed under the guidance of CT scan.

   1) The catheter is used both for drainage of the lymphatic fluid and subsequent injection of the sclerosing agent.

c. Depending on clinical response and tumor regression, additional injections of the sclerosing agent can be repeated at appropriate intervals.[21,31,34,35]

5. Laser technology, specifically CO_2 laser vaporization, has been successful in the treatment of cystic hygroma.[36]

SURGICAL MANAGEMENT

A. Optimal treatment is meticulous, complete excision of the lesion; this is often impossible because of the thin-walled, multilocular nature of the tumor.[22]

B. Several factors affect the timing of surgical excision.
   1. Excision should be immediate in the presence of airway obstruction or threatened airway compromise.
   2. Excision may be performed at 4–12 months of age in asymptomatic infants.[29,35]
   3. Conservative management with observation in symptomatic patients is possible and is advocated by some surgeons because of the documented spontaneous regression of some hygromas.[36]
   4. Surgical excision should be delayed at least three months following acute infection.[21]

C. Surgical procedure:
   1. The skin incision is made directly over the entire mass to allow complete excision of the lesion.[22]
   2. Communicating tumors should be excised separately from separate incision sites to allow optimal visualization for the tumor's complete excision.[21,24]
   3. If a tumor is to be left behind, it is important to leave no fluid-filled cysts.[22]
   4. Any structures that suggest lymphatic trunks should be ligated or cauterized to minimize postoperative fluid accumulation; if all gross lesion and fluid-filled cysts are not excised, the recurrence rate is up to 100 percent.[21,24]
   5. Extreme care is taken to avoid rupturing the cysts during dissection:[21,24]
      a. Cysts are thin walled; when empty, the margins of the lesions become obscure.
   6. Normal structures should not be sacrificed in the course of tumor removal because cystic hygroma is not a malignant tumor.[24]
   7. Care is taken to avoid damaging the nerves and vascular structures that surround the mass.
      a. Adherent mass is freed from the hyoid bone and submandibular gland.
      b. If the submandibular gland requires removal, then the facial artery must be sacrificed.
      c. The inferior borders of the mass may be adherent to portions of the brachial plexus, thus complicating removal.
         1) Recurrence rate is directly related to incomplete removal.
   8. Closed suction drainage is used to drain the mass postoperatively.
   9. Antibiotic therapy is started within one hour of the initial incision and continued for approximately five days postoperatively.[36]

COMPLICATIONS

A. Muscle weakness[21]
B. Nerve damage
   1. Horner syndrome (such as sinking in of the eyeball or ptosis of the eyelid, caused by interruption of the descending sympathetic nerves on the ipsilateral side)[21]

2. Paralysis
   a. 12–33 percent
   b. Risk of permanent nerve injury related to size and extent of tumor, not age at operation[36,37]
3. Nerve damage to the seventh, ninth, tenth, eleventh, and twelfth nerves as well as to the sympathetic system and brachial plexus
C. Damage to vascular structures
D. Airway obstruction
E. Infection
F. Fistula formation[21]
G. Greater risk for recurrence and long-term complications of suprahyoid cystic hygromas than infrahyoid cystic hygromas[38]
H. Cosmetic deformity
I. Mortality: 2–6 percent.[24,25,34–36]

POSTOPERATIVE NURSING CARE

A. Monitor
   1. Vital signs
   2. Hemodynamic stability
   3. Surgical site
      a. Note integrity and condition of wound site.
         1) Postoperative positioning to maintain alignment and avoid tension on the suture line as well as allow adequate viewing of the surgical site
      b. Note amount and type of drainage.
      c. Apply surgical dressing for drainage and bleeding.
      d. Use closed system drainage device(s).
         1) Jackson Pratt drain(s) are most often used.
         2) Note and replace drainage volume as ordered by the medical or surgical team.
B. Pain management
C. Frequent intubation for several days postoperatively to maintain a stable and patent airway around the surgical site until tissue edema resolves
   1. Care for the intubated infant per unit protocol.
   2. Assess and note the state of tissue edema resolution.

OUTCOMES

A. Recurrence is most likely within a year following resection.[21]
B. Recurrence rates are as follows:[21,24]
   1. Approximately 6–10 percent if all macroscopic tumor is resected
   2. Fifty-two percent with incomplete excision
   3. One hundred percent if any fluid-filled cyst remnants have not been removed
C. High-dose steroids and antibiotics can be useful in treating recurrence.[21]

Retinopathy of Prematurity (ROP)

DEFINITION

A. ROP is the disrupted or aberrant growth of the blood vessels in the still developing retina of a premature infant.
B. The effect ranges from mild visual impairment to blindness, depending on the severity of the disease.

C. This disease is classified into distinct stages that progress in a sequential and typical manner.[39]

D. ROP was first described in 1942 by Terry as retrolental fibroplasia.[40] In 1984, the name was changed to retinopathy of prematurity by an international committee established for the purpose of providing uniform classification for the disease.[41]

PATHOPHYSIOLOGY[42-46]

A. Vasculogenesis of the retina begins at 16 weeks gestation and is complete by around 40 weeks gestation.

B. Developing retinal capillaries are susceptible to injury from many risk factors including: hyperoxia, hypoxia, variations in light, certain medications, acidosis, and oxygen exposure.

C. Neovascularization is the end result of the pathologic process of ischemic injury to the developing vascular system of the retina that causes ROP.

ETIOLOGY

A. Vasoconstriction interrupts normal developmental migration of the retinal blood vessels from the anatomically central optic nerve to the peripherally located ora serráta (Figure 1-4).

B. Multiple risk factors in the premature infant population are believed to contribute to retinopathy of prematurity.

   1. Known causes of vasoconstriction of the retinal vasculature are:

      a. Hyperoxia

      b. Lability of blood oxygen content

FIGURE 1-4 ■ **How the ICROP shows the extent and posterior extension of ROP.**

Stage 3 retinopathy is shown in both retinal sketches made on the diagrams of the three zones in the retina. On the left, however, the disease is in Zone III and covers only two clock hours, whereas on the right the disease is in Zone II and extends for 12 clock hours.

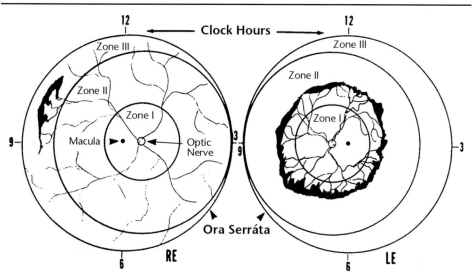

INCIDENCE

A. Peak incidence of ROP occurs in low birth weight infants exposed to high oxygen concentrations for prolonged periods.

B. The more premature the infant, the more likely he is to manifest this disease.

C. The occurrence rate of blindness secondary to ROP in the U.S. is approximately 500–600 annually.[42,47] Approximately 1,300 infants per year are treated for threshold ROP.[48]

D. Specific incidence varies according to birth weight.
   1. Infants <1 kg, 82 percent incidence ROP, 9.3 percent progress to vision-threatening sequelae.[43,44,49]
   2. Infants 1–1.5 kg, 47 percent incidence ROP, 2 percent progress to vision-threatening sequelae.[47,49]

CLINICAL PRESENTATION

A. Premature infants with ROP are identified during a scheduled screening exam.

ASSOCIATIONS

A. The lower the infant's gestational age at birth and the more complicated the NICU course, the greater the risk of developing ROP.

DIAGNOSIS

A. Classification system for ROP (Figure 1-5)
   1. The purpose of this system is to accurately describe the extent of vascular injury in a particular eye using internationally accepted criteria.[50]
   2. Three descriptive dimensions are used: location (zones), stage, and extent.

B. Zones (See Figure 1-4)
   1. Zone I: most posterior region; a circle centered on the optic nerve with a radius two times the distance from the optic nerve to the fovea; potentially the most dangerous zone to be affected
   2. Zone II: extends from the edge of Zone I to the ora serráta on the nasal side and to the anatomic equator on the temporal side
   3. Zone III: a peripheral crescent on the temporal side; the least concerning zone to be affected

C. Staging
   1. Stage 1: A thin demarcation line seen as an abrupt change in the color of the retina indicates where normal vascularization stops.
   2. Stage 2: The demarcation line extends anteriorly from the retinal plane as a ridge into the vitreous humor.
   3. Stage 3: Extraretinal fibrovascular tissue begins to grow on the top of the ridge or posterior to the ridge and extends into the vitreous.
   4. Stage 4: The retina begins to detach from the posterior wall because of the traction exerted by the extraretinal fibrovascular tissue or from serous fluid developing behind it.
      a. Stage 4a: The macula remains attached; the visual prognosis remains hopeful.
      b. Stage 4b: The macula detaches; the visual prognosis is markedly decreased.
   5. Stage 5: The retina detaches completely, folding in on itself and becoming funnel or tulip shaped.
   6. Plus disease: Tortuosity and dilation develop in the posterior pole region of the fundus. Such changes usually indicate an arteriovenous shunt in the

FIGURE 1-5 ■ International classification of retinopathy of prematurity (ICROP) Stages of ROP.

Stage	Description	Picture
Stage 1 ROP	A demarcation line exists between the vascularized and avascularized portion of the retina.	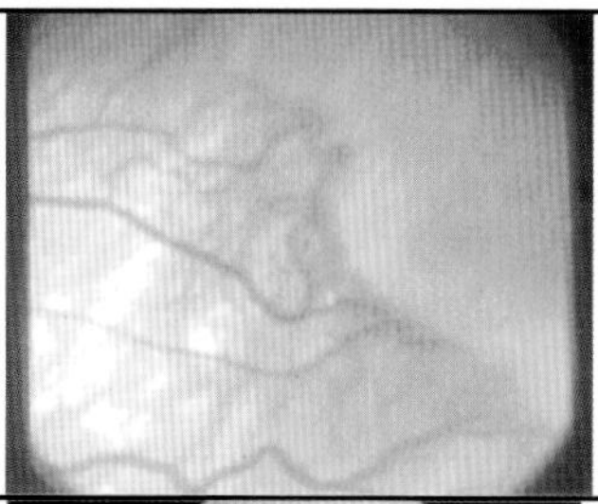
Stage 2 ROP	Demarcation line is present as in Stage 1, but now it has height, width, and volume: a ridge.	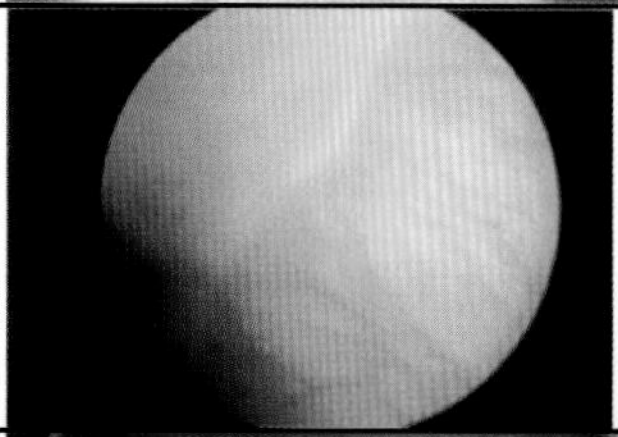
Stage 3 ROP	A ridge is present as in Stage 2, but now there is exraretinal fibrovascular proliferation that may be mild, moderate, or severe.	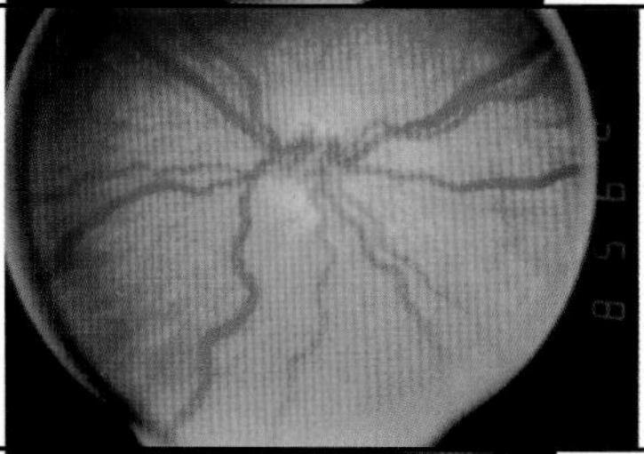
Stage 4 ROP	Partial retinal detachment is present. Stage 4A is extrafoveal retinal detachment.	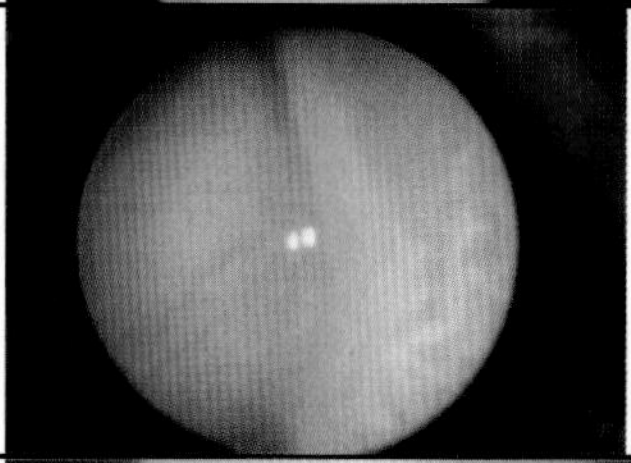
Stage 4B ROP	Stage 4B is retinal detachment that includes the point of keenest vision (the macula).	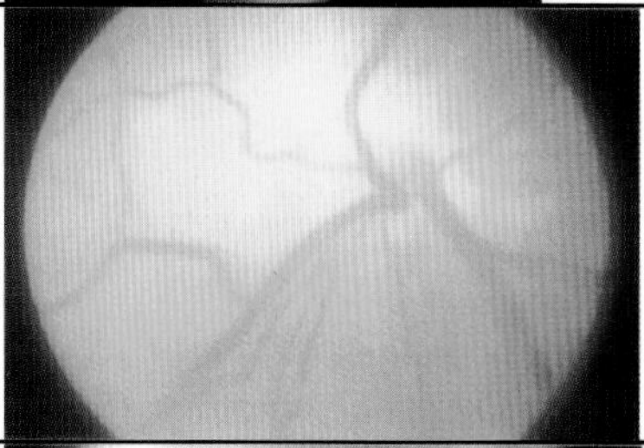
Stage 5 ROP	Total retinal detachment.	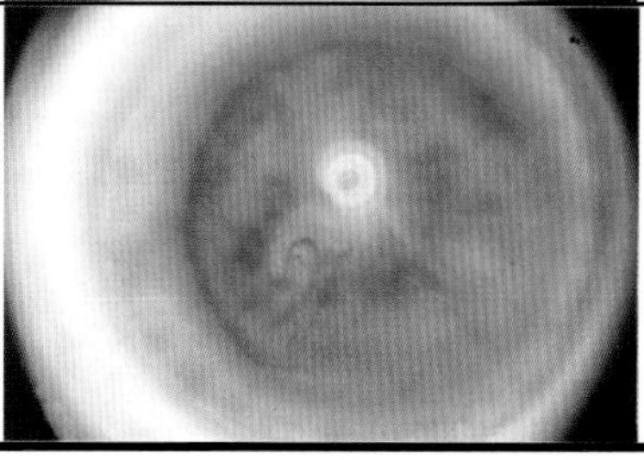

From: Ertzbischoff LM. 2004. A systematic review of anatomical and visual function outcomes in preterm infants after scleral buckle and vitrectomy for retinal detachment. *Advances in Neonatal Care* 4(1): 12. Reprinted with permission from The National Association of Neonatal Nurses.

TABLE 1-2 ■ Surgical Treatment Options for ROP

Procedure and Description	Indications	Advantages and Disadvantages
Cryotherapy Liquid nitrogen is applied to the eye via a prove. The abnormal vessels are frozen, halting vascular growth and reducing the traction on the retina.	Threshold ROP is defined as 5 contiguous or 8 cumulative hours of Stage 3 plus ROP in Zone 1 or 2.[115]	This procedure has been largely replaced by laser therapy. Due to its limited precision, it is used infrequently in modern NICU environments. Preterm infants undergoing cryotherapy with only topical anesthesia had more protracted and severe cardiorespiratory complications than those who received intubation, artificial ventilation, sedation, and analgesia.[116]
Laser Therapy High energy, concentrated in the form of a beam of light, is used to destroy the abnormal vessels.[53]	Threshold ROP is defined as 5 contiguous or 8 cumulative hours of Stage 3 plus ROP in Zone 1 or 2.[53]	Enhanced precision allowing treatment at the vascular edges. Decreased risk of vitreous hemorrhage. Requires no incisions. Enhanced access for treatment of posterior zones (Zone 1). Decreased intraoperative pain and less postoperative inflammation.[60,115]
Scleral Buckle Mechanically reattaches a detached retina by placement of a silicone band around the eye, counteracting the forces putting traction on the retina.[115]	Stage 4 or 5 ROP.	Extreme care must be taken to avoid pulling the band too tight as this can easily impair the infant's retinal and choroidal circulation by increasing intraocular pressure. Within 1 year of intervention, the eye must be evaluated for growth of the globe and orbit. if the silicone band is impinging on growth, it will need to be divided and removed.[60]
Vitrectomy Access to the vitreous cavity is made via incisions through the eye wall, typically posterior to the lens and anterior to the retina. The vitreous and associated scar tissue is removed, preventing further retinal detachment or placing the retina back against the eye wall.	Stage 4 and 5 ROP. Sheets of collagen form within the vitreous cavity causing traction of the retina from the wall of the eye.	**Closed Vitrectomy** More commonly used. Advantage of less globe manipulation and enhanced control of intraocular pressure making corneal surgery unnecessary. **Open-sky Vitrectomy** Advantages include surgical ease due to direct access and better relief of retinal traction. The fluid that is taken out of the vitreous cavity is usually replaced with an air bubble. If the retinal detachment has occurred, a lensectomy may be performed.[115] If an air bubble was placed, the infant should be positioned prone for 24 hours and then upright in a 90° position in a car seat to facilitate proper air bubble placement and enhance retinal attachment. Careful monitoring of infant tolerance of this position using pulse oximetry is required.

From: Ertzbischoff LM. 2004. A systematic review of anatomical and visual function outcomes in preterm infants after scleral buckle and vitrectomy for retinal detachment. *Advances in Neonatal Care* 4(1): 13. Reprinted with permission from The National Association of Neonatal Nurses.

extraretinal fibrovascular tissue on top of the ridge. The clinical significance is that ROP is progressing more rapidly; thus, this is a sign of a poorer prognosis.

D. Extent

    1. The circumferential extent of the disease is noted in clock hours.

    2. One clock hour equals 30 degrees; an entire eye is composed of 12 clock hours.

E. Cicatricial changes[45]

    1. Refer to fibrotic changes. **(See C. Staging, Stage 3, above.)**

    2. The classification of cicatricial changes is not yet universally accepted.

    3. These changes usually arise in eyes that reach acute Stage 3, but have not progressed to significant retinal detachment.

    4. Retinal vessels are pulled laterally by the cicatrization (scar formation), distorting the optic nerve; the fovea is pulled laterally, and a retinal fold may occur. Vision can be significantly reduced by such changes.

TREATMENT OPTIONS/SCREENING[48,51]

A. Screening may vary somewhat by nursery, region, and practicing physician.
   1. Most eye centers recommend that the first eye examination be done at approximately 4–6 weeks after birth and that infants with a birth weight of <1,500 gm or a gestational age of <28 weeks be followed for ROP.
   2. Those who weigh 1,500–2,000 gm, who have had a complicated neonatal course, and are believed to be at high risk by their care provider should also be followed.[52]
B. Screening examination of premature infants for ROP should occur on the following schedule:[52]
   1. The first examination should occur at approximately 32 weeks postconceptional age because vision-threatening ROP has been known to arise at 33–41 weeks postconceptional age; median age of 37 weeks.[51]
   2. Subsequent examinations are scheduled according to the results of the previous examinations.[53]
      a. If Stage 2 disease is present or the retina is immature, the examination should be repeated every one to two weeks.
      b. Stage 3 ROP requires weekly evaluation.
      c. If plus disease is noted, ROP may be progressing faster; repeat exams should occur every three to four days.
C. Examinations are continued until one of the following occurs:
   1. Retinal vascularization has reached Zone III (the risk for ROP has passed).
   2. The threshold for treatment is reached.
   3. The disease has definitively regressed (regression is demonstrated on two sequential exams).
D. Standard of practice is surgical intervention when the prognosis for spontaneous regression is believed to be <50 percent (Table 1-2). This is defined as threshold ROP, which is Stage 3 ROP in five adjacent clock hours or eight cumulative clock hours in Zone I or II.[47,53] A study published in 1998 demonstrated that clinical practice among those who examine and treat ROP use earlier treatment before threshold criteria are met, with the hope that visual outcome will be better with earlier intervention.[54]
   1. Prethreshold ROP has a[45]
      a. 1 in 3 chance of progressing to threshold ROP
      b. 1 in 6 chance of extreme visual loss if not treated promptly when threshold criteria are reached
      c. 1 in 12 chance of extreme visual loss with appropriate treatment
   2. When threshold ROP is reached, there is a 50 percent chance of blindness in the affected eye.
   3. With or without treatment, once threshold disease is reached, fewer than 20 percent of eyes will develop visual acuity of 20/40 or better.[55]

SURGICAL MANAGEMENT

A. Cryotherapy[42,53,56,57]
   1. This treatment decreases the incidence of severe visual impairment by 50 percent.
   2. The process freezes the peripheral avascular region of the retina 360 degrees, reducing or eliminating the signal from the ischemic, avascular tissue to the retina that stimulates neovascularization.

3. Tissue is frozen from the periphery to the center of the avascular region.

4. A retinal probe is applied continuously to the outside of the eye until freezing extends posteriorly to the retinal region.

5. Cryotherapy is the preferred treatment, over laser surgery, in cases where the retina cannot be visualized because of hemorrhage or other circumstances that can prevent transpupillary viewing of the retina.

B. Laser photocoagulation[42,53,54,57–59]

   1. Laser photocoagulation is generally preferred over cryotherapy because infants better tolerate this procedure for the following reasons:

      a. It is less painful. It requires only topical anesthesia and mild sedation as opposed to the general anesthesia with heavy sedation required for cryotherapy.

      b. It is considered less invasive than cryotherapy because the retinal ridge and vessels are specifically targeted for ablative therapy by the laser ray.

      c. It is technically easier because it can be performed at the bedside using lasers attached to an indirect ophthalmoscope that is mounted on the head of the surgeon.

   2. Laser light is directed through the pupil onto the retina to cause photocoagulation (light rays cause coagulation of protein material).

   3. Heat is absorbed by the pigmented tissue of the retina and causes tissue destruction, halting the progression of ROP.

C. Scleral buckle[42,53,60]

   1. Recommended for Stage 4 ROP (partial retinal detachment).

   2. The goal is to reattach the retina and halt or reduce the progression from Stage 4a or 4b to Stage 5 ROP.

   3. The following procedure is used:

      a. A 360-degree silicone band is temporarily placed under the rectus muscle, circumferentially around the external eye, to reshape it in such a way that the posterior intraocular surface is positioned close to the detached retina to create anatomic proximity to allow for spontaneous retinal reattachment.

      b. This procedure is done under direct visualization of the retinal vessels. The surgeon can then observe the choroidal and retinal vessels for blanching, which would indicate that the band is too tight and retinal circulation could be impaired.

      c. Cryotherapy or laser photocoagulation can be performed on the avascular retina at this time if ROP is active.

      d. After approximately one year, the band is divided or removed to allow growth of the globe and orbit. If risk of detachment is identified because of the high elevation of the retina on the ridge of the buckle, the procedure may be deferred.

D. Vitrectomy[42,54,60]

   1. Closed vitrectomy

      a. This procedure is used to treat complete retinal detachment in which the macular region remains intact.

      b. Fibrotic tissue and vascular debris from the posterior retina are removed under direct visualization via a surgical incision with the intent of spontaneous or surgical reattachment of the retina.

      c. Depending on the site of detachment, the lens may be removed during the procedure.

      d. The site of retinal detachment determines the specifics of the procedure.

      e. The advantages of the closed procedure over open-sky vitrectomy is that intraocular pressure is controlled and there is less manipulation of the globe of the eye.

  2. Open-sky vitrectomy[60]

    a. Alternative to closed vitrectomy, this is used when there is complete detachment of the retina and macular region.

      1) The macular region is the most central portion of the retina.

      2) Reattachment is more complicated if the macular region is detached because the retina is free floating and becomes curled.

    b. Technically more challenging, this procedure involves restructuring and shaping the generally free-floating tulip- or funnel-shaped retina.

    c. A scleral support ring is sewn to the globe of the eye for stabilization.

    d. The lens and corneal button are removed to allow visualization and cleaning of fibrous debris from the retina and the area behind or posterior to the retina.

    e. Hyaluronic acid and a glass contact lens are used to temporarily open the funnel-shaped retina, allowing for complete removal of the retrolental membrane and fibrous tissue from the retina itself.

    f. The iridotomy incisions are sutured closed, and the corneal button is sewn back into place.

    g. Hyaluronic acid is injected into the vitreous cavity to re-form the anterior chamber, restore intraocular pressure, and push the retina back into its proper anatomic position.

    h. If the retina remains elevated from the posterior ocular region, external drainage of posterior retinal fluid, rather than direct internal drainage, is done to avoid tearing the friable retina by stretching.

    i. If the retina remains detached and it is believed unlikely to reattach spontaneously, additional surgery can be performed in an attempt to achieve retinal reattachment.

      1) Additional surgery may include reattempts at retinal attachment using either the same surgical procedure or an alternate surgical procedure.

    j. The advantages of open-sky vitrectomy over closed vitrectomy include the following:

      1) There is wide exposure of the operative field.

      2) The retrolental membrane is directly approachable for the procedure of membrane peel.

      3) The much larger work area allows for more complete dissection of scar tissue and relief of peripheral retinal traction.

COMPLICATIONS

A. Success of anatomic reattachment does not correlate with functional vision.

B. The risk of retinal detachment remains for years following surgical reattachment, but becomes less likely each year.

POSTOPERATIVE NURSING CARE

A. General care includes the following:

  1. Medicate for pain and sedate infant as needed.

B. Specific postoperative management depends on the type of anesthesia used.

TABLE 1-3 ■ Development of First Four Branchial Arches

	First Arch	Second Arch	Third Arch	Fourth Arch
Ectoblast (clefts)	External auditory canal	Platysma		
Mesoblast (arches)	Cartilage/bone: mandible, head and neck of malleus, incus body	Cartilage/bone: malleus handle, incus long process, stapes superstructure, styloid, lesser cornus and upper part of body of hyoid bone	Cartilage/bone: greater cornus and lower part of body of the hyoid bone	Cartilage/bone: thyroid, arytenoids
Nerves	CN V2, CN V3	CN VII	CN IX	Superior laryngeal nerve (branch of the vagus nerve [CN X])
Muscles	Mastication muscles	Skin muscles of the face	Stylopharyngeal muscle	Cricothyroid muscle
Arteries		Stapedial artery	Internal carotid artery	Aortic arch (left), subclavian artery (right)
Entoblasts (pouches)	Middle ear Eustachian tube	Palatine tonsil	Inferior parathyroid, thymus, upper part of piriform sinus	Superior parathyroid, C-cells of thyroid, lower part of piriform sinus

CN = cranial nerve; V2 = maxillary nerve; V3 = mandibular nerve

Adapted from: Nicollas R, et al. 2000. Congenital cysts and fistulas of the neck. *International Journal of Pediatric Otorhinolaryngology* 55(2): 117. Reprinted by permission.

C. Postoperative interventions vary and are also specific to the operative procedure.
   1. Cryotherapy
      a. Postoperatively, patients are generally treated with a cycloplegic agent to maintain papillary dilation; intravenous (IV) pain medication; sedation as needed; an intraocular steroid, as well as topical steroids; and, possibly, topical antibiotics.
      b. Cryotherapy produces a significantly greater amount of swelling and redness than laser photocoagulation and also seems to cause significantly greater discomfort postoperatively.[42]
   2. Laser photocoagulation
      a. Postoperatively, infants may require mild pain medication such as topical drops and acetaminophen. Topical steroids and dilation are also prescribed, and patients are typically re-examined after one week.
   3. Scleral buckle
      a. General postoperative care is provided.
   4. Vitrectomy
      a. Closed
         1) General postoperative care is provided.
      b. Open-sky
         1) Postoperatively, patients are generally treated with antibiotics, a cycloplegic, and topical antibiotics.

OUTCOMES[42–44,47,55]

A. Many eyes that develop ROP will improve without treatment to the extent that few or no remnants of the disorder are evident later.
   1. Regression occurs if excessive vessels resorb and normal vascularization reestablishes itself in the central retina.

B. Children with regressed ROP who have an intact retina and macula have been shown to be more susceptible to other visual disorders, including:
   1. Myopia
   2. Amblyopia
   3. Strabismus
   4. Nystagmus
C. Children with a history of cicatricial retinal changes with good visual outcomes remain at risk for retinal problems, including detachment, and therefore require retinal examination at least annually throughout their lives or at least until they are mature and can articulate visual changes.
D. The success rate for scleral buckle are as follows:
   1. Success rates of 8–94 percent have been reported for anatomic reattachment, overall.[61,62] Approximately 20 percent functional success (perception of large forms) has been reported.[48,54,61]
   2. There was a 50 percent higher rate for reattachment when surgery was performed at 2–9 months compared to 7–11 months.[61]
E. The anatomic success rate for retinal reattachment is 47–74 percent.[63,64]

Pharyngeal (Branchial) Arch Anomalies

DEFINITION

A. *Branchial* is derived from the Greek word for gill.[65] During embryologic development, the branchial apparatus resembles gill slits of primitive organisms.[21,66]
B. The branchial apparatus is comprised of five pairs of mesodermal arches, four pairs of ectodermal invaginations known as clefts, and endodermal invaginations known as branchial pouches (Tables 1-1 and 1-3; also see Figure 1-1).[21,66]
C. The only definitive external structure retained from the branchial arches is the dorsal portion of the first branchial arch that becomes the external auditory canal.[66]

PATHOPHYSIOLOGY

A. Although isolated anomalies of the branchial arches do exist, they rarely present in the neonatal period because they are abnormalities of internal structures.
   1. These anomalies frequently present in older infants and children.
   2. Some types of branchial anomalies present most frequently in the second to fourth decades of life.[66]
B. When diagnosed in the neonatal period, branchial arch anomalies present as prominent features in several neonatal syndromes.[67]

ETIOLOGY

A. Embryologic development of the branchial apparatus begins in the fourth week of gestation.
B. Each of the branchial arches contains the following:[66,67]
   1. Nerve
   2. Artery
   3. Cartilaginous rod
   4. Muscular component
C. These structures begin to differentiate between the sixth and seventh week of gestation and eventually give rise to the internal structures of the head and neck.[65,66]

D. Branchial anomalies are believed to result from abnormal persistence of branchial apparatus remnants.

INCIDENCE

A. Approximately 8 percent of isolated branchial arch anomalies are of the first branchial cleft.[68]

B. Most isolated branchial arch anomalies are of the second branchial cleft and are most frequently not noted in the neonatal period, but often present in infancy or childhood.[69]

CLINICAL PRESENTATION

A. With the possible exception of DiGeorge syndrome, in which the physical anomalies can be subtle, major syndromic anomalies that involve the branchial apparatus are usually obvious at the time of birth.

B. There are four categories of these anomalies:
1. Ectopic ear tissue
2. Branchial sinus
3. Branchial fistula
4. Branchial cyst

ASSOCIATIONS[21,67]

A. Most common syndromic associations:
1. Treacher Collins syndrome
    a. Symmetric abnormalities of the first and second branchial arch
    b. Characterized by hypoplasia of the bony and muscular structures of the face and inner ear
    c. Varying degrees of hypoplastic ossicular formation and middle ear hypoplasia that result in conductive hearing loss and malformed or absent external ears
2. DiGeorge syndrome
    a. Congenital disorder of the third and fourth branchial pouches
    b. Results in abnormal development of the thymus and parathyroid glands
    c. High association with conotruncal (outflow tract) cardiac defects
3. Robin sequence
    a. Abnormality in fetal mandibular development
    b. The mandible is a first arch derivative
4. Goldenhar syndrome and hemifacial microsomia
    a. Multiple causative factors that disrupt the mesoderm of the first and second branchial arches
    b. Broad pattern of disorders resulting in a cluster of anomalies that include:
        1) Preauricular appendages and sinuses
        2) Auricular malformations
        3) Facial asymmetry
        4) Ocular abnormalities
        5) Associated findings, including vertebral and cardiac anomalies

DIFFERENTIAL DIAGNOSIS[70]

A. Anomalies of the first branchial arch present in varied ways and are therefore difficult to diagnose.

B. They most commonly present as an area of recurrent inflammation or drainage immediately beneath the mandible.[69]
1. Auricular anomalies
   a. Preauricular sinus
2. Skin tags
3. Lymphadenopathy
C. The second branchial arch is involved in the development of the palatine tonsils and sometimes persists as an internal sinus; so drainage, inflammation, and infection from other causes need to be ruled out.
D. Failed development of the third and fourth branchial pouches results in absence of the thymus and parathyroid glands; thus, other causes of neonatal tetany and impaired cellular immunity could mimic these anomalies.

FIGURE 1-6 ■ A child with a cleft lip and remnants of the first three branchial systems.

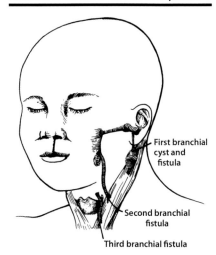

First branchial cyst and fistula

Second branchial fistula

Third branchial fistula

From: Welch KJ, et al., eds. 1986. *Pediatric Surgery,* 4th ed. Chicago: Year Book Medical, 543. Reprinted by permission.

DIAGNOSIS

A. Definitive diagnosis is made by:
1. A geneticist
2. Chromosome studies
3. Diagnostic testing specific to each syndrome

TREATMENT OPTIONS AND NURSING CARE

A. Clinical management of associated anomalies
B. Appropriate consultations for diagnostic purposes
C. Appropriate referrals to optimize long-term outcome
D. Surgical treatment when appropriate

SURGICAL MANAGEMENT

A. Simple branchiogenic anomalies (Figure 1-6)
1. First branchial cleft anomalies
   a. The surgical approach and management is focused on preservation of the facial nerve.
   b. If the area is infected, incision and drainage should be performed, followed 3–6 weeks later by complete surgical excision of the healed sinus or fistula.[69]
2. Second branchial cleft anomalies
   a. Ectopic ear tissue
      1) Simple surgical excision
   b. Branchial sinus fistula
      1) This is the most common lesion of branchial origin seen in the neck.
      2) Fifty percent are noted to be fistulous at the time of surgery.
      3) Infrequently present in infancy, cysts are most commonly seen in late childhood or adulthood.
      4) Surgical procedure is as follows:[69]
         a) The infant is positioned with the neck extended and the head rotated to the opposite side.
         b) The head and chest are slightly elevated.

      c) Neck creases are identified by having the operative assistant flex the neck and turn the head anteriorly; a short transverse ellipse is drawn over the lesion and includes the sinus opening.

      d) A second incision line is marked parallel to a neck fold at the junction of the middle and upper third of the sternocleidomastoid muscle.

      e) The head is returned to the rotated, extended position.

      f) A fine probe is passed into the sinus, and the tract is dissected proximally along the anterior border of the sternocleidomastoid muscle.

      g) A second incision is made, and dissection of the tract below the incision continues to the end of the tract, which is often between the internal and external carotid arteries and below the hypoglossal nerve.

      h) The sinus is excised with its ellipse of skin.

      i) Complete excision of the sinus or fistula is necessary to avoid recurrence; recurrence is more common following cyst excision.

B. Syndromic anomalies

    1. Early middle ear surgery is performed to correct conductive hearing loss.[21,67]

    2. Craniofacial reconstruction is coordinated to coincide with facial growth patterns and psychosocial development.[21,66,67]

      a. If craniofacial reconstructive facial surgery is required, it is often performed in multiple stages.

COMPLICATIONS

A. Facial nerve injury is the most frequent complication, with clefts of the first branchial arch, particularly after infection or surgical intervention.[68]

B. This fistula or sinus may recur.

    1. Fistula recurrence is more common because fistula margins are not as well defined as cystic margins, and incomplete excision can lead to recurrence.

POSTOPERATIVE NURSING CARE

A. General postoperative care is provided.

B. Infants rarely require repair in the neonatal period.

OUTCOMES

A. Outcomes are primarily dependent on associated anomalies.

Choanal Atresia

DEFINITION

Choanal atresia is a congenital obstruction of the posterior nasal choanae that may be bony or membranous, unilateral or bilateral.[71-73]

PATHOPHYSIOLOGY

A. Failure, during development, of the nasopharynx to communicate with the posterior nasal cavity

ETIOLOGY

A. Choanal atresia usually occurs during the fourth week of embryonic life when the mesenchymal plate fails to atrophy. It then ossifies and occludes the posterior nasal aperture.[74,75]

INCIDENCE[74,76]

A. Although choanal atresia is rare, it is the most common congenital anomaly of the nose.

B. It occurs in about 1/5,000–8,000 births.

C. Choanal atresia is twice as common in females as in males.

D. Approximately 70 percent of patients have mixed, both bony and membranous, atresias; 30 percent of patients have bony atresia alone.

E. Choanal atresia is bilateral in about one-third of infants.

F. Unilateral choanal atresia is more common than bilateral choanal atresia.
  1. Unilateral choanal atresia may not be identified for years.

CLINICAL PRESENTATION[75–77]

A. Bilateral choanal atresia is a life-threatening condition. The infant presents with gasping respirations and cyanosis immediately after birth.

B. Unilateral choanal atresia does not usually produce severe symptoms and may be diagnosed only after an increase in watery discharge from the affected side is noted.

ASSOCIATIONS[78,79]

A. Approximately 50 percent of cases have associated anomalies:
  1. CHARGE association (coloboma, heart defects, atresia of the choanae, retardation of growth and development, genital and urinary abnormalities, ear abnormalities and/or hearing loss)
  2. Kabuki syndrome
  3. Pfeiffer syndrome

DIFFERENTIAL DIAGNOSIS[74,75]

A. Congenital narrowing
  1. Choanal stenosis
  2. Piriform aperture stenosis
  3. Binder syndrome (nasal/midface hypoplasia and nasal passage stenosis)[80]
B. Congenital tumors
  1. Nasolacrimal duct cyst
  2. Hemangioma
  3. Dermoid cyst
C. Genetic factors
  1. Fetal alcohol syndrome
  2. CHARGE association
  3. Treacher Collins syndrome
  4. Crouzon syndrome
  5. Apert syndrome
D. Inflammation
  1. Upper respiratory tract infection
  2. Respiratory syncytial virus infection
  3. Gastroesophageal reflux disease
  4. Allergic rhinitis (cow milk or soy protein)
  5. Congenital syphilis (snuffles)
  6. Chlamydia nasopharyngitis
E. Trauma
  1. Intrauterine pressure on the nasal tip (positional asymmetry)

    2. Nasal septum dislocation

F. Malignancy

    1. Lymphoma

    2. Nasopharyngeal rhabdomyosarcoma

G. Laryngeal or tracheal obstruction

H. Iatrogenic factor: Nasal suctioning

DIAGNOSIS[74,76,81,82]

A. Choanal atresia can be diagnosed by the failure of a catheter to pass through either of the nasal passages to the nasopharynx.

B. Because infants are obligate nose breathers, choanal atresia is suspected if the neonate's respiratory distress disappears whenever he begins to cry.

C. Direct examination by fiberoptic nasopharyngoscopy can aid in diagnosis.

D. Confirmation requires a nasal contrast study or CT scan using a high-resolution axial with bone windows to determine the nature and thickness of the atretic plate.

TREATMENT OPTIONS AND NURSING CARE[74,76]

A. Initially treat symptomatic choanal atresia by placing the infant in a prone position and keeping his mouth open with a large open nipple (McGovern nipple) taped or tied in place.

B. An oropharyngeal or endotracheal tube is usually sufficient for emergency control of the airway if a hypoxic episode is observed.

C. Intragastric feedings may be the most effective way to maintain nutrition in the preoperative and acute postoperative periods.

D. Some infants with bilateral choanal atresia do well enough that definitive therapy can be delayed for months or even years.

SURGICAL MANAGEMENT[76,82,83]

A. Early repair is advocated because of the following:

    1. Perforation of the soft bony plate is relatively easy in the first few months of life.

    2. Early repair decreases the risk of fatal asphyxia.

    3. It is less complicated in younger patients, which may decrease length of hospital stay.

B. Surgical management involves removal of the bony atretic plate with a carbon-dioxide laser or high-speed drill or by bone curettage.

C. The most frequent surgical approach in the neonate involves a direct excision through transnasal and transpalatal routes and placement of stents in the posterior choanae.

    1. This procedure carries minimal risk of facial growth disturbance.

    2. This surgery can be performed within the first week of life.

    3. Adequate bony resection, mucosal flaps to cover bony edges, and stents are techniques advocated for prevention of restenosis.

D. Both carbon dioxide and holmium:yttrium-aluminum-garnet (Ho:YAG) lasers have been used to vaporize the atretic plate and cover soft tissues.

    1. Laser resection has been effective for membranous obstructions, but less so for bony occlusions.

E. Topical mitomycin-C can be used after the procedure to decrease fibroblastic activity and to reduce the incidence of re-stenosis by discouraging the formation of scar tissue. Mitomycin-C is an antineoplastic antibiotic that inhibits DNA and protein synthesis.[84]

COMPLICATIONS

A. Stent occlusion
B. Premature/inadvertent stent removal
C. Midface growth changes
D. Other major complications of a repair of choanal atresia:
   1. Cerebrospinal fluid (CSF) leak
   2. Midbrain trauma
   3. Gradenigo syndrome
   4. Palatal perforation
   5. Granuloma formation
   6. Injury to the nasal alae or columella

POSTOPERATIVE NURSING CARE

A. Monitor closely for signs and symptoms of respiratory distress.
B. Adequately sedate the infant in the acute postoperative period to avoid dislodging or inadvertent removal of stents.
C. Suction gently but frequently to maintain patency of nasal stents.
D. Instruct the parents.
   1. Infants will often go home with nasal stents in place.

OUTCOMES

A. Postoperative restenosis can be a problem with all approaches.[76]

Cleft Lip and Palate

DEFINITION

A congenital anomaly that can range from a minor notch of the lip or uvula to complete unilateral or bilateral clefts of the lip, alveolus, and palate.[71,72,85–88]

PATHOPHYSIOLOGY

A. Defects are classified on the basis of embryology:
   1. Clefts anterior to the incisive foramen are clefts of the primary palate. The primary palate, lip, and alveolus fail to fuse around the third week of embryologic development.
   2. Clefts posterior to the incisive foramen are clefts of the secondary palate. These occur when hard and soft palates do not fuse between weeks 7–11.

ETIOLOGY

A. Cleft lip and palate are among the most common craniofacial abnormalities.
   1. Clefting can occur:
      a. As part of an associated syndrome
      b. Through familial inheritance
      c. As an isolated defect
B. Clefts may be the result of maternal use of warfarin or phenytoin during pregnancy.

INCIDENCE[75,85]

A. In Caucasians, cleft lip and palate occur in approximately 1/1,000 births.
B. The incidence in the Asian population is twice that of caucasians, whereas occurrence in African-Americans is approximately 0.4/10,000 live births.

FIGURE 1-7 ■ Cleft palate.

A. Complete cleft of the secondary palate. **B.** Unilateral complete cleft of the primary and secondary palates.

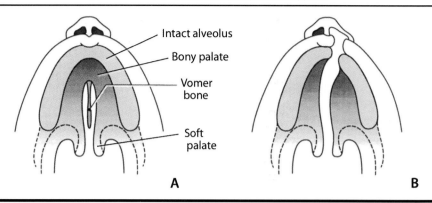

From: Dionisopoulos T, and Williams HB. 1997. Congenital anomalies of the mouth, palate, and pharynx. In *Congenital Anomalies of the Ear, Nose, and Throat*, Tewfik TL, and Der Kaloustian VM, eds. New York: Oxford University Press, 248. By permission of Oxford University Press, Inc.

C. The incidence of clefts of the secondary palate alone is similar in all ethnic groups, 0.5/1,000 live births.

D. Cleft lip is more common in males and occurs more frequently on the left side.

CLINICAL PRESENTATION[71,72,77,86,88]

A. In infants with isolated secondary cleft palate, obstruction of the upper airway may present shortly after birth.

B. Aerophagia and nasopharyngeal reflux are commonly seen.

C. Inability to form an airtight seal around the nipple may generate a negative intraoral pressure.

1. Almost 25 percent of newborns with cleft lip and palate experience early feeding difficulties that can result in poor weight gain during the first month of life.

2. Using soft, easily squeezable bottles and experimenting with nipples of different construction can usually manage the problem.

ASSOCIATIONS

A. Cleft lip and palate are associated with many neonatal syndromes.

B. Isolated cleft of the hard or soft palate is found in approximately 80 percent of newborns with Robin sequence.

DIFFERENTIAL DIAGNOSIS

A. None

DIAGNOSIS[77,88]

A. Cleft lip is an obvious defect noted at birth; cleft palate can be noted upon inspection of the palate (Figures 1-7 and 1-8).

1. Prenatal diagnosis is possible as early as 17–20 weeks gestation.

2. Occasionally, small clefts of the soft palate are undiagnosed at birth, but diagnosed later after repeated ear infections secondary to the abnormal angle of the Eustachian tubes, making these infants more vulnerable to inner ear infections.

TREATMENT OPTIONS AND NURSING CARE[86,88]

A. For prenatally-diagnosed cleft lip and palate, some authors have proposed intrauterine fetal surgery.[89] The benefit of the fetal repair would be the lack of scar formation and resultant dentoalveolar and midface growth deformities seen during wound healing, thereby potentially reducing the number of reconstructive procedures postnatally.

B. In infants with cleft lip and palate, treatment is initiated soon after birth and continues to the age of 18 in those with complex defects.

C. Despite numerous advances in surgical techniques, many unanswered questions remain regarding the optimal timing and surgical procedure that profoundly influence:
1. Facial aesthetics and subsequent psychological impact
2. Maxillary growth
3. Dental development
4. Speech

SURGICAL MANAGEMENT[71,77,86,88]

A. Although numerous techniques are used to repair cleft lip and/or palate, one thing that is consistent throughout the literature is the importance of a multidisciplinary team approach to long-term management. This team should include the plastic and oromaxillofacial surgeons, otolaryngologists, audiologists, orthodontists, speech and language therapists, geneticists, pediatricians, and social workers.[90]

B. Primary closure of the lip is performed between 2 and 3 months of age, and primary closure of the palate is done at approximately 18 months of age.

C. Operative repair of complete clefts of the lip and palate are frequently performed as a simultaneous procedure in infancy.
1. Simultaneous repair is believed to be the best approach because freeing the nose from the maxilla is essential for proper nasal growth.[90]

D. Repair techniques for cleft lip and cleft palate include the following:
1. Unilateral lip repair
   a. Skin and mucosa are dissected away from the labial muscle on each side of the cleft.

FIGURE 1-8 ■ Types of clefts.

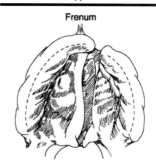

Frenum

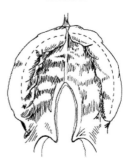

Unilateral

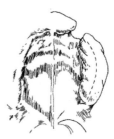

Isolated cleft of palate

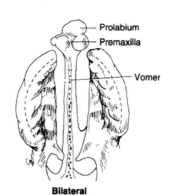

Alveolar cleft

Prolabium
Premaxilla
Vomer

Bilateral

From: Mueller WA. 2004. Oral medicine and dentistry. In *Current Pediatric Diagnosis and Treatment*, 17th ed., Hay WW, et al., eds. New York: McGraw-Hill, 451. Reprinted by permission.

b. The anterior palate is repaired by turning up the lateral and medial vomer mucoperiosteal flaps from the cleft to reconstruct the nasal floor from the posterior part of the hard palate to the nostril sill. These flaps can also be used in repair of the cleft lip.

2. Bilateral lip repair
   a. Bilateral cleft lip is often repaired in two stages using a vomer flap technique.
   b. An interval of five weeks between operations is necessary to avoid the potential complication of atrophy of the premaxilla because a bilateral vomer flap could interfere with the blood supply to the area.
   c. The premaxilla receives its blood supply through the posterior septal arteries, which run along the sides of the nasal septum.

3. Palatal repair
   a. Timing of the palatal closure varies among centers and is decided based on optimizing:
      1) Speech
      2) Maxillary growth
      3) Hearing
   b. The technique used for palatal repair includes reconstruction of the palatal muscles.
   c. The muscles are dissected away from their anomalous insertion on the sides of the gaping cleft, then used as a sling across the cleft, thereby creating a functional soft palate.
   d. Special care is taken to preserve the integrity of the neurovascular palatine bundles.
   e. Tissue layers are closed utilizing absorbable suture material.

4. Secondary surgeries (Figure 1-9) (may have to be done later, depending on the extent of the cleft)
   a. Columella lengthening in bilateral complete clefts
      1) By three or four years of age, children with a history of bilateral cleft lip will have a short columella, broad nose, and flaring nostrils caused by facial growth and inadequate tissue. By four to five years of age, there has been considerable growth with plenty of available tissue for repair.
      2) Repair is achieved using the Millard forked flap procedure, whereby the prolabium is reconstructed (Figure 1-10).

5. Nose reconstruction
   a. Nose deformity, most often seen in patients with complete cleft lip and palate includes the following:
      1) Septum deviation
      2) Alar cartilage asymmetry
      3) Deficient alar base support
      4) Broad nostril sill on the cleft side
      5) Deviation of the columella

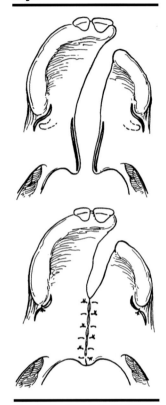

FIGURE 1-9 ■ In the Schweckendiek repair the soft palate only is closed in the first stage.

From: Senders CW, and Sykes JM. 1993. Cleft palate. In *Pediatric Facial Plastic and Reconstructive Surgery*, Smith JD, and Bumsted R, eds. New York: Raven Press, 159. Reprinted by permission.

FIGURE 1-10 ■ Millard forked flap procedure.

We elevate the medial crura, columella, and prolabium as a composite flap using the retrograde approach. To facilitate alar cartilage manipulation and lengthen the columella, we perform bilateral marginal rim incisions extended laterally inside the nostril rim.

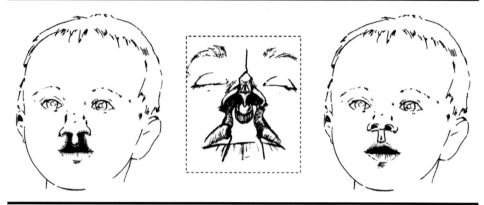

From: Morovic CG, and Cutting C. 2005. Combing the Cutting and Mulliken methods for primary repair of the bilateral cleft lip and nose. *Plastic & Reconstructive Surgery* 116(6): 1614. Reprinted by permission.

    b. If extra cartilage is needed for grafting, chondral cartilage grafts are taken from the crease behind the ear.[91]

6. Pharyngeal flap/pharyngoplasty

    a. Five to 20 percent of patients will have velopharyngeal dysfunction (VPD) following cleft palate repair. A secondary operation to narrow the pharyngeal space can be performed.

    b. VPD is characterized by hypernasal resonance and nasal air escape, which can impair speech.

7. Bone grafting

    a. To achieve complete dental rehabilitation, bone grafting to the alveolar cleft is performed between 8 and 11 years of age. There is no need for dental bridges or prosthetics in approximately 90 percent of the cases.

    b. An autologous cancellous bone fragment, most frequently taken from the anterior iliac crest, is used for this repair.

COMPLICATIONS[92–94]

A. Nasal airway obstruction; more common in bilateral cleft lip
B. Cleft palate fistula
C. Speech problems
D. Problems with dentition and orthodontics
E. Hearing loss
F. Psychological implications

POSTOPERATIVE NURSING CARE[92]

A. Monitor vital signs closely.
B. Administer IV fluids to maintain hydration.
C. Slightly elevate the infant's head during the postoperative period to:
    1. Reduce postoperative swelling
    2. Decrease the risk of aspiration of mucus
D. Closely observe the infant for signs/symptoms of respiratory distress and hemorrhage; these are the major complications in the acute postoperative period.

E. Prevent disruption of the suture line.
   1. Manage pain and sedation as needed.
   2. Use restraints as needed.
F. Observe the suture line closely for bleeding or separating.
G. Provide care in such a way that the infant will avoid crying as much as possible to prevent tension on the suture line.
H. Judiciously and gently suction only when necessary.
   1. Use particular care to avoid trauma to the suture line.
I. Administer prophylactic antibiotics as ordered.
   1. These are usually discontinued two to seven days postoperatively.
J. If incision care or antibacterial ointment is ordered, a gentle rinse or dabbing technique should be used.
   1. Rubbing can cause friction and tension on the suture line that can interfere with healing.
K. Feedings are generally restarted 24 hours postoperatively.
   1. A cleft lip/palate feeder should be used for approximately three weeks postoperatively to avoid pressure on the suture line.
L. Provide parent teaching with special attention to:
   1. Avoiding tension on the suture line
   2. Early recognition of the signs and symptoms of:
      a. Infection of the suture line
      b. Otitis media

OUTCOMES[77,88]

A. Complete cleft lip and palate is a severe malformation that has long-term effects on:
   1. The infant's:
      a. Breathing
      b. Appearance
      c. Speech
      d. Hearing
      e. Facial growth
      f. Feeding
         1) Mastication
   2. The psychological well-being of the child and parents
B. The outcome of surgical repair is directly related to:
   1. The surgical techniques used
   2. The skill of the individual surgeon
      a. Primary surgical repair by a surgeon who is well experienced in cleft palate repair is critical to ensuring the optimal outcome.
      b. Poorly performed surgery may cause subsequent orofacial growth and development problems, increasing the risk of secondary facial and dental deformities and speech impairment.
   3. The timing of the procedure
      a. Timing of operations is balanced between optimal physical and developmental predicted outcomes.
         1) Early closure of the palate greatly enhances speech development, but from an orthodontic standpoint, early closure increases the risk of interference with maxillary growth. Therefore, the prevailing philosophy for surgical management of palate repair is early (one-stage) palatoplasty,

focusing on advantages for speech and hearing, and delayed (two-stage) hard palate closure to allow maxillary growth.[93]

Robin Sequence

DEFINITION[85,88,95,96]

A. Robin sequence is commonly known as the classic triad:
1. Micrognathia (small mandible)
2. Glossoptosis (displacement of the tongue into the pharynx, causing partial or complete obstruction)
3. U-shaped cleft soft palate
B. It is often incorrectly referred to as *Pierre Robin syndrome.*

PATHOPHYSIOLOGY

A. The primary defect, mandibular hyperplasia, causes a cascade of secondary developmental anomalies that result in:
1. Posterior displacement of the tongue
2. Relative hyperglossia
3. Subsequent impairment of palatal shelves from fusing midline; the result can range from:
   a. Minor (a bifid uvula or a submucous cleft palate) *to*
   b. Severe (a complete cleft palate)
B. A submucous cleft palate is a defect of either the bone or muscle layer or of both, with normally intact oral mucosa giving the appearance of an intact palate. This defect can usually be detected through palpation.

ETIOLOGY

A. Mandibular hypoplasia is caused by a single gene defect that is expressed between the seventh and eleventh weeks of gestation.
B. The origin of the mandibular hypoplasia is heterogenous and variable.
1. It may include a genetic syndrome with intrinsic mandibular hypoplasia.
   a. Stickler syndrome has been reported to occur in one of every three Robin sequence cases.
   b. Intrinsic hypoplasia, a hypoplastic mandible associated with a syndrome, would be expected to remain hypoplastic throughout life.
2. Other reported etiologies are:
   a. Teratogenic exposure
      1) The three well-known teratogenic agents that can cause craniofacial abnormalities such as micrognathia are
         a) Alcohol
         b) Isotretinoin (Accutane)
         c) Tobacco
   b. Mechanical factors, which include but are not limited to
      1) Intrauterine fibroids
      2) Bicornate uterus
      3) Transverse positioning of the fetus
      4) Twinning
      5) Oligohydramnios
   c. Hypoplasia of the mandible caused by uterine constraint, which has an excellent prognosis for catch-up growth during the first few years of life

INCIDENCE

A. Robin sequence occurs in 1/8,850 live births.[77,85,95,96]

CLINICAL PRESENTATION[74]

A. Newborns with respiratory obstruction may present with:
1. Apnea
2. Stridor
3. Cyanosis
B. These infants experience feeding difficulties caused by glossoptosis or by other mechanisms of airway collapse related to a syndrome airway abnormality.

ASSOCIATIONS

A. Up to 83 percent of cases of Robin sequence are associated with other syndromes. Ocular anomalies and mental retardation are common. A geneticist should evaluate infants identified with Robin sequence.

DIFFERENTIAL DIAGNOSIS[75,77]

A. Micrognathia is also a classic feature of Treacher Collins syndrome and Hallermann-Streiff-Francois syndrome.
B. Macroglossia may be due to Beckwith-Wiedemann syndrome, Down syndrome, glycogen storage disease, and congenital hypothyroidism.

DIAGNOSIS[96]

A. A careful physical assessment of the infant and detailed pregnancy and family histories are steps to diagnose and determine the etiology of micrognathia in a given patient.
B. Genetic consultation is recommended.

TREATMENT OPTIONS AND NURSING CARE

A. Maintain an open airway while decisions are made regarding care.
1. Prone positioning to maintain anterior displacement of tongue
2. Nasopharyngeal airway, also known as a nasal trumpet, with or without nasal continuous positive airway pressure (NCPAP).
B. Neonates with continued respiratory distress and failed initial temporary measures of prone positioning and nasopharyngeal airway with or without the use of NCPAP may require placement of an endotracheal tube for temporary treatment of obstructive apnea.

SURGICAL MANAGEMENT[75,85,88,95,96]

A. Nonemergency surgical procedures to treat obstructive apnea include:
1. Glossopexy, in which the tongue is sutured to the lower lip
2. Hyomandibulopexy, in which the larynx is anteriorly anchored to proximal structures
3. Subperiosteal release of the floor of the mouth musculature on the mandible
4. Tracheostomy **(See Appendix A: Tracheostomy.)**

OUTCOMES[75]

A. A favorable outcome is best achieved at a center where a multidisciplinary approach is available.
B. Death may be caused by airway obstruction or by other anomalies, such as congenital heart disease.

FIGURE 1-11 ■ **Laryngomalacia.**

A. Note the omegoid shape of the epiglottis and the elongation of the arytenoid cartilages. B. This is the larynx during inspiration. Note that the forces of the inspired air lead to collapse of the laryngeal inlet. Infolding of the epiglottic surfaces and the arytenoid cartilages causes partial airway obstruction.

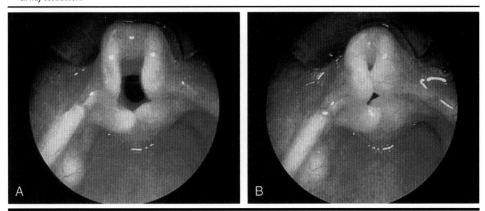

From: Yellon RF, McBride TP, and Davis HW. 2002. Otolaryngology. In *Atlas of Pediatric Physical Diagnosis,* 4th ed., Zitelli BJ, and Davis HW, eds. St. Louis: Mosby, 863. Reprinted by permission.

Laryngomalacia

DEFINITION

Also known as congenital laryngeal stridor, laryngomalacia is a flaccidity of the tissues of the larynx leading to collapse of the supraglottic structures and some airway obstruction with inspiration (Figure 1-11).[72,75,97]

PATHOPHYSIOLOGY

A. Medial and inferior displacement of the arytenoids and epiglottis cause partial obstruction of the supraglottic airway.

ETIOLOGY[98,99]

A. The etiology of laryngomalacia remains unclear; however, the following have all been suggested. No single theory is widely accepted.
 1. Primary disorders of cartilage formation
 2. Nutritional deficiencies
 3. Abnormal embryogenesis
B. Most have attributed laryngomalacia to altered embryologic development, which results in abnormal anatomic development. However, histologic studies failed to demonstrate any inherent cartilaginous abnormality that causes an increase in flaccidity and abnormal collapse of the supraglottic larynx in laryngomalacia.

INCIDENCE[98,100]

A. Laryngomalacia is the most common congenital anomaly of the larynx.
B. Males are affected twice as often as females.
C. This condition accounts for 60–75 percent of laryngeal anomalies in neonates.
D. The vast majority of cases will resolve over a period of weeks to months, with only 10–15 percent requiring surgical intervention.[101]
E. Five to 10 percent of infants with laryngomalacia have a severe form with:
 1. Chronic dyspnea

2. Failure to thrive
3. Obstructive sleep apnea

CLINICAL PRESENTATION[72,91,98,99,102]

A. Stridor is the most frequent symptom of laryngomalacia.
   1. It typically develops within the first two weeks of life and progresses in severity over a period of a few months.
   2. Stridor is described as high pitched and fluttering. In severe cases, stridor can be associated with:
      a. Sternal retraction
      b. Respiratory distress
      c. Feeding difficulties
   3. Stridor is exacerbated by:
      a. Exertion
      b. Feeding
      c. Agitation
      d. Supine positioning
B. Approximately 80 percent of cases are associated with gastroesophageal reflux (GER). GER also may be associated with failure to thrive.
C. Although some cases are self-limiting and resolve over time—usually within 12 to 18 months when tracheal diameter increases and cartilage matures—the symptoms may be so severe that this condition warrants surgical intervention.

ASSOCIATIONS

A. Laryngomalacia frequently is associated with GER, adding to the theory of abnormal neurologic function of the upper airway.

DIFFERENTIAL DIAGNOSIS[75,99]

A. Subglottic stenosis
B. Vocal cord paralysis
C. Bifid epiglottis
D. Saccular cyst
E. Brachial cleft cysts
F. Thyroglossal duct remnants
G. Intraluminal webs
H. Tumors of the larynx
I. Hypoplasia of the mandible
J. Hemangioma
K. Lymphangioma
L. Congenital goiters

DIAGNOSIS[77,99]

A. The gold standard in diagnosis for laryngomalacia is flexible fiberoptic laryngoscopy performed while the infant is awake and demonstrating spontaneous respiratory effort for optimal visualization of the structures of the upper airway.
B. The diagnosis can also be made by using radiographic studies of the tissues of the neck and airway fluoroscopy; however, flexible laryngoscopy is the best adjunct tool to evaluate associated laryngotracheal anomalies.
C. In severe cases where operative intervention is considered, rigid endoscopy is warranted.

Treatment Options and Nursing Care[77,98,103]

A. In the majority of patients, laryngomalacia resolves and no surgical intervention is needed.
  1. Management consists of:
      a. Parent teaching and support because patients are frequently managed at home and followed on an outpatient basis
      b. Appropriate positioning
        1) To help relieve stridor, infants can be placed in the prone position with the neck extended.
      c. Close follow-up

Surgical Management[77,98,99]

A. About 5–10 percent of infants affected with laryngomalacia require surgical intervention. These infants demonstrate:
  1. Severe respiratory distress
  2. Failure to thrive
  3. Severe obstructed apnea
  4. Other severe symptomatology
B. In the past, tracheostomy had been advocated to relieve airway obstruction.[102]
C. More recently, an endoscopic surgical approach to perform epiglottoplasty or supraglottoplasty has shown great success with few complications.[104]
  1. The procedure is performed using suspension laryngoscopy.
  2. Excessive supraglottic tissue that causes airway obstruction such as aryepiglottic folds, lateral epiglottis, and supra-arytenoid tissue is typically trimmed or resected, with a bilateral surgical resection approach using a carbon dioxide laser or sharp dissection instrument.
  3. Controversy exists over the preferred approach of unilateral versus bilateral supraglottic surgical resection. The more conservative unilateral approach has fewer severe complications such as subglottic stenosis (adhesions secondary to scarring) or aspiration, but this approach is also noted to be less successful, with approximately 17 percent of patients requiring a contralateral procedure.[101,105]
D. If symptoms persist and are not adequately relieved, revision procedures may be required. If these are not successful, other interventions may be necessary, such as:
  1. NCPAP
  2. Oxygen therapy
  3. Nasogastric feedings
  4. Tracheostomy **(See Appendix A: Tracheostomy.)**

Complications

A. Granuloma
B. Supraglottic stenosis, secondary to adhesions postprocedure

Postoperative Nursing Care

A. The infant remains intubated for approximately 24 hours postprocedure.
B. Closely monitor:
  1. Vital signs
  2. For signs and symptoms of respiratory distress postextubation

C. Administer as ordered:
1. Antibiotic therapy for approximately five days postoperatively to prevent supraglottic infection
2. Steroid therapy as ordered
3. Pain medication and sedation as needed
D. Minimize the effect of acidity on raw mucosa by:
1. Positioning:
a. With the head of the bed elevated >30 degrees
b. Prone
c. Side-lying
2. Administering antireflux medications as ordered
E. Teach parents to observe for changes in respiratory status.

OUTCOMES[101,105]

A. Overall operative success rate of approximately 80 percent
1. Approximately 90 percent success in isolated laryngomalacia
2. Approximately 50 percent success in laryngomalacia associated with other anomalies

Laryngeal Web

DEFINITION

Congenital malformation involving mucous membrane–covered connective tissue of varying thicknesses between the vocal folds

PATHOPHYSIOLOGY[103]

A. Laryngeal webs are classified according to the scheme proposed by Cohen.[81,106]
1. Type I
a. This anterior web involves 35 percent or less of the glottis.
b. The true vocal cords are visible within a web.
c. There is little or no subglottic extension.
2. Type II
a. This anterior web involves 35–50 percent of the glottis.
b. Subglottic involvement stems more from anterior webbing than from cricoid abnormalities.
3. Type III
a. This anterior web involves 50–75 percent of the glottis.
b. The web is thick anteriorly; the true vocal cords may not be visible.
c. There may be associated cricoid abnormalities.
4. Type IV
a. This web occludes 75–90 percent or more of the glottis.
b. It is uniformly thick both anteriorly and posteriorly.
c. The true vocal cords are not identifiable.
d. The subglottic region is narrowed.

ETIOLOGY

A. Laryngeal webs occur secondary to failed recanalization of the laryngeal lumen during the first trimester of gestation.[75,97–99]

INCIDENCE[97,98,103]

A. Laryngeal webs are uncommon and occasionally familial.

B. About 75 percent of laryngeal webs occur at the level of the glottis or between the vocal cords.

C. Supraglottic webs are very rare and account for less than 2 percent of all congenital laryngeal webs.

CLINICAL PRESENTATION[75,99,103]

A. Stridor may be present.

B. Thin webs limited to the glottis may present with minimal airway obstruction, demonstrating exclusively with hoarseness and weak voice (Types I and II).

C. More extensive webs involving the glottis can be associated with aphonia accompanied by significant airway obstruction that requires an immediate artificial airway (Types III and IV).

D. There is high incidence of cricoid abnormality with Types III and IV; more severe obstruction anomalies are more likely to have abnormalities of the underlying structures that arise embryologically, at approximately the same time as the defect.

ASSOCIATIONS

A. Chromosomal and cardiovascular anomalies are common in patients with a congenital laryngeal web.
   1. Velocardiofacial syndrome may be present.
   2. A chromosome 22q11 deletion is particularly common, as the cardiovascular anomalies associated with the chromosome 22q11 deletion syndrome.
   3. Accordingly, patients with a congenital laryngeal web should undergo genetic screening, including evaluation for a chromosome 22q11 deletion, and a thorough cardiovascular evaluation, including imaging of the aortic arch.
   4. Particular attention should be paid to identifying patients with the triad of a congenital laryngeal web, a chromosome 22q11 deletion, and cardiovascular anomalies, particularly a vascular ring.[107]

DIFFERENTIAL DIAGNOSIS[75]

A. Laryngeal webs always should be considered in children with a congenital history of hoarseness and recurrent croup presenting before six months of age.

B. A laryngeal cyst usually contains mucus from minor salivary glands.

C. Laryngocele arises as a dilation of the saccule of the laryngeal ventricle.

DIAGNOSIS[75,97,103]

A. Immediate diagnosis of a complete or nearly complete web is essential in preventing asphyxiation of the newborn.

B. The diagnosis is suspected with the clinical presence of fixed biphasic stridor.[98]

C. Direct operative laryngoscopy is required for prompt diagnosis and treatment.

D. Although the diagnosis is frequently clear on flexible laryngoscopy, a good quality lateral radiograph of the airway taken at high voltage can aid in the diagnosis of an associated cricoid abnormality.

TREATMENT OPTIONS AND NURSING CARE[102]

A. Treatment options depend on the thickness of the membrane.
   1. Thin, translucent webs can be divided endoscopically using a knife or a laser.
   2. Thick membranes or those with inferior extension into the subglottis most often require:
      a. Open surgical repair

      b. Keel placement

      c. Temporary tracheostomy

SURGICAL MANAGEMENT[98,99]

A. The choice of surgical options depends on the extent and thickness of the web and the degree of associated congenital cricoid malformation.

    1. Treatment using an endoscope

    2. Open laryngotracheal reconstruction

B. Thin membranous webs classified as Type I, which produce minimal symptoms, can be observed until the child is three to four years of age and divided either with a cold instrument (freezing apparatus) or with a carbon dioxide laser.

C. Type II webs can be managed by incising the web along one vocal cord and then proceeding with either staged dilations or by incising the web on the other cord two weeks later.

    1. Keel placement, through either an open or an endoscopic approach, is generally necessary for optimum healing of the anterior commissure after surgical repair and for the best possible voice results postoperatively.

    2. A tracheostomy is often necessary while the keel is in position. **(See Appendix A: Tracheostomy.)**

D. Treatment of Type III and Type IV webs is postponed until the child is three to four years of age.

    1. The standard treatment for significant anterior webbing involves:

      a. A temporary tracheostomy

      b. Laryngotomy

      c. Keel insertion

    2. An alternative treatment is an early single-stage laryngotracheal reconstruction with submucosal resection of the abnormal cricoid cartilage, mucosal flap elevation, and rotation onto the anteromedial aspect of the vocal cords.

      a. An endotracheal tube is inserted for 10–14 days. A great advantage of this approach is the elimination of a tracheostomy.

    3. Posterior glottic webbing is typically a thin membranous sheet between the posterior vocal cords with or without interarytenoid involvement and vocal cord fixation.

      a. Webs involving the interarytenoid region may require laryngofissure, a posteriorly placed costal cartilage graft, and stenting.

COMPLICATIONS

A. Persistent laryngomalacia and poor voice quality

    1. Additional procedures to maximize voice quality:

      a. Laryngeal dilations

      b. Laser procedures for further division or membrane tissue removal

POSTOPERATIVE NURSING CARE

See Appendix A: Tracheostomy.

OUTCOMES[97]

A. Residual anterior webbing may need further treatment.

B. Treatment of thicker subglottic or intralaryngeal webs that require incision, excision, and subsequent dilation may be unsuccessful because of re-formation of the web.

C. Lysis with a carbon dioxide laser is frequently successful.

D. Some surgically treated patients may need a tracheostomy for a prolonged period of time. **(See Appendix A: Tracheostomy.)**

Vocal Cord Paralysis

DEFINITION

Loss or impairment of motor function of the vocal folds, which can be unilateral or bilateral

PATHOPHYSIOLOGY

A. Paralysis of one or both of the vocal cords may be congenital or present at birth due to stretching of the recurrent laryngeal nerves during the birth process.[99,108]

ETIOLOGY[75,98,99]

A. **Unilateral** dysfunction may result from:
   1. Birth trauma
   2. Trauma during thoracic surgery (patent ductus arteriosus ligation)
   3. Compression by mediastinal masses of various origins:
      a. Cardiac
      b. Pulmonary
      c. Esophageal
      d. Thyroid
      e. Lymphoid

B. **Bilateral** vocal cord paralysis is more commonly associated with central nervous system problems, including:
   1. Perinatal asphyxia
   2. Cerebral hemorrhage
   3. Hydrocephalus
   4. Bulbar injury
   5. Arnold-Chiari malformation

C. Most cases of vocal cord paralysis are idiopathic. In these cases, there are no other detectable anomalies, and spontaneous resolution often occurs.

INCIDENCE[75,98]

A. Vocal cord paralysis accounts for 10 percent of all congenital laryngeal abnormalities.

B. It is the second most common cause of neonatal stridor after laryngomalacia.

C. Unilateral vocal cord paralysis occurs more often on the left side; the longer course of the recurrent laryngeal nerve makes it more vulnerable to injury.

CLINICAL PRESENTATION[75,108]

A. **Unilateral** vocal cord paralysis typically presents with a weak, breathy cry and feeding difficulties; however, there is usually no respiratory distress.

B. **Bilateral** vocal cord paralysis typically presents as high-pitched inspiratory stridor with a normal cry or possibly a mildly hoarse cry, but with marked respiratory distress.

C. Feeding difficulties may manifest as aspiration, resulting from inability of the vocal cords to approximate to protect the airway.

D. Airway obstruction from bilateral vocal cord paralysis presents immediately after birth and may be severe, requiring emergency airway interventions such as intubation and possibly tracheostomy. **(See Appendix A: Tracheostomy.)**

ASSOCIATIONS

A. Multiple cranial nerve deficits are common in neonates with congenital vocal cord paralysis, resulting in a high incidence of dysphagia and chronic aspiration.

DIFFERENTIAL DIAGNOSIS[99]

A. Laryngomalacia
B. Laryngotracheal esophageal clefts
C. Laryngotracheal stenosis
D. Tracheoesophageal fistulae
E. Laryngeal and subglottic cysts
F. Tracheomalacia
G. Tracheal stenosis
H. Tracheal compression

DIAGNOSIS[77,98,109]

A. The diagnostic workup should include laryngoscopy, performed either with a flexible endoscope while the patient is awake or with a rigid endoscope under light anesthesia. Operative direct laryngoscopy is usually necessary to confirm the diagnosis.
  1. To assess vocal cord mobility, it is best to perform the examination while the infant is breathing spontaneously and, if possible, crying.
B. Bronchoscopy and esophagoscopy also should also be part of the evaluation.
C. MRI or CT scan of the head should be obtained to rule out any central nervous system abnormalities.

TREATMENT OPTIONS AND NURSING CARE

A. Supportive treatment may be given.
  1. Unilateral:
     a. Surgical intervention rarely required.
     b. Reduce the risk of aspiration by positioning the infant with paralyzed vocal cord superior during feeding and by thickening feedings.
     c. To reduce stridor, position the infant with the paralyzed vocal cord down during periods of rest.
  2. Bilateral:
     a. A tracheostomy is frequently required.
B. Observation for a minimum of one to two years may allow for spontaneous recovery.
  1. In cases of failed spontaneous recovery, the surgical procedures listed below can be considered.

SURGICAL MANAGEMENT[98,109]

A. Tracheostomy **(see Appendix A: Tracheostomy)** is indicated for infants:
  1. With bilateral vocal cord paralysis and severe airway obstruction
  2. With unilateral vocal cord paralysis if there is a significant aspiration
B. In cases in which bilateral vocal cord paralysis does not resolve in one to two years, a vocal cord medullization such as arytenoidectomy is performed endoscopically or using an open procedure.

COMPLICATIONS
A. Aspiration and feeding difficulties
B. Weak cry
C. Failed spontaneous recovery of vocal cord function

POSTOPERATIVE NURSING CARE
See Appendix A: Tracheostomy.

Tracheomalacia

DEFINITION
Tracheomalacia is characterized by abnormal flaccidity of the trachea. During the respiratory cycle, this can lead to abnormal tracheal collapse on expiration, which can result in >10–20 percent obstruction of the airway.[81,98]

PATHOPHYSIOLOGY
A. Two types of tracheomalacia are recognized:
 1. Primary (intrinsic)
 2. Secondary (extrinsic)
B. In the **intrinsic type,** collapse of the trachea, especially during high airflow, is caused by:
 1. The weakness of the supporting tracheal cartilage
 2. Widening of the posterior membranous wall
C. In the **extrinsic type:**
 1. Double aorta is the most common vascular ring that results in tracheal compression.
 2. The most common vascular sling causing airway compression is the innominate artery.
 3. Conditions such as the following may contribute to or precipate the development of a vascular sling.
   a. Tracheoesophageal fistula (TEF)
   b. Localized tracheomalacia associated with tracheostomy
   c. Laryngotracheal esophageal cleft

ETIOLOGY[75,98,99]
A. Primary tracheomalacia is caused by the following:
 1. An inherent weakness of the tracheal cartilaginous rings
 2. Inadequate cartilaginous and myoelastic elements supporting the trachea
B. In secondary tracheomalacia, collapse on expiration may be caused by extrinsic compression of the trachea by a mass or vasculature structure.
C. Iatrogenic causes include the following:
 1. Prolonged intubation
 2. Traumatic intubation

INCIDENCE
A. Specific incidence depends on:[83]
 1. Type (intrinsic or extrinsic)
 2. Causative factors (extrinsic)

CLINICAL PRESENTATION[75,88,98]

A. Often tracheomalacia is not symptomatic until the infant becomes active or agitated or contracts a respiratory tract infection.

B. Patients with tracheomalacia can present with minimal symptomatology to severe, life-threatening airway obstruction.

C. The classic expiratory stridor of tracheomalacia may be present at birth. Other symptomatology includes recurrent cough, apnea, and recurrent bronchopulmonary infection.

D. Infants with tracheomalacia secondary to vascular ring compression typically present earlier and with more severe airway symptomatology than infants with vascular slings. A condition known as "reflex apnea" or "dying spells" has been reported to be associated with innominate artery compression.

ASSOCIATIONS[98]

A. The condition also may involve the bronchi; this involvement is known as bronchomalacia.

B. Tracheomalacia may also occur with laryngomalacia.

DIFFERENTIAL DIAGNOSIS[99]

A. Tracheal stenosis

B. Compression of the trachea by mediastinal masses

DIAGNOSIS[88,98,99]

A. The assessment of a child with tracheomalacia should include airway fluoroscopy and a barium swallow to assess the airway dynamic conditions radiographically and to demonstrate evidence of vascular compression.

B. Rigid bronchoscopy should be performed to completely assess the airway.
   1. It should be used to:
      a. Evaluate the degree of the collapse of the tracheobronchial tree
      b. Assess for the presence of other associated congenital airway lesions
   2. Rigid bronchoscopy allows for better control of the airway and the opportunity for therapeutic intervention, but does require the use of general anesthesia.

C. Endoscopy should be performed during spontaneous respiratory effort to allow optimal visualization of airway dynamics.

D. In cases of suspected vascular compression or cardiac abnormalities contributing to tracheomalacia, MRI and echocardiography may also be warranted before surgery.

TREATMENT OPTIONS AND NURSING CARE[83]

A. The treatment of tracheomalacia depends on the severity of the symptomatology.

B. Mild cases of tracheomalacia often resolve within one to two years of age with no intervention.

C. Early surgical intervention to relieve airway obstruction is often necessary for infants with double aortic arch.
   1. In the majority of patients with double aortic arch, the left arch is smaller and even may be atretic or nonpatent.

D. Surgical intervention is required in many cases for a less constricting vascular ring that includes a right aortic arch with a descending right aorta associated with an aberrant left subclavian artery and persistent ligamentum arteriosum.
   1. This situation usually results in less airway compromise than a true double aortic arch.
E. In infants with associated GER, an upper gastrointestinal series and a pH probe study also may be warranted, especially in children who have secondary conditions such as TEF.

Surgical Management[88,98]

A. In cases of severe airway obstruction and tracheal collapse, tracheostomy with long-term positive airway pressure ventilation may be required. **(See Appendix A: Tracheostomy.)**
B. In cases of vascular compression of the trachea, surgical decompression of the trachea may lead to significant improvement.
   1. Innominate artery compression of the trachea can be relieved by arteriopexy.
      a. An innominate artery is suspended from the sternum to relieve compression on the trachea.
   2. The innominate artery also may be divided and reimplanted more proximally on the aorta to the right side so that it does not cross and compress the trachea.
C. Surgical procedures that have also been considered include placement of internal stents, segmental resection, cartilage grafting of the trachea, and external tracheal stents.[83]

Complications

A. Complications are reported as rare and usually not significant.
B. The most commonly reported complication is minor wound infection.[83]

Postoperative Nursing Care

A. Arteriopexy
   1. Postoperative management as for an infant who has undergone general anesthesia
   2. Thoracic incision postoperative care, including pulmonary toilet and pain management
   3. Chest tube management
   4. Postoperative bronchoscopy when the infant has recovered from general anesthesia to ensure that tracheal collapse during breathing is no longer present
B. Tracheostomy **(See Appendix A: Tracheostomy.)**
C. External tracheal stenting procedures, to treat patients with tracheal and/or bronchomalacia that has not responded to aortopexy or who are not candidates for aortopexy because a long or diffuse segment of airway is involved (varying degrees of success)[83]

Craniosynostosis

Definition

Craniosynostosis is skeletal malformation of the cranium involving premature fusion of one or more of the cranial sutures. Compensatory growth occurs perpendicular to the fused suture, resulting in an abnormally shaped skull.

FIGURE 1-12 ■ Categories of craniosynostosis and the sutures involved.

In synostotic scaphocephaly, the sagittal suture is prematurely synostosed. In synostotic brachycephaly and synostotic anterior plagiocephaly, the coronal suture is closed either bilaterally or unilaterally. In synostotic trigonocephaly, the metopic suture is prematurely closed. In the rarely occurring synostotic posterior plagiocephaly, the lambdoid suture is closed unilaterally. This condition is frequently confused with deformational posterior plagiocephally (bracketed) in which all the sutures are patent. The degree of alteration in cranial shape depends on the timing of synostosis. It may be congenital or develop during infancy, resulting in less severe cranial distortion. Furthermore, cranial shape can be modified when two or more sutures are involved. This figure specifically uses the adjective *synostotic* to describe the cranial shape because brachycephaly, dolichocephaly, and trigonocephaly are known to occur *without* synostosis.

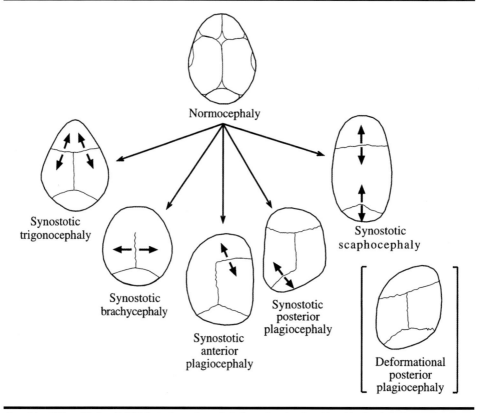

From: Cohen MM Jr, and MacLean RE. 2000. Anatomic, genetic, nosologic, diagnostic, and psychosocial considerations. In *Craniosynostosis: Diagnosis, Evaluation, and Management*, 2nd ed., Cohen MM Jr, and MacLean RE, eds. New york: Oxford University Press, 122. Reprinted by permission of the authors.

PATHOPHYSIOLOGY

A. **Primary:** synostosis without underlying abnormality
   1. Isolated or nonsyndromic
B. **Simple:** fusion of one suture, with growth occurring at a right angle to the stenotic suture[110]
C. **Complex or compound:** fusion of two or more sutures.
   1. Syndromic
D. **Secondary:** cerebral atrophy as the primary occurrence leading to failed cranial growth and premature fusion
E. **Deformational:** cranial deformations attributable to prenatal compression, which should resolve by two months of life[111]

F. **Positional:** increasingly more common secondary to current American Academy of Pediatrics recommendations to position sleeping infants on their back to decrease the risk of sudden infant death syndrome (SIDS)[112]

FIGURE 1-13 ■ Frontal bossing.

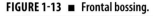

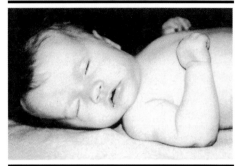

From: De Meirleir L, et al. 1993. Pyruvate dehydrogenase deficiency: Clinical and biochemical diagnosis. *Pediatric Neurology* 9(3): 216. Reprinted by permission.

ETIOLOGY

A. **Primary:** abnormal development of the calvarial sutures with premature closure or agenesis

B. **Secondary:** often due to a structural cerebral abnormality or metabolic derrangement or a rare hematologic condition:[110]

1. Microcephaly secondary to brain atrophy
2. Premature suture fusion secondary to lack of brain growth
3. Thalassemia
4. Mucopolysaccharidosis

INCIDENCE

A. Isolated or nonsyndromic occurrences have the following characteristics:
   1. The incidence is 1/2,000–10,000 births.
   2. They affect males four times more often than females.
   3. Most are sporadic, with a 2–4 percent familial association.[110–112]
   4. In primary or synostotic cases, the deformity is present at birth. Craniosynostosis, the predominant abnormality, requires surgical correction and is categorized according to the affected suture (Figure 1-12).
      a. Sagittal synostosis (scaphocephaly or dolichocephaly) (1/4,200–8,500) accounts for approximately 50 percent of all forms of synostosis.[110–112]
      b. Coronal (plagiocephaly) accounts for approximately 35 percent.
      c. Metopic (trigonocephaly) accounts for approximately 10 percent.
      d. Lambdoidal (brachycephaly) accounts for approximately 5 percent.

B. The incidence of the syndromic class of craniosynostosis is dependent on syndrome incidence.
   1. The following are the most common syndromes involving craniosynostosis:
      a. Saethre-Chotzen
      b. Apert
      c. Crouzon
      d. Pfeiffer
      e. Jackson-Weiss
      f. Carpenter
   2. All are autosomal dominant in inheritance pattern with the exception of Carpenter syndrome, which is autosomal recessive.[111,112]

CLINICAL PRESENTATION

A. Sagittal synostosis (scaphocephaly or dolichocephaly) (see Figure 1-12) results in
   1. Skull elongated by excessive anteroposterior growth away from the complete or partial synostotic sagittal suture[111]

2. Complete sagittal synostosis: occipital bulging, biparietal narrowing, and frontal bossing
3. Anterior sagittal fusion: frontal bossing (Figure 1-13), bicoronal overgrowth.
4. Posterior sagittal fusion: overgrowth of the occipital region and minimal frontal bossing

B. Coronal synostosis (acrobrachycephaly) results in high, short head
C. Metopic synostosis (trigonocephaly) is characterized by a narrow forehead with a midline ridge.
D. Figure 1-14 shows four malformed head shapes resulting from premature closure of sutures.

ASSOCIATIONS

A. Increased intracranial pressure[113]
   1. Fourteen percent incidence
   2. Rare in single-suture synostosis
B. Contralateral ocular torticollis
   1. Fourteen percent incidence
   2. Head tilt toward normal side
C. Shortening of the neck muscles[113]
D. Torticollis[114]
   1. Sixty-four percent deformational plagiocephaly
   2. Head tilt toward abnormal side

DIFFERENTIAL DIAGNOSIS[112]

A. Benign cranial molding
B. Torticollis
C. Primary/nonsyndromic—isolated
D. Syndromic. Most commonly associated syndromes are:
   1. Apert
   2. Crouzon
   3. Jackson-Weiss
   4. Pfeiffer

DIAGNOSIS

A. Differentiating positional deformation from structural deformation is important for treatment and prognosis.
   1. Physical examination: palpable bony ridge over suture location

FIGURE 1-14 ■ **Various malformed head shapes resulting from premature closure of sutures.**

Typical patterns of craniofacial morphology associated with craniosynostosis. **A.** Turribrachycephaly (short, flat head). **B.** Plagiocephaly (slanted head). **C.** Trigonocephaly (triangular head). **D.** Scaphocephaly (keel shaped head).

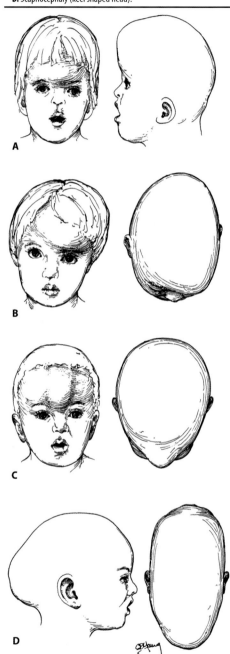

From: Jurkiewicz MJ, et al. 1990. *Plastic Surgery: Principles and Practice.* St. Louis: Mosby, 119. Reprinted by permission.

2. CT scan with three-dimensional reconstruction (preferable) or skull radiograph for definitive diagnosis of involved suture(s)[111,112]
3. Possibly CT, MRI, and electroencephalogram if there are signs of neurologic involvement[112]
4. Funduscopic examination to rule out papilledema and optic atrophy[113]

TREATMENT OPTIONS AND NURSING CARE

A. Surgical correction is needed.
1. Goals
   a. Normalize intracranial pressure.
   b. Permit normal growth of brain and skull.
   c. Correct complications of midfacial hypoplasia.
      1) Ocular
      2) Phonetic
      3) Dental
2. Timing
   a. **Involvement of a single suture:**
      1) Surgery at approximately six weeks of life, following the period of neonatal physiologic anemia
      2) Surgery as soon as possible because satisfactory remodeling of the skull with optimal cosmetic outcome is dependent on the period of rapid brain growth in the first six months
   b. **Involvement of two or more sutures:**
      1) Initial surgery should be performed immediately if there is increased intracranial pressure or potential for this; otherwise, surgical repair should occur as noted above.
      2) When associated with midfacial hypoplasia, multiple, staged procedures with the first surgery at two to six months, a second procedure at approximately four years of age, and a third procedure in early adolescence is frequently the pattern of surgical repair for children with complex craniosynostosis.
3. Directed donor blood
   a. Blood loss can be significant. Because this is a nonemergency procedure, it is possible to prepare the parents for the possibility of transfusion and offer them the option of providing directed donor blood.

SURGICAL MANAGEMENT[110–115]

A. The role of surgery in craniosynostosis remains controversial. Treatment in the neonatal period should be directed to:[115]
1. Preventing a progressive increase in intracranial pressure
2. Preventing local brain distortion
3. Limiting cosmetic deformity
B. The goals of single suture craniosynostosis are:
1. Resecting the affected suture
2. Elevating opposing cranial bones
3. Manual shaping of any other deformities or depressions
C. Multiple suture craniosynostosis is:
1. Staged operative repair with cranial decompression, including orbital decompression as needed

2. Surgical intervention for midface hypoplasia initially performed at 2–6 months of age and then again at 6–10 years of age, timed to follow the emergence of secondary dentition

D. Calvarial vault remodeling is done to achieve normal remodeling of the skull. With regard to head shape, cosmetic outcome is improved by earlier intervention.
  1. Procedure time is 2–3 hours (actual surgical procedure averages 126 minutes).[111] Surgery is performed by a neurosurgeon.

COMPLICATIONS[110–112] (TABLE 1-4)

A. Intraoperative
  1. Blood loss
  2. Anesthesia risks
B. Postoperative
  1. Infection, greatly reduced by postoperative antibiotic coverage
  2. Anemia
  3. Syndrome of inappropriate antidiuretic hormone, panhypopituitarism
  4. Meningocele and/or CSF leakage
  5. Subdural hematoma, subgaleal hemorrhage
  6. Intravascular air
  7. Pressure necrosis of skin
  8. Ocular complications
     a. Retinal damage
     b. Corneal drying
     c. Strabismus from damage to trochlea or canthal tendons
  9. Side effects of anesthesia

TABLE 1-4 ■ Complications of Surgery to Correct Craniosynostosis
Complication
Blood loss
Subdural hematoma
Subgaleal hemorrhage
Cerebrospinal fluid leak
Meningocele
Infection
Intravascular air
Pressure necrosis of skin
Retinal damage
Corneal drying
Strabismus from damage to trochlea or canthal tendons
Syndrome of inappropriate antidiuretic secretion
Panhypopituitarism
Risks from anesthesia

From: Liptak GS, and Serletti JM. 1998. Pediatric approach to craniosynostosis. *Pediatrics in Review* 19(10): 357. (Published erratum in *Pediatrics in Review*, 1999, 20[1]: 20.) Reprinted by permission.

POSTOPERATIVE NURSING CARE[110,112]

A. Follow hematocrit:
  1. Blood loss during the procedure results in an average of 357 ml of packed red blood cells transfused during this procedure.
  2. The goal is for the infant to have a hematocrit of 45 percent at the time of incision closure intraoperatively.
  3. An exiting hematocrit of 45 percent has been shown to reduce the need for postoperative transfusions.
B. Follow procedures to provide postoperative warming secondary to intraoperative heat loss.
C. Administer prophylactic antibiotics as ordered for 24 hours postoperatively.
D. Control pain.

E. Support parents.
   1. Reassure parents that swelling and a misshapen skull in the immediate postoperative period will resolve to become more normal over the first few weeks and will eventually heal to normal configuration.
   2. Postoperative stay is four to five days; encourage parents to return the infant to normal activity once discharged, but to avoid getting the dressing wet.
F. Perform neurosurgical follow-up one and eight weeks postoperatively to assess healing and to evaluate skull defects and bone regrowth.

OUTCOMES

A. Primary craniosynostosis
   1. In general, it is a predominantly cosmetic defect.
   2. Early surgical intervention has an excellent long-term outcome.
B. Syndromic: depends on associated abnormalities

REFERENCES

1. Han H, Patel PK, and Kang NH. 2002. Head and neck embryology. *eMedicine.* Accessed September 27, 2005, from www.emedicine.com/plastic/topic216.htm.

2. Odaci E, and Schaitkin BM. 2005. Face embryology. *eMedicine.* Accessed September 27, 2005, from www.emedicine.com/ent/topic30.htm.

3. Moore KL, and Persaud TVN. 2003. *The Developing Human: Clinically Oriented Embryology,* 7th ed. Philadelphia: Saunders, 201–240, 241–253, 375–380, 465–483, 485–501.

4. Sadler TW. 2004. *Langman's Medical Embryology,* 9th ed. Philadelphia: Lippincott Williams & Wilkins, 363–402, 403–414, 415–426.

5. Moore K, and Persaud TVN. 2003. *Before We Are Born: Essentials of Embryology and Birth Defects,* 6th ed. Philadelphia: Saunders, 152–186, 306–321, 324–328, 344–370, 372–386.

6. Gupta AK, and Varma DR. 2004. Vein of Galen malformations: Review. *Neurology India* 52(1): 43–53.

7. Barr LL. 1999. Neonatal cranial ultrasound. *Radiologic Clinics of North America* 37(6): 1127–1146.

8. Raybaud CA, Strother CM, and Hald JK. 1989. Aneurysms of the vein of Galen: Embryonic considerations and anatomical features relating to the pathogenesis of the malformation. *Neuroradiology* 31(2): 109–128.

9. Volpe JJ. 2001. *Neurology of the Newborn,* 4th ed. Philadelphia: Saunders, 841–856.

10. Truwit CL. 1994. Embryology of the cerebral vasculature. *Neuroimaging Clinics of North America* 4(4): 663–689.

11. Lylyk P, et al. 1993. Therapeutic alternatives for vein of Galen vascular malformations. *Journal of Neurosurgery* 78(3): 438–445.

12. Ciricillo SF, et al. 1990. Interventional neuroradiological management of vein of Galen malformations in the neonate. *Neurosurgery* 27(1): 22–27.

13. Mitchell PJ, et al. 2001. Endovascular management of vein of Galen aneurysmal malformations presenting in the neonatal period. *American Journal of Neuroradiology* 22(7): 1403–1409.

14. Borthne A, et al.1997. Vein of Galen malformations in infants: Clinical, radiological, and therapeutic aspect. *European Radiology* 7(8): 1252–1258.

15. Leff SL, Kronfeld G, and Leonidas JC. 1989. Aneurysm of the vein of Galen. Ultrasound, MRI and angiographic correlations. *Pediatric Radiology* 20(1-2): 98–100.

16. Mickle JP, and Quisling RG. 1986. The transtorcular embolization of vein of Galen aneurysms. *Journal of Neurosurgery* 64(5): 731–735.

17. Lasjaunias P, et al. 1991. Deep venous drainage in great cerebral vein (vein of Galen) absence and malformations. *Neuroradiology* 33(3): 234–238.

18. Dowd CF, et al. 1990. Transfemoral venous embolization of vein of Galen malformations. *American Journal of Neuroradiology* 11(4): 643–648.

19. Carasco A, et al. 1991. Percutaneous transvenous catheterization and embolization of vein of Galen aneurysms. *Neurosurgery* 28(2): 260–266.

20. Halbach W. 1998. Endovascular treatment of mural-type of vein of Galen malformations. *Journal of Neurosurgery* 89(1): 74–80.

21. Kelley DJ, and Meyer CM III. 1997. Congenital anomalies of the neck. In *Congenital Anomalies of the Ear, Nose, and Throat,* Tewfik TL, and Der Kaloustain VM, eds. New York: Oxford University Press, 331–360.

22. Albanese CT, and Wiener ES. 1995. Cystic hygroma. In *Rob and Smith's Operative Surgery: Pediatric Surgery,* 5th ed., Spitz L, and Coran AG, eds. Philadelphia: Lippincott Williams & Wilkins, 94–99.

23. Brown RL, and Azizkhan RG. 1998. Pediatric head and neck lesions. *Pediatric Clinics of North America* 45(4): 889–905.

24. Strigel G. 2000. Hemangiomas and lymphangiomas. In *Pediatric Surgery,* 3rd ed., Ashcraft KW, et al., eds. Philadelphia: Saunders, 977–979.

25. Lewis JM, and Wald ER. 1984. Lymphedema praecox. *Journal of Pediatrics* 104(5): 641–648.

26. Brock ME, et al. 1987. Lymphangioma. An otolaryngologic perspective. *International Journal of Pediatric Otorhinolaryngology* 14(2-3): 133–140.

27. Pijpers L, et al., 1988. Fetal cystic hygroma: Prenatal diagnosis and management. *Obstetrics and Gynecology* 72(2): 223–224.

28. Cohen MM, et al. 1989. Antenatal detection of cystic hygroma. *Obstetrical & Gynecological Survey* 44(6): 481–490.

29. Hartman GE, et al. 1999. General surgery. In *Neonatology: Pathophysiology, and Management of the Newborn,* 5th ed., Avery GB, Fletcher MA, and MacDonald MG, eds. Philadelphia: Lippincott Williams & Wilkins, 1005–1044.

30. Weintraub AS, and Holzman IR. 2000. Neonatal care of infants with head and neck anomalies. *Otolaryngologic Clinics of North America* 33(6): 1171–1189.

31. Cullen MT, et al. 1990. Diagnosis and significance of cystic hygroma in the first trimester. *Prenatal Diagnosis* 10(10): 643–651.

32. Molitch HI, et al. 1995. Percutaneous sclerotherapy of lymphangiomas. *Radiology* 194(2): 343–347.

33. Mettler FA, and Stazzone MM. 2004. Pediatric radiation injuries. In *Nelson Textbook of Pediatrics,* 17th ed., Behrman RE, Kliegman RM, and Jenson HB, eds. Philadelphia: Saunders, 2349–2353.

34. Fonkalsrud EW. 1994. Congenital malformations of the lymphatic system. *Seminars in Pediatric Surgery* 3(2): 62–69.

35. Smithers CJ, and Fishman SJ. 2005. Lymphatic malformations. In *Pediatric Surgery*, 4th ed., Ashcraft KW, Holcomb GW, and Murphy JP, eds. Philadelphia: Saunders, 1044–1046.

36. Kennedy TL. 1989. Cystic hygroma-lymphangioma: A rare and still unclear entity. *Laryngoscope* 99(10 part 2, supplement 49): S1–S10.

37. Stal S, Hamilton S, and Spira M. 1986. Hemangiomas, lymphangiomas, and vascular malformations of the head and neck. *Otolaryngologic Clinics of North America* 19(4): 769–796.

38. Emery PJ, Bailey CM, and Evans JN. 1984. Cystic hygroma of the head and neck: A review of 37 cases. *Journal of Laryngology and Otology* 98(6): 613–619.

39. Whitfill CR, and Drack AV. 2000. Avoidance and treatment of retinopathy of prematurity. *Seminars in Pediatric Surgery* 9(2): 103–105.

40. Terry TL. 1942. Extreme prematurity and fibroblastic overgrowth of persistent vascular sheath behind each crystalline lens. Part I: Preliminary report. *American Journal of Ophthalmology* 25: 203–204.

41. Committee for the Classification of Retinopathy of Prematurity. 1984. An international classification of retinopathy of prematurity. *Archives of Ophthalmology* 102(8): 1130–1134.

42. Lee S. 1999. Retinopathy of prematurity in the 1990s. *Neonatal Network* 18(2): 31–38.

43. Isenberg S. 1999. Eye disorders. In *Neonatology: Pathophysiology and Management of the Newborn*, 5th ed., Avery G, Fletcher M, and MacDonald M, eds. Philadelphia: Lippincott Williams & Wilkins, 1295–1298.

44. Bennett FC. 1999. Developmental outcomes. In *Neonatology: Pathophysiology and Management of the Newborn*, 5th ed., Avery G, Fletcher M, and MacDonald M, eds. Philadelphia: Lippincott Williams & Wilkins, 1486–1487.

45. Graeber JE. 2004. Retinopathy of prematurity. In *Neonatology: Management, Procedures, On-call Problems, Diseases, and Drugs*, 5th ed., Gomella TL, et al., eds. New York: McGraw-Hill, 559–562.

46. Guttentag SH. 1991. Retinopathy of prematurity. In *Manual of Neonatal Care*, 3rd ed., Cloherty JP, and Stark AR, eds. Boston: Little, Brown, 595–598.

47. Miller KM, and Apt L. 2003. The eyes: Retinal vascular diseases. In *Rudolph's Pediatrics*, 21st ed., Rudolf CD, et al., eds. New York: McGraw-Hill, 2393–2395.

48. Good WV, and Gendron RL. 2001. Retinopathy of prematurity. *Ophthalmology Clinics of North America* 14(3): 513–519.

49. Palmer EA, et al. 1991. Incidence and early course of retinopathy of prematurity. *Ophthalmology* 98(11): 1628–1640.

50. Flynn JT, et al. 1987. Retinopathy of prematurity. Diagnosis, severity and natural history. *Ophthalmology* 94(6): 620–629.

51. American Academy of Pediatrics, American Association for Pediatric Ophthalmology and Strabismus, and American Academy of Ophthalmology. 1997. A joint statement: Screening examination of premature infants for retinopathy of prematurity. *Pediatrics* 100(2): 273–274.

52. American Academy of Pediatrics, Section on Ophthalmology. 2001. Screening examination of premature infants for retinopathy of prematurity. *Pediatrics* 108(3): 809–811.

53. Sears J, and Capone A. 1999. Retinopathy of prematurity. In *Ophthalmology*, Yanoff M, Duker JS, and Augsburger JJ, eds. St. Louis: Mosby, 8.19.1–8.19.8.

54. Devine C, and Charles S. 1998. Retinopathy of prematurity. *Ophthalmology Clinics of North America* 11(4): 517–524.

55. Cryotherapy for Retinopathy of Prematurity Cooperative Group. 1996. Multicenter trial of cryotherapy for retinopathy of prematurity. Snellen visual acuity and structural outcome at 5½ years after randomization. *Archives of Ophthalmology* 114(4): 417–424.

56. DeJonge MH, Ferrone PJ, and Trese MT. 2000. Diode laser ablation for threshold retinopathy of prematurity: Short-term structural outcome. *Archives of Ophthalmology* 118(3): 365–367.

57. Cryotherapy for Retinopathy of Prematurity Cooperative Group. 1990. Multicenter trial of cryotherapy for retinopathy of prematurity. Three month outcome. *Archives of Ophthalmology* 108(2): 195–204.

58. D'Amico DJ, et al. 1996. Initial clinical experience with an erbium:YAG laser for vitreoretinal surgery. *American Journal of Ophthalmology* 121(4): 414–425.

59. Hunter DG, and Repka MX. 1992. Diode laser photocoagulation for threshold retinopathy of prematurity: A randomized study. *Ophthalmology* 100(2): 238–243.

60. Andrews AP, Hartnett ME, and Hirose T. 1999. Surgical advances in retinopathy of prematurity. *International Ophthalmology Clinics* 39(1): 275–290.

61. Erzbischoff LM. 2004. A systematic review of anatomical and visual function outcomes in preterm infants after scleral buckle and vitrectomy for retinal detachment. *Advances in Neonatal Care* 4(1): 10–19.

62. Moshfeghi AA, et al. 2004. Lens-sparing vitrectomy for progressive tractional retinal detachments associated with grade 4A retinopathy of prematurity. *Archives of Ophthalmology* 122(12), 1816–1818.

63. Hartnett ME, et al. 2004. Comparison of retinal outcomes after scleral buckle or lens-sparing vitrectomy for Stage 4 retinopathy of prematurity. *Retina* 24(5): 753–757.

64. Kono T, Oshima K, and Fuchino Y. 2000. Surgical results and visual outcomes of vitreous surgery for advanced stages of retinopathy of prematurity. *Japanese Journal of Ophthalmology* 44(6): 661–667.

65. Wilson DB. 1979. Embryonic development of the head and neck. Part 2: The branchial region. *Head and Neck Surgery* 2(1): 59–66.

66. Drumm AJ, and Chow JM. 1989. Congenital neck masses. *American Family Physician* 39(1): 159–163.

67. Mandell DL. 2000. Head and neck anomalies related to the branchial apparatus. *Otolaryngologic Clinics of North America* 33(6): 1309–1332.

68. Triglia JM, et al. 1998. Fist branchial cleft anomalies: A study of 39 cases and a review of the literature. *Archives of Otolaryngology—Head Neck Surgery* 124(3): 291–295.

69. Lindsey WK. 1988. The neck. In *Plastic Surgery in Infancy and Childhood*, 3rd ed., Mustarde JC, and Jackson IT, eds. Edinburgh: Churchill Livingston, 435–449.

70. Azizkhan RG, and DeCou JM. 2003. Head and neck lesions. In *Operative Pediatric Surgery*, Ziegler MM, Azizkhan RG, and Weber TR, eds. New York: McGraw-Hill, 221–240.

71. Avery GB, Fletcher MA, and MacDonald MG. 1999. *Neonatology: Pathophysiology and Management of the Newborn*, 5th ed. Philadelphia: Lippincott Williams & Wilkins.

72. Deacon J. and O'Neill P. 1999. *Core Curriculum for Neonatal Intensive Care Nursing*, 2nd ed. Philadelphia: Saunders.

73. Pulito AR. 2004. Surgical diseases of the newborn. In *Neonatology: Management, Procedures, On-Call Problems, Diseases and Drugs*, 5th ed. Gomella TL, et al., eds. New York: McGraw-Hill, 575–576.

74. Olnes SQ, Schwartz RH, and Bahadori RS. 2000. Consultation with the specialist: Diagnosis and management of the newborn and young infant who have nasal obstruction. *Pediatrics in Review* 21(12): 416–420.

75. Leung AKC, and Cho H. 1999. Diagnosis of stridor in children. *American Family Physician* 60(8): 2289–2296.

76. Keller JL, and Kacker A. 2000. Choanal atresia, CHARGE association, and congenital nasal stenosis. *Otolaryngologic Clinics of North America* 33(6): 1343–1351.

77. Weintraub AS, and Holzman IR. 2000. Neonatal care of infants with head and neck anomalies. *Otolaryngologic Clinics of North America* 33(6): 1171–1189.

78. Ming JE, et al. 2003. Coloboma and other ophthalmologic anomalies in Kabuki syndrome: Distinction from charge association. *American Journal of Medical Genetics. Part A* 123(3): 249–252.

79. Oyamada MK, Ferreira HS, and Hoff M. 2003. Pfeiffer syndrome type 2—case report. *Sao Paulo Medical Journal* 121(4): 176–179.

80. Jaillet J, et al. 2005. Biliary lithiasis in early pregnancy and abnormal development of facial and distal limb bones (Binder syndrome): A possible role for vitamin K deficiency. *Birth Defects Research. Part A, Clinical and Molecular Teratology* 73(3): 188–193.

81. Cohen LF. 2000. Stridor and upper airway obstruction in children. *Pediatrics in Review* 21(1): 4–5.

82. Park AH, Brockenbrough J, and Stankiewicz J. 2000. Endoscopic versus traditional approaches to choanal atresia. *Otolaryngologic Clinics of North America* 33(1): 77–90.

83. Puri P. 2003. *Newborn Surgery*, 2nd ed. London: Arnold, 259–265.

84. Mukesh BN, et al. 2002. Five-year incidence of open-angle glaucoma: The visual impairment project. *Ophthalmology* 109(6): 1047–1051.

85. Kenner C, Lott JW, and Flandermeyer AA. 1998. *Comprehensive Neonatal Nursing: A Physiologic Perspective*, 2nd ed. Philadelphia: Saunders.

86. Kirschner RE, and LaRossa D. 2000. Cleft lip and palate. *Otolaryngologic Clinics of North America* 33(6): 1191–1215.

87. Siberry GK, and Iannone R. 2000. *Harriet Lane Handbook*, 15th ed. St. Louis: Mosby.

88. Spitz L, and Coran AG, eds. 1995. *Rob and Smith's Operative Surgery: Pediatric Surgery*, 5th ed. London, England: Chapman & Hall Medical.

89. Lorenz HP, and Longaker MT. 2003. *In utero* surgery for cleft lip/palate: Minimizing the "ripple effect" of scarring. Journal of Craniofacial Surgery 14(4): 504–511.

90. Christie FB. 1988. Orthodontics in cleft lip and palate. In *Plastic Surgery in Infancy and Childhood*, 3rd ed., Mustarde JC, and Jackson IT, eds. Edinburgh: Churchill Livingston, 41–60.

91. Jeffery SL, Boorman JG, and Dive DC. 2000. Use of cartilage grafts for closure of cleft palate fistulae. *British Journal of Plastic Surgery* 53(7): 551–554.

92. Kenner C. 1988. Cleft palate and lip. In *Neonatal Surgery: A Nursing Perspective*, Kenner C, Harjo J, and Brueggemeyer A, eds. New York: Gruen & Stratton, 91–93.

93. Silvera Q AE, et al. 2003. Long-term results of the two-stage palatoplasty/Hotz' plate approach for complete bilateral cleft lip, alveolus and palate patients. *Journal of Cranio-maxillo-facial Surgery* 31(4): 215–227.

94. Witt PD. 1997. Cleft lip and palate. In *Surgery of Infants and Children: Scientific Principles and practice*, Oldham KT, Colombani PM, and Foglia RP, eds. Philadelphia: Lippincott Williams & Wilkins, 814–824.

95. Hall D. 2004. Common multiple congenital anomaly syndromes. In *Neonatology: Management, Procedures, On-Call Problems, Diseases and Drugs*, 5th ed. Gomella TL, et al., eds. New York: McGraw-Hill, 376–377.

96. Prows CA, and Bender PL. 1999. Beyond Pierre Robin sequence. *Neonatal Network* 18(5): 13–19.

97. Holinger LH. 2003. Congenital anomalies of the larynx. In *Nelson Textbook of Pediatrics*, 16th ed., Behrman RE, Kliegman RM, and Jenson HB, eds. Philadelphia: Saunders, 1409.

98. Mancuso RF. 1996. Stridor in neonates. *Pediatric Clinics of North America* 43(6): 1339–1356.

99. Wiatrak BJ. 2000. Update on the pediatric airway: Congenital anomalies of the larynx and trachea. *Otolaryngologic Clinics of North America* 33(1): 91–110.

100. Denoyelle F, et al. 2003. Failures and complications of supraglottoplasty in children. *Archives of Otolaryngology—Head & Neck Surgery* 129(10): 1077–1080.

101. Reddy DK, and Matt BH. 2001. Unilateral vs bilateral supraglottoplasty for severe laryngomalacia in children. *Archives of Otolaryngology—Head & Neck Surgery* 127(6): 694–699.

102. Willging JP, and Cotton RT. 1997. Congenital anomalies of the neck. In *Congenital Anomalies of the Ear, Nose, and Throat*, Tewfik TL, and Der Kaloustian VM, eds. New York: Oxford University Press, 383–391.

103. Hartnick CJ, and Cotton RT. 2000. Congenital laryngeal anomalies. Laryngeal atresia, stenosis, webs, and clefts. *Otolaryngologic Clinics of North America* 33(6): 1293–1308.

104. Holinger LD, and Konior RJ. 1989. Surgical management of severe laryngomalacia. *Laryngoscope* 99)2): 136–142.

105. Kelly SM, and Gray SD. 1995. Unilateral endoscopic supraglottoplasty for severe laryngomalacia. *Archives of Otolaryngology—Head & Neck Surgery* 121(12): 1351–1354.

106. Wyatt ME, and Hartley BE. 2005. Laryngotracheal reconstruction in congenital laryngeal webs and atresias. *Otolaryngology—Head and Neck Surgery* 132(2): 232–238.

107. McElhinney DB, et al. 2002. Chromosomal and cardiovascular anomalies associated with congenital laryngeal web. *International Journal of Pediatric Otorhinolaryngology* 66(1): 23–27.

108. Gilmore M. 2004. Traumatic delivery. In *Neonatology: Management, Procedures, On-Call Problems, Diseases and Drugs*, 5th ed. Gomella TL, et al., eds. New York: McGraw-Hill, 315–319.

109. de Jong AL, et al. 2000. Vocal cord paralysis in infants and children. *Otolaryngologic Clinics of North America* 33(1): 131–149.

110. Johnston SA. 2001. Calvarial vault remodeling for sagittal synostosis. *AORN Journal* 74(5): 632–647.

111. Lessard ML, and Mulliken JB. 1997. Major craniofacial anomalies. In *Congenital Anomalies of the Ear, Nose, and Throat*, Tewfik TL, and Der Kaloustain VM, eds. New York: Oxford University Press, 301–308.

112. Liptak GS, and Serletti JM. 1998. Pediatric approach to craniosynostosis. *Pediatrics in Review* 19(10): 352–359. (Published erratum in Pediatrics in Review, 1999, 20[1]: 20.)

113. Renier D, et al. 1982. Intracranial pressure in craniosynostosis. *Journal of Neurosurgery* 57(3): 370–377.

114. Bruneteau RJ, and Mulliken JB. 1992. Frontal plagiocephaly: Synostotic, compensational, or deformational. *Plastic and Reconstructive Surgery* 89(1): 21–31.

115. Stout AU, and Stout JT. 2003. Retinopathy of prematurity. *Pediatric Clinics of North America* 50(1): 77–87.

116. Haigh PM, Chiswick ML, and O'Donoghue EP. 1997. ROP: Systemic complications associated with different anaestetic techniques at treatment. *British Journal of Ophthalmology* 81(4): 283–287.

Notes

Notes

2

Neonatal Pulmonary Disorders

Annette Carley, RN, MS, PNP, NNP

Congenital lung malformations are rare and vary considerably in their presentation, complexity, and severity of impact. Neonatal effects may be subtle or overt and often necessitate prompt diagnosis and management. The impact of developmental pulmonary disorders is related to gestational age at occurrence and may manifest as impaired structural integrity of the pulmonary system, including reduced bronchial generations, alveolar number and size, or vascular supply.[1] Consequences of these disorders may pose substantial challenges to medical, surgical, and nursing management.

Precise incidence rates for many congenital lung disorders are difficult to determine because some may spontaneously regress in the prenatal period and others, asymptomatic in the immediate newborn period, may escape detection. Advances in early prenatal and postnatal diagnosis, however, and refined medical and surgical techniques have made it feasible to detect, ameliorate, or correct many of these disorders.[2]

Embryology

A. Development of the upper respiratory tract structures is described in Chapter 1.
B. Development of the lower respiratory tract proceeds as follows.
   1. The larynx, trachea, bronchi, and lungs originate as outgrowths of the primitive embryonic foregut.
      a. In the third week of gestation, a small groove at the cranial end of the foregut tube (laryngotracheal groove) develops a ridge (primitive trachea); two blind pouches (i.e., respiratory diverticulum or lung buds) form caudally.[3]
      b. By the fifth week of gestation, the trachea and esophagus become separated by a mesoderm-derived septum, creating distinct ventral respiratory primordium and dorsal esophagus.[4,5]
      c. The epithelium of the larynx, bronchi, and pulmonary bed originates from endoderm.[5,6]

FIGURE 2-1 ■ **Lung development during the embryonic (A–F) and pseudoglandular (G, H) stages of organogenesis.**

The overall branching pattern of the primitive lung (left panels) results in the development of the bronchial tree. The histologic organization of the fetal lung becomes more complex as branching morphogenesis progresses through these stages (right panels).

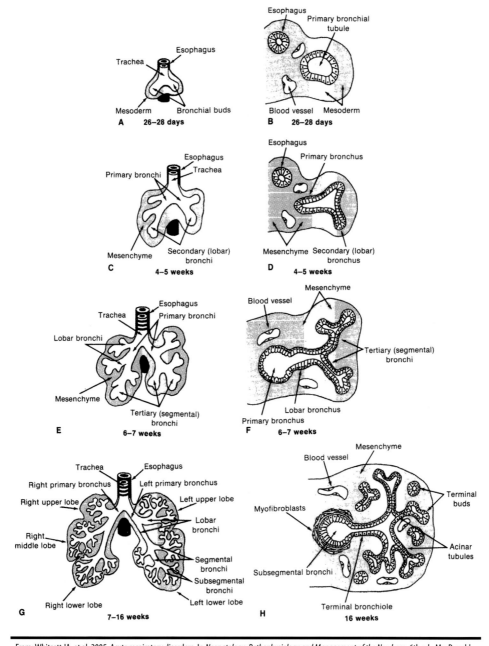

From: Whitsett JA, et al. 2005. Acute respiratory disorders. In *Neonatology: Pathophysiology and Management of the Newborn,* 6th ed., MacDonald MG, Mullett MD, and Seshia MMK, eds. Philadelphia: Lippincott Williams & Wilkins, 554. Reprinted by permission.

    d. Cartilage, muscle, connective tissue, blood vessels, and lymphatics originate from mesoderm.[5,6]

    e. Bronchial and pulmonary development is a result of a cascade of molecular signals involving multiple hormonal growth factors.[5,7]

2. The larynx develops.

    a. As mesenchymal tissue at the cranial end of the laryngotracheal tube proliferates, it creates paired arytenoid swellings that grow toward the tongue into a T-shaped laryngeal outlet.[5,6]

    b. Endodermally derived epithelium forms at the cranial end of the laryngotracheal groove; mesenchyme derived from fourth and sixth pairs of the pharyngeal pouches creates cartilaginous laryngeal support.[6]

    c. Rapid epithelial proliferation temporarily occludes the laryngeal lumen; once recanalized (by week 10), paired recesses (laryngeal ventricles) form, which develop into vocal cords.[5,6]

    d. The epiglottis is created by mesenchymal proliferation at the caudal end of the hypopharyngeal eminence in proximity with the ventral portion of the third and fourth pharyngeal arches; the rostral portion of the hypopharyngeal eminence develops into the posterior tongue.[6]

    e. Myoblastic ingrowth of the fourth and sixth pharyngeal arches favors innervation by the laryngeal branches of the vagus nerve (cranial nerve X).[5]

3. The trachea develops.

    a. The tracheal bud develops at the distal end of the respiratory diverticulum by the fourth gestational week; within one week, it has enlarged into paired outpouchings (bronchial buds), which will develop into the right and left main bronchi.[5]

    b. At the same time, on day 35, the trachea and esophagus are separated by the mesodermally derived septum, which will develop into the cricoid and arytenoid cartilages.[3,4]

    c. The endodermal lining of the laryngotracheal tube distal to the larynx develops into epithelium and glands of both the trachea and pulmonary bed.[6]

    d. Splanchnic mesenchyme differentiates into cartilage, connective tissue, and tracheal muscular support; the cartilage is fully developed by the 24th week of gestation.[3,6]

    e. Cilia are present on the surface epithelium of the trachea by the tenth week of gestation.[3]

    f. Smooth muscle and mucous glands develop in the trachea by the sixteenth week.[3]

4. The bronchi, lungs, and pleura develop during five overlapping developmental periods.

    a. Embryonic period (3–6 weeks gestation)

        1) At the fourth week of gestation, two paired primary bronchial buds develop at the caudal end of the laryngotracheal groove; these grow laterally into the pericardioperitoneal canals, where, in contact with enveloping mesenchyme, they differentiate into bronchi (Figure 2-1A and B).[3,6]

        2) Mesodermally derived, the esophagotracheal septum separates the foregut into the dorsal esophageal and ventral tracheal segments.[4,5]

3) By the fifth week of gestation, the right and left mainstem bronchi have formed; these divide subsequently into lobar and segmental branches (Figure 2-1C and D).[5]

4) The preacinar blood vessels appear.

5) The pulmonary arteries develop from the sixth pair of aortic arches, and pulmonary veins develop from the atrial portion of the heart.[3]

b. Pseudoglandular period (6–16 weeks gestation) (Figure 2-1E–H)

1) This period is characterized by branching morphogenesis and creation of terminal bronchioles.

   a) The first 20 generations of conducting airways develop, consisting of epithelial cells supported by a thin basement membrane and loosely enveloped by mesenchyme.[3,6]

2) All major elements of the lower respiratory tract (except those participating in gas exchange) have formed by the sixteenth week of gestation.[6]

3) Lymphatics appear in the hilum by the eighth week of gestation and in the lung itself by the tenth week.[3]

4) Cilia appear on surface epithelium of the mainstem bronchi at ten weeks gestation and on peripheral airways three weeks later.[3,4]

c. Canalicular period (16–26 weeks gestation) (Figure 2-2A and B)

1) By the seventeenth week of gestation, the acini (gas-exchanging units) and generations 21–23 of the respiratory bronchioles have formed.

2) Intra-acinar capillaries develop and align with air spaces.[4]

3) Alveolar ducts develop and bronchial and bronchiolar lumen enlarge.[6]

4) The surrounding mesenchyme gives rise to bronchial smooth muscle, connective tissue and capillaries, and visceral and parietal pleural layers that will encapsulate the developing lungs, line the thoracic cavity, and create the pleural cavity between layers.[5]

5) By the twentieth week of gestation, cuboidal cells that line acinae develop lamellar bodies, which are the sites of surfactant synthesis and release.[3]

6) By the 24th week of gestation, each terminal bronchiole has developed dual respiratory bronchioles and three to six alveolar units.[5,6]

7) Extrauterine survival is possible at the end of this period.[4]

d. Terminal saccular period (26–40 weeks gestation) (Figure 2-2B–D)

1) The acini are refined into rudimentary, primary saccules; these further differentiate into subsaccules and alveoli.

2) There is a marked decrease in interstitial tissue, with capillary invasion; this increases alveolar-to-blood surface area and enhances extrauterine gas exchange.[3,6]

3) Type II epithelial cells appear, the surfactant system is activated, and storage units (tubular myelin) are seen in air spaces.[6]

4) Type I cells line terminal saccules by the 26th week of gestation.[6]

5) Extrauterine survival is probable.

e. Alveolar period (32 weeks gestation to 8 years of age) (Figure 2-2B–D)

1) Alveoli proliferate and mature from subsaccules.

2) Alveoli attain a polyhedral shape.[3]

3) A secondary alveolar septal partitioning creates true alveoli and alveolar ducts.

4) Approximately 50 million alveoli are present at term.

   a) This represents a sixth of the adult complement.

FIGURE 2-2 ■ Lung development during the canalicular (A), saccular (B), and alveolar stages of organogenesis (C, D).

Dramatic histologic changes in tissue organization occur during these periods. The adult alveolar epithelium is composed of squamous Type I cells and cuboidal Type II cells (inset).

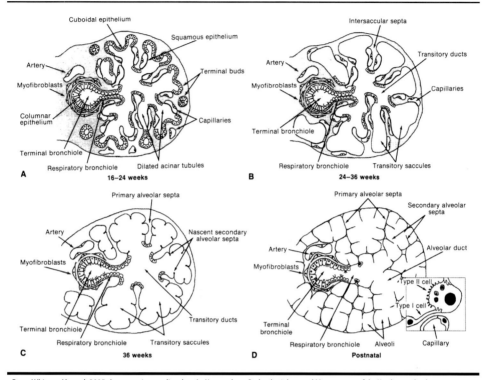

From: Whitsett JA, et al. 2005. Acute respiratory disorders. In *Neonatology: Pathophysiology and Management of the Newborn,* 6th ed., MacDonald MG, Mullett MD, and Seshia MMK, eds. Philadelphia: Lippincott Williams & Wilkins, 556. Reprinted by permission.

    b) After birth, most increased lung size is due to an increased number of bronchioles and alveoli, not to an increase in individual alveolar size.[3,5]

C. Development of the diaphragm proceeds as follows.

1. The diaphragm represents a composite structure, derived from four embryonic components.
   a. Septum transversum
   b. Pleuroperitoneal membranes
   c. Dorsal esophageal mesentery
   d. Body wall muscle
2. The diaphragm is composed of somatic and splanchnic mesoderm.[5,6]
3. A specific chromosomal locus, 15q, is believed to be involved in development of the diaphragm.[6]
4. In the fourth week of gestation, the following occurs.[6]
   a. The intraembryonic coelom gives rise to:
      1) The pericardial cavity
      2) The peritoneal cavity
      3) Two pericardioperitoneal canals on either side of esophagus
   b. The septum transversum (mesodermal tissue):[5,6]

1) Is first noted at the end of the third week of gestation, positioned caudally to the pericardial cavity
2) Partitions the pericardial cavity from the peritoneal cavity
3) Develops into the central tendon of the diaphragm
4) Grows dorsally from the ventrolateral body wall to separate the heart from the liver and partially separate the thoracic cavity from the abdominal cavities

   c. The primitive diaphragm is created after fusion of the pericardioperitoneal canal and the pleuroperitoneal membrane with the dorsal mesentery of the esophagus and the septum transversum.[5]

   d. The crura (median muscular bundle) is formed after myoblast invasion of the dorsal mesentery of the esophagus.[6]

5. By the fifth week of gestation, innervation by the third, fourth, and fifth cervical spinal nerves is achieved as myoblasts and nerve fibers migrate to the developing diaphragm.[5,6]
6. By the ninth to twelfth week of gestation, the enlarging lungs and pleural cavities invade the lateral body walls, splitting them into two layers.[6]
   a. External (definitive abdominal wall)
   b. Internal (peripheral diaphragm)
7. Further extension of this division creates the right and left costodiaphragmatic recesses, which contribute to the dome shape of the mature diaphragm.[6]

Lung Parenchyma Disorders

CONGENITAL LOBAR EMPHYSEMA

Definition
Massive overinflation of one or more lung lobes, which creates symptoms due to compression of pulmonary and mediastinal structures[7–10]

Pathophysiology
A. Congenital lobar emphysema is usually unilobar and most commonly affects the upper lobes.[10,11] The reported distribution of affected lobes is: Left upper lobe, 47–50 percent; right upper lobe, 18–20 percent; right middle lobe, 4–28 percent.[12,13]
B. The space-occupying nature of the lesion creates ipsilateral and contralateral alveolar atelectasis, diaphragmatic compression, and mediastinal shift.[10,14] Bronchial obstruction impairs normal expiration and static recoil of the lung and thus creates distal hyperinflation of otherwise normal lung tissue.[13] The net effect of these features is the creation of an overdistended, noncollapsible lobe, which interferes with normal ventilation efforts.[14] It also creates progressive respiratory distress.

Etiology
A. Up to 50 percent of cases of congenital lobar emphysema have no apparent cause.[8,9,14]
B. Approximately 25 percent of cases are thought to result from a congenital bronchial cartilage defect such as hypoplastic, dysplastic, flaccid, or absent cartilage that occurs during the fourth to sixth weeks of gestation.[8,11,15]

C. Another 25 percent are due to endobronchial obstruction, as a result of redundant mucosal folds or extrinsic bronchial compression. Extrinsic causes include anomalous cardiopulmonary vasculature, diffuse bronchial abnormalities, or an intrathoracic mass.[8–11]

Incidence

A. Though rare, congenital lobar emphysema is the most common neonatal cystic lung malformation, occurring two to three times more frequently in males.[8,10–12,16]

Clinical Presentation

A. Symptoms may present from one week to one month of age.
  1. Decreased breath sounds over the affected side[10,14–16]
  2. Progressive respiratory distress, paralleling the degree of emphysema[8,10,14,15]
  3. Recurrent respiratory distress or infection[15]
  4. Respiratory distress aggravated by feeding[14]
  5. Obstructive symptomatology, including cough, wheeze, and stridor[10,14]
  6. Tachypnea[10,11,14,16]
  7. Intermittent cyanosis,[8,10,11,14,16] though possibly unpredictable as a symptom[12]
  8. Chest wall retractions[11]
  9. Thoracic bulging over the affected side[10,14]
  10. Tracheal or cardiac shift toward the unaffected side[14]
  11. Hyperresonant percussion sounds over the affected side[11,14–16]
  12. Hypotension or other symptoms of inadequate cardiac preload caused by impaired venous return[15]

Associations

A. Associated anomalies are common, occurring in up to 10–30 percent of cases.[9,14]
  1. Patent ductus arteriosus[12,15]
  2. Ventricular septal defect[12,15]
  3. Tetralogy of Fallot[12,15]
  4. Total anomalous pulmonary venous return[15]
  5. Polyalveolar lobe[9]
  6. Pectus excavatum[10]
  7. Diaphragmatic and hiatal hernia[10]
  8. Chondroectodermal dysplasia[10]
  9. Renal aplasia[10]
  10. Cleft palate[10]
  11. Pyloric stenosis[10]
  12. Mediastinal defects[10]

Differential Diagnosis

A. Alternate causes of radiologic or clinical findings that may mimic congenital lobar emphysema:
  1. Atelectasis, with compensatory emphysema[8,14,16]
  2. Congenital diaphragmatic hernia[8–10,14]
  3. Cystic adenomatoid malformation[8–11,16]
  4. Foreign body, creating ball-valve obstruction[10,11]
  5. Pneumatocele[8,10–12,14]
  6. Pulmonary agenesis or hypoplasia with compensatory emphysema[8,10,14]
  7. Tension pneumothorax[8,10–16]
  8. Bronchopulmonary sequestration[9]
  9. Bronchogenic cyst[9]

Diagnosis

A. Lateral chest x-ray: Translucent anterior mediastinum, suggesting lung herniation (Figure 2-3)[14,16]

B. Anteroposterior (AP) chest x-ray (Figure 2-4)

   1. Large, space-occupying hyperlucent lobe, usually in the left upper region, with indistinct lung and vessel markings[8,10,14]

   2. Ipsilateral lobar or segmental atelectasis[8,10,14]

   3. Flattened ipsilateral diaphragm[8,10,14]

   4. Widened rib interspaces[8,10,14]

   5. Mediastinal shift toward the unaffected side[8,10,13,14,16,17]

   6. Herniation of the emphysematous lobe into the mediastinum[8,10]

   7. Solid or opaque mass, which represents trapped fluid within the cyst, present during the first few days of life[14,17]

C. Lateral decubitus chest x-ray: Persistence of a radiographic lucency despite dependent patient positioning[14]

D. Computed tomography (CT) scan: May demonstrate features of the involved lobe, such as a hypodense enlargement with thinned vascular structures[17] or intrinsic or extrinsic bronchial obstruction (Figures 2-5 and 2-6)[8]

E. Fluoroscopy: May identify emphysematous area(s) that remain constant in size despite the phases of respiration[14]

F. Ventilation-to-perfusion scan: May demonstrate diminished ventilation coupled with absent perfusion in ipsilateral lobe and may allow evaluation of the function of adjacent compressed pulmonary tissue[10]

Treatment Options and Nursing Care

A. Congenital lobar emphysema rarely resolves spontaneously.[14] It may do so when caused by a mucus plug. Therefore, the defect is more commonly managed surgically.

B. Immediate maneuvers for stabilization may include:

   1. Selective bronchial intubation with acute pulmonary toilet where the suspected cause is inspissated mucus[9]

   2. Intubation and cautious mechanical ventilation with the lowest possible pressures to minimize lobar distention and avoid increased air trapping, greater mediastinal shift, or possible pneumothorax[9,11]

FIGURE 2-3 ■ Lateral chest x-ray of congenital lobar emphysema depicting retrosternal overinflation of emphysematous lobe.

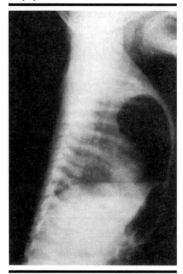

From: Karnak I, et al. 1999. Congenital lobar emphysema: Diagnostic and therapeutic considerations. *Journal of Pediatric Surgery* 34(9): 1348. Reprinted by permission.

FIGURE 2-4 ■ Chest x-ray depicting right-sided hyperexpansion and mediastinal shift to the left.

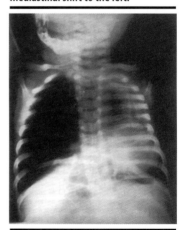

From: Ozcelik U, et al. 2003. Congenital lobar emphysema: Evaluation and long-term follow-up of thirty cases at a single center. *Pediatric Pulmonology* 35(5): 384. Reprinted with permission of Wiley-Liss, Inc., a subsidiary of John Wiley and Sons, Inc.

3. High-frequency ventilation as a strategy to limit excess ventilatory pressures[9]
4. Gastric decompression to decrease diaphragmatic impedance of ventilation efforts
5. Intravascular access for hemodynamic monitoring and acid-base and oxygenation assessments[18]
6. Echocardiography to assess for coexisting cardiac anomalies because 15–30 percent of infants may have associated cardiac defects[12,16]

Surgical Management

A. Bronchoscopy may identify and/or remove the source of obstruction. This procedure must be used cautiously to avoid further compromise of respiratory status from procedural trauma.[8,15] Flexible bronchoscopy may offer advantages over rigid bronchoscopy in evaluation of airway dynamics.[10]
B. Endoscopic decompression of the affected lobe may be performed.[9]
C. Thoracentesis and evacuation of lobar contents by aspiration may be used as a temporizing procedure until a thoracotomy is feasible.[14]
D. Thoracotomy with lobectomy[8,10,16] or segmental resection[8,9,13] can be accomplished as early as day 1 of life and carries a low operative mortality. These procedures may incorporate the use of a thoracotomy drainage tube for postoperative assessment of residual air and fluid. Postsurgical evaluation includes a perfusion scan, which will assess perfusion to the affected lobe and function of both affected and contralateral lobes.[16]

Postoperative Nursing Care

A. Infants undergoing surgical management of congenital lobar emphysema need vigilant nursing assessments postoperatively. In addition to general nursing care **(as noted under Nursing Considerations for Neonatal Pulmonary Disorders later in this chapter),** strategies and considerations specific to lobar emphysema include:
1. Judiciously remove secretions and provide adequate humidification of

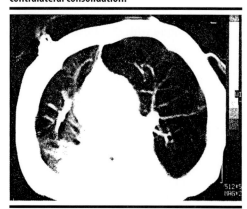

FIGURE 2-5 ■ CT scan of congenital lobar emphysema with left upper lobe hyperaeration and contralateral consolidation.

From: Karnak I, et al. 1999. Congenital lobar emphysema: Diagnostic and therapeutic considerations. *Journal of Pediatric Surgery* 34(9): 1348. Reprinted by permission.

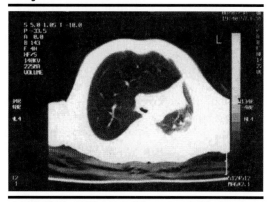

FIGURE 2-6 ■ CT scan depicting both hyperinflation on the right and mediastinal shift.

From: Ozcelik U, et al. 2003. Congenital lobar emphysema: Evaluation and long-term follow-up of thirty cases at a single center. *Pediatric Pulmonology* 35(5): 384. Reprinted with permission of Wiley-Liss, Inc., a subsidiary of John Wiley and Sons, Inc.

ventilator circuitry to decrease the tenacity of secretions (especially in cases in which the cause is inspissated mucus).

2. Monitor volume and character of chest tube drainage if drains are employed following lobectomy or segmentectomy and aseptically maintain closed drainage with careful attention to prescribed suction pressures if suction is indicated.

3. Because of the risks of infection posed by both thoracentesis and thoracotomy, assess the site regularly to determine adequacy of healing and volume and character of drainage. Skin site and attendant dressings should be managed aseptically.

Outcomes

A. Untreated lobar emphysema has high mortality and morbidity risks associated with progressive compression of normal lung lobes or recurrent pneumonia affecting these adjacent compressed lung areas.[7,13,14] The severity of symptoms at the time of diagnosis will dictate management strategies.[10] In a small study, patients managed under a conservative protocol showed no significant difference on follow-up in pulmonary function or symptomatology from surgically managed patients.[8]

B. Postsurgical outcomes include low operative mortality (<5 percent),[11,14] relief of symptoms,[13] and excellent long-term prognosis for normal growth and development if the remaining lung is normal.[11,12] Even for patients treated surgically during infancy, the outcome is good with normal lung volume, normal ventilation:perfusion matching, and normal x-ray and spirometry findings. X-ray and spirometry results in infants with good outcomes suggest postlobectomy compensatory ipsilateral lung growth occurs and adequate overall pulmonary function is achieved.[19]

BRONCHOGENIC CYST

Definition

Cystic airway malformation that creates airway or upper gastrointestinal (GI) tract compression[11]

Pathophysiology

A. The classic depiction of bronchogenic cyst involves absent or atretic bronchial communication with production of space-occupying, mucus-producing cysts that do not participate in ventilation.[20]

B. Cysts vary in size and contain trapped clear, turbid, serous, or viscous secretions. These sequestered secretions may account for the frequently encountered symptoms suggesting infection.[12,15,21]

C. Cysts may occur in either intra- or extrathoracic locations and are most commonly located retro-carinally. If intrapulmonary, they are usually right sided.[11,22,23]

D. There may be no neonatal symptoms unless the cyst is located near a major airway or is rapidly increasing in size and creating tracheal, bronchial, or esophageal compression and distortion.[11,22]

Etiology

A. Bronchogenic cyst represents a bronchopulmonary foregut malformation occurring early in gestation.

B. Centrally located cysts, generally asymptomatic in presentation, result from anomalous budding of the ventral or tracheal foregut during the sixth gestational week, prior to formation of the bronchus.[13,22]

C. Peripherally located cysts, more precisely termed pulmonary parenchymal cysts, are frequently symptomatic because of established bronchial connections. These cysts represent a disorder of bronchial growth and occur as a later (sixth to sixteenth week of gestation) developmental anomaly.[13,22]

Incidence

A. Bronchogenic cyst is the most common foregut duplication lung cyst, represents 5–10 percent of mediastinal masses, and occurs more commonly is males.[12,15,16,22]

Clinical Presentation

A. Bronchogenic cyst may be asymptomatic and present beyond the neonatal period.[12,22,24] Symptoms include:
1. Progressive respiratory distress[14,15]
2. Tachypnea[14]
3. Wheezing[15,22,24]
4. Stridor[14,15,24]
5. Cough[7,24]
6. Tachycardia[14]
7. Cyanosis[15,24]
8. Hyperresonance over the affected lung[14,15]
9. Mediastinal shift toward the contralateral side[14,15]
10. Dysphagia[24]
11. Hemoptysis[24]
12. Substernal or back pain[24]

Associations

A. Associated conditions are rare, but may include pulmonary sequestration,[22] congenital heart defects, and cystic fibrosis.[24]

Differential Diagnosis

A. Alternate causes of radiologic or clinical findings may mimic bronchogenic cyst.
1. Congenital lobar emphysema[13,14,16]
2. Congenital cystic adenomatoid malformation[13]
3. Congenital diaphragmatic hernia[13,14,24]
4. Pneumatocele[11,14,24]
5. Tension pneumothorax[13,14,24]
6. Bronchopulmonary dysplasia for later presenting cases[20]

Diagnosis

A. The AP chest x-ray is notable for a fluid-filled, space-occupying lesion with smooth, rounded, and homogeneous edges[23] or a round or ovoid soft tissue density adjacent to the carina (Figure 2-7).[12]

B. CT scan may confirm the cyst location, define cyst features such as wall thickness and internal contents, and identify associated anomalies that may dictate management options or outcome.[21]

C. Esophageal contrast or scintigraphy may detect compression caused by the defect and differentiate the lesion from other causes of obstruction.[24]

Treatment Options and Nursing Care

A. Surgical treatment is recommended.[25]
B. For symptomatic patients, immediate maneuvers for pulmonary stabilization include intubation and ventilation with the lowest possible pressures to avoid the risk of air trapping.[25]

Surgical Management

A. Excise the entire lesion with cautery of any epithelial remnants. The lesion is generally approached via a right posterolateral thoracotomy incision to optimize operative exposure of the carina and right mainstem bronchus. Lesions >3 cm distal to the carina or at the left mainstem bronchus are approached from a left thoracotomy incision.
B. If the trachea is encountered during dissection, a pericardial patch may be utilized for repair.[7]
C. The extent of the surgical excision depends on the cyst location and degree of accompanying inflammation.
D. Surgical excision is recommended in asymptomatic patients due to the risk of subsequent infection or malignancy such as squamous metaplasia.[7,13,16,23,24]

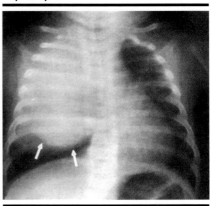

FIGURE 2-7 ■ Large, fluid-filled, bronchogenic cyst (arrows) in this infant with respiratory distress.

From: Swischuk LE. 2004. *Imaging of the Newborn, Infant, and Young Child, 5th ed.* Philadelphia: Lippincott Williams & Wilkins, 161. Reprinted by permission.

Postoperative Nursing Care

A. Infants who have undergone surgical management of bronchogenic cyst will need vigilant nursing assessments postoperatively. In addition to general nursing care **(as noted under Nursing Considerations for Neonatal Pulmonary Disorders later in this chapter),** strategies and considerations specific to bronchogenic cyst include:
   1. Judicious removal of secretions and optimized humidification of ventilator circuitry during mechanical ventilation
   2. Close monitoring for postoperative bleeding as a consequence of resection and cautery procedures (Bleeding may be directly noted at operative sites and indirectly surmised by decreased hematocrit, altered perfusion, or other indicators of depleted intravascular volume.)

Outcomes

A. Though most cases are asymptomatic, the risk of recurrent pulmonary infections or later malignancy may affect ultimate patient outcome. Additionally, in cases with bronchial communication, sudden enlargement of the lesion may result in acute respiratory symptoms.[7,13,23]
B. The prognosis after surgical resection is good.[12]

CONGENITAL CYSTIC ADENOMATOID MALFORMATION (CCAM)

Definition

Dynamic, benign, cystic hamartoma (embryologic overgrowth) of lung tissue, which creates respiratory distress by compressing pulmonary and mediastinal structures[26,27]

Pathophysiology

A. Stocker classified congenital cystic adenomatoid malformation into morphologic types, of which Types I–III account for 95 percent of cases.[3]

1. Type I, the most common, accounts for 50–70 percent of cases.[17,22,28,29] Eleven percent of these lesions have associated anomalies. Despite this, prognosis is good and the survival rate is 90 percent. The lesion consists of a single dominant or multiple large, fluid- or air-containing cysts, which communicate with the bronchial tree and are surrounded by mesenchymal tissue. Elastic tissue is more abundant than normal, but blood vessels are normal. Mucus-secreting cells are not present.[12,17,29]

2. Type II accounts for up to 15–40 percent of cases.[1,12,17,22,28] Mortality is high due to coexisting anomalies in half of the cases. The lesion consists of multiple medium-sized, evenly spaced, fluid- or air-containing cysts, which communicate with normal bronchi. The cysts resemble dilated terminal bronchioles. Blood vessels are normal; however, mucus-secreting cells and elastic tissue are not present.[12,29]

3. Type III accounts for 8–10 percent of cases.[17,22,28] No anomalies are commonly associated with this type; however, mortality is high due to the presence of mediastinal shift or hydrops at the time of diagnosis. The lesion is large and bulky, with evenly distributed, small-sized cysts. No cartilage or mucus-producing cells are present.[12,28–30]

4. Less frequently described are Types 0 and IV.

   a. Type 0, also known as "acinar dysplasia," represents an abnormality of the proximal tracheobronchial tree. The lungs appear small, firm, and granular; this condition is incompatible with life.

   b. Type IV, which accounts for 10–15 percent of cases, represents a distal acinus malformation. Clinically, this produces a large cyst usually confined to the periphery, which may create no symptoms or mild to moderate respiratory distress.[3,17,31]

5. *Congenital pulmonary airway malformation* has recently been proposed as the new term for the disorder, to encompass both cystic and noncystic forms.[32]

B. An alternate anatomic and ultrasonographic classification was proposed by Adzik and associates.[33]

1. Macrocystic lesions, the more common type, contain single or multiple echolucent, fluid-filled cysts. These lesions are not usually associated with hydrops.

2. Microcystic lesions, less commonly encountered, contain solid, bulky echogenic cysts. These lesions are frequently associated with hydrops and pulmonary hypoplasia.

C. A histologic classification was proposed by Morotti and associates.[34]

1. Subtype I, corresponding to Stocker Types I, II, and III, consists of bronchiolar type tissue and likely develops early during the pseudoglandular stage of lung development.

2. Subtype II, corresponding to Stocker Type IV, consists of acinar-alveolar tissue and likely occurs during the saccular stage of lung development.

D. An additional histologic classification was proposed by Cha and colleagues.[27]

1. Pseudoglandular type, resembling the pseudoglandular lung developmental stage at the 6th to 16th week, consists of tightly packed tubules and scattered bronchiolar structures, as seen in Stocker Type III lesions.

2. Canalicular type, resembling the canalicular stage of lung development at the 17th to 28th week, consists of bronchioles, alveolar ducts, and branched alveolar spaces. This classification resembles Stocker Type II lesions.

Etiology

A. Congenital cystic adenomatoid malformation results from failed maturation of bronchiolar structures prior to the development of cartilage, as early as the fifth to sixth gestational week, and resulting in proliferation of terminal bronchiolar-type tissue that lacks mature alveoli.[11,21,23,30,35–37]

B. Less commonly encountered lesions, for example, Stocker Type IV, may arise later in gestation.

C. There are additional proposed explanations of lesion development.
    1. Disruption of normal regulatory hormonal influence or growth processes, such as local underproduction of keratinocyte growth factor or other hormonal growth factors normally produced by the lung that regulate its development[27]
    2. Disruption of the normal apoptosis (programmed cell death) process in the fetal lung[36]

Incidence

A. Recent estimates suggest that CCAM occurs in 9/100,000 births, which represents 25 percent of all congenital lung malformations.[38,39]

B. Precise incidence figures for the lesion are difficult to determine because an estimated 6–25 percent of lesions undergo spontaneous *in utero* regression due either to ischemia of the lesion itself or relative decrease due to increased size of the adjacent lung.[1,28,37,40] However, more routine utilization of prenatal ultrasound has likely increased overall case finding, including these regressed lesions.[41]

C. Males are more frequently affected than females, at a rate of approximately 1.8 to 1.[12,29]

D. The lesion occurs with equal frequency in right and left lungs and is unilobar in 80–95 percent of cases.[1,22,35,37]

Clinical Presentation

A. The clinical expression of CCAM varies, depending upon the amount of parenchyma replaced by the malformation and/or compression of normal lung structures by the lesion.[14,33,42]

B. If the cysts are small and the defect is unilateral, CCAM may be asymptomatic.[28,40]

C. Progressive respiratory distress occurs, with 50–85 percent of cases presenting in the neonatal period.[11,22,37,43] Features of respiratory distress include tachypnea, cyanosis, grunting, and retractions.[28,42]

D. Breath sounds decreased.[28]

E. Heart sounds become distant or shift.[28]

F. There is prominent contour of the affected chest side.[28]

G. Ipsilateral hyperresonance appears.[28]

H. There is hepatosplenomegaly due to thoracic hyperexpansion.[28]

I. There is hypotension or other evidence of poor cardiac preload due to compromised venous return.[28]

J. Symptomatology is attributed to the specific lesion type.
    1. Progressive respiratory distress, mediastinal shift, contralateral atelectasis, and decreased ipsilateral breath sounds are more common for Type I lesions.

2. Severe respiratory distress within 12 hours of postnatal life is more common for Type II lesions.

3. Severe respiratory distress, with marked mediastinal shift and dull percussion sounds over the affected lung, is more common for Type III lesions.[29]

K. The older child may present with recurrent localized pulmonary infection.[31,32]

Associations

A. Prenatal conditions associated with CCAM:
1. History of spontaneous abortions or stillbirths[12,29]
2. Polyhydramnios, in up to 50 percent of cases,[28] caused by decreased swallowing due to esophageal occlusion or overproduction of fetal lung fluid by the abnormal lung tissue[33,35,44]
3. Fetal hydrops due to cardiac compression from the mass, decreased venous return, and impaired lymphatic drainage[29,33,35,43,45]
4. Maternal mirror syndrome: a poorly understood preeclampsia-like phenomenon that creates endothelial injury in the maternal host[17,37,46]

B. Neonatal conditions associated with CCAM:
1. Prematurity[12,29]
2. Renal malformations, such as renal agenesis[10,28,29,44]
3. Gastrointestinal malformations, such as atresias[29]
4. Skeletal malformation, such as pectus excavatum or cervical spine deformities[29,41]
5. Central nervous system malformations, such as hydrocephalus[3]
6. Low birth weight (LBW)[28,29]
7. Pulmonary malformations, such as sequestration, hypoplasia, or diaphragmatic hernia[28,29,35]
8. Sirenomelia[12]

Differential Diagnosis

A. Alternate causes of radiologic or clinical findings may mimic congenital cystic adenomatoid malformation.
1. Congenital diaphragmatic hernia[11,12,14,15,28,35,37,42,47]
2. Bronchopulmonary sequestration[17,28,33,35,40,47]
3. Bronchogenic cyst[28,35,37,40,47]
4. Mediastinal cystic hygroma or teratoma[28,33,35,37,40]
5. Brain heterotopia[33,37,40]
6. Congenital lobar emphysema[12,14,28]
7. Pneumatocele[28]
8. Pneumothorax[12]

Diagnosis

A. The definitive diagnosis of CCAM is confirmed through histologic examination and suggested through imaging studies.[31]
1. Prenatal ultrasound (Figure 2-8) shows a solid or cystic lung mass, coupled with absent systemic vascular Doppler signals and mediastinal shift or hydrops.[37] Hydrops may be evident as ascites, skin or scalp edema, or placental enlargement.[26] Fetal ultrasound may be able to distinguish between lesion types.[41] Though a sensitive test in the prenatal period, approximately half of suspected lesions may not be positively predicted, due to either lesion regression or radiographic similarities with other fetal thoracic lesions.[38]

2. Chest x-ray reveals multicystic, fluid- or air-filled lucencies surrounded by nonhomogeneous lung tissue,[29] or multiple, progressively enlarging cysts creating mediastinal shift toward the contralateral side (Figure 2-9).[15,28]

3. CT scan demonstrates mediastinal shift created by the lesion and the extent of lobe(s) involvement. Lesion types can be identified (Figure 2-10).[16,28] Because the initial chest x-ray may be normal, CT scan has been suggested as an essential tool in aiding a diagnosis of CCAM.[48]

Treatment Options and Nursing Care

A. Prenatal management:
1. Gestational age at detection of the defect will dictate management strategies.[37]
2. Newborn infants with a history of prenatally detected lesions, despite *in utero* regression, will need careful postnatal followup, including CT and/or magnetic resonance imaging (MRI) scans.[28,37]

B. Neonatal management:
1. Delivery should occur in a tertiary level perinatal center, with staff adequately prepared to deal with respiratory compromise at birth.[37,38,49] Presence of the lesion is not an absolute indication for cesarean section delivery.[40]

FIGURE 2-8 ■ Serial ultrasound images at (A) 23, (B) 30 4/7, and (C) 33 4/7 weeks gestation consistent with Type I CCAM.

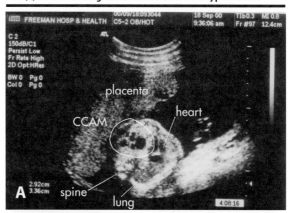

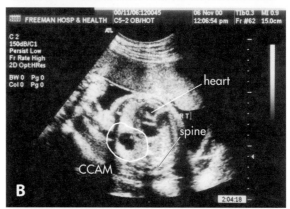

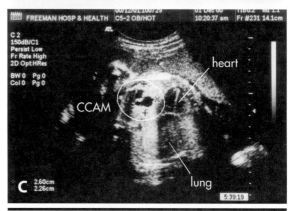

Courtesy of Dr. Howard Thompson and Freeman Hospital, Joplin, Missouri.

2. Immediate maneuvers for pulmonary stabilization include:

  a. Thoracotomy with chest tube drainage for macrocystic lesions causing hemodynamic compromise or in the presence of pleural effusions[43,44]

  b. Endotracheal intubation and mechanical ventilation to treat respiratory failure

  c. Cautious positive pressure ventilation to avoid an increase in gas trapping[25,28]

  d. Selective endotracheal intubation of the contralateral side in cases of unilateral disease[37]

  e. High-frequency ventilation if the patient's ventilatory requirements dictate high peak inspiratory or positive end-expiratory pressures[28]

  f. Extracorporeal membrane oxygenation (ECMO)[43]

  g. Nitric oxide therapy[43]

FIGURE 2-9 ■ AP x-ray of CCAM over the left chest.

Note the mediastinal shift. A large air-filled dominant cyst appears lucent over the lung field.

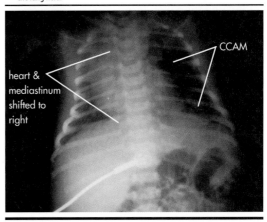

Courtesy of Dr. Howard Thompson and Freeman Hospital, Joplin, Missouri.

Surgical Management

A. Complete resection of the lesion is typically by lobectomy.[1,28,37,48] Bilateral disease may dictate resection of multiple lung lobes.[37]

B. Partial lung resection is discouraged because of the potential for re-expansion of smaller daughter cysts or persistent air leak.[11,28]

C. Postoperatively, one or more chest tubes is utilized to drain residual air or fluid.[11]

Complications

A. Immediate postoperative period:[20,25]

  1. Pulmonary hypertension

  2. Pulmonary edema

Postoperative Nursing Care

A. Infants undergoing surgical management of CCAM need vigilant nursing assessments postoperatively. In addition to general nursing care (**as noted under Nursing Considerations**

FIGURE 2-10 ■ CCAM in a newborn with respiratory distress.

A. Chest radiograph shows mottled lucency within the left upper lung. There is mediastinal shift to the right. **B.** CT scan shows left upper lobe mass containing multiple air-filled cysts of varying sizes.

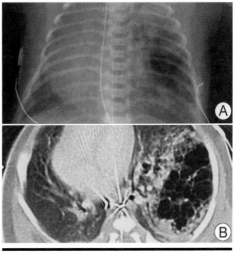

From: Donnelly LF. 2002. Chest. In *PocketRadiologist–Pediatrics: Top 100 Diagnoses*, Donnelly LF, et al., eds. Salt Lake City: Amirsys, 16. Reprinted by permission of the author.

for **Neonatal Pulmonary Disorders later in this chapter),** strategies and considerations specific to CCAM include the following:

1. Judicious removal of secretions and optimized humidification of ventilator circuitry must be provided when mechanical ventilation is employed.
2. A chest tube is typically in place postoperatively. Therefore, ongoing assessments of the character and volume of the drainage is important to detect potential accumulation of air or fluid, which may impair ventilation.[48]
3. Ventilatory management includes cautious application of positive pressure and avoidance of hypoxemia, which may potentiate pulmonary hypertension.[50]
4. Pulmonary vasodilators such as nitric oxide may be continued postoperatively and will require careful monitoring and weaning.

FIGURE 2-11 ■ Illustrations of (A) intralobar and (B) extralobar sequestration.

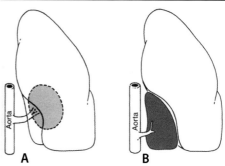

From: Sylvester KG, and Albanese CT. 2005. Bronchopulmonary malformations. In *Pediatric Surgery*, 4th ed., Ashcraft KW, Holcomb GW, and Murphy JP, eds. Philadelphia: Saunders, 281. Reprinted by permission.

Outcomes

A. Outcomes are variable and determined by such features as the presence of hydrops, the lesion type and size, the extent of surgical treatment required, and the impact of coexisting anomalies.[28] The overall mortality rate for congenital cystic adenomatoid malformation is approximately 28 percent.[40]
B. Short-term outcomes of the three most common types, are reported as:[12]
   1. Type I, approximately 90 percent survival
   2. Type II, 56 percent survival
   3. Type III, 60 percent survival
C. The presence of hydrops with either microcystic or macrocystic lesions results in a poor prognosis.
D. When either microcystic or macrocystic lesions occur without hydrops and are managed in a tertiary setting, the chance of survival is good.[33]
E. Long-term expected outcome in surgical survivors is good and dictated by the amount of residual lung after resection and effects of any coexisting anomalies.
F. Subsequent development of neoplasia in retained lesion areas has been reported; therefore, resection in the neonatal period or careful ongoing pulmonary assessments in nonsurgically managed cases is warranted.[37,40,49]

BRONCHOPULMONARY SEQUESTRATION

Definition

A group of defects involving nonfunctional, parenchymal tissue lacking normal airway communication that create variable pulmonary symptomatology[16,37,51,52]

Pathophysiology

A. The sequestered mass consists of nonfunctional lung tissue with a blood supply derived from anomalous systemic vascular connections. The natural history of the lesion is to show relative regression over time and thus may be asymptomatic in some cases.[17]

B. The lesion may be solid or cystic, homogeneous or nonuniform.[53] Although no direct or normal airway connection exists, the sequestered tissue may be partially aerated via collaterals, such as the pores of Kohn, creating the potential for repeated infections.[23,54] Additionally, there may be gastrointestinal tract communication creating symptomatology involving that system.[23] Some authors have subclassified this type of defect as communicating bronchopulmonary foregut malformation.[55]

C. Two classic types of sequestration are described in the literature (Figure 2-11):

  1. Intralobar sequestration (ILS), which accounts for 75 percent of cases, describes a mass embedded within normal lung tissue without a separate pleural membrane. This defect is usually situated in the lower lobes, at the left and posterior basilar segments. Blood supply to the mass arises from the left gastric or adrenal arteries, and venous drainage occurs into the pulmonary vein.[55,56]

  2. Extralobar sequestration (ELS), which accounts for 25 percent of cases, describes a mass that has no normal bronchial or arterial connections. It develops separately from the pleura and adjacent normal lung.[55,57] The lesion, usually left-sided, often contains multiple small blood vessels, with venous drainage occurring into the azygous or hemiazygous vein. This lesion type is generally asymptomatic and is often discovered incidentally.[3,21,56,58]

D. Scimitar variant, also known as "hypogenetic lung syndrome" and "congenital venolobar syndrome," refers to a hypoplastic lung lobe possessing an anomalous blood supply via an arteriovenous malformation.

  1. Venous return occurs via a dominant vein into the right atrium or inferior vena cava and creates a large left-to-right vascular shunt.[13]

  2. The *scimitar* name refers to the swordlike image produced radiographically by the anomalous vessels in the medial aspect of the right lower lung (Figures 2-12 and 2-13).[3,21,59]

Etiology

A. Sequestration represents a spectrum of bronchopulmonary foregut malformations that occur as early as the fifth to seventh week of gestation.

  1. The classic description of the intralobar defect is abnormal caudal lung budding, which dissociates from the tracheobronchial tree, yet retains its primitive systemic vascular connection.[22] As this occurs prior to pleural development, the lesion becomes incorporated in the adjacent lung.[1]

  2. The extralobar defect, presumed to occur later in gestation after development of the visceral pleura, forms separately within its own pleural encasement.[1,60]

B. Reports of both intralobar and extralobar types occurring simultaneously in some patients supports a common embryologic origin.[61] However, differences in presentation are attributed to the timing within a spectrum of the overall disease.[51,62]

C. Evidence suggests an acquired, infectious etiology for the development of most intralobar sequestrations. Stocker and Malczak have proposed that pulmonary infection creates inflammatory and cystic parenchymal changes and potentiates hypertrophy of aberrant systemic blood vessels, thus creating the defect.[51,57,63,64]

D. Additional theories of the origin of sequestration include entrapment, adhesion and traction of the embryonic lung by the diaphragm or other organs, and idiopathic cystic changes.[51,57,65]

Incidence

A. Sequestration represents 0.15–6.4 percent of all congenital pulmonary malformations, which account for approximately 0.1 percent of hospital admissions.[60,61]

1. This makes it the second most common congenital pulmonary malformation.[55]

2. The intralobar type occurs slightly more frequently in males, approximately 1.5:1.[57]

3. The extralobar type is three to four times more common in males.[54]

FIGURE 2-12 ■ Scimitar syndrome.

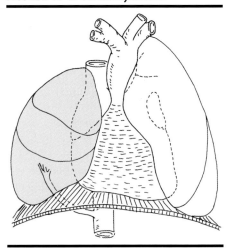

From: Luck SR, Reynolds M, and Raffensperger J. 1996. Congenital bronchopulmonary malformations. *Current Problems in Surgery* 23(4): 300. Reprinted by permission.

B. Intralobar lesions account for 75 percent of all sequestrations; however, the fact that intralobar lesions are more commonly symptomatic enhances their case finding and so may increase their reported frequency.[1,52,54]

1. Intralobar lesions can occur in either hemithorax; 80 percent of extralobar defects occur on the left side.[58,61]

C. Scimitar lesions are estimated to occur in 1–3/100,000 live births.[66]

Clinical Presentation

A. Sequestration may be asymptomatic if the lesion is extralobar or small and not impairing ventilation.[54]

B. Recurrent pneumonia caused by poor lobe drainage occurs more commonly in lesions with GI tract communication.[14,22,57]

1. Suggestive clinical features may include:[11,13,14,21]
   a. Purulent sputum
   b. Cough
   c. Fever

C. Respiratory distress is caused by the mass effect on mediastinal or lung structures.[17,52] Symptoms of this may include wheezing or tachypnea.[23,54]

D. Pleural effusion may occur.[1,15,58]

E. Cardiac murmur may be present.[23]

F. Symptoms of congestive heart failure, such as tachycardia, respiratory distress, feeding intolerance, irritability, or hepatosplenomegaly, may be caused by associated cardiac lesions[13] or large vascular shunts created by the abnormal blood vessel communications.[13,15,23,51,52]

G. Clinical findings associated with scimitar lesions include:[66]

1. Shift in heart sounds or cardiac impulse to the right

2. Systolic murmur, and diminished breath sounds on the right

3. Dextroposition of the heart is common due to right-sided lung hypoplasia

Associations

A. Associated anomalies are common, including prenatal findings of polyhydramnios, pleural effusion, and hydrops.[1,52,67] These findings are likely caused by the mass effect of the lesion and subsequent lymphatic obstruction.[1]

B. Fourteen percent of intralobar lesions have associated anomalies, including:[61]

1. Esophageal diverticula
2. Diaphragmatic hernia
3. Skeletal anomalies
4. Cardiac and pericardial anomalies
5. Renal malformations
6. Cerebral anomalies

C. Approximately 50–65 percent of extralobar lesions have associated anomalies, usually more serious, including:[52,61,64]

FIGURE 2-13 ■ Chest x-ray of scimitar malformation.

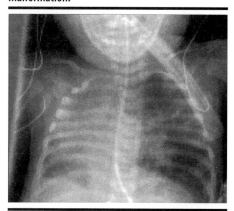

From: Westra SJ. 2002. Chest. In *PocketRadiologist–Pediatrics: Top 100 Diagnoses,* Donnelly LF, et al., eds. Salt Lake City: Amirsys, 98. Reprinted by permission of the author.

1. GI malformations, such as duplications, cysts, and fistulas[1,52,54,55,61,65]
2. Vertebral or skeletal defects, including pectus excavatum[12,16,55,57,61]
3. Cardiac and pericardial defects, including atrial and ventricular septal defects, tricuspid atresia, aortic stenosis, truncus arteriosus, and transposition of the great vessels[1,11,12,16,52,55]
4. Diaphragmatic defects in up to 30 percent of cases[1,51,53,55,57,65,67–69]
5. Congenital cystic adenomatoid malformation[16,53,55,65]
6. Esophageal cysts[67]
7. Bronchogenic cysts[16,53,55,57]
8. Pleural effusions, due to dilated subpleural lymphatics[58]
9. Pulmonary agenesis,[11] or hypoplasia[55]
10. Congenital lobar emphysema[55]

D. Approximately 25 percent of scimitar lesions have associated defects, including:[13,70]

1. Pulmonary hypoplasia
2. Horseshoe lung
3. Cardiovascular anomalies, including:[59,66]
   a. Atrial septal defect
   b. Patent ductus arteriosus
   c. Pulmonary artery hypoplasia
   d. Pulmonary venous obstruction
   e. Hypoplastic left ventricle
   f. Tetralogy of Fallot
   g. Aortic arch obstruction

E. Forty percent of ILS or ELS with GI tract communication have associated anomalies, including rib and vertebral defects, esophageal and gastrointestinal defects (such as duplications and malformation), thoracic defects (such as diaphragmatic hernia and bronchogenic cyst), duodenal and anorectal malformations, and Goldenhar syndrome.[55]

Differential Diagnosis

A. Alternate causes of radiologic or clinical findings may mimic sequestration.
1. Arteriovenous fistula.[51,60]
2. Bronchogenic cyst[1,55,60,61,65,67]
3. Congenital cystic adenomatoid malformation[1,16,17,22,53,55,60,65]
4. Congenital diaphragmatic hernia[1,22,51,53,61,65,67]
5. Pneumonia and empysema[60]
6. Intestinal duplication cysts[55,65]
7. Lobar emphysema[60]
8. Neuroblastoma[1,17,55,65]
9. Pulmonary or mediastinal neoplasia[60]
10. Renal dysplasia[65]
11. Teratoma[1,55,65]
12. Adrenal hemorrhage[55,65]
13. Hemangioma and lymphangioma[55]

B. Alternate causes of radiographic findings of scimitar syndrome include:[66]
1. Dextrocardia
2. Atelectasis
3. Pulmonary hypoplasia
4. Tension pneumothorax
5. Congenital lobar emphysema

Diagnosis

A. The definitive diagnosis of sequestration is made on surgical inspection, but it can be suggested by imaging studies.[51]
1. Prenatal ultrasound:
   a. Polyhydramnios, because of esophageal obstruction[52]
   b. Fetal hydrops with massive pleural effusion, because of lymphatic or venous obstruction or large arteriovenous (A-V) pressure gradient[52]
   c. Homogenous, hyperechoic, triangular, or conical mass in lower lung lobes[1,16,55]
      1) Sequestrations large enough to be detected on prenatal ultrasound are usually extralobar, though it is not always possible to distinguish between intralobar and extralobar types.[1,17]
      2) Decreasing echogenicity of the lesion with advancing gestational age can create difficulty in differentiating the lesion from normal parenchyma.
   d. Doppler documentation of the anomalous arterial supply[1]
      1) The arterial and venous supply to the mass is not always evident prenatally; therefore, the diagnosis of sequestration may not be fully confirmed or excluded on the basis of this study alone.[52]
2. Postnatal ultrasound:
   a. Echogenic lung mass[55] (The hyperechoic appearance of the mass is believed to be created from dilated or mucus-filled bronchioles.[52] This finding is considered by most authors to be pathognomonic of sequestration. However, demonstration of a pulmonary mass supplied by systemic vessels is suggestive, not specific, of pulmonary sequestration and warrants further evaluation.[53])
   b. Demonstrably abnormal vascular supply, which is essential for diagnosis and will facilitate surgical management[1,16]

1) Color Doppler ultrasound can demonstrate an aberrant vascular supply and distinguish sequestration from other mass lesions.[53]

3. Chest x-ray:
   a. Triangular mass or cluster of cysts in the left lower lobe encroaching the mediastinum or posterior mediastinal mass, suggesting an extralobar lesion with traction exerted by an anomalous vascular connection (Figure 2-14).[11,21,57,60,68]
   b. Cystic cavity or left lower lobe consolidation, suggesting an intralobar lesion.[11]

4. CT scan: This may demonstrate a lesion with an abnormal blood supply.[17] Additionally, CT scan may distinguish sequestration from an adrenal or mediastinal mass and determine the extent of parenchymal involvement.[25,55] In cases of scimitar, CT scan may reveal the anomalous pulmonary vein or associated pulmonary defects such as horseshoe lung.[66]

5. MRI scan:
   a. This may depict intrathoracic and extrathoracic masses and vascular connections and thus aid in the diagnosis of lesion type.
      1) Specifically, tracheal, esophageal, diaphragmatic, and renal sites of anomalous connections and soft tissue masses and abnormal vessels arising from the aorta can be documented.[51,56]
   b. As with CT scan, in cases of scimitar, MRI may assist with visualization of anomalous venous drainage or pulmonary defects.[66]

6. Bronchogram: This can show a lesion with no demonstrable contrast filling, indicating a mass sequestered from normal airway communication.[57]

7. Bronchoscopy:
   a. This can depict purulent matter emanating from the orifice of the affected lobe region or detect an aspirated foreign body.[21]
   b. Bronchoscopy is felt to be of limited use in diagnosing sequestration.[51] However, in cases of scimitar, bronchoscopy may reveal bronchial branch abnormalities.[66]

8. Barium swallow: This can show an abnormal GI communication with the tracheobronchial tree.[51]

9. Angiography:
   a. Once considered essential in the determination of the aberrant vascular connections encountered in sequestration, this has now been supplanted by the use of noninvasive studies that include CT, MRI, and ultrasound.[13,22]
   b. However, some authors suggest that angiography remains superior to MRI techniques in its ability to demonstrate complex pathology.[51]

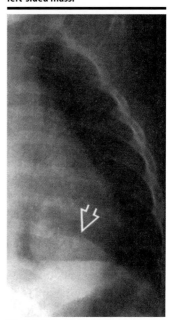

FIGURE 2-14 ■ Sequestration. Chest x-ray image demonstrates a left-sided mass.

From: Donnelly LF. 2002. Cardiac. In *PocketRadiologist–Pediatrics: Top 100 Diagnoses*, Donnelly LF, et al., eds. Salt Lake City: Amirsys, 25. Reprinted by permission of the author.

10. Echocardiogram:
    a. In cases of scimitar, this may depict the anomalous venous drainage and associated cardiovascular anomalies.
        1) Up to 75 percent of infants with a symptomatic scimitar presentation will have additional anomalies.[66]
11. Cardiac catheterization: In cases of scimitar, this will confirm the diagnosis, quantify the degree of pulmonary hypertension, and delineate the anatomy.[66]

Treatment Options and Nursing Care

A. Prenatal management
    1. Up to 70 percent of cases of sequestration may regress prenatally, likely due to torsion of the defect on its vascular stalk with subsequent ischemia and absorption.[1,23]
    2. Fetal therapy is indicated in the presence of hydrops or large pleural effusion.[23]
B. Neonatal management
    1. The risk of concurrent pulmonary hypoplasia warrants delivery and postnatal management in a tertiary level perinatal center.[1]
    2. Imaging studies such as echocardiography are suggested because of the increased risk of associated cardiovascular anomalies.[1]
    3. Controversy exists regarding optimal management of the asymptomatic infant, especially when the lesion involved is small.[1,23,55] An uninfected extralobar lesion without demonstrable symptoms may be followed clinically.[13] Additionally, no consensus exists regarding management of lesions that have undergone *in utero* regression.[1] However, symptomatic and large asymptomatic lesions should be resected.[54]
    4. Immediate maneuvers for stabilization in the symptomatic infant include the following.
        a. Pulmonary support with supplemental oxygen and/or mechanical ventilation as needed to maintain normal acid-base and oxygenation status (Infants with sequestration are at risk for conditions such as pneumonia, pleural effusion, and pulmonary edema because of the large vascular shunt that can compromise ventilation.[1])
        b. Tube thoracostomy to drain large pleural effusions if present[1]
        c. Cardiovascular support: diuretics, pressors, and cardiotonics as needed to treat congestive heart failure resulting from a large vascular shunt or associated cardiac defects[13,15,66]
        d. Antibiotic therapy as indicated to treat acute or chronic infection created by poor lobe drainage[15]
        e. Pulmonary vasodilators such as nitric oxide to manage pulmonary hypertension, as in cases of scimitar[66]

Surgical Management

A. Intralobar lesions
    1. Surgical resection of the lesion with ligation and division of the anomalous systemic vascular connections may be performed.
    2. Excision may be surgically complex, depending on the degree of adjacent lung inflammation.
    3. Segmentectomy, the removal of only the involved lung area, is technically feasible.
        a. Careful attention must be paid to ensure that all inflamed tissue is removed.
        b. Lobectomy is generally advocated.[55,57,64]

B. Extralobar lesions
  1. Simple surgical excision of the affected lobe is usually recommended.[16,57,67]
C. Scimitar variant lesions
  1. These are treated according to the complexity of the defect.
    a. Ligation or embolization of systemic arterial collateral vessels to control left-to-right shunting
    b. Local resection with reanastomosis of anomalous veins to the atrium
    c. Pneumonectomy of the entire involved lung[13,66]
  2. Immediacy of surgical management is dictated by the presence or absence of pulmonary hypertension. Infants without this finding may not warrant immediate surgical intervention.[66]

Postoperative Nursing Care

A. Infants undergoing surgical management of bronchopulmonary sequestration need vigilant nursing assessments postoperatively. In addition to general nursing care **(as noted under Nursing Considerations for Neonatal Pulmonary Disorders later in this chapter),** strategies and considerations specific to sequestration include:
  1. Extralobar lesions
    a. These are typically treated by lobectomy and ligation of vascular connections and so pose risks of postoperative bleeding.
    b. Infants require careful monitoring of intravascular volume status, including:
      1) Heart rate
      2) Blood pressure
      3) Perfusion
  2. Intralobar lesions
    a. These may require obligate parenchymal loss during resection, which can impair postoperative pulmonary stabilization.
    b. Infants require careful monitoring to detect and appropriately manage the potential complications of:
      1) Hypoxemia
      2) Hypercarbia
      3) Acidosis
  3. Scimitar lesions
    a. These are surgically managed with intricate vascular ligation, which poses a substantial risk for postoperative hemorrhage.
    b. Pulmonary hypertension can be exacerbated by:
      1) Acidosis
      2) Hypoxemia
      3) Hypercarbia
      4) Hypothermia
    c. Careful ventilatory weaning is indicated.
    d. Suction cautiously.
    e. Handle gently.
    f. Myocardial dysfunction may be a feature of the postoperative period.
      1) It may necessitate the use of inotropic support.
      2) Carefully assess:[66]
        a) Heart rate
        b) Blood pressure
        c) Perfusion

Outcomes

A. Mortality rates for ILS and ELS are reported to be 13–25 percent, primarily as a consequence of pulmonary hypertension or coexisting life-threatening anomalies.[55]

B. The presence of hydrops at the time of diagnosis is the most prognostically significant factor.[1,23] Lesions without accompanying hydrops have a good outcome, and it has been suggested that some cases might be managed conservatively without mandated surgical intervention.[13]

C. Anatomic intricacies of the vascular supply to the lesion may complicate surgical resection efforts and pose both intraoperative and postoperative bleeding risks to the infant.[1,23] Therefore, for all lesion types, preoperative identification of vascular connections is advocated to limit this risk.[54,68]

D. Following surgical management of sequestration, some authors have reported improved cardiac output and exercise tolerance.[57]

   1. Intralobar sequestration

      a. Surgical resection is generally curative, though parenchymal loss because of resection may compound the effects of preexisting pulmonary hypoplasia.[1]

   2. Extralobar lesions

      a. The prognosis depends on the impact of associated anomalies.

      b. In surgically managed cases, because the resection involves no parenchymal loss, an excellent pulmonary outcome is expected.[1,17]

   3. Scimitar lesions

      a. Poor surgical outcome is expected if there is evidence of preexisting pulmonary hypertension.

      b. Some management success has been reported with arterial embolization techniques to control the degree of vascular shunting.[61,66]

      c. Lung transplant can be done when other surgical options have been exhausted.[61,66]

      d. Infants symptomatic due to coexisting anomalies have a surgical mortality rate of 50 percent.[59]

PULMONARY LYMPHANGIECTASIA

Definition

An obstructive lymphatic disorder that creates bulky and inelastic lungs and presents with immediate respiratory distress[14]

Pathophysiology

A. Pulmonary lymphangiectasia refers to a diffuse overgrowth of the entire lung lymphatic system, which creates bulky, inelastic, and noncompressible lungs.[3,14]

   1. Although not an intrinsic lung abnormality, failed normal regression of lymphatics allows lymphatic fluid accumulation.[71]

   2. Grossly, the lungs are lobulated and contain abnormal subpleural, septal, and perivascular lymph vessels.

   3. The entire lung surface is covered with a dense mesh of serous-filled cystic lymphatics.

   4. The net clinical effect of these features is compromised ventilation caused by:

      a. Decreased pulmonary compliance

      b. Increased work of breathing[68]

B. Three types of lymphangiectasia are described in the literature. These have been referred to as "Noonan's classifications."[72]

    1. Isolated or primary pulmonary lymphangiectasia[71,73]

        a. A primary developmental defect isolated to the pulmonary lymphatics.

        b. This condition generally involves both lungs and carries a poor prognosis.

    2. Secondary, or acquired lymphangiectasia[73]

        a. A defect secondarily caused by venous obstruction

        b. Has a poor prognosis for cases symptomatic in the newborn period

    3. Generalized lymphangiectasia

        a. Lymphatic overgrowth throughout the body

        b. Prognostically superior, due to less severe pulmonary involvement[72]

Etiology

A. The cause of pulmonary lymphangiectasia is unknown for the majority of cases.[71,74] It is postulated to result from failed regression of the pulmonary lymphatics at approximately the twelfth to sixteenth week of gestation, leading to an accumulation of lymphatic fluid.[71,75]

B. This lesion may also occur as a result of obstructive pulmonary venous or cardiovascular lesions.[72]

C. A familial tendency has been described, owing to either an autosomal recessive or dominant inheritance trait with variable penetrance.[72]

Incidence

A. A rare disorder, more commonly affecting males[76]

Clinical Presentation

A. Symptoms of pulmonary lymphangiectasia, should they occur, are present in the immediate neonatal period. They may appear following or exacerbated by a pulmonary infection.[71]

    1. Progressive respiratory distress.[68,71,75]

    2. Tachypnea[74]

    3. Cyanosis[74]

    4. Pneumothorax[68]

    5. Pericardial effusions[71]

    6. Pleural effusions[68,71]

Associations

A. Prenatally, lymphangiectasia has been associated with:

    1. Polyhydramnios[45]

    2. Chylothorax

    3. Pulmonary hypoplasia[72]

    4. Hydrops[75]

B. Neonatal anomalies and conditions associated with pulmonary lymphangiectasia include:

    1. Congenital heart disorders, particularly those with obstructed pulmonary venous flow. Associated lesions include:

        a. Hypoplastic left heart syndrome

        b. Total anomalous pulmonary venous return

        c. AV canal and septal defects[3,76]

    2. Renal malformations, including dysplasia [3,72]

    3. Noonan syndrome[72,75,77]

    4. Turner syndrome[72,75]

5. Down syndrome[72,75]
6. Yellow nail syndrome[77]
7. Ichthyosis congenita neonatorum[3,75]
8. Fryn syndrome[75]

Differential Diagnosis

A. Alternate causes of radiologic or clinical findings may mimic pulmonary lymphangiectasia.
   1. Wilson-Mikity syndrome[14]
   2. Pneumonia[66]
   3. Hyaline membrane disease[68]
   4. Pulmonary interstitial emphysema[3,72,78]
   5. Pulmonary cystic lesions[72]
   6. Cyanotic heart disease[74]
   7. Emphysema[72]
   8. Asthma[72]
   9. Chylothorax or pleural effusion[74]

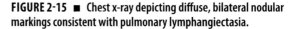

FIGURE 2-15 ■ Chest x-ray depicting diffuse, bilateral nodular markings consistent with pulmonary lymphangiectasia.

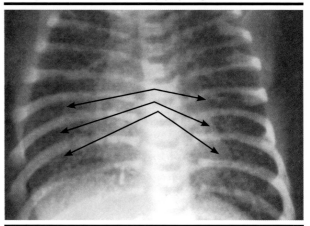

From: Singleton EB, and Wagner ML. 1971. *Radiologic Atlas of Pulmonary Abnormalities in Children.* Philadelphia: Saunders, 52. Reprinted by permission.

Diagnosis

A. The diagnosis is histologically proven, yet suggested by laboratory and imaging findings.[72,75]
   1. Pleural fluid aspiration and evaluation, in the presence of associated effusion or chylothorax[73]
   2. Chest x-ray, which may be notable for features including (Figure 2-15):
      a. Diffuse, coarse, reticulonodular lung markings, which suggest dilated lymphatics
      b. Generalized mottling and hyperinflation, with focal cystic areas
      c. Interstitial infiltration or pleural effusions[73]
      d. Kerley B lines: Prominent interstitial and subpleural lymphatics[3]
   3. High-resolution CT scan, which can confirm prominent, thickened, interlobular septae[73]

Treatment Options and Nursing Care

A. No specific therapy is advocated.[76]
B. Supportive pulmonary therapy is indicated, including diuretics, mechanical ventilation with positive end-expiratory pressure, and supplemental oxygen to treat accompanying pulmonary edema and pleural effusions.[79]
C. Drainage of pleural and pericardial effusions may be employed; however, because of fluid reaccumulation, this remains solely a temporizing maneuver.[71]

Surgical Management

A. For localized disease, surgical resection may be possible.[71,77] Lung transplantation has been proposed as a therapy.[71]

Postoperative Nursing Care

A. Infants with a diagnosis of pulmonary lymphangiectasia are not typically managed surgically; however, they may have undergone temporizing procedures such as thoracotomy drainage of pleural or pericardial effusions. In addition to general nursing care **(as noted under Nursing Considerations for Neonatal Pulmonary Disorders later in this chapter)**, strategies and considerations specific to pulmonary lymphangiectasia include:

1. Careful ongoing assessments of chest tube or pericardial tube drainage character and volume
2. Accurate assessments of intake and output, especially in cases in which medical management includes diuretics
3. For patients managed with mechanical ventilation and supplemental oxygen, careful ongoing assessments of oxygenation and acid/base balance and careful weaning

Outcomes

A. Mortality is high, with rare reported survival beyond the newborn period, especially in symptomatic cases and primary pulmonary or acquired types with pulmonary involvement.[68,73,74,77]
B. A report published in 2003 suggests some management success with supportive care in a premature infant.[75]

Diaphragmatic Disorders

CONGENITAL DIAPHRAGMATIC HERNIA (CDH)

Definition

Developmental defect of the diaphragm that allows migration of abdominal viscera upward into the chest cavity, impairing pulmonary development and creating respiratory distress[20]

Pathophysiology

A. The diaphragmatic defect, usually situated at the posterolateral foramen of Bochdalek, allows herniation of abdominal cavity contents into the thorax. The three most commonly reported sites of the diaphragmatic defect are:[80,81]

1. Posterolateral (Bochdalek, 85–90 percent)
2. Retrosternal (Morgagni, 2–15 percent)
3. Esophageal hiatal (<5 percent)

B. Compression of the herniated abdominal organs causes a maturational arrest of bronchial branching that ultimately leads to decreased bronchial divisions, decreased airway size, and decreased size and number of saccules and alveoli.

1. Both lungs are affected, although the effect is greatest on the side of the diaphragmatic defect.[81–84]

C. Paralleling the pulmonary branching defect, there is a decreased number of pulmonary arterioles with increased medial arterial wall size.[81–84]

1. Persistent, high pulmonary vascular resistance after birth enhances right-to-left shunting, creating postnatal hypoxemia and acidosis.[45]

Etiology

A. The classic Bochdalek hernia results from failure of development of the posterolateral retrosternal portion of the diaphragm prior to the twelfth gestational week, with persistence of the pleuroperitoneal canal or foramen of Bochdalek; this allows upward migration of abdominal viscera.

B. The less commonly encountered Morgagni hernia results from failed fusion of the sternal and costal segments of the diaphragm.[80,85]

Incidence

A. The reported incidence is 1/2,000–5,000 live births.[80,86]

B. The defect occurs more commonly in males and carries a 2 percent recurrence risk in subsequent pregnancies.[87]

C. The left side is involved in 85–90 percent of all cases. This has been attributed to liver impedance to right-sided herniation.[88] Most Morgagni hernias are right-sided.[14,85]

D. Perinatally, 30 percent of infants with diaphragmatic hernia will be delivered stillborn, and an estimated 30–50 percent of prenatal survivors will die prior to transfer to a Level III neonatal care unit.[80]

Clinical Presentation

A. Up to 10 percent of cases may present beyond the neonatal period.[80] However, symptoms generally present in the first hours of life.[11]

1. Scaphoid abdomen[11,20,80,87–90]
2. Barrel chest—increased anterior-posterior chest diameter or asymmetric chest contour[14,88–90]
3. Mediastinal shift or shift of point of maximal cardiac impulse[80,87,88,90]
4. Variable degree of respiratory distress, including grunting, tachypnea, pallor, cyanosis, and retractions[80,87,89]
5. Poor lung expansion[90]
6. Decreased breath sounds on the affected side, though this may occur bilaterally[20,80,87,88,90]
7. Bowel sounds audible in the chest[80]
8. Signs of diminished cardiac output due to decreased venous return caused by a shift of mediastinal structures[90]

Associations

A. Polyhydramnios is a commonly associated prenatal finding[88,91]

B. Other associated major anomalies occur in 25–50 percent of cases, including:[37,86,92]

1. Pulmonary defects:[14,89]
   a. Pulmonary hypoplasia
   b. Sequestration
2. Cardiovascular defects:[14,20,81,85,92,93]
   a. Atrial and ventricular septal defects (Morgagni)
   b. Tetralogy of Fallot (Morgagni)
   c. Coarctation of the aorta
   d. Hypoplastic left heart syndrome
3. Central nervous system defects,[92] including neural tube defects[20,89,93]
4. Skeletal defects[20,93]
5. Gastrointestinal defects,[92] including malrotation[14,89,93] and omphalocele[14]
6. Chromosomal anomalies,[92] including trisomies 13,18, and 21[20,85,89,93]
7. Genitourinary tract defects[20,92,93]

8. Craniofacial defects[20]
9. Fryn syndrome[87,92]
10. Pallister-Killian syndrome[92]

Differential Diagnosis

A. Alternate causes of radiologic or clinical findings may mimic congenital diaphragmatic hernia.
  1. Bronchogenic cyst[83,89]
  2. Congenital cystic adenomatoid malformation[14,80,88–90]
  3. Congenital lobar emphysema[88–90]
  4. Diaphragmatic paralysis or eventration[88,89]
  5. Pulmonary sequestration[80]
  6. Cystic teratoma[80]
  7. Neurogenic tumor[80]
  8. Lung sarcoma[80]
  9. Pneumatocele[14,89,90]
  10. Pneumothorax[88]
  11. Pleural effusion[88]

Diagnosis

A. Diagnosis is confirmed with imaging studies.
  1. Prenatal ultrasound may show:
     a. Polyhydramnios, though this represents a nonspecific marker of obstruction[90]
     b. Fluid-filled retrocardiac mass[88]
     c. Deviation of cardiac axis or mediastinal shift[89,90]
     d. Bowel and/or stomach in thorax, best viewed in relation to the inferior margin of the scapula or the four-chamber view of the heart[37,88]
     e. Intrathoracic peristalsis of bowel loops[37]
  2. Postnatal AP chest x-ray (Figure 2-16), which may be notable for:
     a. Hemithorax filled with mass that is either air-filled bowel loops or opaque[20,80,88,89]
     b. Cardiac displacement away from the side of herniation[20,88,90]
     c. Abdomen devoid of air[88]
     d. Diaphragmatic line not appreciable[90]
     e. Coiling of a radiopaque nasogastric tube in chest, if utilized as a radiographic marker[88]
     f. Right-sided and Morgagni lesions that are more difficult to appreciate, possibly presenting as consolidation or a fluid density on x-ray[80,85] (A lateral x-ray may aid in the diagnosis of these defects.[85])
  3. Contrast studies contraindicated[80]

FIGURE 2-16 ■ Postnatal AP chest x-ray depicting left hemithorax filled with bowel loops, consistent with left-sided congenital diaphragmatic hernia.

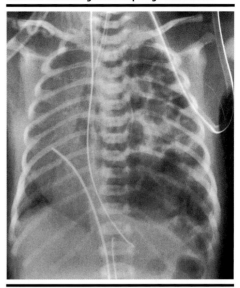

From: Clark DA. 2000. *Atlas of Neonatology*. Philadelphia: Saunders, 106. Reprinted by permission.

Treatment Options and Nursing Care

A. Fetal therapy in some prenatally diagnosed cases[42]

B. Neonatal management

   1. Delivery should occur in a tertiary perinatal center, with perinatal and neonatal staff adequately prepared to deal with respiratory compromise at birth.[25,37,92]

   2. Immediate maneuvers for pulmonary stabilization include:

     a. Immediate intubation and mechanical ventilation (Bag and mask ventilation is contraindicated because of the risk of air distention of displaced abdominal organs and subsequent impeded lung expansion.[42,80,87–89,92])

     b. Positive pressure ventilation with lowest pressures and rate necessary so as to avoid barotrauma[80]

     c. Oxygen-enriched environment, with preductal oxygen saturation maintained >90 percent[25,89]

     d. "Permissive hypercarbia/hypercapnia" ventilatory strategy, which allows elevated $PaCO_2$ as long as pH is maintained, utilizing buffer as needed to correct acidosis[42,80,89] (Spontaneous ventilatory efforts by the infant are acceptable.[87])

     e. Buffer, such as sodium bicarbonate or tromethamine (THAM), and appropriate fluids to correct metabolic acidosis, which may potentiate pulmonary hypertension[25,88]

     f. Nasogastric tube to decompress the stomach[42,80,87–89,92]

     g. Arterial and central venous access to monitor blood pressure, acid-base and oxygenation status, and for medication administration[18,42,80,87,88,92]

     h. Side-lying position, with hernia side dependent[7,90]

   3. Preoperative and postoperative pulmonary management, including administration as necessary of:

     a. Mechanical ventilation, with a goal of maintaining oxygenation while minimizing barotrauma[80,87]

       1) Conventional mechanical ventilation to provide oxygen, pressure, and rate so that:[80,89]

         a) Preductal saturation is maintained ≥85 percent

         b) Preductal PaO_2 ≥60 mmHg

         c) Postductal PaO_2 ≥40 mmHg

       2) Protective pulmonary strategies, including:[80,94]

         a) Reduced tidal volumes

         b) Pressure-limited "permissive hypercapnia" ventilation

       3) High-frequency ventilation (HFV) and high-frequency oscillatory ventilation (HFOV) for hypoxia and/or hypercarbia unresponsive to conventional ventilation techniques[80]

       4) Attention to the potential need for increased ventilatory support in the event of postoperative decrease in chest compliance[90]

     b. ECMO[42,80,87]

       1) To provide cardiopulmonary support and modify hypoxic or metabolic factors that can aggravate pulmonary hypertension

       2) Used for infants with severe pulmonary hypertension refractory to conventional management

       3) Shown to improve survival in congenital diaphragmatic hernia by up to 15–20 percent

  c. Inhaled nitric oxide
  1) To provide for selective pulmonary vasodilation in cases of severe pulmonary hypertension[89]
  2) Inconclusive evidence of specific benefit in cases of congenital diaphragmatic hernia[80,94]
  d. Exogenous surfactant
  1) Infants with congenital diaphragmatic hernia may have both quantitative and qualitative decreases in surfactant amount and function.[84]
  2) Surfactant may:[80,81]
    a) Improve oxygenation
    b) Decrease the potential for air leak
    c) Decrease the need for ECMO
  3) The specific benefits of the use of surfactant in the management of congenital diaphragmatic hernia are inconclusive. (Some data suggest a worsened outcome in selected infants treated with surfactant.[87,92])
  e. Intratracheal pulmonary ventilation with direct oxygen delivery at the tip of the endotracheal tube (Shown in limited studies to effectively enhance carbon dioxide elimination.[94])
  f. Perfluorocarbons, as a technique of either total or partial liquid ventilation (Shown in limited studies to both enhance gas exchange and pulmonary mechanics and foster postnatal pulmonary growth.[94])
C. Consideration of a lung transplant, including segmental grafts in cases of CDH with chronic respiratory insufficiency[94]

Surgical Management

A. Congenital diaphragmatic hernia "represents a physiologic emergency, rather than a surgical emergency" (p. 696).[25] This is not the case if bowel integrity is a concern.[20]
  1. Urgent surgical repair has not been definitively shown to improve survival.
  2. Emphasis is now placed on preoperative pulmonary stabilization and treatment of pulmonary hypertension prior to undertaking corrective surgical repair.[87]
  3. Infants may undergo surgical correction of diaphragmatic hernia while on ECMO.[37]
B. A primary closure technique may be employed.
  1. A transabdominal approach and subcostal incision can be used to bring the involved organs down into the abdomen.[87] The volume of herniated organs varies with the type of diaphragmatic defect. Left-sided defects may involve the stomach, colon, small intestine, spleen, and occasionally the liver. Right-sided defects generally involve only the liver.[7]
  2. Small defects may be corrected by primary closure with permanent sutures. Large defects may be treated by primary closure; however, this may result in a residual flattened diaphragm and subsequent poor air excursion.[80]
  3. Chest tube placement is optional and used primarily for assessment of postoperative drainage and bleeding.[87] If utilized, the tube is placed to a water seal because suction may adversely shift the mediastinum and create a pneumothorax.[25,80]
C. A prosthetic patch may be utilized for closure if tension is created as the muscle edges are approximated.[80]
  1. If little or no diaphragmatic remnant is evident

    2. To avoid the risk of diaphragmatic flattening

D. Postoperative complications include the following.

    1. Kinking of the hepatic vein and superior vena cava, especially with right-sided defects

    2. Postoperative bleeding, which can occur either from manipulation of the liver or when the repair is done with the patient on ECMO and anticoagulant therapy[80]

E. Postoperatively, infants may experience a honeymoon phase with stabilized oxygenation and ventilation status.[37,89] However, the risk of pulmonary hypertension remains, and strategies to limit this risk should be incorporated.

Postoperative Nursing Care

A. Infants undergoing surgical management of congenital diaphragmatic hernia need vigilant nursing assessments postoperatively. In addition to general nursing care **(as noted under Nursing Considerations for Neonatal Pulmonary Disorders later in this chapter)**, strategies and considerations specific to CDH include the following.

    1. A chest tube may be in place postoperatively for residual fluid drainage. This must be maintained with water seal drainage without the use of suction to:[80]

        a. Avoid uncontrolled mediastinal shift

        b. Allow gradual ipsilateral lung inflation

        c. Limit contralateral lung hyperexpansion

    2. Chest tube drainage must be carefully assessed for:

        a. Volume

        b. Character

    3. Substantial pulmonary hypoplasia may accompany this disorder, warranting careful ventilatory adjustments.

    4. Infants with CDH may have refractory pulmonary hypertension. Avoid hypoxemia and acidosis.

Outcomes

A. Mortality for diaphragmatic hernia is high, reported at 30–60 percent.[80,93]

B. Survival is dependent upon the age at presentation, degree of pulmonary hypoplasia, presence of pulmonary hypertension, and access to optimal perinatal management. Those patients presenting with severe respiratory symptoms within the first six hours of life have approximately a 50 percent chance of survival.[88] A metanalysis of multiple outcome studies reveals the median mortality for the fetus diagnosed prenatally to be 58 percent, the infant born live has a mortality of 48 percent, and the infant who survives until operative repair has a mortality of 33 percent.[86]

C. Other indicators may have prognostic significance.

    1. Prenatal findings of polyhydramnios,[1,81] intrathoracic stomach or liver,[80,81] mediastinal shift,[81] left ventricular hypoplasia, and reduced lung-to-head ratio,[80] all of which may correlate to pulmonary hypoplasia and suggest poor outcome[87]

    2. Presence of other life-threatening anomalies[93]

    3. Minimum lung volume of 45 percent of expected age-matched controls, in post-ECMO cases[83]

    4. Ability to achieve a preoperative pH ≥ 7.25 or $PaCO_2$ <40–50 mmHg, proposed as clinical indicators of a successful outcome[11,93] (However, the lack of patient uniformity and practice variation related to ventilation techniques, timing

of surgical repair, and access to ECMO limit the clinical application of these measures.[80])

D. The pulmonary outcome of CDH is dependent upon the degree of pulmonary hypoplasia and lung injury sustained during the neonatal period.[80,95]

  1. Greater than 50 percent of those survivors who required substantial ventilatory support in the neonatal period have some residual pulmonary impairment, such as:[80,81]

    a. Bronchial reactivity

    b. Chronic lung disease

  2. CDH survivors may have ongoing evidence of pulmonary hypertension, warranting ongoing follow-up and potential treatment.[87,92]

  3. Postoperative complications such as chylothorax and recurrent hernia may adversely affect pulmonary outcome.[80]

E. Nonpulmonary complications of congenital diaphragmatic hernia and its treatments include the following.

  1. Gastroesophageal reflux (GER)[80,81,89,96]

    a. This may be due to impaired esophageal motility caused by:[89]

      1) Obstruction and dilation of the esophagus

      2) Abnormal anatomy at the gastroesophageal junction

      3) Absence of all or part of the perihiatal diaphragm

    b. Reflux occurs as a complication in the majority of patients treated with ECMO and may result in:[88,96]

      1) Recurrent bronchitis

      2) Aspiration pneumonia

      3) Worsening chronic lung disease

    c. GER treatment options include:[89,96]

      1) Nursing maneuvers such as:

        a) Small-volume frequent feedings

        b) Prone, elevated positioning

      2) Medical/surgical maneuvers such as:

        a) Increased density feedings

        b) Prokinetics

        c) H_2 blockers

        d) Fundoplication

  2. Failure to thrive

    a. This is due to poor growth from inadequate oral intake or increased caloric requirement caused by increased work of breathing.[81,96] Despite optimized nutritional management:

      1) Greater than half of CDH survivors have suboptimal growth[92]

      2) Up to 50 percent of patients treated with ECMO are at less than the fifth percentile for weight at age two[88]

  3. Neurologic and developmental impairment with increased risk of motor, verbal, and neurocognitive delays

    a. Decreased cerebral perfusion resulting from hyperventilation or alkalinization therapy may enhance this risk.

    b. ECMO has been associated with increased risks of:[87,92,96]

      1) Developmental delay

      2) Progressive sensorineural hearing loss

      3) Vision loss

      4) Seizure disorders

4. Musculoskeletal growth abnormalities, which may be caused by the inherent increased work of breathing or adhesions developing postoperatively[80,96]
   a. Anterior chest wall deformities
   b. Pectus deformities, such as pectus excavatum[96]
   c. Scoliosis
5. Small bowel obstruction, due to postoperative adhesions[96]
6. Recurrent hernia, especially following prosthetic patch repair of the initial defect, which can necessitate additional surgery[80,87,92,96]

EVENTRATION OF THE DIAPHRAGM

Definition

Abnormal elevation of all or part of the diaphragm, which creates paradoxical motion during the phases of respiration[80,97]

Pathophysiology

A. Poorly developed or controlled muscle allows for paradoxical diaphragmatic movement during the phases of respiration. During inspiration, the hemidiaphragm rises cephalad, and the mediastinum shifts toward the unaffected side, impeding lung expansion and thus gas exchange.[20]

B. Pulmonary hypoplasia caused by compression by deviated structures can occur because of eventration, though pulmonary hypertension as a sequela is uncommon.[80,97]

C. All or part of the diaphragm may be affected in congenital cases.
   1. Additionally, the phrenic nerve may be hypoplastic.
   2. Total eventration occurs more commonly on the left, though a partial eventration is more commonly on the right.
   3. The pleura and peritoneum are normal, but they may touch or be separated merely by a small fibrous rim.[14]
   4. For cases in which the affected diaphragm is a thin membrane, the functional impact may be identical to congenital diaphragmatic hernia.[80]

Etiology

A. Congenital abnormality or an acquired defect
   1. Congenital eventration: Improper development of the diaphragmatic muscle, with complete or partial absence of muscle or tendon in the septum transversum[80]
   2. Acquired eventration: Phrenic nerve interruption or injury following birth trauma or surgical thoracic manipulation[20]

Incidence

A. Congenital diaphragmatic eventration is rare, occurring in 5 percent of diaphragmatic anomalies. Congenital diaphragmatic abnormalities, including hernia, agenesis, and eventration, occur in 1/2,000–3,000 births.[97]

Clinical Presentation

A. The clinical expression of eventration is variable, and some cases may be asymptomatic. Symptoms, when they occur, include:
   1. Dyspnea due to mediastinal shift affecting the contralateral side[14,20,80]
   2. Tachypnea[14,80]
   3. Cyanosis[14]
   4. Pallor[80]
   5. Tracheal and cardiac shift[14,80]

6. Dull percussion sounds over the affected side[14,80]
7. Diminished breath sounds on the affected side or bilaterally[14,80]
8. Scaphoid abdomen[14]
9. Inability to wean from ventilator support because of impaired diaphragmatic function affecting spontaneous respiratory efforts[80]
10. Possible recurrent pneumonia or gastrointestinal symptoms, including vomiting, flatulence, and dyspepsia, in the older child[14,80]

Associations

A. Associated anomalies
    1. Pulmonary sequestration[14,80]
    2. Congenital heart disease[80]
    3. Tracheomalacia[80]
    4. Cerebral agenesis[80]
    5. Chromosomal abnormalities, including trisomy 13 and 18[80]
    6. Renal ectopia[14]

Differential Diagnosis

A. Alternate causes of radiologic or clinical findings may mimic eventration.
    1. Congenital diaphragmatic hernia[14,97]
    2. Phrenic nerve paralysis[11,14]
    3. Pleural effusion[14,80]
    4. Bronchogenic cyst[80]
    5. Pulmonary sequestration[80]
    6. Pulmonary consolidation[80]
    7. Mediastinal tumors[14,80]

FIGURE 2-17 ■ Eventration: AP chest x-ray demonstrating elevated left hemidiaphragm consistent with eventration.

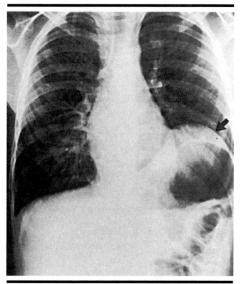

From: Arensman RM, Bambini DA, and Chiu B. 2005. Congenital diaphragmatic hernia and eventrations. In *Pediatric Surgery*, 4th ed., Ashcraft KW, Holcomb GW, and Murphy JP, eds. Philadelphia: Saunders, 317. Reprinted by permission.

Diagnosis

A. Prenatally, suspected cases must be distinguished from CDH, because immediate clinical management for these conditions may be quite different.[97]
B. Prenatal ultrasound suggests lung or abdominal organ displacement. Precise prenatal diagnosis may be hindered by sonographic similarities between this and diaphragmatic hernia. For this reason, MRI has been suggested as a superior prenatal diagnostic tool.[97]
C. Prenatal MRI will depict organ displacement, though an evident hemidiaphragm.[97]
D. Postnatal ultrasound may document mediastinal shift and paradoxical movement of the diaphragm during respiratory phases.[80]
E. Chest x-ray may be notable for an elevated hemidiaphragm on both AP (Figure 2-17) and lateral views.[11,20,80]

F. Fluoroscopy may show paradoxical motion of the hemidiaphragm during respiratory phases.[14,20]

Treatment Options and Nursing Care

A. Infants with eventration may be managed medically; however, failure of conservative maneuvers will warrant surgical management.

B. Eventration caused by birth injury may resolve spontaneously, although the clinical course of eventration is often unpredictable.[14]

C. Pulmonary stabilization in symptomatic patients includes the use of positive end-expiratory pressure to help control paradoxical diaphragmatic movement.[14]

D. Some authors recommend initial conservative management, including:[14,80]
1. Upright positioning
2. Supplemental oxygen
3. Mechanical ventilation
   a. Mechanical ventilation may be needed to support adequate gas exchange for several weeks.
4. Optimized nutrition

Surgical Management

A. Surgical management is indicated when the infant:
1. Has persistent respiratory distress requiring prolonged mechanical ventilation
2. Has recurrent pulmonary infections
3. Fails to thrive

B. Plication of the diaphragm, involving imbrication (overlapping) and flattening of the diaphragm muscle with suture, is the procedure of choice.

Postoperative Nursing Care

A. Following plication of the diaphragm:[80]
1. The diaphragm is immobilized
2. Paradoxical movement is reduced
3. Tidal volume and maximal breathing capacity are increased

B. In addition to general nursing care **(as noted under Nursing Considerations for Neonatal Pulmonary Disorders later in this chapter)**, strategies and considerations specific to eventration include:
1. Ongoing pulmonary assessments
2. Cautious ventilatory weaning postoperatively as spontaneity of pulmonary effort improves
3. Protracted mechanical ventilation, which will warrant:
   a. Judicious removal of secretions
   b. Optimized humidification of ventilatory circuitry
   c. Later initiation of oral enteral feedings
   d. Ongoing oral care and stimulation, including:
      1) Strategies such as nonnutritive pacifier use to augment efforts to ultimately establish oral feedings and avoid oral aversion

Outcomes

A. Surgical outcome is generally favorable.
1. Perioperative mortality and morbidity are usually related to complications of protracted mechanical ventilation.

2. If phrenic nerve function remains intact, the following is expected.[14]
   a. Mortality is low.
   b. Symptoms will be relieved.
   c. Immediate improvement in pulmonary mechanics ensues.
3. Despite surgical manipulation, diaphragmatic function is maintained.[80]
B. Outcome may be complicated by the following.[14,80]
   1. The presence of chronic infection
   2. Diaphragmatic rupture
   3. Injury to organs such as the stomach
   4. The presence of major anomalies
C. Following surgery, the following occurs.
   1. Long-term pulmonary function is expected to be excellent.
   2. Some follow-up data of cases of diaphragmatic hernia and large eventration defects suggests an increase in:[98]
      a. Thoracic rigidity
      b. Recurrent paradoxical diaphragmatic motion
      c. Excess bronchial reactivity in adult survivors

Acquired or Associated Pulmonary Disorders

CHYLOTHORAX

Definition

Abnormal collection of chylous lymphatic fluid, which may create respiratory compromise from lung compression and nutritional and immune deficiencies[99]

Pathophysiology

A. Chyle is lymphatic fluid that has been enriched with secreted chylomicrons and lymphocytes.
   1. It is normally collected and transported via the thoracic duct into the circulation.[100]
   2. Although chyle itself does not create pleural inflammation, pulmonary symptoms may result from lung compression due to large chylous collections.[99]
B. Prenatally, large pleural effusions may increase intrapleural pressure, invert the diaphragm, obstruct venous return, compress the heart, and lead to cardiac failure. Additionally, the intrathoracic presence of a large fluid collection may create pulmonary hypoplasia.[16,101]
C. Acute or chronic loss of chyle poses the risk of:
   1. Malnutrition
   2. Fluid and electrolyte imbalances
   3. Acid-base disturbances
   4. Immune deficiency from loss of T cells[102]

Etiology

A. Chylothorax may occur as either a congenital or an acquired disorder.
   1. Congenital chylothorax
      a. This is idiopathic in the majority of cases[14,103]
      b. Known causes include thoracic duct atresia, congenital fistula of lymphatic channels, and generalized lymphatic malformations.[103]

2. Acquired chylothorax
   a. Direct trauma to the thoracic duct, such as a complication of a cardiothoracic surgical procedure or birth trauma[14,103,104]
   b. Elevated superior vena caval pressure, such as from thrombotic obstruction to the thoracic duct orifice, creating increased intravascular pressure and chyle leakage from the lymphatics[104,105]
   c. Neoplasia or other inflammatory processes[104]

Incidence

A. The estimated incidence of fetal chylothorax is 1/10,000–15,000 pregnancies, and the condition occurs with equal frequency in males and females.[1]
B. Congenital chylothorax is the most common cause of pleural effusions in the neonate.[103] Fifty percent present during the first week of life.[104]

Clinical Presentation

A. The neonatal presentation of chylothorax depends on the volume and rate of chylous loss; hence, symptom onset may be immediate or weeks after birth.[103]
   1. Dyspnea due to atelectasis and mediastinal shift[14]
   2. Tachypnea[14]
   3. Cyanosis[14]
   4. Ipsilateral percussion dullness[7,14]

Associations

A. Chylothorax may be associated with the prenatal finding of polyhydramnios and accounts for up to a 15–30 percent perinatal mortality rate.[1,103]
   1. Associated anomalies include trisomy 21, Noonan and Turner syndromes, lymphangiectasia, and neuroblastoma.[100,103,104]

Differential Diagnosis

A. Alternate causes of radiologic or clinical findings that can mimic chylothorax include:
   1. Atelectasis[106]
   2. Lymphatic defect, such as cystic hygroma[79]
   3. Hydrops fetalis[79]
   4. Congenital cystic adenomatoid malformation[1]

Diagnosis

A. The diagnosis of chylothorax is suggested on imaging findings and confirmed with the analysis of the chylous fluid.
   1. The chest x-ray (Figure 2-18) can be notable for opacity on the affected side or mediastinal shift.[14]
   2. Postthoracotomy fluid assessment can be notable for a massive volume of chylous fluid and milky fluid appearance. Of note is the fact that fluid will be clear and light yellow and not milky if there has been no enteral fat intake.[7] On laboratory analysis, confirmation of chylothorax is made by:
      a. Absolute cell count of >1,000/ml[100,104,106]
      b. >70 percent of cells lymphocytes,[100,104] which persists despite any enteral intake
      c. Protein >20 gm/liter[104]
      d. Triglyceride level >100 mg/dl (>1.1 mmol/liter)[100,104]
      e. Sterile culture (because chyle is naturally bacteriostatic)[99,104]

Treatment Options and Nursing Care

A. Prenatally detected pleural effusion and chylothorax, if creating fetal distress and hydrops, may suggest the need for *in utero* therapy.[103]

B. The management of chylothorax is controversial.[103] Conservative protocols have been advocated because 75–90 percent of cases may resolve spontaneously during the first 7–14 days. Conservative strategies include:

1. Mechanical ventilation, including high-frequency ventilation, to reduce the risk of barotrauma which has been advocated for cases involving pulmonary hypertension or hypoplasia[101]

2. Dietary strategies

  a. Breast milk or formula trial or substitution of medium-chain triglycerides (MCT) for the dietary fat source is possible.

  b. MCT will bypass the intestinal lymphatics and be directly absorbed into the portal venous system. Though MCT may still increase lymphatic flow through the thoracic duct, it does so to a lesser extent than regular formula.

  c. Parenteral hyperalimentation may be utilized to provide nutrition temporarily, thus bypassing the enteral route. It has been suggested that because central venous catheter use for hyperalimentation poses the risk of thrombosis, which may worsen the chylothorax, peripheral access may be the preferred route of delivery.[103]

FIGURE 2-18 ■ Chylothorax. AP chest x-ray demonstrating bilateral opacification and blunting of costophrenic margin, consistent with right-sided bilateral chylothorax.

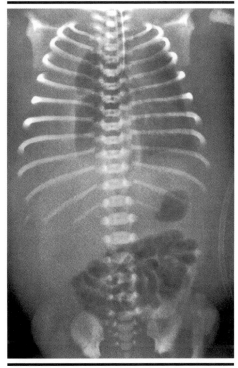

From: Clark DA. 2000. *Atlas of Neonatology.* Philadelphia: Saunders, 105. Reprinted by permission.

Surgical Management

A. Surgical management may be indicated for failure of a conservative trial or if the volume of chylous fluid is excessive and creating respiratory symptomatology. Chylous losses >15 ml/kg/day warrant surgical intervention.[102]

1. Thoracostomy drainage: An indwelling chest tube can be inserted for both diagnostic and therapeutic indications.

  a. Placed under ultrasound guidance, connected to closed water seal drainage, and utilized with the patient positioned fluid-dependent, this will permit full lung expansion and apposition of the visceral and parietal pleura.

  b. Continuous drainage decreases the risk of pneumothorax, hemothorax, or chylous loculations more effectively than intermittent drainage.[103,107]

2. Pleurodesis: Utilizes sclerosing agents or fibrin glue to create pleural adhesion and subsequent obliteration of the chylous leak.
   a. This procedure requires a fully expanded lung to allow apposition of the pleural surfaces and even distribution of the sclerosing agent within the pleural space.
   b. In cases of high-volume chylous leak, this may be an ineffective strategy.[108]
3. Thoracic duct ligation:
   a. This may be accomplished endoscopically.
   b. It is primarily utilized for posttraumatic chylothorax or failure of conservative measures.[102–104]
4. Pleuroperitoneal shunt:
   a. An afferent pleural catheter is bluntly inserted through the intercostal muscles into the thorax.
   b. An efferent catheter is drawn into the peritoneal cavity.
   c. A pumping chamber, tunneled subcutaneously, is utilized to manually overcome peritoneal pressures and drain pleural fluid.
   d. Success rates as high as 92 percent have been reported with this technique.[99]

Postoperative Nursing Care

A. Infants with congenital chylothorax may be managed medically or surgically.
   1. Infants managed conservatively will need:
      a. Frequent assessment of volume and character of thoracostomy drainage
      b. Replacement of thoracostomy drainage volume as needed with colloid and immunoglobulins to prevent complications of:[103]
         1) Hypovolemia
         2) Hyponatremia
         3) Lymphopenia
         4) Metabolic acidosis
         5) Hypoproteinemia
      c. Ongoing nutritional assessments so that they can maintain optimal caloric and elemental intake
         1) Infants with chylothorax may be treated with specialized enteral formulas and/or hyperalimentation, which warrant attention to accurate, consistent delivery.
   2. Surgically managed cases will need careful attention to ventilatory weaning postoperatively.

Outcomes

A. Survival from congenital chylothorax, regardless of etiology, is estimated at 85 percent.[79,103]
B. Successful outcome is primarily related to good nutritional and ventilatory management of the neonate.[103]
C. Chronic conditions that may overall impact a successful outcome are:[14]
   1. Bronchopulmonary dysplasia
   2. Malnutrition
   3. Postsurgical complications
      a. Sepsis
      b. Persistent chylothorax

Pulmonary Air Leak

PNEUMOTHORAX, PULMONARY INTERSTITIAL EMPHYSEMA, PNEUMOMEDIASTINUM, AND PNEUMOPERICARDIUM

Definition

Extrapulmonary extravasation of air, which may create respiratory and cardiovascular compromise

Pathophysiology

A. Following alveolar rupture, air may remain trapped in the interstitium, creating pulmonary interstitial emphysema (PIE) or may dissect along the perivascular and peribronchial connective tissue sheath to the mediastinum.

B. Air remaining within the mediastinum creates a pneumomediastinum. Rupture and dissection of mediastinal air into the pleural space creates a pneumothorax. Mediastinal air that ruptures into the pericardial space creates a pneumopericardium.[76,109]

C. In cases of pneumothorax, if the air collection within the pleural space sufficiently increases intrapleural pressure, a tension pneumothorax results. The lungs become poorly compliant, and ventilation of both lungs is impaired. Vena cava compression may interfere with venous return and cardiac output, leading to pulmonary and cardiovascular compromise and clinical deterioration.[109,110]

D. Pneumopericardium, a rare event, is generally preceded by other forms of air leak. Air that has tracked along the vessels to the mediastinum may dissect into the pericardium when under enough pressure. When the gas volume is sufficiently large, it will compress the heart and decrease cardiac output.[111]

Etiology

A. The usual neonatal cause of pulmonary air leak is rupture of alveoli into the perivascular and peribronchial spaces, either because of high transalveolar pressure or abnormal gas distribution with subsequent alveolar overdistention.[109,110] A much less common cause of air leak is rupture of surface blebs on the lung itself.[109]

B. Pneumothorax may be either spontaneous or acquired.
1. Spontaneous pneumothorax may occur because of high initial spontaneous inflation pressures overdistending previously ventilated lung areas.
2. Acquired pneumothorax generally occurs after the presence of significant pulmonary disease and/or artificial ventilation therapy.[110]
3. An uncommon cause of pneumothorax is a bronchopleural fistula, caused by procedural trauma from intubation or airway suctioning.[112]

Incidence

A. Pulmonary air leak is estimated to occur in 1–2 percent of all newborns, but symptoms are evident in only approximately 0.05–0.07 percent.

B. Of all intensive care nursery admissions, 2–8 percent will have a documented air leak.[109]

C. The frequency of air leak increases with decreasing gestational age at birth.
1. Data from the early 1980s suggest that 35 percent of infants weighing <1,000 gm at birth will develop pulmonary interstitial emphysema, 20 percent will develop pneumothorax, 3 percent will develop pneumomediastinum, and 2 percent will develop pneumopericardium during the neonatal period.[109]

2. More recent data, however, suggest the incidence of air leak such as pneumothorax has decreased, attributed to the introduction of postnatal therapies that include exogenous surfactant and gentler ventilation techniques.[73]

Clinical Presentation

A. Neonatal conditions such as meconium aspiration syndrome, congenital diaphragmatic hernia, pulmonary hypoplasia, and urinary tract anomalies are often complicated by air leak.[109,110]

B. Pulmonary air leak may be asymptomatic if it is small and does not create cardiovascular or respiratory compromise. Onset of symptoms may be sudden or gradual.

  1. Grunting[109]
  2. Tachypnea[109]
  3. Cyanosis[109,113]
  4. Chest wall retractions[109]
  5. Shift of point of maximal cardiac impulse due to heart displacement away from the collection of air[109,110,113]
  6. Increased ventilatory needs to support oxygenation and acid-base balance[109,113,114]
  7. Abrupt fall in blood pressure, heart rate, and/or respiratory rate[7,114]
  8. Hyperresonance and diminished breath sounds on the ipsilateral side[113]
  9. Muffled heart sounds caused by the superimposed collection of air[110]
  10. Irritability and restlessness caused by hypoxemia[114]
  11. Asymmetry of chest contour or movement[114]
  12. Decreased compliance, hypercarbia, and hypoxia[110]
  13. Increased diastolic pressure, decreased systolic pressure, tachycardia, bradycardia, and decreased peripheral pulses caused by obstructed venous return and diminished cardiac output[110]

Associations

A. Use of mechanical ventilation[109,110]

B. Use of continuous positive airway pressure (CPAP)[109]

C. Presence of underlying lung disease

  1. Data from the presurfactant era suggest that, in infants with documented respiratory distress syndrome, 12 percent of cases will develop air leak, even in the absence of mechanical ventilation. When mechanical ventilation or CPAP is utilized, 26 percent and 11 percent, respectively, develop air leak.[109]
  2. More recent data suggest the incidence of air leak, such as pneumothorax, in the preterm infant population <33 weeks gestation to be <10 percent and approximately 4 percent when treatment strategies such as surfactant and gentle ventilation are utilized.[115,116]

D. High morbidity and mortality for pneumopericardium[109]

Differential Diagnosis

A. Alternate causes of radiologic and clinical symptoms that may mimic pulmonary air leak include:

  1. Congenital cystic adenomatoid malformation[12,22]
  2. Bronchopulmonary dysplasia[22,106]
  3. Skin fold[73]
  4. Respiratory distress syndrome[106]

Diagnosis

A. Imaging findings to confirm a diagnosis based on clinical symptoms

B. Transillumination of the thorax

   1. The affected side transmits excess or asymmetric light. This may be presumptively diagnostic, as well as useful in determining adequate treatment.[109,110]

   2. Although considered a highly sensitive and specific tool for the diagnosis of pneumothorax, its accuracy can be affected by:

      a. Small air collections or increased skin thickness obstructing light transmission leading to underdiagnosis of pneumothorax

      b. Subcutaneous air collections or edema leading to overdiagnosis

      c. Decreasing ambient external light

         1) Position the light perpendicular to the chest.

         2) Avoid obstructions such as tape and monitor leads to enhance success with this technique.[112]

C. Chest x-ray

   1. Pneumothorax

      a. This condition is notable for a radiolucent collection within the pleural space.

      b. As pleural air accumulates in the anterior chest, AP, lateral, and/or decubitus views may be needed to document the abnormal air collection and differentiate it from pneumomediastinum.[114]

      c. In cases in which the air collection is under tension, there will be displacement of lung and mediastinal structures away from the involved side, allowing the collapsed lung edge to become radiographically evident (Figure 2-19).[113]

   2. Pneumomediastinum

      a. This condition is notable for highlighting and elevating the thymus, commonly referred to as the "sail sign" or "angel wings."[110] Hyperlucency around the heart border and between the sternum and the heart border may be present (Figure 2-20).[109]

   3. Pneumopericardium

      a. This condition is notable for highlighting and encircling the heart.[110]

      b. A lucent halo with narrowing of the cardiac silhouette may be present (Figure 2-21).[111]

   4. PIE

      a. PIE results in a "salt and pepper" pattern of lung parenchyma juxtaposed with lucent interstitial air.[109]

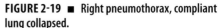

FIGURE 2-19 ■ Right pneumothorax, compliant lung collapsed.

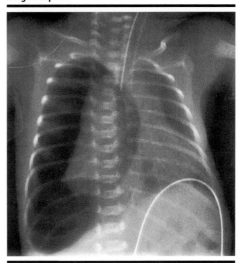

From: Clark DA. 2000. *Atlas of Neonatology*. Philadelphia: Saunders, 91. Reprinted by permission.

b. Tortuous ovoid or linear lucencies may be present on x-ray, extending from the hilum to the periphery in a nonarborizing pattern that does not diminish on expiratory views (Figure 2-22).[22,73]

Treatment Options and Nursing Care

A. Clinical management of air leak is often complicated by simultaneous decreased pulmonary compliance, which necessitates increased ventilatory support.[117]

1. In cases of PIE, strategies that may be effective in managing symptoms or preventing progression of air leak include:

   a. Positioning of the patient with the affected side down in an effort to decompress the overdistended areas

   b. Selective bronchial intubation of the contralateral side, with subsequent selective ventilation of the unaffected lung[109]

   c. Ventilatory techniques that limit peak and mean airway pressures and inspiratory time,[110] such as HFOV and HFV[109,117]

B. Simple pneumothorax, without tension or evidence of cardiovascular compromise, may be treated with the nitrogen-washout technique of inhalation of 100 percent oxygen for up to a 24 to 48 hour period.[109,118]

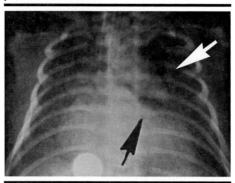

FIGURE 2-20 ■ Pneumomediastinum. AP chest x-ray image of "sail sign" consistent with pneumomediastinum.

From: Carey BE. 1999. Neonatal air leaks: Pneumothorax, pneumomediastinum, pulmonary interstitial emphysema, pneumopericardium. *Neonatal Network* 18(8): 83. Reprinted by permission.

FIGURE 2-21 ■ Pneumopericardium: (A) Lateral and (B) anteroposterior chest x-ray images of pneumopericardium depicting a well-encased halo of air surrounding the heart.

A. Lateral: air confined to pericardium   B. Anteroposterior film: pericardium distinct

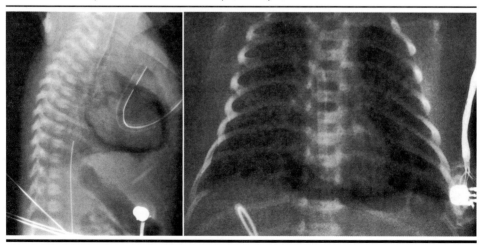

From: Clark DA. 2000. *Atlas of Neonatology.* Philadelphia: Saunders, 96. Reprinted by permission.

1. This strategy promotes reabsorption of free pleural air into the blood at the expense of nitrogen.
2. Caution must be exercised with this therapy, however, because of the potential risks of oxygen toxicity.[109,110]

C. Tension pneumothorax warrants immediate drainage of accumulated air.[109,110,112] Needle aspiration utilizes a 22- to 25-gauge butterfly or angiocatheter device, inserted over the superior aspect of the rib in the midclavicular line. Suction is applied manually, utilizing a 10–20 ml syringe and three-way stopcock.
   1. This therapy is generally meant to be temporizing until a thoracotomy tube can be placed.[110]
   2. Care must be exercised to avoid inadvertent procedural complications, including lung perforation, myocardial perforation, or intercostal laceration.[113]

Surgical Management

A. For tension pneumothorax, a thoracostomy (chest) tube is placed utilizing a #8 to #12 French catheter following needle aspiration.
   1. The approach is from either the first to third intercostal space at the midclavicular line or the sixth to seventh intercostal space at the mid-axillary line, avoiding the breast and areolar tissue, with tip ideally positioned between the lung and the anterior chest wall.[110]
   2. After placement of the indwelling tube, a closed chest drainage system is utilized to provide a water seal and drainage collection chambers and a port for application of continuous negative suction.[107,112]

B. Pneumomediastinum is generally not under tension or symptomatic in presentation. It therefore may usually be managed with observation[110] or inhaled oxygen as for simple pneumothorax.[109]

C. Pneumopericardium commonly presents with symptoms suggesting tension and tamponade.
   1. This condition is life threatening and must be immediately drained surgically.[109]
   2. Temporizing therapy with an 18- to 20-gauge catheter as a pericardial drain, approached substernally,[112] may be utilized until the more definitive cutdown can be operatively undertaken.[110]

D. PIE may require surgical lung resection, such as bullectomy or pneumonectomy, for intractable cases.[73]

Complications

A. Bronchopulmonary dysplasia is a frequent complication of pulmonary interstitial emphysema.[109] This is likely due to prolonged mechanical ventilation.[73]

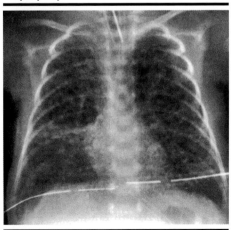

FIGURE 2-22 ■ PIE. Anteroposterior chest x-ray image of bilateral pulmonary interstitial emphysema depicting linear lucencies extending to the periphery.

From: Clark DA. 2000. *Atlas of Neonatology.* Philadelphia: Saunders, 99. Reprinted by permission.

Postoperative Nursing Care

A. In addition to general nursing care, infants who have undergone medical or surgical management of air leak need careful ongoing assessments.

B. Care of chest tubes.

    1. Complications associated with chest tubes include:[119]

        a. Infection

        b. Bleeding

        c. Nerve damage

        d. Diaphragmatic trauma

    2. Chest tubes must be placed using sterile technique and maintained aseptically to reduce the risk of infection.

        a. Bleeding may occur:

            1) During placement, caused by:

                a) Vessel or organ perforation

            2) During maintenance, perhaps caused by:[42]

                a) Inappropriate suction

                b) Manipulation

                c) Migration

        b. Site assessments for drainage or bleeding are important.

        c. Ongoing assessments of indicators of infection may include:

            1) Respiratory or cardiovascular deterioration

            2) Temperature instability

            3) Changes in hematologic, gastrointestinal, or central nervous system assessments **(See Nursing Considerations for Neonatal Pulmonary Disorders later in this chapter.)**

C. Thoracotomy incisions and placement of drainage devices may be a source of pain and agitation for the infant, warranting:

    1. Judicious use of anesthetic and analgesic agents

    2. Ongoing assessments of the efficacy of pain management

Outcomes

A. Most infants with a history of pneumothorax will have an uneventful recovery.[110]

B. LBW infants experiencing air leak may have a three- to fourfold greater risk of death. This risk is created from pulmonary complications, such as air embolization and bronchopulmonary dysplasia, or nonpulmonary complications, such as intraventricular hemorrhage, likely due to the effects of venous stasis or hypercarbia-induced cerebral blood flow changes[110] in a brain with limited autoregulatory capability.[112]

Nursing Considerations for Neonatal Pulmonary Disorders

IMMEDIATE AND PREOPERATIVE MANEUVERS FOR STABILIZATION

Resuscitation, stabilization, and ongoing management of the neonate with a pulmonary disorder demand expert nursing assessment and timely interventions.

Airway Protection

A. Ensuring adequate oxygenation and ventilation while limiting lung injury[25]

    1. Remove oral or endotracheal secretions[120]

    2. Position the infant.

a. Elevate the head of the bed to:[44]
  1) Enhance pulmonary inflation when pressure from abdominal contents may cause respiratory embarrassment
  2) Augment management of secretions
b. Consider prone positioning with appropriate monitoring if this facilitates enhanced gas exchange.
3. Provide cautious oxygen and ventilatory support as needed to promote acid-base balance and adequate oxygenation.
  a. Certain conditions such as congenital diaphragmatic hernia mandate direct endotracheal ventilation when such support is needed because bag and mask ventilation poses the risk of further respiratory compromise from gaseous abdominal distention.
  b. For defects such as congenital cystic adenomatoid malformation and congenital diaphragmatic hernia, ventilatory support strategies that avoid overdistending cystic areas or poorly developed parenchyma are advocated.[25]
4. Avoid hypoxemia, which may exacerbate pulmonary hypertension.[44]

Fluid and Electrolyte Support

A. Ongoing assessments of indicators of fluid and electrolyte balance should be made.
  1. Infants tolerate operative intervention more optimally if they are adequately hydrated.
  2. Thus, prevention of fluid and electrolyte disturbances is important.[121]
B. Although ensuring adequate fluid intake is critical, equal attention must be paid to the possibility of pulmonary or body wall edema created from volume overload.[25,44]
C. Clinical indicators of hydration status and electrolyte balance include:[44,121]
  1. Blood pressure
  2. Heart rate
  3. Body weight
  4. Skin turgor
  5. Edema
  6. Urine output
  7. Urine concentration and indices
  8. Serum electrolytes
D. Accurate measurement and recording of intake and output is critical.[44]

Thermoregulation

A. Decrease heat loss through the routes of convection, conduction, radiation, and evaporation.[25] Body heat loss may increase oxygen consumption and lead to acidosis.[120]
B. Newborns, because of their larger relative body surface area and limited brown fat and glycogen stores, are at particular risk for heat loss from exposure.[25,121]
C. Specific maneuvers to limit heat loss include:
  1. Clothing, including hats[25]
  2. Impermeable plastic wraps and shields[25]
  3. Overhead radiant heat warmers with preheated linens when incubator use is precluded[25]
  4. Incubators with preheated linens
  5. Warmed intravenous solutions and ventilator mist

Gastric Decompression

A. Indwelling or intermittent gastric suction may be needed.

B. Decompression of the stomach will limit potential impedance of diaphragmatic excursion and reduce the risk of aspiration.[44,120,121]

C. For certain conditions such as congenital diaphragmatic hernia, gastric decompression is critical to optimizing pulmonary management.

POSTOPERATIVE STABILIZATION

Airway Protection

A. This includes the previous strategies of secretion removal, ventilatory and oxygen support, and positioning.

B. Despite an initial postoperative honeymoon period of pulmonary stability, especially with defects such as congenital diaphragmatic hernia, infants remain at risk for complications such as pulmonary hypertension.

   1. Strategies such as minimal handling protocols and noninvasive monitoring, as well as prompt recognition and treatment of hypoxemia, should be employed to limit these potential sequelae.[89]

Cardiovascular Support

A. Perform ongoing assessments of heart rate, blood pressure, and perfusion.

   1. Cardiotonics and vasopressors may be prescribed to support blood pressure or optimize cardiac contractility.[121]

      a. Nursing responsibilities when these agents are employed include cautious, accurate delivery and ongoing assessment of efficacy.

   2. Capillary filling time of two to three seconds indicates adequate perfusion.[2]

Fluid, Electrolyte, and Nutritional Support

A. The previously described indicators of hydration status must be noted.

   1. Urine output of 1.5–3 ml is the goal of fluid therapy and indicates adequate cardiac output and intravascular volume.[120]

   2. Surgical manipulation of organs and structures often creates "third spacing" of fluids, which may be clinically evident as edema or depleted intravascular volume.

   3. Fluid support in the form of crystalloid, such as dextrose in water, normal saline, or Ringer's lactate, is generally indicated.

   4. Colloid support, in the form of albuminated saline or fresh frozen plasma, may additionally be indicated in the presence of depleted intravascular volume.[122]

   5. Although ensuring adequate intravascular volume is essential, edema complicating ventilation may necessitate the use of diuretics.

   6. Strict intake and output measurements and assessments of perfusion and hydration therefore become critical nursing responsibilities.

   7. Vascular access may be obtained utilizing umbilical, percutaneous, or peripheral arterial or venous sites for both monitoring and providing fluid, electrolytes, and nutrition.

   8. Postoperative fluid shifts and catecholamine surges may deplete available stores of calcium and glucose and alter electrolyte balance. Therefore, frequent assessment of these parameters is indicated.[2,18,25]

Thermoregulation

A. This includes providing a neutral thermal environment to decrease oxygen and caloric consumption and strategies to prevent or modify the effects of heat loss as previously described.

Gastric Decompression

A. Continued postoperatively until pulmonary stability and GI function are assured, gastric decompression may create the need for nonenteral sources of nutrition such as parenteral alimentation.

Pain and Agitation Relief

See Chapter 10: Assessment and Management of Postoperative Pain; section on Pharmacologic Approaches to Pain Management

Infection Control and Management

A. These include ongoing assessments of both subtle and overt indicators of sepsis.
   1. The neonatal patient is immune disadvantaged due to factors such as decreased levels of immunoglobulins and decreased neutrophil numbers and kinetics.[25]
B. Surgical manipulation and the use of indwelling drainage devices and central vascular catheters create additional immune risks.[121]
   1. Careful and timely administration of antimicrobials and attention to aseptic technique for procedures is critical.
   2. Surgical wounds require vigilant assessments to ensure optimal healing and limit the risk of secondary infections.
   3. Drains such as thoracotomy tubes require ongoing monitoring of volume and character of output.[2]
   4. Indicators of sepsis are often nonspecific.
      a. Respiratory changes, such as apnea, tachypnea, grunting, flaring, or changes in breath sounds
      b. Cardiovascular changes, including increases or decreases in heart rate or blood pressure or decreased perfusion
      c. Hematologic changes, such as abnormal clotting, increased or decreased white blood cell count, or decreased number of platelets or anemia
      d. GI changes, such as distention, decreased bowel sounds, or emesis
      e. Central nervous system changes, such as lethargy, irritability, or tone changes
      f. Temperature instability, including hyperthermia or hypothermia[2,123]

Outcomes

A. Specialized equipment and resources may be required in the home setting.
B. Pulmonary sequelae such as chronic lung disease may dictate the use of equipment, such as supplemental oxygen or medications.
C. Developmental delays resulting from hypoxia, acidosis, or intracranial hemorrhage may necessitate specialized support services such as physical or vocational therapy.
D. Ongoing nutritional needs or complications such as GERD may dictate the use of specialized formulas, feeding strategies, or secondary surgeries.
E. Detailed family education and training related to these issues will be critical to the success of postdischarge care.[89]

REFERENCES

1. Devine P, and Malone F. 2000. Non-cardiac thoracic anomalies. *Clinics in Perinatology* 27(4): 865–900.

2. Wong D, et al. 1999. Conditions caused by defects in physical development. In *Whaley & Wong's Nursing Care of Infants and Children,* 6th ed., Wong D, et al., eds. St. Louis: Mosby, 475–558.

3. Stocker JT. 1994. Congenital and developmental diseases. In *Pulmonary Pathology,* 2nd ed., Dail D, and Hammar S, eds. New York: Springer-Verlag, 155–190.

4. Blackburn ST. 2003. *Maternal, Fetal, & Neonatal Physiology: A Clinical Perspective,* 2nd ed. Philadelphia: Saunders, 310–369, 412–470.

5. Sadler TW. 2004. *Langman's Medical Embryology,* 9th ed. Philadelphia: Lippincott Williams & Wilkins, 211–221, 275–284.

6. Moore KL, and Persaud TVN. 2003. *The Developing Human: Clinically Oriented Embryology,* 7th ed. Philadelphia: Saunders, 188–200, 241–253.

7. Raffensperger J. 1990. Congenital malformations of the lung. In *Swenson's Pediatric Surgery,* 5th ed., Raffensperger J, ed. Norwalk, Connecticut: Appleton & Lange, 743–753.

8. Karnak I, et al. 1999. Congenital lobar emphysema: Diagnostic and therapeutic considerations. *Journal of Pediatric Surgery* 34(9): 1347–1351.

9. Olutoye O, et al. 2000. Prenatal diagnosis and management of congenital lobar emphysema. *Journal of Pediatric Surgery* 35(5): 792–795.

10. Ozcelik U, et al. 2003. Congenital lobar emphysema: Evaluation and long-term follow-up of thirty cases at a single center. *Pediatric Pulmonology* 35(5): 384–391.

11. Bagwell CE. 1993. Surgical lesions of pediatric airways and lungs. In *Neonatal and Pediatric Respiratory Care,* 2nd ed., Koff P, Eitzman D, and Neu J, eds. St. Louis: Mosby, 128–154.

12. Johnson K, and Cooper T. 1998. Congenital diseases affecting the lung parenchyma: Cystic malformations of the lung. In *Contemporary Diagnosis and Management of Neonatal Respiratory Diseases,* 2nd ed., Hansen T, Cooper T, and Weisman L, eds. Newtown, Pennsylvania: Handbooks in Health Care, 171–177.

13. Hebra A, Othersen HB, and Tagge E. 2000. Bronchopulmonary malformations. In *Pediatric Surgery,* 3rd ed., Ashcraft K, et al., eds. Philadelphia: Saunders, 273–286.

14. Krummel T. 1998. Congenital malformations of the lower respiratory tract. In *Kendig's Disorders of the Respiratory Tract in Children,* 6th ed., Kendig E, Chernick V, and Boat T, eds. Philadelphia: Saunders, 287–328.

15. Haller J, et al. 1978. Surgical management of lung bud anomalies: Lobar emphysema, bronchogenic cyst, cystic adenomatoid malformation, and intralobar pulmonary sequestration. *Annals of Thoracic Surgery* 28(1): 33–43.

16. Burge D, and Samuel M. 1998. Structural anomalies of the airway and lungs. In *Paediatric Surgery,* Atwell J, ed. New York: Oxford University Press, 170–186.

17. Schwartz D, Reyes-Mugica M, and Keller M. 1999. Imaging of surgical diseases of the newborn chest: Intrapleural mass lesions. *Radiologic Clinics of North America* 37(6): 1067–1078.

18. Turner C. 2000. Vascular access. In *Pediatric Surgery,* 3rd, ed., Ashcraft K, et al., eds. Philadelphia: Saunders, 108–114.

19. McBride J, et al. 1980. Lung growth and airway function after lobectomy in infancy for congenital lobar emphysema. *Journal of Clinical Investigation* 66(5): 962–970.

20. Hartmen G, et al. 1999. General surgery. In *Neonatology: Pathophysiology and Management of the Newborn,* 5th ed., Avery G, Fletcher M, and MacDonald M, eds. Philadelphia: Lippincott Williams & Wilkins, 1005–1044.

21. Luck S, Reynolds M, and Raffensperger J. 1986. Congenital bronchopulmonary malformations. *Current Problems in Surgery* 23(4): 251–314.

22. Hernanz-Schulman M. 1993. Cysts and cystlike lesions of the lung. *Radiologic Clinics of North America* 31(3): 631–649.

23. Lazar E, and Stolar C. 1995. Congenital pulmonary and chest wall malformations. In *Perinatal and Pediatric Respiratory Care,* Barnhart S, and Czervinski M, eds. Philadelphia: Saunders, 526–535.

24. Tireli GA, et al. 2004. Bronchogenic cysts: A rare congenital cystic malformation of the lung. *Surgery Today* 34(7): 573–576.

25. Chahine A, and Ricketts R. 1999. Resuscitation of the surgical neonate. *Clinics in Perinatology* 26(3): 693–715.

26. Howell LJ, and Dunphy PM. 1999. Fetal surgery: Exploring the challenges in nursing care. *Journal of Obstetric, Gynecologic, and Neonatal Nursing* 28(4): 427–432.

27. Cha I, et al. 1997. Fetal congenital cystic adenomatoid malformations of the lung: A clinicopathologic study of eleven cases. *American Journal of Surgical Pathology* 21(5): 537–544.

28. Sittig S, and Asay G. 2000. Congenital cystic adenomatoid malformation in the newborn: Two case studies and review of the literature. *Respiratory Care* 45(10): 1188–1195.

29. Stocker JT, Madewell J, and Drake R. 1977. Congenital cystic adenomatoid malformation of the lung: Classification and morphologic spectrum. *Human Pathology* 8(2): 155–171.

30. Gilbert E, and Opitz J. 1989. Malformations and genetic disorders of the respiratory tract. In *Pediatric Pulmonary Disease,* Stocker J, ed. New York: Hemisphere, 29–100.

31. Tastan Y. 2000. Pathological case of the month: Congenital cystic adenomatoid malformation of the lung. *Archives of Pediatric and Adolescent Medicine* 154(6): 633–634.

32. Laberge JM, Bratu I, and Flageole H. 2004. The management of asymptomatic congenital lung malformations. *Paediatric Respiratory Reviews* 5(supplement A): S305–S312.

33. Adzik NS, et al. 1985. Fetal cystic adenomatoid malformation: Prenatal diagnosis and natural history. *Journal of Pediatric Surgery* 20(5): 483–488.

34. Morotti R, et al. 1999. Congenital cystic adenomatoid malformation of the lung (CCAM): Evaluation of the cellular components. *Human Pathology* 30(6): 618–625.

35. Revillon Y, et al. 1993. Congenital cystic adenomatoid malformation of the lung: Prenatal management and prognosis. *Journal of Pediatric Surgery* 28(8): 1009–1011.

36. Cass D, et al. 1998. Increased cell proliferation and decreased apoptosis characterize congenital cystic adenomatoid malformation of the lung. *Journal of Pediatric Surgery* 33(7): 1043–1047.

37. Crombleholme T. 1996. Prenatal diagnosis and management of surgical pulmonary problems. *Neonatal Respiratory Diseases* 6(5): 1–12.

38. Gornall AS, et al. 2003. Congenital cystic adenomatoid malformation: Accuracy of prenatal diagnosis, prevalence and outcome in a general population. *Prenatal Diagnosis* 23(12): 997–1002.

39. Laberge J, et al. 2001. Outcome of the prenatally diagnosed congenital cystic adenomatoid lung malformation: A Canadian experience. *Fetal Diagnosis and Therapy* 16(3): 178A–186A.

40. Bunduki V, et al. 2000. Prognostic factors associated with congenital cystic adenomatoid malformation of the lung. *Prenatal Diagnosis* 20(6): 459–464.

41. Neilson I, et al. 1991. Congenital adenomatoid malformation of the lung: Current management and prognosis. *Journal of Pediatric Surgery* 26(8): 975–981.

42. Pulito AR. 2004. Surgical diseases of the newborn. In *Neonatology: Management, Procedures, On-Call Problems, Diseases, and Drugs,* 5th ed., Gomella TL, et al., eds. New York: Lange Medical Books, 572–584.

43. Seo T, et al. 1999. Acute respiratory failure associated with intrathoracic masses in neonates. *Journal of Pediatric Surgery* 34(11): 1633–1637.

44. Wilson J, and Maenner V. 1993. Congenital cystic adenomatoid malformation. *Neonatal Network* 12(6): 15–20.

45. Jona J. 1998. Advances in fetal surgery. *Pediatric Clinics of North America* 45(3): 599–604.

46. Adzik NS, et al. 1993. Fetal surgery for cystic adenomatoid malformation of the lung. *Journal of Pediatric Surgery* 28(6): 806–812.

47. VanLeeuwen K, et al. 1999. Prenatal diagnosis of congenital cystic adenomatoid malformation and its postnatal presentation, surgical indications, and natural history. *Journal of Pediatric Surgery* 34(5): 794–799.

48. Khosa JK, Leong SL, and Borzi PA. 2004. Congenital cystic adenomatoid malformation of the lung: Indications and timing of surgery. *Pediatric Surgery International* 20(7): 505–508.

49. Miller J, Corteville J, and Langer J. 1996. Congenital cystic adenomatoid malformation in the fetus: Natural history and predictors of outcome. *Journal of Pediatric Surgery* 31(6): 805–808.

50. Pittman L. 2002. Congenital cystic adenomatoid malformation of the lung. *Neonatal Network* 21(3): 59–66.

51. Spinella P, Strieper M, and Callahan C. 1998. Congestive heart failure in a neonate secondary to bilateral intralobar and extralobar pulmonary sequestrations. *Pediatrics* 101(1-1): 120–124.

52. May D, et al. 1993. Perinatal and postnatal chest sonography. *Radiologic Clinics of North America* 31(3): 499–516.

53. Newman B. 1990. Real-time ultrasound and color-Doppler imaging in pulmonary sequestration. *Pediatrics* 86(4): 620–623.

54. Piccione W, and Burt M. 1990. Pulmonary sequestration in the neonate. *Chest* 97(1): 244–246.

55. Corbett HJ, and Humphrey GM. 2004. Pulmonary sequestration. *Paediatric Respiratory Reviews* 5(1): 59–68.

56. Vegunta R, and Teich S. 1999. Preoperative diagnosis of extralobar pulmonary sequestration with unusual vasculature: A case report. *Journal of Pediatric Surgery* 34(8): 1307–1308.

57. Buntain W, et al. 1977. Pulmonary sequestration in children: A twenty-five year experience. *Surgery* 81(4): 413–420.

58. Boyer J, et al. 1996. Extralobar pulmonary sequestration masquerading as a congenital pleural effusion. *Pediatrics* 97(1): 115–117.

59. Park MK. 2002. Miscellaneous congenital cardiac conditions. In *Pediatric Cardiology for Practitioners,* 4th ed. St. Louis: Mosby, 256–267.

60. Engelke S, et al. 1987. What is your diagnosis? *Perinatology–Neonatology* 11(1): 29–30.

61. Savic B, et al. 1979. Lung sequestration: Report of seven cases and review of 540 published cases. *Thorax* 34(1): 96–101.

62. Laurin S, and Hagerstrand I. 1999. Intralobar bronchopulmonary sequestration in the newborn: A congenital malformation. *Pediatric Radiology* 29(3): 174–178.

63. Stocker JT, and Malczak HT. 1984. A study of pulmonary ligament arteries. Relationship to intralobar pulmonary sequestration. *Chest* 86(4): 611–615.

64. Nicolette L, et al. 1993. Intralobar pulmonary sequestration: A clinical and pathological spectrum. *Journal of Pediatric Surgery* 28(6): 802–805.

65. Carpentieri D, et al. 2000. Subdiaphragmatic pulmonary sequestration: A case report with review of the literature. *Journal of Perinatology* 20(1): 60–62.

66. Mordue BC. 2003. A case series of five infants with scimitar syndrome. *Advances in Neonatal Care* 3(3): 121–132.

67. Tolkin J, MacAdam C, and Moody S. 1987. Radiological case of the month: Extralobar pulmonary sequestration. *American Journal of Diseases of Children* 141(11): 1223–1224.

68. Stern R. 1996. Congenital anomalies. In *Nelson Textbook of Pediatrics,* 15th ed., Nelson W, et al., eds. Philadelphia: Saunders, 1198–1201.

69. Schwartz M, and Ramachandran P. 1997. Congenital malformations of the lung and mediastinum: A quarter century of experience from a single institution. *Journal of Pediatric Surgery* 32(1): 44–47.

70. Salmons S. 2000. Pulmonary sequestration. *Neonatal Network* 19(7): 27–31.

71. Antonetti M, et al. 2000. Congenital pulmonary lymphangiectasia: A case report of thoracic duct agenesis. *Pediatric Pulmonology* 32(3): 184–186.

72. Bouchard S, et al. 2000. Pulmonary lymphangiectasia revisited. *Journal of Pediatric Surgery* 35(5): 796–800.

73. Newman B. 1999. Imaging of medical disease of the newborn lung. *Radiologic Clinics of North America* 37(6): 1049–1065.

74. Huber A, et al. 1991. Congenital pulmonary lymphangiectasia. *Pediatric Pulmonology* 10(4): 310–313.

75. Scott C, et al. 2003. Primary pulmonary lymphangiectasis in a premature infant: Resolution following intensive care. *Pediatric Pulmonology* 35(5): 405–406.

76. Koenig J, and Cooper T. 1998. Congenital diseases affecting the lung parenchyma: Other lung malformations. In *Contemporary Diagnosis and Management of Neonatal Respiratory Diseases,* 2nd ed., Hansen T, Cooper T, and Weisman L, eds. Newtown, Pennsylvania: Handbooks in Health Care: 177–185.

77. Stringel G. 2000. Hemangiomas and lymphangiomas. In *Pediatric Surgery,* 3rd ed., Ashcraft K, et al., eds. Philadelphia: Saunders, 965–986.

78. Rettwitz-Volk W, et al. 1999. Congenital unilobar pulmonary lymphangiectasis. *Pediatric Pulmonology* 27(4): 290–292.

79. Welty W, and Hansen T. 1998. Pulmonary edema. In *Contemporary Diagnosis and Management of Neonatal Respiratory Diseases,* 2nd ed., Hansen T, Cooper T, and Weisman L, eds. Newtown, Pennsylvania: Handbooks in Health Care, 110–116.

80. Arensman R, Bambini D, and Chiu B. 2005. Congenital diaphragmatic hernia and eventration. In *Pediatric Surgery,* 4th ed., Ashcraft K, et al., eds. Philadelphia: Saunders, 304–323.

81. Katz A, Wiswell T, and Baumgart S. 1998. Contemporary controversies in the management of congenital diaphragmatic hernia. *Clinics in Perinatology* 25(1): 219–248.

82. O'Toole S, et al. 1996. Pulmonary vascular abnormalities in congenital diaphragmatic hernia. *Clinics in Perinatology* 23(4): 781–794.

83. Thibeault D, and Haney B. 1998. Lung volume, pulmonary vasculature and factors affecting survival in congenital diaphragmatic hernia. *Pediatrics* 101(2): 289–295.

84. Wilcox D, et al. 1996. Pulmonary parenchymal abnormalities in congenital diaphragmatic hernia. *Clinics in Perinatology* 23(4): 771–779.

85. Soylu H, et al. 2000. Morgagni hernia: An unexpected cause of respiratory complaints and a chest mass. *Pediatric Pulmonology* 30(5): 429–433.

86. Beresford M, and Shaw N. 2000. Outcome of congenital diaphragmatic hernia. *Pediatric Pulmonology* 30(3): 249–256.

87. Doyle NM, and Lally KP. 2004. The CDH Study Group and advances in the clinical care of the patient with congenital diaphragmatic hernia. *Seminars in Perinatology* 28(3): 174–184.

88. Guillory C, and Cooper T. 1998. Diseases affecting the diaphragm and chest wall: Diseases of the diaphragm. In *Contemporary Diagnosis and Management of Neonatal Respiratory Diseases*, 2nd ed., Hansen T, Cooper T, and Weisman L, eds. Newtown, Pennsylvania: Handbooks in Health Care, 188–197.

89. Juretschke L. 2001. Congenital diaphragmatic hernia: Update and review. *Journal of Obstetric, Gynecologic, and Neonatal Nursing* 30(3): 259–268.

90. Theorell C. 1990. Congenital diaphragmatic hernia: A physiologic approach to management. *Journal of Perinatal and Neonatal Nursing* 3(3): 66–79.

91. Moreno CN, and Iovanne BA. 1993. Congenital diaphragmatic hernia: Part 1. *Neonatal Network* 12(1): 19–27.

92. Downard CD, and Wilson JM. 2003. Current therapy of infants with congenital diaphragmatic hernia. *Seminars in Neonatology* 8(3): 215–221.

93. Kaiser J, and Rosenfeld C. 1999. A population-based study of congenital diaphragmatic hernia: Impact of associated anomalies and preoperative blood gases on survival. *Journal of Pediatric Surgery* 34(8): 1196–1202.

94. Ivascu FA, and Hirschl RB. 2004. New approaches to managing congenital diaphragmatic hernia. *Seminars in Perinatology* 28(3): 185–198.

95. Sakurai Y, et al. 1999. Pulmonary barotrauma in congenital diaphragmatic hernia: A clinicopathological correlation. *Journal of Pediatric Surgery* 34(12): 1813–1817.

96. Nobuhara K, et al. 1996. Long-term outlook for survivors of congenital diaphragmatic hernia. *Clinics in Perinatology* 23(4): 873–887.

97. Tsukahara Y, et al. 2001. Prenatal diagnosis of congenital diaphragmatic eventration by magnetic resonance imaging. *American Journal of Perinatology* 18(5): 241–244.

98. Vanamo K, et al. 1996. Long-term pulmonary sequelae in survivors of congenital diaphragmatic defects. *Journal of Pediatric Surgery* 31(8): 1096–1100.

99. Murphy M, Newman B, and Rodgers B. 1989. Pleuroperitoneal shunts in the management of persistent chylothorax. *Annals of Thoracic Surgery* 48(2): 195–200.

100. Buttiker V, Fanconi S, and Burger R. 1999. Chylothorax in children: Guidelines for diagnosis and management. *Chest* 116(3): 682–687.

101. Kugelman A, Gonen R, and Bader D. 2000. Potential role of high-frequency ventilation in the treatment of severe congenital pleural effusion. *Pediatric Pulmonology* 29(5): 404–408.

102. Stringel G. 2000. Hemangiomas and lymphangiomas. In *Pediatric Surgery*, 3rd ed., Ashcraft K, et al., eds. Philadelphia: Saunders, 965–986.

103. Al-Tawil K, et al. 2000. Congenital chylothorax. *American Journal of Perinatology* 17(3): 121–126.

104. Beghetti M, et al. 2000. Etiology and management of pediatric chylothorax. *Journal of Pediatrics* 136(5): 653–658.

105. Kurekci E, Kaye R, and Koehler M. 1998. Chylothorax and chylopericardium: A complication of a central venous catheter. *Journal of Pediatrics* 132(6): 1064–1066.

106. Cooper T. 1998. X-ray patterns in neonatal lung disease. In *Contemporary Diagnosis and Management of Neonatal Respiratory Diseases*, 2nd ed., Hansen T, Cooper T, and Weisman L, eds. Newtown, Pennsylvania: Handbooks in Health Care, 58–63.

107. Stillwell P. 1995. Disorders of the pleura. In *Perinatal and Pediatric Respiratory Care*, Barnhart S, and Czervinske M, eds. Philadelphia: Saunders, 537–547.

108. Tuggle D. 2000. Acquired pulmonary and pleural disorders. In *Pediatric Surgery*, 3rd ed., Ashcraft K, et al., eds. Philadelphia: Saunders, 287–299.

109. Whitsett J, et al. 1999. Acute respiratory disorders. In *Neonatology: Pathophysiology and Management of the Newborn*, 5th ed., Avery G, Fletcher MA, and MacDonald M, eds. Philadelphia: Lippincott Williams & Wilkins, 485–508.

110. Cooper T. 1998. Subacute and chronic acquired parenchymal lung diseases. In *Contemporary Diagnosis and Management of Neonatal Respiratory Diseases*, 2nd ed., Hansen T, Cooper T, and Weisman L, eds. Newtown, Pennsylvania: Handbooks in Health Care, 139–149.

111. Carey B. 1999. Neonatal air leaks: Pneumothorax, pneumomediastinum, pulmonary interstitial emphysema, pneumopericardium. *Neonatal Network* 18(8): 81–84.

112. Carroll P. 1991. Pneumothorax in the newborn. *Neonatal Network* 10(2): 27–34.

113. Wyatt T. 1995. Pneumothorax in the neonate. *Journal of Obstetric, Gynecologic, and Neonatal Nursing* 24(3): 211–216.

114. Gregory SEB. 1987. Air leak syndromes. *Neonatal Network* 5(5): 40–46.

115. Koivisto M, et al. 2004. Changing incidence and outcome of infants with respiratory distress syndrome in the 1990s: A population-based survey. *Acta Paediatrica* 93(2): 177–184.

116. Hobar JD, et al. 2002. Trends in mortality and morbidity for very low birth weight infants, 1991–1999. *Pediatrics* 110(1 part 1): 143–151.

117. Wood B. 1993. The newborn chest. *Radiologic Clinics of North America* 31(3): 667–676.

118. Sistoza L. 2004. Air leak syndromes. In *Neonatology: Management, Procedures, On-Call Problems, Diseases, and Drugs*, 5th ed., Gomella TL, et al., eds. New York: Lange Medical Books, 524–530.

119. Gomella T, et al. 2004. Chest tube placement. In *Neonatology: Management, Procedures, On-Call Problems, Diseases, and Drugs*, 5th ed., Gomella TL, et al., eds. New York: Lange Medical Books, 169–171.

120. Hamm CR. 2004. Respiratory management. In *Neonatology: Management, Procedures, On-Call Problems, Diseases, and Drugs*, 5th ed., Gomella TL, et al., eds. New York: Lange Medical Books, 44–68.

121. Shaw N. 1990. Common surgical problems in the newborn. *Journal of Perinatal and Neonatal Nursing* 3(3): 50–65.

122. Engle WD, and LeFlore JL. 2002. Hypotension in the neonate. *NeoReviews* 3(8): 157–162.

123. Tappero E. 2004. Clinical and laboratory evaluation of neonatal infection. In *Infection in the Neonate: A Comprehensive Guide to Assessment, Management, and Nursing Care*, Askin DF, ed. Santa Rosa, California: NICU Ink, 129–141.

NOTES

3

Neonatal Cardiovascular Surgical Conditions

Katherine M. Jorgensen, RNC, MSN/MBA, HonD

Congenital heart disease, the most common of all major congenital anomalies, is diagnosed in 4–9/1,000 live born infants.[1-3] Not all of these alterations are life threatening; however, prompt diagnosis and treatment are crucial in the more complex, life-threatening cardiac conditions that present at birth. For early recognition, one must understand the etiology and presentation because one alteration in development may provide a variety of resulting events and clinical findings (Table 3-1).

Diagnostic measures provide a means of differentiating between a cardiac problem and one that is based in another organ system. Diagnostics allow the health care provider to distinguish between the various lesions that cause acyanotic and cyanotic heart disease. Acyanotic lesions permit a mixing of oxygenated and deoxygenated blood via a left-to-right shunt while providing oxygenated blood systemically. These include patent ductus arteriosus (PDA), the most common, especially in preterm infants; atrial and ventricular septal defects (ASD and VSD); aortic stenosis; coarctation of the aorta; interrupted aortic arch; and endocardial cushion defect. Cyanotic or ductus-dependent lesions are defects that provide deoxygenated blood to the systemic circulation due to right-to-left shunting, which bypasses the pulmonary system. These include transposition of the great arteries, tricuspid atresia, truncus arteriosus, and tetralogy of Fallot.

Prompt diagnosis facilitates the medical and surgical care that will address both primary and secondary events, where there may be high rates of morbidity and mortality. During this critical diagnostic and treatment period, comfort of both the infant and the parent must be addressed as all parties traverse this very stressful journey in the intensive care setting. The diagnosis, treatment, and nursing care of infants who present with patent ductus arteriosus, tetralogy of Fallot, D-transposition of the great arteries, hypoplastic left heart syndrome, and total anomalous pulmonary venous connection are discussed.

TABLE 3-1 ■ Fetal Cardiac Development and Associated Abnormalities[3,13,28]

Gestational age	Development	Associated Defect
Day 18 to 19	Beginning heart development	
Day 21	Fusion into one heart tube	
Day 22	Circulation (ebb and flow)	
Day 23	Rotation to right into bulboventricular loop	Dextrocardia
Week 4	Head fold bringing pericardial cavity ventral to foregut and caudal to oropharyngeal membrane	
Week 4–end	Coordinated contractions with unidirectional flow	
Week 4 to 5 starts Week 8 completed	Partitioning of atrioventricular canal and atria and ventricle partitioning	AV canal ASD VSD
Week 4 to 5 Week 6 to 8 Week 5	Brachial/aortic arches Adult configuration of aortic arch Septal partitioning of bulbous cordis and truncus arteriosus and spiraling of septum	Double aortic arch with vascular ring Coarctation of the aorta Truncus arteriosus Transposition of great arteries Aorticopulmonary septal defect Aortic stenosis/atresia Pulmonary stenosis/atresia
Week 5 to 8	Pulmonary vein development and integration into left atrium	Anomalous pulmonary venous connections
Week 8	Vena cava formation	Vena cava abnormalities
Week 8	Cardiac development completed	

Embryology

A. The cardiovascular system is the first system to function in the embryo, with blood circulation commencing by the third week after conception.[3]
B. The cardiovascular system is required early in the developing embryo because supply and function are limited in the early development of the yolk sac.
  1. Deliver oxygen and nutrients to all tissues in the body
  2. Remove waste from the body tissues
  3. Provide overall homeostasis
C. Cardiac development proceeds as follows.
  1. The heart originates as cells that aggregate to form two longitudinal cellular strands called cardiogenic cords.[3–5]
    a. The cardiogenic cords migrate to each other and fuse as canalization occurs within these structures to form the endocardial heart tubes. These tubes fuse to form a single heart tube.
    b. This single heart tube then bends to the right and forms the bulboventricular loop.
    c. This loop will later contribute to the ventricular chambers of the heart.
D. During the first month of development, the following occurs.
  1. Blood begins to circulate by day 22 of gestation.[3]
  2. Circulation consists of bidirectional movement due to the peristaltic activity of this primitive organ.
  3. By the end of week 4, coordinated contractions are established, thus contributing to a unidirectional blood flow pattern.[3]

FIGURE 3-1 ■ Development of the heart, gestational weeks 4–5.

A to C. Sagittal sections of the heart during the fourth and fifth weeks, illustrating blood flow through the heart and division of the atrioventricular canal. **D.** Coronal section of the heart at the plane shown in C. Note that the interatrial and interventricular septa have started to develop.

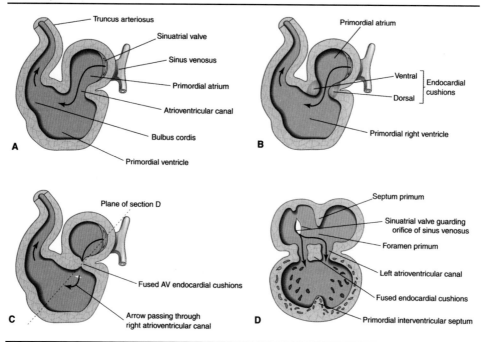

From: Moore KL, and Persaud TVN. 2003. *The Developing Human: Clinically Oriented Embryology,* 7th ed. Philadelphia: Saunders, 341. Reprinted by permission.

E. During the fourth and fifth weeks of development, the following occur.
   1. Atrial and ventricular partitioning begin (Figure 3-1).
     a. Formation of atrioventricular (AV) endocardial cushions
   2. The cushions fuse in week 5, causing the formation of right and left AV canals.
   3. These two canals freely communicate between the atria and ventricles until the valves between these chambers form and begin to regulate flow. Further partitioning is accomplished by the atrial and ventricular septums, separating the chambers from right and left.[3,5]
F. The atrial wall develops.
   1. A result of the formation and ultimate fusion of the septum primum and septum secundum
   2. Septum primum
     a. It extends from the "roof" of the atria to the endocardial cushion.
     b. To support flow from the right to the left side of the atria, the area closest to the origin of this tissue will perforate, providing what is later known as the foramen ovale.
   3. Septum secundum
     a. Grows ventrally next to the septum primum
     b. Becomes integral in the closure to the foramen ovale after birth as blood flow changes from right-to-left to left-to-right[3,5]

G. The ventricular septum develops.
    1. This occurs concurrently with the atrial septum changes.
    2. The membranous portion of the septum originates as a ridge or fold in the "floor" of the common ventricular chamber.
    3. As the ventricles dilate, this tissue elongates.
    4. By the end of the seventh week, growth has encouraged the muscular portion of the septum to reach up to and fuse with the endocardial cushion.
    5. By the eighth week of gestation, a four-chambered heart is evident with the development and fusion of the atrial and ventricular septums and the endocardial cushion.[3–5]

H. The great vessels develop.
    1. During weeks 4 and 5, the brachial arches form.
    2. These integrate with arteries from the aortic arches to create the adult version of the aortic arch by week 8 of gestation.
    3. There is a series of six pairs of arches present at various times during embryologic development.
    4. Only the fourth and sixth pairs are important in cardiac development.
        a. The fourth pair evolves into a portion of the arch as seen after fetal development is complete.
        b. The sixth pair of arches evolves into the ductus arteriosus and a portion of the pulmonary artery.
        c. The other pairs either degenerate or go on to form other vessels within the circulatory system.

I. Differentiation of the aorta and pulmonary artery proceeds.
    1. Appropriate articulation within the system is achieved during week 5 with the development of the aorticopulmonary septum that divides the bulbous cordis and truncus arteriosus.
    2. This septum, once in place, spirals to twist the pulmonary trunk around the ascending aorta.
    3. These vessels interface with the cardiac structure as outflow from the right ventricle goes to the pulmonary bed via the pulmonary artery.
    4. The aorta carries oxygenated blood from the left ventricle to the systemic circulation.
    5. The pulmonary veins also develop during this period.
    6. The vessels are integrated into the left atria to permit flow of oxygenated blood from the pulmonary circulation.[3,5]

J. During week 8 of development, the following occurs.
    1. The cardiac structure and the major vessels of circulation are formed and provide circulation of blood volume throughout the developing embryo.
    2. Disruption of any of the steps in development prior to this time by the following will cause defects and abnormalities based upon the actual timing of the noxious event.[6]
        a. Environmental factors
        b. Drugs
            1) Alcohol
            2) Dilantin
            3) Progesterone
            4) Lithium
        c. Maternal viral infections
            1) Rubella

   2) Coxsackievirus
d. Maternal diseases
e. Unusual radiation exposure
f. Chromosomal defects

Prenatal Diagnosis of Congenital Heart Disease

A. The diagnosis of congenital cardiovascular disease can be made *in utero* using two-dimensional echocardiography.
  1. Movement of the heart is visible by week 6 of gestation.
  2. The greatest visualization opportunity is between weeks 18 and 24 of gestation.[7]
  3. Indications for a fetal echocardiogram include the following.
    a. Abnormal fetal findings by other modes of assessment
      1) Fetal arrhythmias
        a) Indicator of other structural anomalies, with a reported risk of 6 to 15 percent[7]
      2) Extracardiac anomalies
        a) High association with cardiac anomalies with a risk of 25 to 45 percent[7]
      3) Chromosomal anomalies
        a) High association with cardiac anomalies with a risk of 30 to 50 percent[7]
      4) Abnormal growth
        a) Associated with fetal hypoxia and congestive heart failure
      5) Fetal distress
        a) Associated with fetal hypoxia and congestive heart failure
    b. Maternal risk factors
      1) Environmental risks
      2) Maternal disease
        a) Lupus
        b) Diabetes
      3) A previous pregnancy in which the fetus had congenital heart disease
        a) The risk of a second child with a congenital heart defect is 2 percent, or double the normal risk of 1 percent in a woman without such a history.[7]
  4. Visible by fetal echocardiogram are the four chambers, valve placement and function, great vessels outlet flow, and aortic arch.
  5. Prenatal or neonatal echocardiography depicts the structural alterations and flow.[8]

Neonatal Diagnosis of Congenital Heart Disease

PHYSICAL EXAMINATION

A. A careful physical examination and assessment must be done on all infants, especially those with an identified increased risk of congenital heart disease.
  1. Observe the infant at rest.
    a. **Color.** The infant with cardiac disease may present with pallor, mottling, or cyanosis, depending on the mix of oxygenated and deoxygenated

blood within the cardiac system and the degree of associated pulmonary compromise.

b. **Respiratory rate and effort.** Respiratory rate is increased in the infant with cardiac disease. This tachypnea is generally not associated with increased work of breathing (WOB), as it would be in an infant with respiratory disease. Thus, the infant presents distress free while breathing rapidly.

c. **General tone.** It may be depressed.

d. **Activity.** Increased activity compromises this infant, so a natural compensation and self-protection from this stress appears go into effect with a low energy state.

2. Auscultate while the infant is undisturbed.

   a. Heart rate
      1) Tachycardia
      2) Bradycardia

   b. Murmurs
      1) Not all cardiac defects produce a murmur.
      2) Murmurs are due to turbulence of flow.
      3) Defects without restriction in flow, while producing abnormal flow patterns, often will not present with a murmur until much later in the evolution of hemodynamic changes caused by the defect.
      4) Murmurs are graded one to six, with one being barely audible and six being extremely loud.[8,9]

   c. Clicks and split sounds
      1) These are associated with valvular involvement.
      2) They cause compromise that can occur in isolation or are associated with other cardiac defects.
      3) Appreciate these alterations in heart sounds by auscultating the apex, upper and lower left sternal borders, upper right sternal border, lower back, and axilla.[8]

   d. Pattern (rhythm)
      1) Arrhythmias are indicative of conduction issues that may or may not be related to structural defects.
      2) Many are recognized during the fetal period, thus requiring increased surveillance and maternal treatment to support the fetus while *in utero*.
      3) Conduction abnormalities require careful investigation upon birth or presentation.

   e. Breath sounds
      1) Generally clear and equal prior to the onset of pulmonary compromise, regardless of the rate of respirations
      2) Can be described as "wet" with coarse rales as pulmonary congestion in conjunction with cardiac compromise progresses

3. Palpate the infant.

   a. Pulses
      1) Compare upper extremities to lower extremities, right to left, and right upper to any lower pulse.
      2) Pulses are especially useful in the assessment of cardiac output and left-sided cardiac function.

    b. Chest

       1) The following findings are abnormal in the newborn and significant in the assessment of cardiac dysfunction.

         a) Thrill

         b) Bruit

         c) Tap

    c. Liver and spleen

       1) Enlargement of the liver is associated with congestive heart failure.

       2) Early assessment of hepatic size prior to increasing compromise can be helpful in the later diagnosis because congestive heart failure and liver engorgement may progress (dependent upon the particular lesion).

  4. Obtain blood pressures in the four extremities.

    a. These provide information regarding left-sided function and distribution of systemic blood flow.

    b. A key component of obtaining reliable data is to keep the infant calm and quiet during this assessment. The use of swaddling, an extra pair of hands, and a pacifier can be of great assistance in avoiding elevated parameters caused by agitation.

    c. Abnormal findings are arm pressures that are higher than leg pressures by 20 mmHg.

Chest X-Rays, Anteroposterior and Lateral

A. Heart size and shape

  1. Increased heart size, cardiomegaly, is indicative of congestive heart failure.

  2. Abnormal boot shape is a diagnostic finding in tetralogy of Fallot.[8]

  3. A snowman-shaped heart is associated with total anomalous pulmonary venous return.[10]

B. Pulmonary markings and expansion

  1. These are important in the differential diagnosis determining cardiac or respiratory etiology for the distress seen.

  2. Increased vascular markings are seen with left-to-right shunting, whereas diminished markings are associated with defects that restrict blood flow to the lungs.

Differential Diagnosis of Cardiovascular Disorders

A. Hyperoxia test

  1. A hyperoxia test consists of obtaining a blood gas first in room air and then again after providing 100 percent oxygen or as high a concentration as is obtainable.

    a. An infant with cardiac disease will have a limited response, with a maximum PaO_2 <200 mmHg.[11]

    b. This is due to intracardiac shunting that does not pass the deoxygenated blood through the pulmonary bed for oxygenation.[12]

    c. With optimal ventilation and oxygenation, most infants presenting with other etiologies of distress and hypoxia will respond with a PaO_2 >300 mmHg.[13] Infants with persistent pulmonary hypertension of the newborn (PPHN) may not respond to a hyperoxia test. An echocardiogram will assist in differentiating PPHN from primary cardiac disease.

  2. This test is used to differentiate between intrapulmonary and intracardiac shunting.

B. Transcutaneous and oximetry monitoring
1. If neonatal echocardiography is readily available, other diagnostic maneuvers may be eliminated and an immediate echocardiogram performed.
   a. Cardiac structure
   b. Ventricular function
   c. Blood flow
   d. M-mode electrocardiograph (provides information regarding chamber size and wall thickness)
   e. Two-dimensional and color flow Doppler (show flow velocity and direction)
2. The increased availability of this technology provides a rapid and definitive diagnosis and decreases the need for more invasive diagnostic procedures.

C. Twelve-lead electrocardiogram (ECG)
1. Assesses cardiac conduction and rhythm
2. Reveals abnormal rate and rhythm or arrhythmias that may alter cardiac output
3. Reveals alteration in ventricular forces suggesting hyper- or hypoplasia

D. Cardiac catheterization by insertion of a radiopaque catheter into the circulatory system
1. This allows the care provider to obtain pressures and oxygen saturations throughout the cardiac structure.
2. It is used much less today for diagnosis. It is often confined to procedures aimed at corrective or palliative repairs of defects previously diagnosed by echocardiogram.[13]

Preoperative Cardiac Stabilization

A. Prostaglandin E_1
1. A continuous infusion of prostaglandin E_1 is used.
2. Prostaglandin E_1 acts as a vasodilator to maintain ductal patency.
3. An initial dose of 0.05 to 0.1 mcg/kg/minute is initiated and titrated to the response.[14,15]
4. Infusion can be via a peripheral intravenous or an umbilical arterial catheter with the tip positioned at or near the ductus.[14,15]
5. A positive response is increased oxygenation and maintenance of the continuous ductal murmur that should occur within 30 minutes of initiating the infusion.[14]
6. Side effects of this potent vasodilator include the following.[14,15]
   a. Systemic vasodilation
   b. Flushing
   c. Hypotension
   d. Hyperthermia
   e. Bradycardia and tachycardia
   f. Seizure-like activity
   g. Apnea
   h. With long-term use, possible bone changes that will resolve slowly after termination of this therapy[14]

B. Digoxin
1. Digoxin is used to provide cardiac augmentation in the treatment of congestive heart failure (CHF) associated with a number of cardiac defects.
2. Its action is to increase contractility and thus increase cardiac output.[14,16]

3. It is primarily given intravenously initially and in acute CHF.
4. In acute CHF, digitalization or a series of loading doses can be initiated to hasten the actions of the medication.
5. The dosage varies depending on gestational age because excretion via the kidneys is dependent on overall renal function.[14,16]
6. For prolonged use, the infant can be treated orally; however, because of GI absorption, this requires an increase in the dose by 25 percent.[14]
7. Adverse effects include the following.[14]
   a. Prolonged PR interval
   b. Bradycardia
   c. Atrial or ventricular arrhythmias
   d. Feeding intolerance
   e. Vomiting and diarrhea
8. There is an increase in these signs of toxicity in association with hypokalemia and the addition of or changes in concurrent diuretic therapy.
9. Careful monitoring is necessary.
   a. Periodic lead II ECGs to assess the PR interval
   b. Electrolyte assessment

C. Balloon septostomy[17]
   1. This is done during cardiac catheterization.
   2. The infant is restrained and sedated during the procedure to maintain proper positioning.
   3. A balloon catheter is inserted through the foramen ovale into the left atrium, guided by cardiac echocardiography.
   4. A tear is made through the atrial septum to facilitate mixing of oxygenated and unoxygenated blood..
   5. Monitoring is done.
      a. Constantly during the procedure
      b. Postprocedure to assess for
         1) Increased arterial oxygen saturation
         2) Vital signs and compare to precatheterization values
         3) Bleeding at insertion site (apply pressure dressing)
   6. Complications may occur.
      a. Perforation and tearing of right or left atrial walls or pulmonary veins
      b. Rupture of tricuspid valves
      c. Atrial dysrhythmias
      d. Cerebral emboli or subarachnoid hemorrhage
      e. Pneumopericardium
      f. Bleeding at insertion site

Patent Ductus Arteriosus

DEFINITION

Continued patency of the ductus arteriosus that permits bypass of the pulmonary bed *in utero* and normally closes at birth in response to increased oxygen and the initiation of pulmonary function and to a decrease in available prostaglandin E_2 with separation from placental circulation[8,12]

PATHOPHYSIOLOGY

A. When normal closure fails to occur, the flow of blood reverses to a left-to-right shunt, increasing pulmonary blood flow.

B. The increased blood volume within the lungs is responsible for increased WOB and varying degrees of congestive heart failure.

   1. CHF signs and symptoms are present, dependent upon the extent of the dysfunction.

      a. Pulmonary venous engorgement

         1) Tachypnea

         2) Intercostal retractions

         3) Other signs of increased WOB

      b. Substernal retractions

      c. Head bobbing using all accessory muscles

      d. Nasal flaring

      e. Look of panic

      f. Systemic engorgement

         1) Hepatic congestion and enlargement occur.

         2) Edema is present.[18,19]

         3) Tachycardia is present as a compensatory mechanism to increase cardiac output.[16] Cardiac output is decreased within this set of findings.

         4) In addition, the infant is either lethargic or irritable and will tire with exertion such as crying or feeding.

         5) Weight gain is poor to nonexistent while this alteration persists.[8,20]

ETIOLOGY

A. Patency occurs in the presence of alterations in oxygenation, systemic and pulmonary resistance gradients, and prematurity.

INCIDENCE[21]

A. Occurs in 45 percent of infants weighing <1,750 gm

B. Occurs in 80 percent of infants weighing <1,200 gm

CLINICAL PRESENTATION[8,20]

A. Tachypnea

B. Intercostal retractions

C. Hypoxia

D. Bounding pulses

E. Widened pulse pressures

F. Murmur

   1. The murmur is described as machinery-like and continuous.

   2. It is best appreciated at the upper left and midsternal borders.[8,20]

ASSOCIATIONS

A. PDA is also associated with compromise of other organs.

   1. Decreased cerebral blood flow

   2. Necrotizing enterocolitis (NEC)

DIFFERENTIAL DIAGNOSIS

A. Respiratory distress syndrome

B. Other cardiac anomalies

DIAGNOSIS

A. Chest x-ray reveals increased pulmonary vascularity and markings, as well as cardiomegaly.

B. Echocardiogram can visualize the ductus and ductal flow.

TREATMENT OPTIONS AND NURSING CARE

A. Treatment is two-dimensional.
   1. Symptomatic
      a. Increased WOB caused by the increased volume load on the pulmonary system
         1) Decreased fluid intake
         2) Increased respiratory support
      b. Increased stress
         1) Positioning support
         2) Environmental control
   2. Pharmacologic
      a. Furosemide (Lasix) or other diuretics are used to treat pulmonary edema.
      b. Indomethacin is a nonsteroidal anti-inflammatory that inhibits prostaglandin synthesis, thus effecting closure of the ductus.
         1) Intravenous (IV) indomethacin is given over 30 minutes in three doses at 12–24 hour intervals, dependent upon clinical presentation and tolerance.[14,15] The course may be repeated once as clinically necessary, if tolerated by the infant.
         2) Indomethacin treatment is most effective in the first two weeks of life and ineffective after four to six weeks of life.[8]
         3) Rapid infusion may have adverse effects on organ blood flow; specifically, cerebral, gastrointestinal, and renal.[14]
         4) Decrease in renal function is a prominent side effect.
            a) Decreased urine output
            b) Increased creatinine
         5) If the urine output falls below 1 ml/kg/hour, do the following.[15]
            a) Temporarily suspend treatment *or*
            b) Lengthen time between doses
         6) This treatment is contraindicated in the presence of active bleeding, altered platelet counts, thrombocytopenia, NEC, hyperbilirubinemia, and renal failure.
         7) Careful monitoring of the following is required.[14,15]
            a) Urine output and function
            b) Abnormal bleeding
            c) Platelet counts
            d) Electrolyte values
            e) Glucose levels
            f) Cardiac status, murmurs, and pulses.

SURGICAL MANAGEMENT

A. Surgical treatment is needed if pharmacologic treatment fails or is contraindicated.
   1. Left thoracotomy and retraction of the left lung to visualize and tie off the ductus without the use of cardiopulmonary bypass may be done.

2. A chest tube may be placed, the incision closed, and the infant returned to the NICU.

3. This short and relatively low-risk procedure is often done at the bedside in the NICU to decrease the morbidity associated with transport to the operating room.

B. Occlusion can be achieved in larger neonates by cardiac catheterization.

COMPLICATIONS

A. Rarely occur

B. Injury to the laryngeal nerve (hoarseness)

C. Atelectasis

D. Left phrenic nerve damage

E. Thoracic duct (chylothorax)

F. Reopening of the ductus[21]

POSTOPERATIVE NURSING CARE

See Postoperative Nursing Care at the end of this chapter.

OUTCOMES

A. The overall mortality risk for surgery is <2 percent.[8,20] Increased mortality is associated with increased severity of illness and pulmonary hypertension.

Tetralogy of Fallot

DEFINITION

A. Tetralogy of Fallot (TOF) is defined as four structural and functional alterations (Figure 3-2)
   1. Large VSD
   2. Pulmonary stenosis or other outflow tract anomaly
   3. Overriding aorta
   4. Right ventricular hypertrophy

PATHOPHYSIOLOGY

A. Four anomalies as stated above in DEFINITION.

B. The severity of the condition depends on the degree of right ventricular outflow obstruction.

C. With increased severity of obstruction, increased shunting occurs across the VSD.

ETIOLOGY

A. TOF arises from the anterior displacement of the infundibular septum during cardiac development.

INCIDENCE

A. TOF accounts for 10 percent of all congenital heart defects.[8]

B. The incidence is slightly higher in males than females.

FIGURE 3-2 ■ Tetralogy of Fallot.

The four components of the defect: Pulmonary stenosis, overriding aorta, interventricular septal defect, and hypertrophy of the right ventricle.

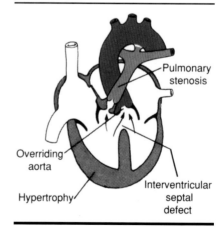

From: Sadler TW. 2006. *Langman's Medical Embryology*, 10th ed. Philadelphia: Lippincott Williams & Wilkins, 178. Reprinted by permission.

CLINICAL PRESENTATION

A. The infant with TOF presents shortly after birth with a loud murmur and/or cyanosis. "Cyanotic," or ductus-dependent, defects require a PDA to shunt oxygenated blood into the system for mixing as well as to provide adequate circulation.
1. Cyanosis and associated hypoxia can be categorized as mild to severe, dependent upon the degree of subpulmonary obstruction.
2. As the ductus and other fetal shunts diminish, increased symptomatology will occur with growing central cyanosis.
3. The systolic ejection murmur is heard at the mid- and upper-left sternal borders; there is also a ventricular tap that is audible at the lower-left sternal border. A systolic thrill and a ductal murmur may be appreciated.
4. Clubbing of the fingers and polycythemia may be present due to chronic hypoxia.

ASSOCIATIONS

A. DiGeorge syndrome
B. Branchial arch abnormalities
C. VACTERL association (an acronym for vertebral anomalies; anal atresia; cardiac defect, most often a ventricular septal defect; tracheoesophageal fistula; renal anomalies; and limb anomalies, most often radial dysplasia)

DIFFERENTIAL DIAGNOSIS

A. Other cyanotic cardiac lesions

DIAGNOSIS

A. Identification of a combination of structural and functional alterations by a three-dimensional echocardiogram (see DEFINITION).

TREATMENT OPTIONS AND NURSING CARE

A. In severe hypoxia and minimal pulmonary blood flow, prostaglandin E_1 can be used to dilate the ductus and increase pulmonary blood flow.[12]
B. Management prior to surgery focuses on fluids and the prevention of polycythemia, hypoxia, and infection.
C. Many centers are now attempting early repair in the newborn period to decrease the sequelae that can be associated with this defect.[22]
D. Some defects can be alleviated with a primary procedure; others will require an immediate palliative procedure and staging of interventions. This is determined by the extent of the defect and other anomalies, as well as the size of the infant. Treatment can be prolonged throughout the first year of life.
E. "Tet" or "blue" spells, periods of severe decompensation that are characteristic of this anomaly, must be treated.
1. A classic "tet" spell includes agitation, hyperpnea, profound cyanosis, and syncope because a large right-to-left shunt causes a decrease in PaO_2, an increase in $PaCO_2$, and a decrease in pH.[8]
2. Unrelieved "tet" spells can lead to loss of consciousness, hypoxia, seizures, and death.[8]
3. The onset and increased frequency of these episodes are indications for immediate intervention.
4. Treatment during a spell is to provide oxygen, sedate with morphine sulfate, and provide volume expansion.

5. Propranolol may be used in an attempt to decrease the spasm within the right ventricular outflow tract.[8,22]

6. If the surgical procedure is to be delayed, discharge teaching for the parents will be critical and support at home, crucial.

7. Parents can manage a "tet" spell at home by placing the infant in a knee-chest position. This maneuver decreases the systemic venous return by trapping the blood in the lower extremities, thus increasing pulmonary blood flow.[8]

F. Preoperative management is directed toward decreasing the risk of adverse outcomes.

1. Address and support each organ system.

2. Cardiovascular and respiratory assessment and support must focus on maintaining perfusion and optimal oxygenation.
   a. Blood pressure, an indicator of proper organ perfusion and function, can be monitored either centrally or peripherally.
   b. Inotropic support may be necessary to optimize perfusion.
   c. Dopamine and dobutamine both work by increasing heart rate and contractility, thus increasing cardiac output.
      1) A low dose of dopamine is used to increase renal function via vasodilation of the renal vasculature, increasing perfusion.

3. Acid/base status must be closely monitored and corrected as acidosis decreases myocardial contractility, thus affecting cardiac output in an infant who is already compromised.[16]

4. Careful monitoring of urine output will assist in maintaining proper fluid management and balance.

5. Hemodilution and vascular volume must be balanced to prevent polycythemia, yet not overburden this very tenuous system.
   a. IV administration of fluids requires an inline air-eliminating filter to prevent microbubbles from entering the circulation.
   b. Because of abnormal shunts and flow patterns, these microbubbles can enter the brain, causing a cerebrovascular accident.

6. Infectious disease considerations and management focus on surveillance and administration of antibiotics as indicated.
   a. Preoperative antibiotics may be a standard of care in many institutions.

7. Treatment of CHF and hypoxic spells is provided as indicated.

8. A supportive environment for the infant will decrease stress and energy expenditure.
   a. Neutral thermal support decreases other organ expenditures regardless of the diagnosis of the infant.
   b. Decreased stimulation and supportive positioning also provide increased comfort and decreased stress, thus assisting the other stabilizing techniques used in the care of the infant.

SURGICAL MANAGEMENT

A. Close the VSD, which eliminates the overriding aorta and increases the pulmonary blood flow; thus decreasing the stress on the right ventricle (evident by hypertrophy).

B. The timing and type of procedure used are determined by the cause of the pulmonary obstruction.

1. If the flow restriction is infundibular (subpulmonic), obstruction within the outflow tract may be removed, and correction may be done using a primary

procedure if the pulmonary artery is of an adequate size.

2. If the decreased flow is caused by pulmonary atresia or stenosis, palliative procedures may be necessary.

   a. Creation of a Blalock-Taussig shunt (Figure 3-3) is indicated in the case of an absent or diminutive pulmonary artery. This increases blood flow from the right ventricle to the pulmonary bed to increase oxygenation by anastomosis of the subclavian and pulmonary arteries.

   b. This shunt can also be accomplished using a GORE-TEX tube graft.

FIGURE 3-3 ■ Diagram of most commonly performed systemic-to-pulmonary artery shunts.

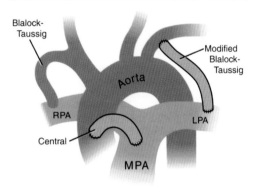

RPA = right pulmonary artery; MPA = main pulmonary artery; LPA = left pulmonary artery.

From: Artman M, Mahony L, and Teitel DF. 2002. *Neonatal Cardiology.* New York: McGraw-Hill, 96. Reprinted by permission.

C. Final corrective surgery consists of patching the ventricular septal defect and ensuring adequate right ventricular outflow patency. The overriding aorta now is properly situated within the left ventricle, and the right ventricular hypertrophy will subside over time.

D. Cardiopulmonary bypass may be performed.

1. Blood is drained from the right side of the heart, oxygenated, and then returned to the ascending aorta for systemic circulation.

2. Blood is diluted and anticoagulation agents added to decrease viscosity and vascular resistance, as well as to prevent extravascular clotting within the pump and circuit.

3. An aortic cross-clamp is placed to prevent backflow into the left ventricle.

4. Myocardial damage is averted with the use of general hypothermia and cardioplegia (injected into the aortic root).[23,24]

5. During the time of bypass, mechanical ventilation is discontinued. In complex procedures, circulation is also discontinued, providing an inert, blood-free site for surgery and clear visualization and access to perform the procedure.

6. At the completion of the procedure, as circulation and ventilatory supports return, the infant is slowly rewarmed, and protamine is given to reverse the anticoagulation effects of heparin.

7. Pacing wires are often placed to assist in potential postoperative arrhythmias.

8. The chest is often left open for later closure after the possibility of capillary leak syndrome has passed.

9. Careful transport back to the NICU must address respiratory and cardiac support, line and tube placement, thermoregulation, and comfort.

COMPLICATIONS

A. Complications of cardiopulmonary bypass include the following.

1. Hemorrhage

   a. This can be caused by the prolonged effect of anticoagulation, sutures, and the invasive devices that are in place.

   b. Carefully assess dressings and chest tube drainage for blood loss.
   c. Replacement fluids, depending on the infant's hematocrit, are provided postoperatively to maintain fluid volume balance.[23]
   d. Evaluate clotting factors periodically to assess the effect of anticoagulation and reversal of the process.
      1) Additional protamine may be indicated.
   e. Periodically monitor ionized calcium, which can become altered because of blood product administration.
   f. Infants at the greatest risk for bleeding include those with cyanosis and polycythemia preoperatively, prolonged pump time, prolonged hypothermia, or poor perfusion.
   g. Assess the infant for signs of tamponade, especially a bleeding infant, who could form extravascular clots within the chest tubes.
B. Postoperative arrhythmias are not uncommon; so pacing wires are put in place during the operative procedure. Careful monitoring of heart rate, rhythm, and pressures is ongoing.
C. Respiratory function may be compromised postoperatively because of the cardiac lesion and the lack of mechanical ventilation during the operative procedure.[23]
   1. Lesions producing a left-to-right shunt and increased pulmonary blood flow as in PDA can cause pulmonary hypertension preoperatively.
   2. Postoperatively, the lungs are stiff and less compliant.
   3. Atelectasis is common following a period of respiratory nonuse in the perioperative period.
   4. Cardiopulmonary bypass and hemodilution affect oncotic pressure, which can increase capillary leak and the potential for pulmonary edema. Preoperative congestive heart failure compounds this problem.
   5. Pulmonary hypertension may be treated with mild hyperventilation.

POSTOPERATIVE NURSING CARE
See Postoperative Nursing Care at the end of this chapter.

OUTCOMES
A. The outcome depends on the degree of pulmonary stenosis and the extent of intervention required to ensure pulmonary flow and decrease the degree of right ventricular hypertrophy.

D-Transposition of the Great Arteries

DEFINITION
This is ventricular-arterial discordance. The systemic and pulmonary circulations are parallel, requiring intracardiac mixing of oxygenated and deoxygenated blood for survival (Figure 3-4).

PATHOPHYSIOLOGY
A. The aorta is transposed into the right ventricle.
   1. Systemic blood returning to the right atrium passes to the right ventricle and is returned to the systemic circulation in a deoxygenated state.
B. The pulmonary artery arises from the left ventricle.
   1. Oxygenated blood from the pulmonary bed enters the left atrium and returns to the pulmonary bed via the left ventricle.

ETIOLOGY

A. Failure of the aortopulmonary trunk to twist causes abnormal communications between the ventricles and great vessels.

B. This occurs during the fifth week of fetal development.

INCIDENCE

A. This is the most common form of cyanotic heart disease.

B. Its prevalence is 5 percent, with a male to female ratio of 3:1.[21]

CLINICAL PRESENTATION

A. The infant will be profoundly cyanotic within hours of birth.

B. There is increased oxygen saturation in the lower extremities when compared to the upper.

C. The infant will demonstrate tachypnea without respiratory distress.

D. A murmur is rarely present.

E. CHF is present.

ASSOCIATIONS

A. Cardiac associations include the following.
   1. VSD
   2. ASD
   3. Coarctation of the aorta
   4. Subvalvular pulmonary stenosis

B. The incidence of association with noncardiac anomalies is low.

DIFFERENTIAL DIAGNOSIS

A. Other cyanotic heart lesions

B. PPHN

DIAGNOSIS

A. Oxygen saturation is higher in the lower extremities due to right-to-left shunting through the ductus arteriosus with an increase in oxygenated blood flowing from the pulmonary artery to the descending aorta.

B. Chest x-ray classically shows an "egg-on-a-string" caused by a narrow mediastinum and malposition of the pulmonary artery.

C. Two-dimensional echocardiogram clearly identifies abnormal ventricular-arterial connections.

D. Right ventricular hypertrophy is evident on ECG after several days.

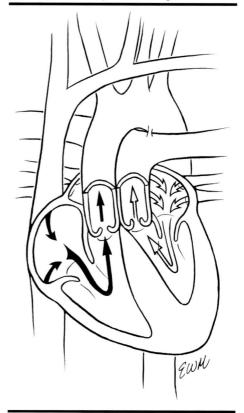

FIGURE 3-4 ■ Transposition of the great arteries.

Illustration by Elizabeth Massari.

TREATMENT OPTIONS AND NURSING CARE

A. It is important to assess the degree of patency of the ductus arteriosus and foramen ovale because the infant will be dependent on them for oxygenated blood.

   1. Maintain patency of the ductus arteriosus with prostaglandin E_1.

B. Volume infusion may be required due to the vasodilating nature of prostaglandin E_1.

C. Balloon septostomy can be done if the foramen ovale is restricted, causing limited flow and communication between right and left atria.

SURGICAL MANAGEMENT

A. Arterial switch procedure (Figure 3-5) using cardiopulmonary bypass[10]

   1. The aorta and pulmonary artery are transected above the valves and sutured to the appropriate ventricle.

   2. Coronary arteries are transferred to the pulmonary artery from the aorta to maintain coronary perfusion.

COMPLICATIONS

A. Anticoagulation caused by cardiopulmonary bypass

B. Hemorrhage from incision line, chest tube, and catheter sites

C. Infection

D. Pulmonary artery hypertension crisis

   1. Acute increase in pulmonary artery pressure, which can precipitate right heart failure as result of:

      a. Acidosis

      b. Hypoxia

      c. Hypercarbia

      d. Cold stress

      e. Agitation caused by pain

E. Arrhythmias

F. Neurologic complications

   1. Cerebral vascular accident

   2. Seizures

POSTOPERATIVE NURSING CARE

See Postoperative Nursing Care at the end of this chapter.

OUTCOMES

A. Early mortality is 2–5 percent.

B. Five-year survival is >80 percent.[21]

FIGURE 3-5 ■ Technique of the arterial switch operation.

A. The great arteries are transected above the sinuses of Valsalva. **B.** The coronaries are excised from the aorta (Ao), transposed posteriorly, and anastomosed to the pulmonary artery (PA) (neoaorta) using a "trap-door technique." **C.** The distal aorta is brought behind the pulmonary artery (Lecompte maneuver) and anastomosed to the neoaorta. **D.** Separate pericardial patches are sutured to fill in the defects in the aorta created by excision of the coronary arteries. **E.** Completed repair. RCA, right coronary artery; LCA, left coronary artery.

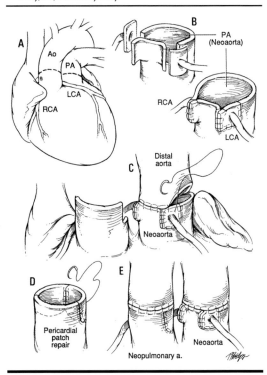

From: Karl TR. 1995. Transposition of the great arteries. In *Critical Heart Disease in Infants and Children*, Nichols DG, et al., eds. Philadelphia: Mosby, 832. Reprinted by permission.

Hypoplastic Left Heart Syndrome

DEFINITION

Hypoplasia of the left ventricle causing inadequate systemic perfusion

PATHOPHYSIOLOGY

A. The dominant right ventricle maintains perfusion via the ductal right-to-left shunt *in utero*.

B. At birth, pulmonary resistance decreases, and systemic resistance increases, reversing the ductal shunt and decreasing systemic perfusion (Figure 3-6).

C. There is a decrease in systemic cardiac output and aortic pressure with circulatory shock and metabolic acidosis (Figure 3-7).

ETIOLOGY

A. Decreased blood flow to the left ventricle during embryologic development due to restriction of blood flow into the left ventricle

INCIDENCE

A. One percent of all cardiac defects[21]

FIGURE 3-6 ■ Hypoplastic left heart syndrome in a 24-hour-old patient with falling pulmonary vascular resistance and a nonrestrictive ductus arteriosus.

FIGURE 3-7 ■ Acute circulatory collapse following constriction of the ductus arteriosus in hypoplastic left heart syndrome.

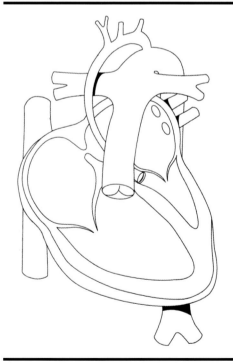

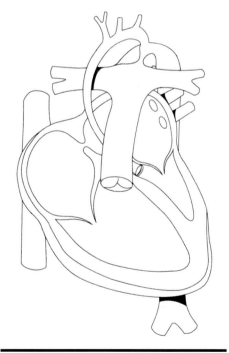

Adapted from: Wechsler SB, and Wernovsky G. 2004. Cardiac disorders. In *Manual of Neonatal Care,* 5th ed., Cloherty JP, Eichenwald EC, and Stark AR, eds. Philadelphia: Lippincott Williams & Wilkins, 428. Reprinted by permission.

Adapted from: Wechsler SB, and Wernovsky G. 2004. Cardiac disorders. In *Manual of Neonatal Care,* 5th ed., Cloherty JP, Eichenwald EC, and Stark AR, eds. Philadelphia: Lippincott Williams & Wilkins, 429. Reprinted by permission.

B. Most common cause of death resulting from congenital heart disease in the first month of life

CLINICAL PRESENTATION

A. Asymptomatic until ductus arteriosus begins to close
B. Respiratory distress with tachypnea
C. Impaired feeding
D. Decreased pulse velocity on palpation
E. Pale skin with poor perfusion
F. No murmur
G. CHF

ASSOCIATIONS

A. Mitral valve stenosis
B. Coarctation of the aorta
C. ASD
D. VSD
E. Hypoplastic aorta

DIFFERENTIAL DIAGNOSIS

A. PPHN
B. Sepsis
C. Other cyanotic heart lesions

DIAGNOSIS

A. ECG shows diminutive to no left-sided forces; right ventricular hypertrophy is present.
B. Echocardiogram shows a diminutive left ventricle.

TREATMENT OPTIONS AND NURSING CARE

A. Intubate the infant to provide adequate oxygenation and ventilation.
B. Manage metabolic acidosis.
C. Administer prostaglandin E_1 as ordered to maintain patency of the ductus arteriosus.
D. Palliative shunts are not effective because of a hypoplastic aorta.
E. Perform a Stage 1 Norwood procedure to provide adequate systemic blood flow.
F. Perform a cardiac transplant.

SURGICAL MANAGEMENT

A. Stage 1 Norwood includes the following (Figure 3-8).
   1. The pulmonary artery is divided and joined with the ascending aorta.
   2. The ductus arteriosus is ligated.
   3. The atrial septum is removed so that there is adequate atrial mixing.
   4. A Blalock-Taussig shunt is placed.
      a. This allows blood from the joined pulmonary artery and aorta to reach the pulmonary bed for oxygenation.[10]
B. Glenn shunt and Fontan procedures can be done later in infancy and childhood.

COMPLICATIONS

See COMPLICATIONS under D-Transposition of the Great Arteries, above.

FIGURE 3-8 ■ Stage I Norwood procedure.

A. Transection points of the main pulmonary artery (PA) and ductus arteriosus. **B.** Atrial septectomy to avoid pulmonary venous hypertension. Patch closure of the distal main PA. Division and ligation of the ductus arteriosus. **C and D.** Construction of a "neoaorta" using the proximal main PA, diminutive ascending aorta, and vascular allograft. **E.** Pulmonary blood flow supplied by a right modified Blalock-Taussig shunt connecting the right subclavian artery to the right PA. Ao, aorta; LV, left ventricle; RV, right ventricle.

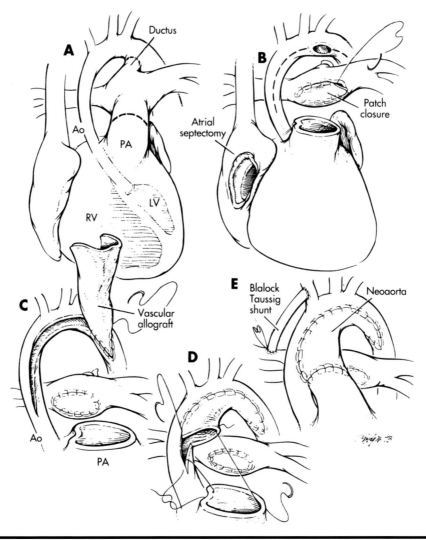

From: Nicolson SC, Steven JM, and Jobes DR. 1995. Hypoplastic left heart syndrome. In *Critical Heart Disease in Infants and Children,* Nichols DG, et al., eds. Philadelphia: Mosby, 870. Reprinted by permission.

POSTOPERATIVE NURSING CARE

See Postoperative Nursing Care at the end of this chapter.

OUTCOMES

A. The mortality rate of the Stage I Norwood is ≥35 percent.[21]
    1. The period of highest mortality is the first six months.
    2. Survival at 12 months is 45 percent.

Total Anomalous Pulmonary Venous Connection

DEFINITION (FIGURE 3-9)

A. Pulmonary veins do not drain into the left atrium. Instead, they drain into the right atrium through an abnormal confluence.[10]

B. A patent foramen ovale or ASD is essential for atrial mixing of blood.

C. There is unobstructed flow when the abnormal connection occurs above the diaphragm.

D. There is obstructed flow when the abnormal connection occurs below the diaphragm via the ductus venosus.

FIGURE 3-9 ■ Total anomalous pulmonary venous connection.

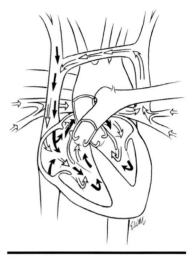

Illustration by Elizabeth Massari.

PATHOPHYSIOLOGY

A. Unobstructed flow
   1. Blood flows preferentially through the patent foramen ovale into the right atrium and crosses into the left atrium, left ventricle, and ascending aorta.

B. Obstructed flow
   1. Blood via the ductus venosus is directed into the right ventricle, across the ductus arteriosus, and into the descending aorta.

ETIOLOGY

A. This defect occurs during pulmonary vein development between weeks 5 and 8 of fetal development.

INCIDENCE[21]

A. One percent of all congenital heart defects
B. Male to female ratio 4:1

CLINICAL PRESENTATION

A. Unobstructed
   1. CHF
   2. Growth restriction
   3. Frequent pulmonary infections
   4. Mild cyanosis
   5. Oxygen saturation increased in the lower half of the body

B. Obstructed
   1. Moderate to severe respiratory distress
   2. Oxygen saturation decreased in the upper half of the body
   3. Narrow pulse pressure
   4. Decreased pulses and perfusion
   5. Split second heart sound (S2)
   6. Cyanosis that worsens with feeding

ASSOCIATIONS

A. Trisomy 22[10]
B. Patent foramen ovale

C. ASD
D. Small left side of the heart
E. PDA

DIFFERENTIAL DIAGNOSIS

A. Respiratory distress syndrome
B. Sepsis
C. Other cyanotic heart lesions

DIAGNOSIS

A. There is a split S2.
B. ECG shows right ventricular hypertrophy.
C. Chest x-ray shows a small to normal sized heart with increased vascular markings.
D. Echocardiogram shows abnormal vasculature and exclusive right-to-left shunting across the patent foramen ovale.

TREATMENT OPTIONS AND NURSING CARE

A. Unobstructed
   1. Assure adequate atrial mixing with a balloon septostomy if the communication between atria is small.
   2. Treat CHF.
   3. Delay surgery until after the neonatal period if possible.
B. Obstructed
   1. Intubate the infant to increase oxygenation and ventilation.
   2. Administer diuretics as ordered for pulmonary edema.
   3. Manage metabolic acidosis.
   4. Administer prostaglandin E_1 as ordered to maintain patency of the ductus arteriosus.
   5. Prepare the infant for corrective surgery.

SURGICAL MANAGEMENT

A. Anastomosis of the anomalous pulmonary veins into the left atrium is done, with closure of atrial communication.
B. Procedures will vary, dependent upon the type of anomalous drainage present.

COMPLICATIONS

A. Pulmonary hypertension
B. Atrial arrhythmias
C. Obstruction at the site of the anastomosis
D. Anticoagulation due to cardiopulmonary bypass
E. Hemorrhage from the incision line, chest tube, and catheter sites
F. Infection
G. Pulmonary artery hypertension crisis
   1. Acute increase in pulmonary artery pressure, which can precipitate right heart failure as a result of the following.
      a. Acidosis
      b. Hypoxia
      c. Hypercarbia
      d. Cold stress
      e. Agitation due to pain

H. Arrhythmias
I. Neurologic complications
   1. Cerebral vascular accident
   2. Seizures

POSTOPERATIVE NURSING CARE
See Postoperative Nursing Care below.

OUTCOMES
A. In infants with this disorder and unobstructed flow, the surgical mortality rate is 5 to 10 percent.
B. The surgical mortality rate can be as high as 20 percent in the obstructed, infracardiac type of defect.[21]

Postoperative Nursing Care

A. Postoperative care concerns are specific to the procedure, the hemodynamics of the repair, and the effects on other organ systems of the following.[23,25]
   1. Anesthetic agents
   2. Bypass time
   3. Aortic cross-clamp time
   4. Hypothermia
   5. Circulatory arrest time
B. Cardiopulmonary bypass in neonates is often poorly tolerated because of the following.[24]
   1. The effect of the priming volume need for the bypass pump
   2. The effects of hypothermia
   3. The duration of the surgical procedure
   4. Capillary leak syndrome due to hemodilution
   5. Bleeding caused by prolonged bypass time
C. The condition of the infant preoperatively, in combination with all of the perioperative factors, impacts the postoperative course.
D. Assessment includes the following.
   1. Respiratory function
   2. Perfusion
   3. Renal function
   4. Chest tube drainage
   5. Hemodynamic measurements
   6. Bleeding
   7. Infection
   8. Neurologic function
E. Invasive monitoring may include the following.
   1. Arterial line
   2. Right atrial catheter to measure central venous pressure
   3. Left atrial catheter for indirect data on systemic ventricular function
   4. Pulmonary artery catheter monitoring pulmonary artery pressure
   5. Temporary transthoracic pacing wires on epicardial surface of atria and/or ventricle
F. Stabilize cardiac function, which may be difficult because of a number of factors.
   1. Stiff cardiac muscle—response to the abnormal anatomic structure and the surgical intervention

2. Effect on cardiac output—preload, afterload, and contractility
3. Hypothermia and electrolyte imbalance[23]
4. Preoperative hypoxia, myocardial ischemia, and acidosis adversely affecting contractility
5. A thermoneutral environment (Prevent hypothermia and hyperthermia, thus decreasing the metabolic demands that are inherent with either condition.)
6. Electrolyte assessment and management
7. Pharmacologic agents used to support cardiac function and output
   a. Nitroglycerin and nitroprusside are vasodilators that act upon the systemic and pulmonary vascular beds to decrease resistance that can decrease afterload.
   b. Dopamine and dobutamine increase the force of the contraction, thus increasing stroke volume and cardiac output.
   c. Vascular volume balance will be critical in achieving normal cardiac function. Assessment and replacement as necessary are required prior to or in conjunction with the use of the pharmacologic agents to ensure the best desired effect.

G. Provide ongoing respiratory support.
   1. Maintain adequate oxygenation and ventilation.
   2. Arterial blood gases, pulse oximetry, and transcutaneous monitoring provide the information necessary to deliver appropriate ventilatory support for oxygenation and gas exchange.
   3. Endotracheal suctioning should be done only when necessary; this will decrease episodes of hypoxic pulmonary vasoconstriction.
   4. Provide chest tube care.

H. The renal system is sensitive to cardiopulmonary bypass, hypothermia, and decreased cardiac output.[23]
   1. Renal function is compromised until cardiac output is optimized.
      a. Assess renal function (serial creatinine and blood urea nitrogen values).
      b. Assess fluid and electrolyte balance.
         1) This may be complicated by capillary leak syndrome and a shift of fluid to the extravascular space, depleting intravascular volume.[23]
         2) Fluid restriction may be necessary if postcardiopulmonary bypass fluid overload is present.
            a) Fluid overload is common postoperatively.
            b) Administer diuretics as ordered.
   2. Urine output must be closely monitored, with a desired minimum output of 0.5 to 1 ml/kg/hour.[23]
      a. A urinary catheter in the acute postoperative period increases the accuracy of urinary output measurement.
      b. Low-dose dopamine may be used to increase renal perfusion, thus affecting urine production.
      c. Furosemide may be used to establish urine flow.
   3. Monitor intake and output meticulously.
      a. Daily weight
      b. Serum electrolytes
      c. Hyperalimentation (Delay this until fluid and electrolyte balance is achieved; then administer parenteral and enteral nutrition as ordered and tolerated.)

I. Care for the infant's skin.
   1. Extravascular displacement of fluid can cause edema and the potential for breakdown.
   2. Assessment must be done and soft bedding and support used to protect the skin from damage and breakdown caused by distention and pressure points.
J. Maintain glucose homeostasis.
   1. Altered due to hypoperfusion of the pancreas and increased levels of circulating catecholamines, or stress hormones, which increase glucose metabolism[23]
   2. May require adjustments of parenteral administration
K. Provide comfort measures and manage pain.
   1. Sedation, analgesia, and environmental considerations are employed to decrease stress and agitation, which can contribute to increased vascular reactivity.
      a. Pharmacologic support with sedation and analgesia is indicated postoperatively, with very careful assessment and management of cardiac, hemodynamic, and respiratory parameters.
      b. Nonpharmacologic comfort measures such as supportive positioning and environmental controls will augment any pharmacologic effects.
         1) Maintain a thermoneutral environment.
         2) Protect the infant from light, sound, and activity.
   2. Circulating stress hormones increase glucose metabolism, thus impacting glucose homeostasis.
   3. Unmanaged pain has deleterious effects.
      a. Hypoxia due to unmanaged pain will affect cardiac function and complicate respiratory management.[26]
      b. Unmanaged pain can have long-lasting effects after the neonatal period. Alterations in perception and response have been noted.[27]
L. Provide support to the parents.
   1. Parents require a great deal of support throughout this admission: during the diagnostic period, preoperatively, and postoperatively because of the complexity of the disease and pathology.
   2. Give frequent, concrete explanations and permit time for questions.
      a. Use visual aids such as drawings and models to assist parents in understanding the pathophysiology of the defect.
      b. Answer questions honestly and in language the family can understand.
      c. Incorporate the parents into the infant's care as soon as possible to provide them with an early relationship with the infant that can either prepare them for discharge or comfort them during loss.
   3. Do discharge teaching.
      a. Begin as early as possible.
      b. During times of stress and crisis, learning and retention of information may be compromised.
      c. Reinforce teaching both verbally and in writing.
      d. Home supports for both reassurance and assistance provide a transition from the acute care setting into the community without the perception of abandonment or loss of support.
      e. Recurrent hospitalization may be a reality for the family. The initial experience in the NICU will have a definite impact on the skills, endurance, and success of the family unit.

REFERENCES

1. Botto LD, Correa A, and Erickson D. 2001. Racial and temporal variation in the prevalence of heart defects. *Pediatrics* 107(3): e32.

2. Goldmuntz E. 2001. The epidemiology and genetics of congenital heart disease. *Clinics in Perinatology* 28(1): 1–10.

3. Moore KL, and Persaud TV. 2003. *The Developing Human: Clinically Oriented Embryology*, 7th ed. Philadelphia: Saunders, 329–380.

4. Watanabe M. 2006. Cardiac embryology. In *Neonatal-Perinatal Medicine: Diseases of the Fetus and Infant*, 8th ed., Martin RJ, Fanaroff AA, and Walsh MC, eds. Philadelphia: Mosby, 1195–1202.

5. Kirby ML. 1998. Development of the fetal heart. In *Fetal and Neonatal Physiology*, 2nd ed., Polin RA, and Fox WW, eds. Philadelphia: Saunders, 793–801.

6. Zahka KG. 2006. Causes and associations. In *Neonatal-Perinatal Medicine: Diseases of the Fetus and Infant*, 8th ed., Martin RJ, Fanaroff AA, and Walsh MC, eds. Philadelphia: Mosby, 1202–1205.

7. Snider AR. 1998. Cardiovascular diagnosis in the fetus and the effects of congenital heart lesions on developing physiology. In *Fetal and Neonatal Physiology*, 2nd ed., Polin RA, and Fox WW, eds. Philadelphia: Saunders, 996–1013.

8. Lott JW. 2003. Assessment and management of cardiovascular system. In *Comprehensive Neonatal Nursing: A Physiologic Perspective*, 3rd ed., Kenner C, Lott JW eds. Philadelphia: Saunders, 376–408.

9. Vargo L. 2003. Cardiovascular assessment. In *Physical Assessment of the Newborn: A Comprehensive Guide to the Art of Physical Examination*, 3rd ed., Tappero EP, and Honeyfield ME, eds. Santa Rosa, California: NICU INK, 81–96.

10. Artman M, Mahony L, and Teitel DF. 2002. *Neonatal Cardiology*. New York: McGraw-Hill.

11. Beekman RH. 1991. Neonatal cardiac emergencies. In *Neonatal Emergencies*, Donn SM, and Faix RG, eds. Mount Kisco, New York: Futura, 345–370.

12. Hsu DT, and Gersony WM. 2005. Medical management of the neonate with congenital heart disease. In *Intensive Care of the Fetus and Neonate*, 2nd ed., Spitzer AR, ed. Philadelphia: Mosby, 929–938.

13. Zahka KG, and Gruenstein DH. 2006. Approach to the neonate with cardiovascular disease. In *Neonatal-Perinatal Medicine: Diseases of the Fetus and Infant*, 8th ed., Martin RJ, Fanaroff AA, and Walsh MC, eds. Philadelphia: Mosby, 1215–1222.

14. Young TE, and Mangum B. 2000. *NeoFax: A Manual of Drugs Used in Neonatal Care*, 13th ed. Raleigh, North Carolina: Acorn.

15. Bell SG. 1998. Neonatal cardiovascular pharmacology. *Neonatal Network* 17(2): 7–15.

16. Kulik LA, Hickey PA, and Lawrence PR. 1991. Pharmacologic interventions for the neonate with compromised cardiac function. *Journal of Perinatal & Neonatal Nursing* 5(2): 71–83.

17. Zahka KG, and Siwik ES. 2006. Principles of medical and surgical management. In *Neonatal-Perinatal Medicine: Diseases of the Fetus and Infant*, 8th ed., Martin RJ, Fanarroff AA, and Walsh MC, eds. Philadelphia: Mosby, 1265–1275.

18. Furdon SA. 1997. Recognizing congestive heart failure in the neonatal period. *Neonatal Network* 16(7): 5–13.

19. Monett ZJ, and Moynihan PJ. 1991. Cardiovascular assessment of the neonatal heart. *Journal of Perinatal & Neonatal Nursing* 5(2): 50–59.

20. Sullivan SE, and Drummond WH. 2005. Ductus arteriosus. In *Intensive Care of the Fetus and Neonate*, 2nd ed., Spitzer AR, ed. Philadelphia: Mosby, 897–908.

21. Park MK. 2002. *Pediatric Cardiology for Practitioners*, 4th ed. Philadelphia: Mosby, 174, 183, 202, 206, 383, 385, 386.

22. Marino BS, Bird GL, and Wernovsky G. 2001. Diagnosis and management of the newborn with suspected congenital heart disease. *Clinics in Perinatology* 28(1): 91–136.

23. Craig J. 1991. The postoperative cardiac infant: Physiologic basis for neonatal nursing interventions. *Journal of Perinatal & Neonatal Nursing* 5(2): 60–70.

24. Karl TR. 2001. Neonatal cardiac surgery. *Clinics in Perinatology* 28(1): 159–185.

25. Merle C. 2001. Nursing considerations of the neonate with congenital heart disease. *Clinics in Perinatology* 28(1): 223–233.

26. Anand KJS, and the International Evidence-Based Group for Neonatal Pain. 2001. Consensus statement for the prevention and management of pain in the newborn. *Archives of Pediatric and Adolescent Medicine* 155(2): 173–180.

27. American Academy of Pediatrics and Canadian Paediatric Society. 2000. Prevention and management of pain and stress in the neonate. *Pediatrics* 105(2): 454–461.

28. Kirby ML. 2004. Development of the fetal heart. In *Fetal and Neonatal Physiology*, 3rd ed., Polin RA, Fox WW, and Abman S, eds. Philadelphia: Saunders, 613–620.

NOTES

NOTES

Neonatal Gastrointestinal Surgical Conditions

Ellen Tappero, RNC, MN, NNP
Catherine Witt, RNC, MS, NNP

Neonatal surgical conditions affecting the gastrointestinal (GI) tract are varied and can be found anywhere from the esophagus to the anus. Many of the conditions cause obstruction only, and there is little chance of intestinal compromise caused by a delay in diagnosis. However, others are more acute, requiring immediate recognition and treatment to avoid devastating sequelae.

All of the surgical conditions of the GI tract present a nursing challenge because of the nonspecific and overlapping clinical symptomatology. Neonatal nurses must have a thorough understanding of the pathophysiology of each anomaly in order to intervene appropriately, in a timely manner, and to provide parental support. Factual information of the infant's condition and plan of care must be communicated so that parents understand the disease process and their infant's ongoing health care needs.

This chapter addresses the major surgical conditions affecting the neonatal GI tract and addresses clinical history, diagnostic evaluation, and therapeutic intervention for each condition.

Embryology

PRIMORDIAL GUT

A. This forms during the fourth week as the head, tail, and lateral folds incorporate the dorsal part of the yolk sac into the embryo.[1-3]
B. The endoderm develops into most of the glands and epithelium of the digestive tract.[1,3]
C. The epithelium at the cranial and caudal ends of the digestive tract is derived from the ectoderm of the stomodeum (mouth) and proctodeum (anal pit).[1,3]
D. The endoderm determines the temporal and positional information, which is important in the development of the gut.[1]
E. The splanchnic mesenchyme surrounding the primordial gut develops into:[1,3]
  1. Connective tissue

2. Muscular tissue
3. Layers of the wall of the digestive system
F. The primordial gut is divided into three separate parts.[1–3]
   1. Foregut
   2. Midgut
   3. Hindgut

FOREGUT

A. Organs formed from the foregut[1,3]
   1. Oral cavity
   2. Pharynx
   3. Tongue
   4. Tonsils
   5. Salivary glands
   6. Upper respiratory system
   7. Lower respiratory system
   8. Esophagus
      a. The respiratory diverticulum (lung bud) develops at four weeks gestation at the ventral wall of the foregut.[1,2]
      b. It develops from the foregut caudally to the pharynx.[1]
      c. The dorsal portion, the esophagus, is separated from the ventral portion, the respiratory primordium (which becomes the trachea), by the tracheoesophageal septum.[2]
      d. The esophagus lengthens quickly as the heart and lungs descend and reaches final length by seven weeks gestation.[1]
      e. The endoderm forms the epithelium and glands. The epithelium initially obliterates the lumen of the esophagus, but recanalization occurs by the end of the embryonic period.[1,3]
      f. Both striated (upper two-thirds) and smooth (lower one-third) muscle tissue develops in the esophagus.[2]
      g. The vagal nerve innervates the striated muscles, and the splanchnic plexus innervates the smooth muscle.[2]
   9. Stomach
      a. The distal part of the foregut begins as a tubular structure and dilates around the site of the stomach at about the fourth week of gestation.[1,2]
      b. It enlarges and broadens ventrodorsally, with the dorsal border of the stomach growing faster than the ventral border, forming the greater curvature of the stomach.[1,3]
      c. The stomach slowly rotates 90 degrees in a clockwise direction around a longitudinal and anteroposterior (AP) axis.[1–3]
         1) The ventral border moves to the right, and the dorsal border moves to the left.
         2) The ventral surface was the original left side; the dorsal surface was the original right side.[1]
         3) The cranial region becomes oriented to the left and slightly inferiorly, and its caudal region becomes oriented to the right and superiorly.[1]
         4) The long axis of the stomach is almost transverse to the long axis of the body in its final position.[1]
         5) The dorsal mesentery suspends the stomach in the abdominal cavity (dorsal mesogastrium).[1]

      6) The ventral mesentery (ventral mesogastrium) attaches the stomach and duodenum to the ventral abdominal wall and developing liver.[1,3]

10. Duodenum

    a. Early in the fourth week the duodenum develops from:[1-3]

      1) The caudal part of the foregut

      2) The cranial part of the midgut

      3) The splanchnic mesenchyme

    b. A C-shaped loop of duodenum:[1-3]

      1) Forms ventrally

      2) Rotates to the right and lies external to the peritoneum

      3) Takes its final position to the left side of the abdominal cavity

    c. The duodenum and pancreas head become fixed in a retroperitoneal position.[2]

    d. During the fifth to sixth weeks of gestation, epithelial cells temporarily obliterate the lumen of the duodenum.[1-3]

      1) It is recanalized by the end of the embryonic period.[1-3]

    e. The duodenum is supplied by branches of the celiac and superior mesenteric arteries.[2]

11. Liver, gallbladder, and biliary apparatus

    a. Development of the liver primordium begins in the middle of the third week of gestation as a ventral outgrowth from the distal end of the foregut.[2,3]

    b. Rapidly growing cells penetrate the septum transversum, the mesodermal plate between the pericardial cavity, and the stalk of the yolk sac.[2,3]

    c. Two cell populations develop into the hepatic diverticulum and the pancreas.

    d. The hepatic diverticulum extends into the splanchnic mesoderm, the area between the developing heart and midgut.[1,3]

      1) It divides into two parts.[2]

        a) The large cranial part of the hepatic diverticulum forms the liver between weeks 5 and 10.[1,3]

          • Interlacing hepatic cords that differentiate into liver cells

          • The epithelial lining of the intrahepatic part of the biliary apparatus

        b) The small caudal part of the hepatic diverticulum becomes the gallbladder.[1,2]

      2) The stalk of the hepatic diverticulum becomes the cystic duct.[1,2]

        a) The bile duct develops from the stalk connecting the hepatic and cystic ducts to the duodenum.[1]

        b) Bile formation begins during week 12 of gestation.[2,3]

        c) Bile enters the duodenum after week 13 of gestation.[1]

    e. Hematopoietic, Kupffer, and connective tissue cells are derived from the mesoderm of the septum transversum.[2,3]

      1) Hematopoiesis begins during week 6.

    f. The ventral mesogastrium is the peritoneal connection between the foregut and the ventral abdominal wall.[2]

      1) As the liver grows, the septum transversum thins, becomes membranous, and forms the lesser omentum.

      2) The falciform ligament also forms and extends from the liver to the ventral abdominal wall.[1,2]

    g. The central tendon of the diaphragm is a portion of the septum that remains and consists of densely packed mesoderm.

    h. The liver is covered by peritoneum, except where it is in direct contact with the diaphragm.[1]

  12. Pancreas

    a. Pancreatic buds arise from endodermal cells between the layers of mesentery.[1–3]

    b. The dorsal pancreatic bud appears first and grows rapidly.[1,3]

    c. The ventral pancreatic bud grows near the entry of the bile duct and rotates with the intestine.[1–3]

      1) The ventral bud lies immediately below and behind the dorsal bud.[1–3]

      2) It later fuses posteriorly with the dorsal bud.[1–3]

    d. At this point, the ducts also fuse and form the following structures.[1,2]

      1) The main pancreatic duct

      2) The accessory pancreatic duct

    e. Tubules form early in fetal life.

      1) Pancreatic islets develop from cells that separate the tubules and lie between acini.[1]

    f. Insulin secretion begins by ten weeks gestation.[1,3]

    g. Glucagon is detected as early as 15 weeks gestation.[1]

  13. Spleen

    a. It begins development from a mass of mesenchymal cells located between layers of the dorsal mesogastrium.[1,3]

    b. The spleen obtains its shape early in the fetal period.[1,3]

    c. The spleen is a hematopoietic center until late in gestation.[1]

B. Omental bursa

  1. Cavities develop in the mesenchyme and eventually form a single cavity known as the omental bursa (lesser peritoneal sac).[1,3]

  2. The bursa enlarges as the stomach rotates.[1]

  3. The superior and inferior recess of the omental bursa form and later disappear.[1]

C. Mesenteries

  1. The mesenteries are double layers of peritoneum that enclose an organ and connect it to the body wall.[2]

  2. Peritoneal ligaments pass from one organ to another or from organ to body wall.[2]

  3. Mesenteries and ligaments become pathways for nerves, vessels, and lymphatics.[2]

  4. A membrane, the greater omentum, overhangs the developing intestines.

  5. The lesser omentum forms from the liver as it grows into the septum and thins. This membrane extends from the stomach and upper duodenum to the liver.

  6. The falciform ligament extends from the liver to the ventral abdominal wall.

MIDGUT

A. Derivatives of the midgut include the following.[1–3]

  1. Small intestine

  2. Ascending colon

  3. A large portion of the transverse colon

  4. Cecum

    a. The cecal diverticulum appears on the caudal limb of the midgut in the sixth week of gestation.[1–3]

5. Appendix
   a. The apex grows slowly and forms the appendix.
   b. This later grows rapidly and is a long tube at the distal end of the cecum by the time of birth.
   c. The position of the appendix in relation to the cecum varies in its final position.[1]
B. The midgut begins distal to the entrance of the bile duct into the duodenum and ends at the junction of the proximal two-thirds of the transverse colon with the distal one-third.[1]
C. Blood flow is supplied by the superior mesenteric artery.[1]
D. The mesentery suspends the U-shaped midgut loop from the dorsal abdominal wall.[1]
   1. The midgut loop has a cranial and caudal limb.[1,2]
      a. The cranial limb elongates quickly and forms small intestinal loops known as the primary intestinal loop.[1,2]
         1) The cephalic (cranial) limb develops into the distal part of the duodenum, the jejunum, and part of the ileum.[2]
      b. The caudal limb grows slowly and forms the cecal diverticulum, which becomes the following.[1,2]
         1) Cecum
         2) Appendix
         3) Ascending colon
         4) Proximal two-thirds of the transverse colon
E. Because of rapid growth and elongation of the intestinal loop and growth of the liver, there is not enough room in the abdomen.[1–3]
   1. Abdominal loops enter the extraembryonic cavity in the umbilical cord during the sixth week of gestation.[1–3]
   2. This is known as physiologic umbilical herniation.[1–3]
F. The midgut loop rotates 90 degrees counterclockwise around the axis of the superior mesenteric artery while it is in the umbilical cord.[1,3]
   1. The caudal limb ends up on the left.[1,3]
   2. The cranial limb ends up on the right.[1,3]
   3. During this time, the midgut continues to elongate and forms coiled loops.[1,3]
G. By week 10 of gestation, the intestines return to the abdomen.[1,3]
   1. This is known as reduction of the physiologic midgut hernia.[1,3]
   2. The small intestine returns first and occupies the central region of the abdomen.[1]
   3. The large intestine rotates 180 degrees counterclockwise and occupies the right side of the abdomen.[1]
   4. The ascending colon becomes more recognizable as the abdominal wall lengthens.[1]
   5. The mesenteries are pressed against the posterior abdominal wall when the intestines assume their final position.
      a. The ascending colon becomes retroperitoneal as the mesentery fuses with the parietal peritoneum.[1]
   6. The mesentery of the colon is absorbed because of the pressure of the duodenum against the abdominal wall.[1,3]
   7. The mesentery of the jejunum and ileum remains attached.[1,3]

Hindgut

A. Hindgut derivatives[1-3]
1. The distal third of the transverse colon (left one-third to one-half)
2. Descending colon
3. Sigmoid colon
4. Rectum
5. The upper part of the anal canal
6. The internal lining (epithelium) of the urinary bladder
7. Urethra
B. Supplied by the inferior mesenteric artery[1]
C. Cloaca[1,3]
1. This is the endoderm-lined terminal part of the hindgut.
2. The cloacal membrane is formed from the endoderm of the cloaca and the ectoderm of the anal pit.[1,3]
3. The cloaca is divided into dorsal and ventral parts by the urorectal septum.[1,3]
   a. The urorectal septum grows toward the cloacal membrane and forms folds.
   b. The cloacal membrane ruptures and creates two openings.[1,3]
      1) Rectum and anal canal (dorsal)
      2) Urogenital sinus (ventral), which forms the urinary bladder and urethra
4. The urorectal septum fuses with the cloacal membrane by week 7, dividing it into the:[1,3]
   a. Anal membrane
      1) At the end of week 8, the anal membrane ruptures and forms the anal canal.
   b. Urogenital membrane
5. The urorectal septum divides the cloacal sphincter into two parts.[1,3]
   a. The anterior part develops into the superficial transverse perineal, bulbospongiosus, and ischiocavernosus muscles.
   b. The posterior part becomes the external anal sphincter.
D. Anal canal[1]
1. The superior two-thirds of the anal canal is derived from the hindgut.
   a. It is supplied by the superior rectal artery.
   b. The superior rectal vein supplies venous drainage.
   c. The inferior mesenteric lymph nodes provide lymphatic drainage.
2. The inferior one-third is derived from proctodeum.
   a. It is supplied by the inferior rectal arteries.
   b. The inferior rectal vein supplies venous drainage.
   c. The superficial inguinal lymph nodes provide lymphatic drainage.

Esophageal Atresia (EA) and Tracheoesophageal Fistula (TEF)

Definition

EA is a malformation of the esophagus. It ends in a blind pouch. TEF is an abnormal connection between the trachea and the esophagus.

Pathophysiology

A. There are five basic esophageal malformations:[4-6]
1. Proximal esophageal atresia with a fistula between the distal esophagus and the trachea (86 percent) (Figure 4-1A)

FIGURE 4-1 ■ Types of esophageal atresia and tracheoesophageal fistula.

A. Esophageal atresia with distal tracheoesophageal fistula. **B.** Pure esophageal atresia (without a tracheoesophageal fistula). **C.** H-type tracheoesophageal fistula. **D.** Esophageal atresia with proximal tracheoesophageal fistula. **E.** Esophageal atresia with proximal and distal tracheoesophageal fistulas. Note that the proximal fistula usually enters the trachea 1 to 2 cm above the blind-ending upper pouch.

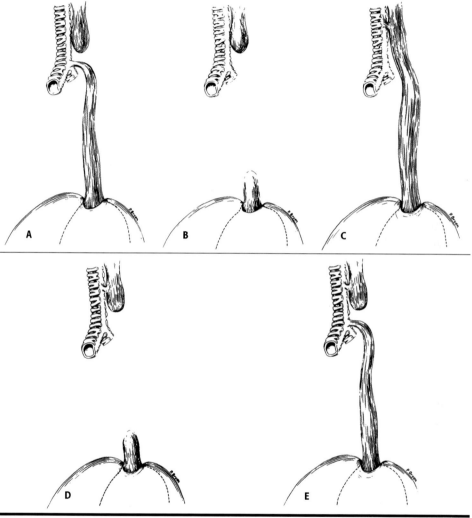

From: Spitz L. 2005. Esophageal atresia and tracheoesophageal malformations. In *Pediatric Surgery*, 4th ed., Ashcraft KW, Holcomb GW, and Murphy JP, eds. Philadelphia: Saunders, 355, 356. Reprinted by permission.

2. Atresia of the esophagus without a fistula (7 percent)—The proximal pouch ends blindly in the neck or is a short stump that extends 2–3 cm above the diaphragm. The long gap between the two esophageal ends usually makes primary anastomosis impossible (Figure 4-1B).

3. Tracheoesophageal fistula without an atresia, or H-type fistula (4 percent)—The fistula usually occurs between the esophagus and the cervical trachea (Figure 4-1C).

4. Esophageal atresia with proximal tracheoesophageal fistula (2 percent)—The fistula is between the upper pouch and the trachea (Figure 4-1D).

5. Esophageal atresia with proximal and distal tracheoesophageal fistula (<1 percent)—Fistulas are between both the upper pouch and lower portion of the esophagus and the trachea (Figure 4-1E).

ETIOLOGY

A. The exact etiology of the disturbed embryogenesis is unknown.

B. A generalized disturbance in embryogenesis is suggested by the association of vertebral defects, anal atresia, and cardiac, renal, and limb abnormalities. The noted occurrence of TEF in monozygotic twins in which only one is affected by EA/TEF further complicates understanding the genetic basis for esophageal anomalies and suggests that developmental events may be more important than genetic factors.[5]

C. The esophagus and trachea develop from a common foregut derivative during the third and fourth weeks of embryogenesis, 34–36 days after fertilization. Separation of the esophagus and trachea takes place with an ingrowth of mesodermal ridges and epithelial proliferation.[4] Failed recanalization of the esophagus may further block esophageal development and result in EA. Improper formation of septal ridges between the esophagus and the trachea may lead to failure of the esophagus to develop and a TEF.[1,7]

INCIDENCE

A. This occurs in 1/3,000–4,500 live births.[5,8]

B. Thirty to 40 percent are born prematurely.

C. This is slightly more common in males than in females.

CLINICAL PRESENTATION

A. Polyhydramnios may have occurred during pregnancy.

B. Postdelivery, symptoms that the infant exhibits may include excessive drooling and frequent coughing or choking as secretions overflow from the esophageal pouch.

C. Aspiration from the upper pouch or through a fistula may result in a cough, tachypnea, and/or hypoxia.

D. There may be intermittent episodes of cyanosis.

E. Attempts at oral feeding are often accompanied by vomiting, coughing, choking, and cyanosis.

F. Scaphoid abdomen may be noted if there is no fistula to the lower esophagus.

G. Respiratory symptoms are most common when diagnosis is delayed and there is aspiration of the secretions from the upper pouch.

H. Abdominal distention can be seen when there is a fistula between the trachea and the distal portion of the esophagus. Crying can lead to rapid distention of the GI tract with air and can cause reflux of gastric contents through the fistula into the trachea.[7]

ASSOCIATIONS

A. Approximately 50 percent of infants with EA have associated anomalies.

B. The most frequent abnormalities are:[7,9]
  1. Musculoskeletal
     a. Musculoskeletal anomalies include:
        1) Vertebral body abnormalities
        2) Rib defects
        3) Defects of the extremities

b. Approximately 15 percent of these defects occur as part of the VATER association (an acronym for **v**ertebral defects, **a**nal atresia, **t**racheoesophageal fistula with **e**sophageal atresia, and **r**adial and renal anomalies).[9]

c. The same cluster of symptoms is found with VACTERL association (VATER plus **c**ardiac defects and **l**imb anomalies).[9,10]

d. Esophageal abnormalities can also be seen in the CHARGE association (an acronym for **c**oloboma, **h**eart disease, choanal **a**tresia, **r**etarded growth and development, **g**enital hypoplasia, and **e**ar anomalies with deafness).[10]

e. The presence of 13 pairs of ribs with a long gap between the proximal and distal portions of the esophagus is a predictor of EA.[11]

2. Cardiovascular

   a. Cardiovascular anomalies (25–40 percent) are especially severe when there are multiple associated anomalies of the skeletal and GI systems.

   b. The most common are:

      1) Ventricular septal defect

      2) Patent ductus arteriosus

      3) Tetralogy of Fallot

3. Gastrointestinal

   a. GI anomalies have been documented in 12 percent of cases and include:[9]

      1) Imperforate anus

      2) Duodenal atresia

      3) Pyloric stenosis

4. Genitourinary (GU)

DIFFERENTIAL DIAGNOSIS

A. Infants presenting with drooling and choking with attempted feedings should have neurologic and feeding disorders ruled out.

B. Anomalies that are identified on initial examination should be further evaluated.

DIAGNOSIS

A. Prenatal diagnosis

1. Absence of a stomach bubble on prenatal ultrasonography carries a positive predictive value of 56 percent for esophageal atresia. However, amniotic fluid may pass into the stomach through a tracheoesophageal fistula, thereby demonstrating a normal stomach bubble on ultrasound, and the EA/TEF can then be missed.

2. Many infants diagnosed prenatally have trisomy 18 or other anomalies and therefore carry a poorer prognosis than those whose prenatal ultrasound is nondiagnostic.[12]

B. Postnatal diagnosis

1. Passing a catheter through the esophagus into the stomach may not be possible.

   a. The catheter meets resistance at 9–13 cm.

   b. If the tube is soft and flexible, it may curl in the upper pouch and give a false sense that it has passed into the stomach.

2. An AP and a lateral radiograph of the chest, neck, and abdomen will confirm the position of the catheter within the upper esophageal pouch. Air in the abdomen confirms the presence of a distal TEF.

3. A contrast study of the upper esophagus is contraindicated in most cases because of the danger of aspiration. However, it may be useful in the diagnosis of H-type fistulas because they are more difficult to diagnose.
4. Bronchoscopy and endoscopy may also be required to allow for direct visualization of the fistula.[5,7]

TREATMENT OPTIONS AND NURSING CARE

A. Preoperative care is focused on the symptoms presented and the maintenance of airway integrity.
  1. Insert a sump catheter into the upper esophageal pouch and attach it to low, intermittent suction. If none is available, repeated suctioning is essential to clear the upper airway and to prevent overflow of secretions.
  2. Elevate the head of the bed 30–45 degrees to decrease the risk of reflux of gastric contents through the distal fistula into the lungs. Flat or head down position may be used if there is no TEF. This position will then facilitate drainage of the esophageal pouch.
  3. Administer intravenous (IV) glucose and fluids.
  4. Administer oxygen as needed.
  5. Provide broad-spectrum antibiotic coverage.
  6. Use comfort measures to reduce crying, which can lead to further abdominal distention and an increased risk of reflux.[9]

SURGICAL MANAGEMENT

A. The surgical option for the management of the infant with esophageal atresia depends on the following.
  1. The underlying medical condition of the infant
  2. The type of defect
  3. The distance between the esophageal segments
B. Initial surgery includes fistula ligation and placement of a gastrostomy tube for decompression and feedings.
C. Primary reanastomosis can be accomplished if the distance between the proximal and distal ends of the esophagus are not so far apart that stretching them to meet will cause excessive tension on the anastomosis. The fistula is ligated, and the ends of the esophagus are attached.
D. Staged repair is the surgical option when a significant distance separates the two ends of the esophagus. Six to 12 weeks are usually required for spontaneous growth of the proximal segment to elongate to the level of the mediastinum, where reanastomosis is possible.[5,13]

COMPLICATIONS

A. Common complications include:[4,5,7,8]
  1. Dysfunctional peristalsis in the distal segment leading to reflux apnea, swallowing difficulties, and episodes of vomiting and gastroesophageal reflux (GER) occurs in 30 to 65 percent of patients.
  2. Recurrent TEF occurs in 5 to 12 percent.
  3. Anastomotic stenosis occurs in 40 to 50 percent.
  4. Anastomotic leaks occur in 15 percent.

POSTOPERATIVE NURSING CARE

A. Extubation should be undertaken when respiratory function has returned to normal.

B. Secretions are often problematic in even the simplest repairs.
1. Careful and frequent suctioning of the posterior pharynx to prevent an accumulation of secretions is imperative to a smooth postoperative course.
2. The suction catheter should be passed to a predetermined depth above the surgical site to avoid disruption of the anastomosis.
C. To prevent trauma to the surgical site, avoid hyperextension or forceful rotation of the head.
D. The infant should be supported with intravenous fluids and total parenteral nutrition until the anastomosis is proven intact and patent.
E. If a gastrostomy is present, feedings may be initiated within 48 hours, but reflux may aggravate an anastomotic leak.
F. Oral feedings are usually withheld for 5 to 10 days, but may be advanced rapidly once the anastomosis has been demonstrated to be intact and patent.[5,9]

OUTCOMES

A. The prognosis depends on the presence or absence of associated anomalies.
B. Infants born with EA with distal TEF, weighing more than 1,500 gm, and with no other life-threatening congenital anomaly, no major chromosomal anomaly, and no major respiratory complication have nearly a 100 percent chance of successful repair and survival.[5,8,13]
C. The main cause of death in all infants with EA is related to the associated congenital anomalies. In premature infants with associated anomalies, a 50 percent survival rate is reported.[8,13]

Gastroesophageal Reflux

DEFINITION

The presence of acidic gastric contents in the esophagus, which cause inflammation of the esophageal tissue and can result in aspiration of the stomach contents into the lungs, causing pneumonia

PATHOPHYSIOLOGY

A. GER is the regurgitation of gastric contents into the:
1. Esophagus
2. Upper airways
3. Tracheobronchial area
B. Severe GER can lead to inflammation and stricture of the esophagus.
C. If GER is left untreated, it can cause:[14]
1. Failure to thrive
2. Esophagitis
3. Anemia
4. Esophageal stricture
5. Inflammatory esophageal polyps

ETIOLOGY

A. Normal anatomic conditions believed to play a role in *preventing* reflux:
1. The distal portion of the esophagus, which lies below the diaphragm, has a higher pressure than the proximal esophagus and the stomach. The pressure helps prevent reflux of the stomach contents into the esophagus.
2. The esophagus enters the stomach at an angle known as the angle of His. This angle is thought to play a role in preventing reflux in humans.[15]

B. Disruptions in anatomic conditions that may contribute to reflux:
1. Premature infants may have a decreased angle of His.
2. Pressure in the proximal esophagus may be decreased because of immaturity.
3. Delayed maturation of the lower esophageal sphincter may also play a role in reflux in preterm infants.
4. Infants with congenital diaphragmatic hernia, gastroschisis, and omphalocele are prone to reflux. It is caused by malposition of the esophagus or stomach and increased intra-abdominal pressure.
5. Poor gastric motility or delayed gastric emptying time can also contribute to reflux.

INCIDENCE

A. GER is reported in 3–10 percent of very low birth weight (VLBW) infants (<1,500 gm).[7]
B. Fifty percent of healthy infants may have symptomatic reflux at two months of age.[7]

CLINICAL PRESENTATION

A. Vomiting is the most common symptom of GER in infants; most emesis occurs with burping during feeding or two or three hours after a feeding.
B. Failure to thrive may occur.
C. "Irritable" behavior may be demonstrated with feeding, such as crying, arching, and aversion to feeding.
D. Signs and symptoms of respiratory distress can indicate aspiration of stomach contents.
E. Apnea may occur.

ASSOCIATIONS

A. More common in infants with small bowel obstruction or other intestinal anomalies as well as in infants with neurologic abnormalities
B. Premature infants, especially those <32 weeks gestation[16]

DIFFERENTIAL DIAGNOSIS

A. Gastroesophageal reflux should be suspected in an otherwise healthy infant with postprandial regurgitation.
B. Regurgitation ranges from effortless spitting to forceful vomiting.
C. An upper GI series is important to rule out anatomic causes of vomiting such as:
1. Esophageal stricture

FIGURE 4-2 ■ Nissen fundoplication.

An operation to sew the top of the stomach (fundus) around the esophagus. Used to stop stomach contents from flowing back into the esophagus (reflux) and to repair a hiatal hernia. **A.** Before surgery. **B.** Sutures. **C.** After surgery.

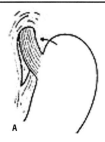

A

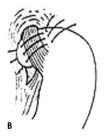

B

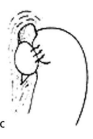

C

From: National Institute of Diabetes and Digestive and Kidney Diseases. 2000. *Dictionary of Digestive Diseases.* NIC Publication No. 00–2750. Bethesda, Maryland: National digestive Diseases Information Clearinghouse. Retrieved December 9, 2005, from http://digestive.niddk.nih.gov/ddiseases/pubs/dictionary/pages/l-p.htm.#N.

   2. Esophageal webs
   3. Volvulus
   4. Meconium ileus/plug
   5. Peptic stricture
   6. Esophageal dysmotility
D. Other causes of vomiting to be ruled out are the following.[7]
   1. Sepsis
   2. Urea cycle defects
   3. Formula intolerance
   4. Increased intracranial pressure
   5. Pancreatic abnormalities
   6. Hydronephrosis
   7. Drug toxicity

DIAGNOSIS

A. Contrast studies of the esophagus and stomach illustrate the presence of anatomic abnormalities and reflux of gastric contents. Use of a technetium isotope allows for evaluation of gastric emptying time.[15]
B. To perform an esophageal pH study, a pH electrode is placed in the lower third of the esophagus and the pH is continuously measured over a 24-hour period. A pH of <4 is diagnostic of GER.[14] Patterns of GER with activity such as sleeping, feeding, and positioning can also be assessed.

TREATMENT OPTIONS AND NURSING CARE

A. Less severe cases may respond to noninvasive intervention such as small, frequent feedings and elevating the head of the bed 30 degrees. Thickening of feedings with rice cereal may decrease frequency of emesis, but is controversial.[16]
B. Infants presenting with more serious symptoms, such as failure to thrive or chronic irritability, may require medications to be prescribed.
   1. H_2 receptor antagonists such as ranitidine or cimetidine may be effective in decreasing the amount of acid produced and aid in the healing of the esophagitis.[15]
   2. Prokinetic agents such as metoclopramide may be useful when delayed gastric emptying contributes to reflux.
   3. However, medications have shown to be of limited value in decreasing the incidence of apnea and bradycardia in premature infants.[17]
C. Documentation of feedings and associated signs and symptoms of reflux are important in determining the severity of the problem and gauging whether medical intervention is successful.
D. Daily weight and an accurate record of intake and output are needed.
E. If medical management fails to control the symptoms or complications of reflux, surgical intervention may be necessary.

SURGICAL MANAGEMENT

A. The most common surgical procedure used to treat reflux is a Nissen's or Thal's fundoplication (Figure 4-2).
   1. The lower esophagus is mobilized, the fundus of the stomach is wrapped from left to right behind the esophagus, and the edges are sutured in front of the esophagus.

2. In the Nissen fundoplication, the stomach is wrapped 360 degrees around the distal esophagus. In the Thal fundoplication, the wrap is 270 degrees, which may decrease gaseous distention of the stomach.[16]

3. The wrap increases the pressure in the lower esophagus and acts as a one-way valve.

B. A gastrostomy tube may be placed as well to ensure adequate nutrition and to provide for a vent for gas.

C. Laparoscopic surgery has been shown to be an effective technique in performing fundoplication and gastrostomy tube placement and results in a decreased length of hospitalization postoperatively.[18,19]

COMPLICATIONS

A. Complications of gastrostomy tube placement:
1. Bleeding or irritation of the skin at the site
2. Leaking around the tube at the insertion site

B. Complications of fundoplication:
1. Gaseous distention of the stomach
2. Retching and difficulty swallowing
3. Failure or overtightness of the wrap
4. Delayed gastric emptying
5. Necessity for revision of the fundoplication in 24 percent of procedures.
6. Highest failure rate is seen in infants with associated anomalies such as:[7]
   a. TEF
   b. Congenital diaphragmatic hernia
   c. Neurologic disorders

POSTOPERATIVE NURSING CARE

A. Infants undergoing fundoplication and gastrostomy tube placement are usually able to restart enteral feedings within 24 to 48 hours after surgery.

B. Proper fit of the gastrostomy tube must be ensured, and effective intragastric and transabdominal seals must be provided.[20]
1. The tube must fit closely against the stomach wall.
2. If a balloon is present, the volume of water used to inflate it must be documented.
3. The length of the tube segment that is visible outside the abdomen should be noted and measured on a regular basis.
4. If leaking occurs, it may be caused by evaporation of water in the balloon or failure of the transabdominal seal.
   a. Replacing water in the balloon and keeping the gastrostomy tube perpendicular to the abdominal wall will increase the effectiveness of the seal.[20]
5. In some cases, a larger tube will need to be placed.

C. Prior to discharge, parents must be taught how to replace the tube should it become dislodged. Parents also need to be instructed in how to care for the skin around the tube and how to handle leaking.

OUTCOMES

A. Most infants can be treated medically with a 75 percent recovery rate.

B. Of those that fail medical treatment at three months of age, 10–15 percent require prolonged medical treatment and 10–15 percent require surgery.

C. Surgical long-term results are reported at 95 percent total clinical cures.[7]

Gastroschisis

DEFINITION

A defect in the abdominal wall lateral to the umbilical cord

PATHOPHYSIOLOGY

A. The defect is usually small (2–4 cm) and is most frequently found to the right of the umbilicus.

B. Abdominal contents, including the small intestine, part of the colon, and occasionally the liver, may herniate through the defect while the fetus is *in utero*.

C. There is no peritoneal sac covering the intestines; therefore, they are exposed to the amniotic fluid *in utero* (Figure 4-3).

FIGURE 4-3 ■ Gastroschisis.

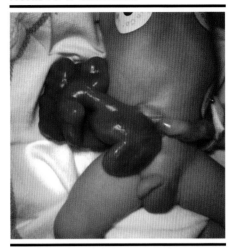

From: Clark DA. 2000. *Atlas of Neonatology,* 7th ed. Philadelphia: Saunders, 192. Reprinted by permission.

ETIOLOGY

A. The most popular theory is that of a vascular accident during embryogenesis causing occlusion of the mesenteric artery. This causes necrosis and rupture of a portion of the abdominal wall.[21,22]

B. A second theory is that the defect occurs secondary to an incomplete infolding of the embryonic disc with incomplete formation of the abdominal wall.[1,7]

INCIDENCE

A. Gastroschisis occurs every 0.3–2/10,000 live births.[23]

B. It occurs more frequently in teen pregnancies and in mothers from low socioeconomic groups and social instability.

C. Alcohol, recreational drugs, and smoking have been shown to increase risk in some studies.[24–26]

CLINICAL PRESENTATION

A. At birth, the herniated bowel is often edematous and may present as a mass of matted intestine rather than distinguishable loops because of prolonged exposure to amniotic fluid.

ASSOCIATIONS

A. Generally, this is an isolated defect without associated chromosomal abnormalities or other anomalies.

B. An association with intestinal atresia is probably secondary to complications of the gastroschisis itself.

DIFFERENTIAL DIAGNOSIS

A. Ruptured omphalocele

B. Cloacal exstrophy

DIAGNOSIS

A. If this defect is suspected or diagnosed, the pregnancy may be monitored with serial ultrasounds to look for increasing intestinal dilation or thickening of the bowel wall.

 1. Some studies have predicted a poor outcome associated with thickened bowel wall or intestinal dilation.[27]

 2. Other studies have not shown such a correlation.[28]

TREATMENT OPTIONS AND NURSING CARE

A. Numerous studies have tried to determine the appropriate management of the delivery of an infant with gastroschisis.

 1. Obstetric management

   a. Preterm delivery was originally believed beneficial, thereby limiting the time the bowel is in contact with the amniotic fluid, but this has not been shown to improve outcome.[29]

   b. Cesarean section may be of some benefit in limiting trauma to the exposed bowel. However, when these infants are compared to those delivered vaginally, neonatal outcome has not been shown to be significantly improved.[29,30]

   c. Minimizing the time between delivery and surgical repair is important. It is recommended that, when possible, these mothers of known affected infants be transferred to the hospital where the surgery will take place.[31]

 2. Following delivery

   a. Care of this defect is focused on the following.

     1) Protecting the bowel from further injury or trauma

     2) Gentle handling of exposed intestines

     3) Avoid placing the baby in a prone position with the bowel draped to one side because this can cause kinking of the superior mesenteric artery and lead to necrosis and ischemic bowel.

     4) Place the infant in a side-lying position (preferably the right side) to facilitate venous return from the bowel.

     5) An orogastric tube should be placed and maintained on low, intermittent suction to provide gastric decompression.

   b. In the delivery room, sterile dressings soaked in warm saline should be applied to the bowel, and the entire lower abdomen is then wrapped in plastic wrap. As an alternative, the entire baby can be placed in a "bowel bag."[32]

   c. Maintain fluid balance.

     1) Infants with abdominal wall defects may require as much as three times the amount of maintenance fluid as a normal neonate prior to surgery and during the first 24–48 hours after surgery.[31]

     2) Intake and output should be accurately monitored. Blood pressure and perfusion status should also be followed to assure adequate intake.

   d. Maintain thermoregulation. The large surface area of the bowel places these infants at high risk for profound hypothermia. Temperature must be monitored closely, and the infant should be maintained on a radiant warmer or other heat source.

   e. Prophylactic broad-spectrum antibiotic therapy should also be initiated.

SURGICAL MANAGEMENT

A. Primary closure. This procedure returns the entire bowel to the abdominal cavity. However, if the defect is large or the bowel is very edematous, it may not be possible to replace all of the bowel at one time.

B. Staged closure. If the extra-abdominal contents cannot be returned at the time of the initial surgery, a silastic silo is created outside the abdominal wall. The silastic is sutured around the abdominal wall defect, and the bowel is supported inside (Figure 4-4). A small portion of the bowel is pushed into the abdomen each day until all the contents of the silo are inside the abdominal wall. This can usually be achieved within five to seven days.[31]

COMPLICATIONS

A. Aggressive attempts at primary closure may create increased abdominal pressure, leading to:
  1. Decreased cardiac output
  2. Respiratory compromise
  3. Decreased perfusion to the intestines, kidneys, and lower extremities
  4. Bowel ischemia and necrosis

B. Complications following gastroschisis repair include sepsis, intestinal atresia, and prolonged ileus. Necrotizing enterocolitis (NEC) may also be seen in these babies.

C. Complications from prolonged parenteral nutrition may include direct hyperbilirubinemia, cirrhosis, and liver failure.

FIGURE 4-4 ■ Gastroschisis with silastic silo closure.

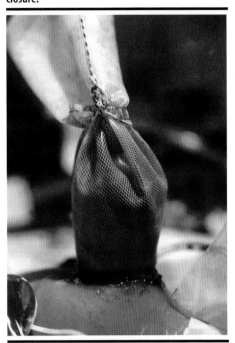

From: Clark DA. 2000. *Atlas of Neonatology,* 7th ed. Philadelphia: Saunders, 192. Reprinted by permission.

POSTOPERATIVE NURSING CARE

A. Monitor the infant closely during reduction of the abdominal contents and in the immediate postoperative period for signs and symptoms of increased abdominal pressure.
  1. The heart may be compressed because of increased intra-abdominal pressure pushing the diaphragm up and decreasing intrathoracic space.
  2. Increased intrathoracic pressure can result in cardiovascular compromise secondary to compression of the inferior vena cava.
  3. Symptoms include decreased blood pressure, decreased renal perfusion, and bowel ischemia.
  4. Careful monitoring of blood pressure, heart rate, urine output, and acid-base status is essential.

B. Sedation and mechanical ventilation are required until the entire bowel has been reduced.

C. Total parenteral nutrition will be required until bowel function returns and enteral feedings can be tolerated. This may be as long as four to six weeks after abdominal closure. A central venous catheter will be essential to provide for adequate parenteral calories.

FIGURE 4-5 ■ Omphalocele.

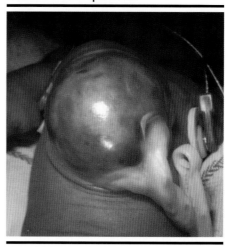

From: Clark DA. 2000. *Atlas of Neonatology,* 7th ed. Philadelphia: Saunders, 190. Reprinted by permission.

OUTCOMES

A. Mortality rate for gastroschisis is less than 5 percent.[7]
B. Mortality is usually caused by associated intestinal atresia.[23,31]
   1. Ten percent of infants with gastroschisis have intestinal atresias.[23,31]

Omphalocele

DEFINITION

An embryologic defect caused by failure of the intestine to return to the abdominal cavity during the tenth week of gestation[1]

PATHOPHYSIOLOGY

A. The defect can range in size from 1–2 cm in diameter, containing a single loop of bowel, to 10–15 cm, containing virtually all of the abdominal contents (Figure 4-5).
B. Development of the abdominal muscle and peritoneal layers is incomplete; the intestines and sometimes the liver herniate into the base of the umbilical cord.
C. A translucent membrane covers the herniated sac, which is part of the umbilical epithelium.
D. The abdominal cavity tends to be small and underdeveloped.

ETIOLOGY

A. Etiology is uncertain. The leading theory is incomplete folding of the embryonic disc, preventing complete closure of the abdominal wall.[1]

INCIDENCE

A. 1–3/10,000 live births[1,23]

CLINICAL PRESENTATION

A. The defect will be apparent at the time of birth as a herniation into the base of the umbilical cord.
B. It is usually covered with a transparent sac, although this sac may rupture, leaving the intestines and other contents loose.
C. Small defects may not be readily apparent, especially those containing only one or two loops of bowel.

Associations

A. Fifty to 70 percent association with chromosomal anomalies or other structural defects,[33,34] including:
   1. Trisomy 13
   2. Trisomy 18
   3. Congenital heart defects (tetralogy of Fallot and atrial septal defects—19–25 percent)[35]
   4. Facial clefts
   5. GU anomalies
B. Beckwith-Wiedemann syndrome
C. Pentalogy of Cantrell

Differential Diagnosis

A. Gastroschisis
B. Patent urachus

Diagnosis

A. Fetal ultrasound
B. Increased maternal serum α-fetoprotein in up to 89 percent of fetuses with an omphalocele[23]

Treatment Options and Nursing Care

A. Immediate care of the infant with an omphalocele is similar to that of one with a gastroschisis.
   1. The defect should be covered with a warm, saline-soaked, sterile dressing and then with a waterproof barrier such as plastic wrap or a bowel bag.
   2. An orogastric tube should be placed to low, intermittent suction to allow for decompression of the stomach and bowel.
   3. IV fluids should be provided.
   4. Intake and output should be monitored closely along with heart rate, blood pressure, and perfusion.
B. The infant should be examined for other defects or signs of chromosomal abnormalities.
   1. An echocardiogram should be done to rule out congenital heart disease.
C. Prophylactic antibiotic therapy may be prescribed preoperatively and for 24–72 hours postoperatively.

Surgical Management

A. Primary repair can usually be done without much difficulty if the defect is small.
B. Staged repair is required when the defect is large, particularly if it includes the liver.
   1. A sheet of silastic is sewn around the defect, and the omphalocele is suspended inside the silo (Figure 4-6).
   2. Gradual manual reduction is performed over a period of several days. Reduction of the liver requires care: The hepatic and portal veins cannot be kinked or occluded.

Complications

A. Gastroesophageal reflux is a common occurrence in these infants.

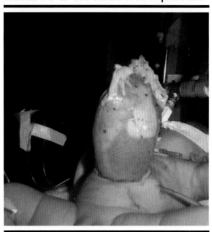

FIGURE 4-6 ■ Silo closure of an omphalocele.

From: Clark DA. 2000. *Atlas of Neonatology,* 7th ed. Philadelphia: Saunders, 191. Reprinted by permission.

POSTOPERATIVE NURSING CARE

A. Mechanical ventilation is required in anticipation of the respiratory compromise that can occur as the abdominal contents are replaced.
   1. In most cases, the infant will remain on mechanical ventilation and sedation until the entire bowel is in place.
B. Monitor for respiratory and cardiovascular compromise.
   1. Following primary and staged reduction, the following must be monitored closely.
      a. Blood gases
      b. Fluid and electrolyte status
      c. Heart rate
      d. Blood pressure
C. Capillary leakage and third spacing are not uncommon.
D. Elevated liver enzymes may indicate decreased hepatic blood flow due to occlusion of the hepatic or portal veins.
E. Total parenteral nutrition will be required.
F. Placement of a central venous catheter will allow for maximum nutrition.
   1. If the defect is small and a primary closure is done, the infant may be able to tolerate enteral feedings fairly quickly.
   2. Infants who had large defects or a staged repair may take several weeks to establish enteral feedings.

OUTCOMES

A. Mortality rates vary depending on:
   1. Associated defects
   2. Chromosomal abnormalities
   3. The size of the omphalocele
B. An isolated omphalocele without heart disease has a mortality rate of approximately 30 percent, depending on the size of the defect.[31,33,34]

Pyloric Stenosis

DEFINITION

Hypertrophic pyloric stenosis is one of the most common conditions requiring surgery in the newborn.[36] It is caused by hypertrophy of the pylorus, which results in stricture of the outlet from the stomach to the small intestine.

PATHOPHYSIOLOGY

A. Constant contraction of the circular and longitudinal pyloric muscle causes it to become longer and thicker, preventing passage of food from the stomach to the intestine.

ETIOLOGY

A. The exact etiology of pyloric stenosis is unknown.
B. It is thought to have a genetic/hereditary component because up to 5 percent of infants with the disease are born to mothers who had the disease.[37]
C. The lesion may be congenital or may be secondary to factors such as increased gastric acid and muscle spasms or abnormal motility.
D. Abnormal nerve innervation has also been suggested as a cause of pyloric stenosis.[38]

E. It may be caused by an inadequate number of receptors in the pyloric muscle that detect nitric oxide and peptides, signaling the pyloric muscle to relax.[8,16]

INCIDENCE

A. Pyloric stenosis occurs in 1–4/1,000 live births.[37]
B. It is more common in males, particularly firstborn.
C. It is more common among Caucasian infants.

CLINICAL PRESENTATION

A. It typically presents at two to six weeks of age with nonbilious vomiting. Onset may be sudden or present gradually with worsening of symptoms, eventually leading to the classic projectile vomiting.
B. Accompanying signs and symptoms of dehydration, weight loss, and jaundice may be present.

ASSOCIATIONS

A. GER is commonly reported, but whether it occurs due to the stenosis or as a contributing factor is unclear.[36]
B. Intestinal malrotation, esophageal atresia, and obstructive uropathy have infrequently been reported.

DIFFERENTIAL DIAGNOSIS

A. GER
B. Obstruction of the small bowel

DIAGNOSIS

A. On physical examination, most infants will have a small, oval-shaped mass palpable in the right upper quadrant below the liver.
  1. This mass may be difficult to palpate if the infant is distressed.
  2. If a mass cannot be felt, the diagnosis may be made by abdominal ultrasound or an upper GI study with contrast solution.[13]

TREATMENT OPTIONS AND NURSING CARE

A. Infants who are not significantly dehydrated can be operated on without delay.
B. Infants who present with dehydration, electrolyte imbalances, or acidosis require fluid resuscitation and correction of acidosis prior to surgical intervention.
C. Attention to blood pressure, urine output, and perfusion is important.
D. A nasogastric tube should be maintained on low, intermittent suction to allow for gastric decompression and to prevent aspiration of stomach contents.

SURGICAL MANAGEMENT

A. Reparative procedure is a pyloromyotomy. An incision is made in the longitudinal and circular muscles of the pylorus, thereby releasing the stricture.
B. Repair can also be performed laparoscopically.

COMPLICATIONS

A. Persistent vomiting the first few days after surgery is not an uncommon complication, and normal stomach emptying may not return until a week after surgery.

POSTOPERATIVE NURSING CARE

A. Maintain fluid and electrolyte balance.
B. Pain control is the main requirement for the first few hours postoperatively.

C. Feedings can be introduced once the infant is extubated and awake.
   1. Usually introduced by about 6–8 hours of age.
   2. Advanced to full feedings by 24–48 hours.
   3. Early feedings have reduced hospital stay significantly in recent years.[36]

Outcomes

A. The disorder is corrected with surgery and generally does not recur.[36]

Intestinal Atresia and Stenosis

Definition

Defect in the continuity of the intestine

Pathophysiology

A. An atresia is a failure of the lumen of the small bowel to form properly, causing an obstruction in the small bowel.
B. Types of atresias include:
   1. Mucosal membranes or webs
   2. Blind ends of intestine separated by fibrous cords or by mesenteric defects
   3. Large gaps of defective mesentery with decreased blood supply to the distal bowel
C. There can be multiple areas of atresia in the intestine.[39]

Etiology

A. Duodenal atresia is thought to be caused by a failure of recanalization during the eighth week of gestation.
   1. This failure may result in complete atresia or stenosis or in formation of a web inside the duodenum, causing an obstruction.
B. Surrounding pancreatic tissue (annular pancreas) can also cause obstruction of the duodenum.
C. Jejunal and ileal atresias are believed to be caused by an interruption of the blood supply and localized ischemia causing necrosis and subsequent reabsorption of the affected bowel.

Incidence

A. Atresia of the bowel is the most common cause of intestinal obstruction in the newborn.
B. The incidence is 1/2,500–5,000 births.[40]
C. Jejunoileal atresias occur in 1/1,000 live births, equally distributed between the ileum and jejunum.[40]
D. Duodenal atresias occur in 1/2,500 live births, with 30 percent of these being associated with trisomy 21.[40]

Clinical Presentation

A. The mother of a fetus with a high intestinal obstruction may present with polyhydramnios.
B. Infants who are not diagnosed prenatally will present with abdominal distention and vomiting.
   1. Emesis may be clear or bilious, depending on the level of the stenosis.
C. An incomplete atresia or stenosis may not present in the immediate newborn period, depending on the ability of food to pass the obstruction.

D. During the first few weeks after birth, these infants may present with dehydration, hyponatremia, jaundice, and failure to thrive.

ASSOCIATIONS

A. Up to one-third of infants with duodenal atresia will have trisomy 21.[40,41]

B. Infants with duodenal atresia may have the following associated anomalies.
   1. Congenital heart disease
   2. Renal anomalies
   3. Esophageal atresia
   4. VACTERL association

C. Jejunoileal atresias usually present as an isolated defect and have a low association with other anomalies.

DIFFERENTIAL DIAGNOSIS

A. Midgut volvulus

B. Malrotation

C. Meconium ileus

D. Meconium plug

E. Hirschsprung's disease

DIAGNOSIS

A. Prenatal
   1. Prenatal ultrasound will be significant for dilated loops of bowel or a large stomach bubble, followed by a large dilated loop of bowel proximal to the obstruction (double bubble).

B. Neonatal
   1. Radiographic studies of a newborn with duodenal atresia will demonstrate the classic double bubble of air in the stomach and in the obstructed duodenum, with no air below the obstructed area.
   2. X-rays of atresias of the jejunum or ileum demonstrate areas of gas or fluid-filled loops of bowel, but scant amounts of gas in the rest of the abdomen.

TREATMENT OPTIONS AND NURSING CARE

A. Bilious vomiting in the newborn is considered a surgical emergency until proven otherwise.
   1. Nothing should be given by mouth (NPO).
   2. Intravenous fluids should be started immediately.
   3. A nasogastric tube should be set to low, intermittent suction to allow for decompression of the stomach and small bowel. (Intermittent suction is the only appropriate suction to use for GI decompression and evacuation of stomach contents. Continuous suction would result in adherence of the stomach wall to the suction catheter and damage to the mucosa.)
   4. A physical examination for associated anomalies should be performed.

SURGICAL MANAGEMENT

A. The atretic portion of the bowel should be removed and, depending on the length of normal bowel, anastomosis of the ends of the bowel may be performed.

B. If gaps of normal bowel are large, the ends may need to be tapered in order to connect a larger lumen segment to a smaller one.

C. In infants with multiple atresias, one or more stomas may be created temporarily, although this has not been shown to improve outcome.[40]

D. Infants with duodenal atresia and anastomosis may require a gastrostomy tube to provide for adequate decompression and to avoid traumatizing the site of the anastomosis.

COMPLICATIONS

A. Short bowel syndrome (SBS) can be seen in infants with numerous atretic areas in the jejunum or ileum that may have minimal normal bowel left following surgical repair.
   1. Lactose intolerance, malabsorption, and diarrhea may be significant in these infants.
   2. Prolonged parenteral nutrition and slow introduction of feedings will be required.
   3. It can take many months and even years before full enteral nutrition is achieved.
B. Strictures or adhesions may develop.

POSTOPERATIVE NURSING CARE

A. Maintain gastric decompression as ordered.
B. Total parental nutrition will be necessary until the return of normal bowel function, which may take as long as one to three weeks. The more proximal the atresia, the longer it takes normal bowel function to return.[7,39]
C. Give antibiotics prophylactically.
D. Leaks of the anastomosis site can occur following surgery. These will present with abdominal distention, vomiting, and pneumoperitoneum.

OUTCOMES

A. Survival is decreased in infants with:
   1. Multiple atresias
   2. Complications such as Down syndrome or cystic fibrosis
   3. Associated abdominal wall defects, intestinal perforation, and peritonitis

Meconium Ileus

DEFINITION

Meconium ileus is a failure to pass meconium, due either to a mechanical obstruction or to the thickness of the meconium. The bowel is obstructed by this accumulation of thick meconium.

PATHOPHYSIOLOGY

A. Hyperviscous secretions from the mucous glands of the small intestine result in meconium that is very thick and tenacious.
   1. The tenacity of the meconium in the ileum results in an inability of the meconium to travel through the small intestine into the colon, causing the ileum to become obstructed.

ETIOLOGY

A. Most infants with meconium ileus are eventually diagnosed with cystic fibrosis.
   1. Lack of the enzymes responsible for fat and protein metabolism causes these infants to produce meconium that is abnormally thick and viscous.[16,41]

INCIDENCE

A. Ten to 15 percent of infants with cystic fibrosis will have meconium ileus.[8]

CLINICAL PRESENTATION

A. Prenatal
1. Perforation and meconium peritonitis may be seen on prenatal ultrasound as abdominal calcifications.
B. Neonatal
1. It may present with signs and symptoms of small bowel obstruction, including abdominal distention, bilious emesis, and failure to pass meconium.
2. The meconium mass may be palpable on physical examination.
3. Obstruction of the ileus with meconium can lead to bowel perforation and meconium peritonitis.

ASSOCIATIONS

A. Cystic fibrosis
1. Cystic fibrosis occurs in approximately 1/1,600 live births.
2. Cystic fibrosis is more common in Caucasian infants.
3. Up to 25 percent of infants with cystic fibrosis will present in infancy with meconium ileus.[8]

DIFFERENTIAL DIAGNOSIS

A. Meconium plug
B. Small bowel atresia
C. Hirschsprung's disease

DIAGNOSIS

A. Abdominal x-ray
1. The x-ray will show dilated loops proximal to the obstruction with a narrowed microcolon distal to the obstruction.
2. The dilated bowel may be hazy in appearance with small bubbles of trapped air mixed with meconium.

TREATMENT OPTIONS AND NURSING CARE

A. The infant should be NPO.
B. The infant should be maintained on IV fluids.
C. A gastric tube is inserted and placed to low, intermittent suction to decompress the bowel.
D. If no perforation is present, water-soluble contrast enemas are administered to soften the meconium and facilitate its passage through the intestine.
E. If prenatal or postnatal perforation is present or if the bowel cannot be evacuated with enemas, surgery is required.

SURGICAL MANAGEMENT

A. A laparotomy is performed, and the affected part of the bowel is resected with anastomosis of the two ends or creation of a stoma.
B. Irrigation of the meconium blockage may be attempted either during the procedure or postoperatively via an ileostomy.[42]

COMPLICATIONS

A. Segments of the bowel may be lost due to the thickness of the meconium.
B. Peritonitis may occur.
C. Infection may occur.
D. If the diagnosis is cystic fibrosis, the infant will need careful follow-up for complications of this disease.

POSTOPERATIVE NURSING CARE

A. Total parenteral nutrition and antibiotics are maintained until the infant is recovered from surgery and enteral feedings are established.

B. Pulmonary toilet with chest physiotherapy, acetylcysteine sodium aerosols, and humidity are important in caring for infants with cystic fibrosis.

C. Genetic counseling and testing to establish the presence of cystic fibrosis are necessary.
  1. DNA testing
  2. Sweat chloride test if the nurse is able to collect enough sweat (If not, the test can be attempted later.)

OUTCOMES

A. Morbidity or mortality associated with meconium ileus is generally due to complications associated with cystic fibrosis and associated pulmonary disease.

B. Surgical mortality is approximately 10 percent.[8]

Malrotation/Volvulus

DEFINITION

Intestinal obstruction caused by knotting and twisting of the bowel (Figure 4-7)

PATHOPHYSIOLOGY

A. Rapid lengthwise growth of the intestines during early gestation requires outward midgut herniation at the umbilical ring; involution and counterclockwise rotation of the intestine and superior mesenteric artery are properly completed with the cecum positioned in the right lower quadrant.
  1. This important sequence in the embryologic development of the gut precedes anatomic fixation of the intestine to the posterior peritoneal wall, thereby holding the intestine in place.

B. When the rotation fails to occur normally, the bowel is free to move around and kink or twist upon itself (volvulus).
  1. This results in intestinal obstruction, vascular compromise, and necrosis of the bowel.[43]

ETIOLOGY

A. The etiology of spontaneous malrotation is not known.

B. Malrotation is a component of gastroschisis, omphalocele, and diaphragmatic hernia.[16]

INCIDENCE

A. The incidence of isolated malrotation is unknown.

B. The incidence of clinical symptoms resulting in a diagnosis of malrotation is approximately 1/6,000 live births. A diagnosis cannot be made in the absence of symptoms.[43]

CLINICAL PRESENTATION

A. Most cases of malrotation present during the first month of life.

B. Bilious emesis, abdominal distention, and tenderness may be present, depending on where the volvulus is located.

C. If a large portion of intestine is involved or if necrosis has developed, the infant may present with hypotension, acidosis, and respiratory failure.

FIGURE 4-7 ■ Anomalies of rotation and fixation.

Anomalies of rotation and fixation. **A.** Normal anatomy: Cecum lies in right lower quadrant; transverse colon overlies duodenum. **B.** Incomplete rotation (Ladd bands): Cecum lies just below and anterior to the duodenum, where it becomes fixed to the posterior wall by abnormal peritoneal bands. The bands cross over, compress, and obstruct the duodenum. **C.** Nonrotation ("left-sided colon"): The entire small intestine lies in the right side of the abdominal cavity, whereas all of the large intestine lies on the left. Volvulus may occur, but the condition is more frequently asymptomatic. **D.** Reverse (clockwise) rotation: Duodenum overlies and may obstruct the transverse colon. **E.** Nonfixation ("midgut volvulus"): Mesentery fails to adhere to the posterior abdominal wall so that the small intestine hangs loosely from the superior mesenteric artery and is free to twist around it or on itself to create a volvulus, typically involving the duodenum.

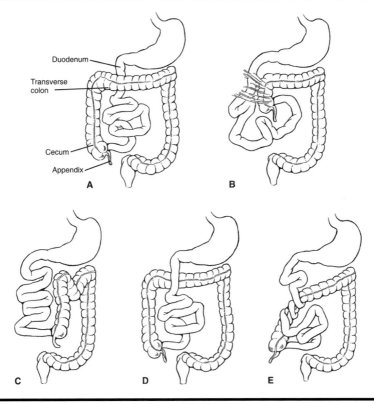

From: Thigpen JL, and Kenner C. 2003. Assessment and management of the gastrointestinal system. In *Comprehensive Neonatal Nursing: A Physiologic Perspective*, 3rd ed., Kenner C, and Lott JW, eds. Philadelphia: Saunders, 476. Reprinted by permission.

ASSOCIATIONS

A. Imperforate anus
B. Intestinal atresia
C. Cardiac anomalies
D. Trisomy 21

DIFFERENTIAL DIAGNOSIS

A. Small bowel atresia
B. Necrotizing enterocolitis

DIAGNOSIS

A. Abdominal x-ray
   1. Malrotation and the presence of a volvulus may not be visible on an abdominal radiograph.

2. Distention of the bowel proximal to the volvulus and decreased amounts of air distal to the site, on abdominal x-ray, are similar to findings with a small bowel atresia.

B. An upper GI with contrast is necessary for diagnosis.

TREATMENT OPTIONS AND NURSING CARE

A. The outcome for patients with a midgut volvulus is dependent on rapid diagnosis, stabilization, and surgical intervention.

B. Gastric decompression, intravenous fluid resuscitation, and correction of acidosis and electrolyte imbalances must occur without delay; infants in respiratory failure will require mechanical ventilation.

C. This is considered a surgical emergency and should be responded to as such.

D. Broad-spectrum antibiotics should be administered.

SURGICAL MANAGEMENT

A. Laparotomy
   1. The entire intestine and mesentery are lifted out to assess completely.
   2. The volvulus is unwound in the opposite direction of the torsion. If the bowel is viable, it will improve in color and appearance with relief of torsion.
   3. Nonviable bowel is resected.
   4. If the entire midgut is infarcted, the infant may be returned from surgery without resection, and hospice care will be approached with the family.
   5. If the retained bowel is viable, the surgeon will dissect the Ladd's bands, which secure the cecum and mesocolon in abnormal positions to the posterior body wall. This increases the base of the mesentery and allows for replacement of the intestine into the abdomen.
   6. Appendectomy is routinely performed, and the bowel is replaced with the small intestine on the right and the large intestine on the left.[43]

COMPLICATIONS

A. If large portions of the intestine are infarcted and thus require removal, the patient will suffer from short-bowel syndrome.
   1. Prolonged parenteral nutrition is required because of the malabsorption and feeding intolerance seen in SBS.
   2. Enteral feedings are introduced gradually with very small amounts of dilute formula.
      a. Hydrolysated or predigested formula may be required.
   3. Tolerance of full enteral feedings may not occur for several months.
   4. Supplementation with fat-soluble vitamins may be necessary.

POSTOPERATIVE NURSING CARE

A. Gastric decompression and fluid and electrolyte support are necessary postoperatively.

B. Hypovolemia and acidosis must be corrected.
   1. These conditions can be present preoperatively and continue postoperatively as well, depending on:
      a. How much bowel was affected
      b. If there were any bowel perforations

OUTCOMES

A. Outcome is dependent upon:
   1. The amount of affected intestine
   2. The degree of acidosis and electrolyte imbalance
   3. The presence of respiratory failure
B. If a large amount of bowel is removed, complications of short-bowel syndrome will add to morbidity and mortality.[43]

Hirschsprung's Disease

DEFINITION

First described by a Denmark pediatrician in the 1880s, Hirschsprung's disease is characterized by the absence of ganglion cells in the distal part of the colon

PATHOPHYSIOLOGY

A. Absence of ganglion cells results in the absence of peristalsis in the affected part of the colon, causing a functional obstruction at and below the level of aganglionosis.
B. The length of bowel affected is variable, and there is a distinct level of aganglionosis beyond which no ganglion cells are found.

ETIOLOGY

A. It is believed to be caused by a failure of neural crest neuroblasts to migrate to the distal part of the colon, thereby resulting in a lack of ganglion cells.[1]
B. Another theory attributes it to destruction of ganglion cells by anoxia or an infectious agent.[7,42]

INCIDENCE

A. It occurs in 1/5,000 births.[39,42]
B. It occurs predominately in white males.[39,42]
C. Predominance in males suggests the possibility of a hereditary component; positive family history has been noted in up to 30 percent of infants.[7]

CLINICAL PRESENTATION

A. In more severe cases, infants present with symptoms of intestinal obstruction:
   1. Abdominal distention
   2. Bilious vomiting
   3. Failure to pass meconium
B. Mild cases may not present in the immediate newborn period and can be unrecognized for a period of time, despite a history of constipation, until abdominal distention or enterocolitis becomes severe.

ASSOCIATIONS

A. Because the ganglion cells present in the colon are derived from the same neural crest as the oral, facial, and cranial ganglia, children with Hirschsprung's disease have a small but statistically significant increased risk of hearing loss and decreased peripheral nerve function.[44]

DIFFERENTIAL DIAGNOSIS

A. Malrotation/volvulus
B. Meconium ileus
C. Small bowel obstruction

DIAGNOSIS

A. Infants who do not pass meconium during the first 36–48 hours of life or who have signs of intestinal obstruction should be investigated with the suspicion of Hirschsprung's disease.
   1. An abdominal x-ray may be of limited use in defining exactly where the obstruction is located, but will be significant for dilated loops of bowel and decreased air in the rectum.
   2. A barium enema will show dilated colon where the ganglion cells are present, followed by a small or narrow distal colon.
   3. Biopsy of rectal tissue looking for the presence or absence of ganglion cells is necessary for definitive diagnosis.

TREATMENT OPTIONS AND NURSING CARE

A. The infant should remain NPO.
B. IV fluid intake and output should be monitored closely.
C. Evaluation of electrolytes should be done every day or more often if results are abnormal.
D. A nasogastric tube should be maintained on low, intermittent suction to allow for decompression of the stomach and intestine.
E. To prevent overwhelming systemic sepsis, antibiotics are started if the infant presents with signs of enterocolitis.
F. Antibiotics may also be started prophylactically if surgery is anticipated.
G. Colonic irrigation may be required prior to surgery to evacuate any stool from the colon and to decrease the risk of peritonitis.[4]
   1. Normal saline or other isotonic solutions are used.

SURGICAL MANAGEMENT

A. A colostomy is placed at the level of the colon at which ganglion cells appear on progressive, intraoperative biopsies.
B. At 6–12 months of age, the normal part of the colon is connected to the anus.
C. An alternative approach is to remove the affected rectal mucosa, retaining the aganglionic rectal muscular cuff.
   1. The ganglion-containing colon is then anastomosed to the anorectum.
   2. Advances in laparoscopic surgery have made this approach more practical in infants.[4,8]

COMPLICATIONS

A. Postoperative stricture formation
B. Dysmotility of the colon

POSTOPERATIVE NURSING CARE

A. The stoma should be examined regularly to ensure good perfusion and integrity of skin around the site.
B. Following a pull-through procedure, some children experience enterocolitis symptoms or constipation, both of which need immediate follow-up, including antibiotics and rectal irrigation.

OUTCOMES

A. Up to 85 percent of patients will have no adverse affects after surgery and will have normal bowel habits.

B. Approximately 15 percent of patients will have occasional problems with constipation or incontinence.
   1. Rarely, patients will experience severe problems with constipation or incontinence requiring:[7,8]
      a. Laxatives
      b. Dietary manipulation
      c. Anal dilation

Necrotizing Enterocolitis

DEFINITION

Partial or full-thickness intestinal ischemia, usually of the terminal ileum

PATHOPHYSIOLOGY

A. Necrotizing enterocolitis is a spectrum of illness that varies from a mild self-limiting process to a severe disorder characterized by necrosis of the mucosa and submucosal layers of the gastrointestinal system with sepsis, organ failure, and potentially death.

B. NEC can be triggered by factors such as:[45–47]
   1. Antenatal maternal cocaine use
   2. Maternal prolonged rupture of membranes
   3. Certain pharmacologic agents
      a. Any drug with high osmolarity (e.g., phenobarbital elixir) given to a neonate
      b. Any drug that may compromise intestinal perfusion (e.g., indomethacin)
   4. Hypoxia
   5. Circulatory disturbances
   6. Umbilical catheters
   7. Shock
   8. Hyperosmolar feedings
   9. Exchange transfusions

ETIOLOGY

A. The precise cause is speculative and probably multifactorial.

B. NEC is thought to result from three major pathologic mechanisms occurring in combination. These mechanisms involve:[45,47]
   1. Mesenteric ischemia/tissue hypoxia
   2. Enteral feedings
   3. Bacterial flora/toxins

INCIDENCE

A. Overall, incidence is between 1 and 8 percent of all newborns admitted to the NICU.[47,48] It is the most common GI emergency encountered in the NICU.

B. The disease occurs both sporadically and in clusters.

C. NEC is equally distributed between males and females.[45]

D. The majority of neonates affected are born prematurely, although approximately 10 percent of those affected are term.[49]

FIGURE 4-8 ■ AP supine x-ray of a 35-week gestational age neonate with pneumatosis intestinalis. Note bubbly and linear appearance of air.

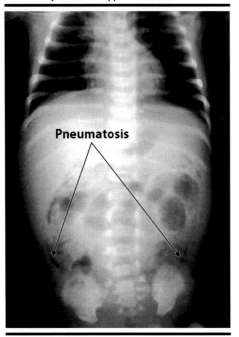

From: Horton KK. 2005. Pathophysiology and current management of necrotizing enterocolitis. *Neonatal Network* 24(1): 44. Reprinted by permission.

FIGURE 4-9 ■ Abdominal x-ray. Gas evident in portal vein and in peritoneal cavity.

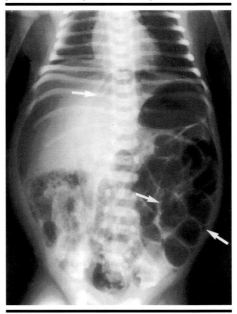

From: Meerstadt PWD, and Gyll C. 1994. *Manual of Emergency X-Ray Interpretation.* Philadelphia: Saunders, 224. Reprinted by permission.

E. The risk of NEC increases as gestational age and birth weight decrease.[47,50]

F. The mortality rate for NEC has been calculated as high as 13/100,000 live births, with ranges of 20–40 percent of cases.[48]

CLINICAL PRESENTATION

A. Early presenting signs are varied, but usually include nonspecific GI compromise or nonspecific signs of sepsis.

B. The typical newborn with NEC is a premature infant who develops gastric aspirates, abdominal distention, vomiting that may or may not be bilious, and bloody stools after enteral feedings have been started.

C. Apnea and bradycardia, lethargy, and poor perfusion may also be prominent findings.

D. Localized abdominal erythema or bluish discoloration with mild to marked abdominal tenderness are other physical signs of an associated peritonitis.

E. Onset usually occurs in the first two weeks of life, but late onset NEC may occur as late as three months of age in the VLBW infant.[46,47]

ASSOCIATIONS

A. Certain risk factors such as prematurity and feedings have been consistently observed in newborns with NEC.

B. There are no reported associated chromosomal abnormalities or other anomalies.

DIFFERENTIAL DIAGNOSIS

A. Diagnosing NEC is a process of elimination.
B. The following should be considered along with other medical and/or surgical conditions when the infant presents with a tender abdomen.
   1. Pneumonia
   2. Urinary tract infection
C. Colitis should also be ruled out.
D. Reaching an accurate diagnosis requires:
   1. Skill in physical assessment
   2. Recognition of characteristic symptoms of common neonatal conditions
   3. The judicious selection of laboratory and radiologic tests

FIGURE 4-10 ■ Intestinal perforation.

Large volume of free air on left lateral decubitus x-ray in a 24-week gestational age neonate.

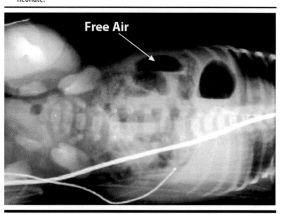

Free Air

From: Horton KK. 2005. Pathophysiology and current management of necrotizing enterocolitis. *Neonatal Network* 24(1): 42. Reprinted by permission.

DIAGNOSIS

A. Diagnosis of NEC starts with a high degree of suspicion in infants at risk.
B. Laboratory findings include:
   1. Electrolyte imbalance
   2. Abnormal blood gases with acidosis, hypoxia, and hypercapnia
   3. Increased white blood cell count with an increased band count or, as the disease progresses, decreased absolute neutrophil count and thrombocytopenia[46]
C. Diagnosis is confirmed by the presence of pneumatosis intestinalis, indicating air within the bowel wall on an abdominal x-ray (Figure 4-8).
   1. There is a spectrum of the disease, with milder cases exhibiting only distention of the bowel loops with bowel wall edema (the bowel wall appears thickened).
D. Pneumoperitoneum on x-ray is indicative of intestinal perforation.
E. Air noted within the portal venous system is seen in near total intestinal necrosis and is associated with a significantly increased mortality rate in medically and surgically treated infants (Figure 4-9).[49]
F. Intestinal perforation accounts for free abdominal air (Figure 4-10). This situation usually requires emergency surgical intervention.

TREATMENT OPTIONS AND NURSING CARE

A. The goal of medical management is to stabilize the infant and to prevent progression of mild NEC to advanced disease.
   1. Infants suspected of having NEC should be made NPO and IV fluids started immediately.
   2. A nasogastric tube should be maintained to low, intermittent suction to allow for decompression of the stomach and prevent restriction of blood flow that

results from increasing intraluminal and extraluminal pressure on the bowel wall.

3. Abdominal girth measurements should be done serially to assess for abdominal distention.
4. Assess cardiac and respiratory status and as well as acid-base and electrolyte balances.
5. The infant's course is monitored by abdominal x-rays taken every six to eight hours, looking for GI complications such as progressive intestinal obstruction and perforation.

B. Respiratory support with intubation and ventilation is often required.
C. Systemic antibiotics should be administered after blood cultures are obtained. Initial therapy includes ampicillin, anaerobic bacterial coverage, and an aminoglycoside. Antibiotic treatment is then modified when culture results are reported.[14]
D. Thrombocytopenia and anemia are frequently seen with NEC. Platelet and red blood cell transfusions are often needed.[7]
E. Progressive disease in spite of maximal medical support requires surgical intervention.

SURGICAL MANAGEMENT

A. A pediatric surgeon should be consulted early in the course of the disease.[51]
B. Indications for surgery include:
    1. Pneumoperitoneum (free air present on a left lateral decubitus film)
    2. A persistently dilated intestinal loop on serial x-rays
    3. Abdominal wall cellulitis
    4. Progressive clinical deterioration despite maximum medical support[45,46,51]
C. Surgery is required in approximately 25–50 percent of newborns with NEC. Ideally, surgery is performed when the bowel is gangrenous but not perforated.[46]
D. If the neonate cannot tolerate surgery, a percutaneous peritoneal drain can be placed and surgery delayed until the infant is more stable.
E. The principles of surgical therapy for NEC include:
    1. Careful examination of the bowel with removal of all necrotic bowel while preserving as much viable bowel as possible
    2. Intestinal decompression
    3. Diversion of fecal material through the creation of ostomies[49]
F. Primary anastomosis is an option if there is only a single segment of necrotic bowel and no distal involvement.
G. If the necrosis is more widespread, a proximal stoma is created, and then a "second look" surgery may be done between 24 and 72 hours later to re-evaluate questionable bowel as necrotic versus viable.
H. Preservation of adequate intestinal length is essential for continued growth and development of the infant and avoiding the consequences of long-term parenteral nutrition.[46]

COMPLICATIONS

A. The most common complication after medical management is stricture of the colon.[46]
B. Approximately half of all infants who undergo surgery have complications, which may include stomal stenosis, stomal prolapse, intestinal strictures, short-bowel syndrome, wound infection, wound dehiscence, and enterocutaneous fistula.[45–47]

POSTOPERATIVE NURSING CARE

A. Clinical condition usually improves following the removal of the necrotic bowel.

B. Postoperative care includes gastric decompression and IV fluids.

C. Feedings are initiated approximately ten days after surgery, when the infant has stabilized and GI function has resumed.[7,45]

D. Antibiotic therapy is continued for 10–14 days after pneumatosis intestinalis has resolved.[7]

E. Infants who are gaining weight and weigh between 2.5 and 5 kg can have their stomas closed at three to five months of age.

F. Timing of the stoma closure depends on several factors.[46]
1. Symptoms of stricture formation
2. Amount of stoma drainage
3. Rate of weight gain
4. Length of time since operative intervention

OUTCOMES

A. Approximately 50 percent of newborns with NEC who are medically treated clinically resolve their disease without surgical intervention.[46]

B. Newborns with NEC who undergo surgical treatment have survival rates of 44–87 percent.[45,46]

C. Long-term prognosis is determined by the amount of intestine lost and removed with surgery.

Anorectal Malformations

DEFINITION

A. Persistent cloaca

B. Anal stenosis

C. Membranous anal atresia

D. Anal agenesis

E. Anorectal agenesis

F. Rectal atresia

PATHOPHYSIOLOGY

A. Anorectal malformations comprise a wide spectrum of abnormalities (Figure 4-11).

B. Low lesions may have normal pelvic anatomy or near normal positioning of the rectum within the pelvic musculature.

C. In high lesions, the rectum has not descended through the pelvic musculature and may communicate via a fistula to the GU tract.

ETIOLOGY

A. The anus and the rectum originate from an embryologic structure called the cloaca.

B. In-growths and folds from the lateral walls of this structure form the urorectal septum at the fourth to sixth week of gestation.

C. This septum separates the rectum dorsally from the urinary tract ventrally.

D. Both systems (rectum and urinary tract) are completely separated by the seventh week of gestation.

FIGURE 4-11 ■ Types of anorectal malformations.

A. Persistent cloaca. Note the common outlet for the intestinal, urinary, and reproductive tracts. B. Anal stenosis. C. Membranous anal atresia (imperforate anus). D and E. Anal agenesis with a perineal fistula. F. Anorectal agenesis with a rectovaginal fistula. G. Anorectal agenesis with a rectourethral fistula. H and I. Rectal atresia.

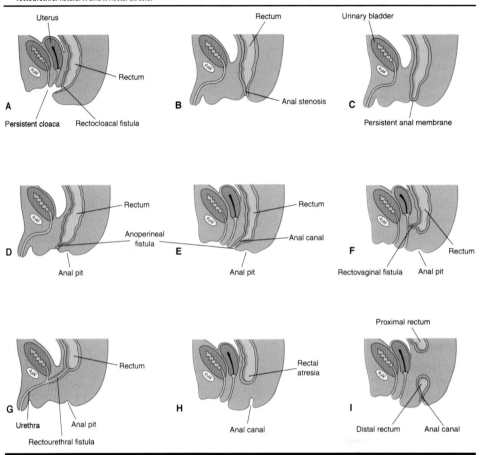

From: Moore KL, and Persaud TVN. 2003. *The Developing Human: Clinically Oriented Embryology,* 7th ed. Philadelphia: Saunders, 283. Reprinted by permission.

E. At this time, the urogenital portion of the cloaca has an external opening, whereas the anal portion is closed by a membrane that opens at the eighth week of gestation.

F. Failure of this complex separation process at any point in embryonic development will result in one of the many anatomic findings associated with imperforate anus abnormalities.[1]

INCIDENCE

A. Imperforate anus occurs in approximately 1/4,000–5,000 births.[1,52]

B. Most types of anorectal anomalies are more common in males than females.[1,53]

C. There is usually no family history of this abnormality.[52]

CLINICAL PRESENTATION

A. Presenting signs and symptoms for anorectal anomalies will vary slightly, depending on the type of defect.

B. Most of the anomalies are obvious at birth or on physical examination when a normal anal opening is noted to be absent.

C. There is a high incidence of fistulas with anorectal defects, and meconium may be passed in the urine (in males) or may be noted at the vaginal outlet (in females). With anal stenosis, the rectum is narrowed but patent, and therefore meconium stools may be passed.

D. A deep anal dimple may hide a complete membrane, and a rectal atresia consisting of a web several centimeters above the anus may be overlooked until it is noted that the infant is distended and has not passed meconium.

E. The atretic type of anorectal malformation is rare, and the infant generally presents with signs and symptoms of intestinal obstruction (failure to pass stool, bilious vomiting, abdominal distention).

ASSOCIATIONS

A. About 50 percent of infants with anorectal anomalies have an associated defect, with GU tract malformations found most frequently (20–54 percent).[52]

B. Urologic abnormalities are seen in 30 percent of infants with high anorectal anomalies.[54]

C. Conversely, infants with perineal fistulas (low defects) have less than a 10 percent chance of having an associated urologic defect.[55]

D. Urologic defects include:
   1. Renal agenesis or dysplasia
   2. Hydronephrosis
   3. Horseshoe kidneys

E. Esophageal atresia with TEF (10 percent) and congenital heart disease (7 percent) have also been noted.[4,7]
   1. When these anomalies are found, the VATER and VACTERL associations should be considered.[7]

DIFFERENTIAL DIAGNOSIS

A. Visual and digital examinations are diagnostic, and anomalies are usually detected early in life.
   1. Some types are harder to detect early on (e.g., anal stenosis, rectal atresia) and may present later in life.

B. In either sex, a flat perineum with a short sacrum and little muscle contraction suggest a high anomaly.

C. Physical examination should be directed toward detecting associated malformations.

D. Rule out a urinary fistula by examining urine for meconium epithelial cells.[7]

DIAGNOSIS

A. Evaluation of anorectal malformations involves the inspection of the entire perineum. All of the following signify a low lesion.
   1. A perineal fistula opening into the vagina
   2. A fistula seen along the median raphe to the tip of the penis
   3. An anal membrane deformity

B. Fistulas are often best observed 12–24 hours after birth, when meconium passage through a fistula is more likely to be seen.[4]

FIGURE 4-12 ■ Algorithm for management of males with anorectal malformation.

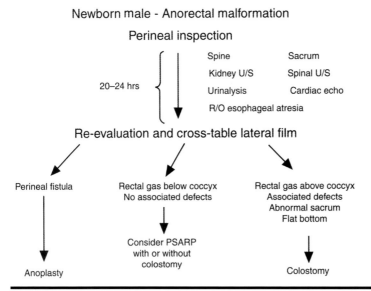

From: Pena A, and Levitt MA. 2005. Imperforate anus and cloacal malformations. In *Pediatric Surgery,* 4th ed., Ashcraft KW, Holcomb GW, and Murphy JP, eds. Philadelphia: Saunders, 501. Reprinted by permission.

C. Examination of the perineum will also provide information about sacral innervation and muscular development.
  1. A flat perineum with no anal dimple and poor muscular response to cutaneous stimulation around the anal area are signs of defective perineal innervation.
  2. A slow dribble of urine or a distended bladder provides proof of poor innervation. It is also a sign that the infant has a high malformation.
D. Signs of ambiguous genitalia, poor development of the labia, and, in the male, undescended testicles are further evidence of a more severe defect.
E. The abdomen is specifically palpated for distention and enlargement of the kidneys or bladder.
F. The urine should be examined for meconium epithelial cells.
G. X-rays of the sacrum, perineal and spinal ultrasonography, magnetic resonance imaging (MRI), and voiding cystourethrogram may all be used to distinguish high lesions requiring colostomy from low lesions that can be repaired immediately. An inverted lateral x-ray study (Wangensteen-Rice technique) may demonstrate air collected in the blind-ending rectum at or near the perineum.
H. Needle aspiration for detecting the rectal pouch involves advancing a needle while attempting to aspirate. If no meconium has been obtained by the time the needle has been advanced 1.5 cm, the defect is assumed to be a high lesion.[4,7,8,14]

TREATMENT OPTIONS AND NURSING CARE

A. As in all of the abnormalities associated with intestinal obstruction, initial management requires establishing IV access and monitoring fluid and electrolyte balance.

FIGURE 4-13 ■ Algorithm for management of a female with anorectal malformation.

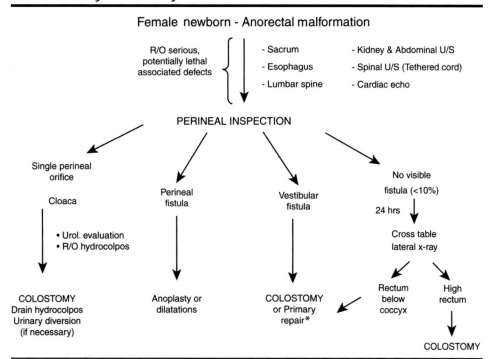

* Depending on the experience of the surgeon and general condition of the patient

From: Pena A, and Levitt MA. 2005. Imperforate anus and cloacal malformations. In *Pediatric Surgery*, 4th ed., Ashcraft KW, Holcomb GW, and Murphy JP, eds. Philadelphia: Saunders, 502. Reprinted by permission.

B. Monitor for bowel complications such as perforation and enterocolitis.

C. Place a gastric decompression sump tube to avoid vomiting and aspiration.

D. Administer antibiotics to sterilize the bowel.

E. Perform serial urinalyses to check for meconium. If positive, this is considered indicative of a rectourinary fistula.[14]

SURGICAL MANAGEMENT

A. Operative management of a newborn with an anorectal malformation varies with the type of defect and determines the immediate future of the infant. An important decision to be made by the surgeon is whether the infant needs a colostomy and whether urinary diversion is necessary to prevent sepsis or metabolic acidosis.

B. Management of male and female infants differs significantly.

   1. Males

      a. Male infants with low malformations do not need a colostomy and can be treated by dilation of the anus or by perineal anoplasty in cases of anal stenosis during the newborn period. Figure 4-12 illustrates a decision-making algorithm for the initial management of male patients. When managed appropriately, these infants have an excellent prognosis. The incidence of associated urologic defects is very low.

      b. All other defects are best managed during the newborn period with a colostomy for decompression and diversion of fecal contents.

    c. Definitive repair is generally done by a posterior sagittal anorectoplasty and is delayed for 3–12 months to allow for growth and pelvic enlargement.[52]

    d. Laparoscopic surgical repair is now being done by pediatric surgeons as a way of decreasing scarring, pain, and the length of the hospital stay.[56]

2. Females

    a. In approximately 95 percent of infants, only a thorough perineal examination is needed to make the diagnosis; therefore, the decision to make a colostomy in female infants is an earlier process. Figure 4-13 illustrates the decision-making algorithm used for female infants.

    b. The presence of a single perineal opening indicates that the infant has a cloaca and an associated urologic condition. Immediate abdominal ultrasound and urologic evaluation are required.

    c. Primary surgery involves a colostomy with reconstruction of the vagina and urinary tract.

    d. With a diverting colostomy in place and urinary diversion where indicated, the infant's recovery is usually uneventful, and the surgeon can wait three to six months before attempting the main repair, called a posterior sagittal anorectovaginourethroplasty.[52]

COMPLICATIONS

A. Severe diaper rash may occur as a result of multiple bowel movements. The diaper rash improves as the number of bowel movements gradually decreases.[7,52]

POSTOPERATIVE NURSING CARE

A. A colostomy requires standard skin care and close monitoring.

B. In infants with rectourethral fistula, a Foley catheter remains in place for 8–14 days. If there is accidental dislodgement of the catheter, the infant must be observed for spontaneous voiding because reintroduction of the catheter can disrupt the repair.

C. IV antibiotics are given for 48–72 hours.

D. Antibiotic ointment is applied topically to the site for eight to ten days.

E. Oral fluids are given soon after surgery, followed by a regular diet.

F. Infants who undergo abdominal surgery may need to be NPO one to two days as well as have a nasogastric tube placed for drainage.

G. During postoperative recovery, the urine should be monitored for signs of meconium, which would indicate a recurrent fistula.

H. Two weeks after corrective surgery, the infant is started on anal dilations.

    1. The parents learn to dilate the anus twice a day. Every week the size of the dilator is increased and passed to stretch the anus to normal size.

    2. Once the anus reaches the desired size, the colostomy can be closed.

    3. Severe strictures may be seen when the dilation program is not done properly or if the blood supply to the rectum has been damaged. Once the dilator passes easily, the frequency of dilations is tapered.[52]

I. Continence varies by malformation.

    1. With low anorectal malformations, 80–90 percent of infants are continent after surgery.

    2. With high malformations, only 30 percent of infants achieve continence.[53]

Outcomes

A. Of significance in the long-term outcome of imperforate anus is the presence of skeletal deformities of the sacrum.

　1. One or several sacral vertebrae may be missing.

　2. Patients with an absent sacrum have major deficits in neural innervation to the musculature responsible for fecal and urinary continence.[55]

B. Other spinal anomalies include:

　1. Tethered cord[57]

　2. Distal cord lipoma

　3. Spina bifida[52]

C. Urinary incontinence is relatively common after cloaca repair. Male infants rarely suffer from urinary incontinence.

D. Constipation is a common sequelae.

E. Twenty-five percent of all infants suffer from fecal incontinence, but they significantly improve their quality of life when enrolled in a bowel management program.[58]

Inguinal Hernia

Definition

Inguinal hernia is the prolapse of a portion of the bowel and gonads through the inguinal ring and into the inguinal canal.

Pathophysiology

A. An inguinal hernia is caused by a failure of the processus vaginalis to close or by a congenital weakness.

B. The bowel enters the scrotal sac in the male or the soft tissue of the labia in the female newborn.[59]

C. A patent processus is seen as a potential hernia. The hernia is produced only when the intra-abdominal contents leave the peritoneal cavity and protrude into the processus vaginalis.

D. If only fluid leaves the peritoneal cavity, the defect is called a communicating hydrocele. A communicating hydrocele is always associated with a hernia.[60]

E. An incarcerated hernia occurs when the prolapsed sac contents (generally bowel in the male and ovary, fallopian tube, or bowel in the female) are caught within the processus, leading to impaired venous and lymphatic drainage, increasing edema and pressure, and eventually leading to obstruction.

F. When the blood supply is cut off to the herniated organs, gangrene and necrosis develop. When these changes occur, the term *strangulation* is used, highlighting the need for immediate surgical intervention.[59]

Etiology

A. Most inguinal hernias in infants are indirect, resulting from a persistent patency of the processus vaginalis.

B. The processus vaginalis is present in the developing fetus at the twelfth week of gestation. The processus is a peritoneal diverticulum that extends through the internal inguinal ring.

　1. As the testis descends at approximately the twenty-eighth week of gestation, a portion of the processus attaches to the testis as it exits the abdomen and is pulled into the scrotum with the testis (Figure 4-14).[61,62]

FIGURE 4-14 ■ Common hernias and hydroceles.

A. Incomplete congenital inguinal hernia resulting from persistence of the proximal part of the processus vaginalis. **B.** Complete congenital inguinal hernia into the scrotum resulting from persistence of the processus vaginalis. Cryptorchidism, a commonly associated anomaly, is also illustrated. **C.** Large cyst or hydrocele that arose from an unobliterated portion of the processus vaginalis. **D.** Hydrocele of the testis and spermatic cord resulting from peritoneal fluid passing into an unclosed processus vaginalis.

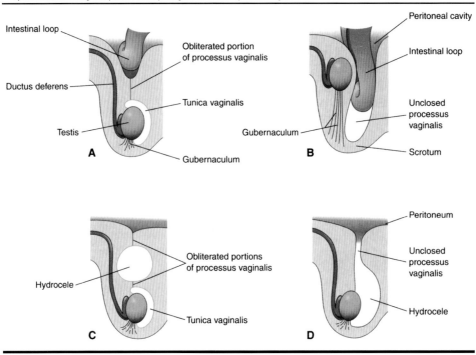

From: Moore KL, and Persaud TVN. 2003. *The Developing Human: Clinically Oriented Embryology,* 7th ed. Philadelphia: Saunders, 325. Reprinted by permission.

    2. The ovaries in the female also descend into the pelvis, but do not leave the abdominal cavity. The processus vaginalis in females extends into the labia majora through the inguinal canal.[61,62]

C. Late in gestation or shortly after birth, the layers of the processus vaginalis fuse and eventually obliterate the entrance of the inguinal canal in the vicinity of the inguinal ring.[60,62]

D. The exact time that obliteration occurs is unknown. In approximately 20 percent of individuals, the processus vaginalis remains patent throughout life but without symptoms of hernias or hydroceles.[60]

INCIDENCE

A. The incidence of inguinal hernia varies and is estimated to be 10–20/1,000 live births. In most studies, male infants with hernias outnumber females by a 6:1 to 10:1 ratio.[60–62]

B. Premature infants are at greater risk than term infants for developing inguinal hernias.

    1. They may be secondary to increased abdominal pressure from feeding and respiratory effort before closure of the processus vaginalis.[63]

    2. Inguinal hernias associated with cryptorchid testes are particularly common.[4,62]

3. Incidences vary and are reported to be close to 30 percent in males and 2 percent in females.[60–62,64]

C. Approximately 50 percent of inguinal hernias present in the first year of life, and most are seen in the first six months.

D. Position is as follows.[60,62,65]
   1. 50–60 percent on the right side
   2. 30 percent on the left side
   3. 10–20 percent bilateral

E. The incidence of incarcerated hernias ranges from 12 to 17 percent.[62] The incidence of incarcerated hernias is higher in females.[61]

CLINICAL PRESENTATION

A. A bulge or lump is found in the groin area.

B. The first sign of an inguinal hernia may be an intestinal obstruction that is a result of incarceration.

ASSOCIATIONS

A. Associated diseases have been found to increase both the incidence of hernia and the risk of recurrence after repair.
   1. Infants with cystic fibrosis have up to a 15 percent incidence of inguinal hernia. This is approximately eight times higher than the normal population.[60]
   2. Infants with disorders of connective tissue formation (Ehlers-Danlos syndrome) and mucopolysaccharidosis (Hunter-Hurler syndrome) are at higher risk for developing hernias.[60,61]

B. Fluid in the peritoneal cavity, because of either a ventriculoperitoneal shunt or peritoneal dialysis, predisposes a patient to inguinal hernia.[60,63,64]

C. There is a high familial incidence of hernia that seems to indicate an inherited defect.[61,65]

D. There is also an increased incidence of indirect inguinal hernia in infants with a family history of congenital dislocation of the hip and congenital abdominal wall defects.[60,63]

DIFFERENTIAL DIAGNOSIS

A. An inguinal hernia should be differentiated from a hydrocele.
   1. An incarcerated hernia may be mistaken for a tense hydrocele.
   2. If the bulge in the groin area is a hydrocele, there will be no history of reducibility, and the swelling will be translucent, smooth, and usually nontender.

B. Torsion of the testicle may also be misdiagnosed as an inguinal hernia. Testicular torsion is revealed as a nontransilluminating, tender mass in the groin region.[59,61]

DIAGNOSIS

A. A diagnosis of a hernia can be made only when a bulge or lump is found on physical examination. Inguinal hernias usually appear as a bulge in the groin region and extend toward or into the scrotum. Occasionally, it can appear as a swelling in the scrotum without a bulge in the inguinal region.

B. It is visible most frequently with crying or straining (increased intra-abdominal pressure). The hernia usually spontaneously reduces when at rest or with relaxation or can be manually reduced with upward and posterior pressure directly on the mass.[59–61]

C. A history of intermittent labial, groin, or scrotal swelling that reduces spontaneously is indicative of an indirect inguinal hernia.[60,62]

D. It may be difficult to distinguish an inguinal hernia from a hydrocele.

    1. In an infant with an inguinal hernia, the scrotal swelling varies, becoming larger with crying and becoming smaller or disappearing during relaxation.

    2. An isolated hydrocele does not change in size during the day and may disappear over the first year of life.

    3. Gentle pressure or squeezing may reduce the fluid in the hydrocele from the scrotum into the peritoneal cavity.

        a. The fluid will abruptly reappear when intra-abdominal pressure is increased, as with crying or straining.[60]

    4. The examiner may be able to differentiate a hernia from a hydrocele by palpating a thickened cord as it crosses the pelvic tubercle.

        a. A finger laid over and parallel to the inguinal structures and then rubbed across the cord at the head of the pubic tubercle imparts the sensation of rubbing two pieces of silk together.

        b. A positive silk sign indicates thicker cord structures in the inguinal canal than in the normal side.[61,62]

    5. Transillumination is of no value in differentiation because gas in the bowel transilluminates a hernia as well as a fluid-filled hydrocele.

    6. An abdominal film demonstrating gas in the hernia sac is diagnostic for an inguinal hernia, but there is limited enthusiasm for this diagnostic technique because of concerns regarding costs and gonad radiation.[59,60,62,65]

E. Ultrasound of the inguinal canal and scrotum is often diagnostic and can be used after difficult or inconclusive physical examinations.[60]

F. The incarcerated hernia occurs when the contents of the hernia sac cannot be reduced back into the abdominal cavity.

    1. Incarceration of organs, usually the intestine, leads to discoloration of the hernia and surrounding area and is associated with signs and symptoms of intestinal obstruction such as:[14,59,61]

        a. Irritability or continuous crying

        b. Vomiting

        c. Abdominal distention

        d. Bloody stools

        e. No stool output

    2. In infant girls, the most common intra-abdominal organ that is incarcerated is the ovary.[4,62]

TREATMENT OPTIONS AND NURSING CARE

A. The focus of nursing care preoperatively is on keeping the infant comfortable and quiet.

B. Manual reduction may be done by guiding the bowel loops back into the abdominal cavity, using gentle pressure in order to detect incarcerations early.[66]

C. Observation of the infant for incarceration or strangulation of the hernia sac contents is an ongoing process until surgery is performed.

D. Oral feedings should be continued if obstruction of the bowel does not occur.

E. If vomiting has occurred, the infant's fluid and electrolyte status should be monitored closely.[59]

SURGICAL MANAGEMENT

A. Unless incarceration occurs, inguinal hernias are not considered emergency surgery and can be performed on an outpatient basis.[14,61]

B. Because the incidence of incarceration approaches 30 percent in the premature infant, elective hernia repair should be considered before discharge from the NICU.[4,60,64]

C. Hospitalization should be limited to infants with cardiac, respiratory, or other medical conditions that place them at risk for apnea and bradycardia after general anesthesia. This is especially true for the anemic infant.[4,59,60]

D. Anesthesia is provided as follows.
1. Most hernia repairs are performed using general anesthesia, but the anesthesia technique used must take into account the general condition and gestational age of the infant.
2. Local or spinal anesthesia is reserved for premature infants or those with associated diseases that make general anesthesia more risky.
3. Spinal anesthesia has been used with success in 80 percent of attempts in infants as small as 1,500 gm.[4,60]
4. Caudal injection of a long-acting local anesthesia is administered to anesthetize all wound layers. Less anesthetic gas and medications are required during the operation, but some complications may arise, and this method is used only by experienced anesthesiologists.[60]

E. Herniorrhaphy proceeds as follows.
1. A 2–4 cm transverse incision is made in the skin in the area overlying the inguinal canal.
2. The external inguinal ring is dissected from the fat of the external oblique muscle.
3. At this point, in both male and female infants, the hernia sac is seen bulging from the external inguinal ring. The sac is found lying within the inguinal canal, anterior and usually medial to the spermatic cord.
4. Great care and gentleness are required during the dissection of the hernia sac to avoid injury to surrounding structures such as the vas deferens artery and spermatic vessels.
5. The hernia sac is opened to observe intra-abdominal structures (bowel, ovary), and the viability of these structures is assessed.
   a. If the sac contents are viable, the structures are reduced into the abdomen, and the processus vaginalis is closed.
   b. If there is incarceration with questionable bowel viability, a separate abdominal incision is used to help in the reduction and to evaluate the extent of the bowel infarction. Frequently, bowel that appears nonviable in a strangulated position shows evidence of viability after reduction into the abdomen.
   c. If nonviable bowel or ovary is visible, a bowel resection or gonadal removal is necessary.[60]

COMPLICATIONS

A. In the premature infant, apnea is a life-threatening complication after hernia repair.
1. Guidelines recommended by pediatric anesthesiologists state that any premature infant less than 60 weeks postconceptional age should have cardiorespiratory monitoring for at least 12–24 hours after surgery.[61]

2. Others suggest delaying repair until the infant is at least 46 weeks postconceptional age.[4]

B. The occurrence of wound infection is approximately 1 percent.[62]

C. The incidence of recurrence of the hernia is less than 1 percent.[60,62]

POSTOPERATIVE NURSING CARE

A. Pain relief in the postoperative period may take on several forms.
   1. Mild oral analgesics may be used, but the delayed onset of action may be a disadvantage.
   2. Acetaminophen suppositories are a good choice for pain relief if emesis occurs.
   3. Pediatric surgeons use injection of the skin wound edges with a long-acting local anesthetic such as bupivacaine. It is safe and effective but does not anesthetize the deeper tissue layers.[60]

B. Monitor infants closely for signs and symptoms of complications postoperatively.

C. Maintain skin integrity at the wound site, and monitor for any drainage, bleeding, or signs of wound infection.[59]

D. Place the infant in a side-lying or supine position with the head turned to the side to avoid disruption of the suture line.

OUTCOMES

A. Inguinal hernias do not resolve spontaneously and must therefore be surgically repaired.
   1. Surgical repair may be done as an outpatient, and 90 percent of complications can be avoided if the surgery is performed within the first month of diagnosis.

B. In premature infants with a reducible hernia, repair is performed just before discharge when the infant weighs between 1,800 and 2,000 gm.[61]

REFERENCES

1. Moore KL, and Persaud TVN. 2003. *The Developing Human: Clinically Oriented Embryology,* 7th ed. Philadelphia: Saunders, 242–253, 256–285.

2. Sadler TW. 2004. *Langman's Medical Embryology,* 9th ed. Philadelphia: Lippincott Williams & Wilkins, 285–319.

3. Moore KL, and Persaud TVN. 2003. *Before We Are Born: Essentials of Embryology and Birth Defects,* 6th ed. Philadelphia. Saunders, 202–227.

4. Hartman GE, et al. 1999. General surgery. In *Neonatology: Pathophysiology and Management of the Newborn,* 5th ed., Avery GB, Fletcher MA, and MacDonald MG, eds. Philadelphia: Lippincott Williams & Wilkins, 1005–1044.

5. Filston HC, and Shorter NA. 2000. Esophageal atresia and tracheoesophageal malformations. In *Pediatric Surgery,* 3rd ed., Ashcraft KW, ed. Philadelphia: Saunders, 348–369.

6. Spitz L. 2005. Esophageal atresia and tracheoesophageal malformations. In *Pediatric Surgery,* 4th ed., Ashcraft KW, Holcomb GW, and Murphy P, eds. Philadelphia: Saunders, 352–370.

7. Thigpen JL, and Kenner C. 2003. Assessment and management of the gastrointestinal system. In *Comprehensive Neonatal Nursing: A Physiologic Perspective,* 3rd ed., Kenner C, and Lott JW, eds. Philadelphia: Saunders, 448–485.

8. Ryckman FC, and Balistreri WF. 2002. The neonatal gastrointestinal tract. Part 2: Upper gastrointestinal disorders. In *Neonatal-Perinatal Medicine: Diseases of the Fetus and Infant,* 7th ed., Fanaroff AA, and Martin RJ, eds. St. Louis: Mosby, 1263–1268.

9. Watson R. 2004. Gastrointestinal disorders. In *Core Curriculum for Neonatal Intensive Care Nursing,* 3rd ed., Verklan MT, and Walden M, eds. Philadelphia: Saunders, 643–702.

10. Jones KL. 2006. *Smith's Recognizable Patterns of Human Malformation,* 6th ed. Philadelphia: Saunders, 276–277, 756–757.

11. Kulkarni B, et al. 1997. 13 pairs of ribs—A predictor of long gap atresia in tracheoesophageal fistula. *Journal of Pediatric Surgery* 32(10): 1453–1454.

12. Stringer MD, et al. 1995. Prenatal diagnosis of esophageal atresia. *Journal of Pediatric Surgery* 30(9): 1258–1263.

13. Jona JZ. 1998. Advances in neonatal surgery. *Pediatric Clinics of North America* 45(3): 605–617.

14. Betz CL, and Sowden LA. 2004. *Mosby's Pediatric Nursing Reference,* 5th ed. St. Louis: Mosby, 177–180, 208–211.

15. Boix-Ochoa J, and Ashcraft KW. 2005. Gastroesophageal reflux. In *Pediatric Surgery,* 4th ed., Ashcraft KW, Holcomb GW, and Murphy JP, eds. Philadelphia: Saunders, 383–404.

16. Vanderhoof JA, Zach TL, and Adrian TE. 1999. Gastrointestinal disease. In *Neonatology: Pathophysiology and Management of the Newborn,* 5th ed., Avery GB, Fletcher MA, and MacDonald MG, eds. Philadelphia: Lippincott Williams & Wilkins, 739–763.

17. Kimball AL, and Carlton DP. 2001. Gastroesophageal reflux medications in the treatment of apnea in premature infants. *Journal of Pediatrics* 138(3): 355–360.

18. Rothenberg SS. 1998. Experience with 220 consecutive laparoscopic Nissen fundoplications in infants and children. *Journal of Pediatric Surgery* 33(2): 274–278.

19. Esposito C, Montupet P, and Reinberg O. 2001. Laparoscopic surgery for gastroesophageal reflux disease during the first year of life. *Journal of Pediatric Surgery* 36(5): 715–717.

20. Bordewick AJ, Bildner JI, and Burd RS. 2001. An effective approach for preventing and treating gastrostomy tube complications in newborns. *Neonatal Network* 20(2): 37–40.

21. DeVries PA. 1980. The pathogenesis of gastroschisis and omphalocele. *Journal of Pediatric Surgery* 15(3): 245–251.

22. Hoyme HE, Jones MC, and Jones KL. 1983. Gastroschisis: Abdominal wall disruption secondary to early gestational interruption of the omphalomesenteric artery. *Seminars in Perinatology* 7(4): 294–298.

23. Robinson JN, and Abuhamad AZ. 2000. Abdominal wall and umbilical cord anomalies. *Clinics in Perinatology* 27(4): 947–978.

24. Torfs CP, et al. 1994. A population based study of gastroschisis: Demographic, pregnancy, and lifestyle risk factors. *Teratology* 50(1): 44–53.

25. Torfs CP, et al. 1996. Maternal medications and environmental exposures as risk factors for gastroschisis. *Teratology* 54(2): 84–92.

26. Nichols CR, Dickinson JE, and Pemberton PJ. 1997. Rising incidence of gastroschisis in teenage pregnancies. *Journal of Maternal and Fetal Medicine* 6(4): 225–229.

27. Abuhamad AZ, et al. 1997. Superiormesenteric artery Doppler velocimetry and ultrasonographic assessment of fetal bowel in gastroschisis: A prospective longitudinal study. *American Journal of Obstetrics and Gynecology* 176(5): 985–990.

28. Luton D, et al. 1997. Prognostic factors of prenatally diagnosed gastroschisis. *Fetal Diagnostic Therapy* 12(1): 7–14.

29. Dunn JC, Fonkalsrud EW, and Atkinson JB. 1999. The influence of gestational age and mode of delivery on infants with gastroschisis. *Journal of Pediatric Surgery* 34(9): 1393–1395.

30. Reinhart BK, et al. 1999. Modern obstetric management and outcome of infants with gastroschisis. *Obstetrics and Gynecology* 94(1): 112–116.

31. Klein MD. 2005. Congenital abdominal wall defects. In *Pediatric Surgery,* 4th ed., Ashcraft KW, Holcomb GW, and Murphy JP, eds. Philadelphia: Saunders, 659–669.

32. Strodtbeck F. 1998. Abdominal wall defects. *Neonatal Network* 17(8): 51–53.

33. Mayer T, et al. 1980. Gastroschisis and omphalocele: An eight year review. *Annals of Surgery* 192(6): 783–787.

34. Nicolaides KH, et al. 1992. Fetal gastrointestinal and abdominal wall defects: Associated malformations and chromosomal effects. *Fetal Diagnostic Therapy* 7(2): 102–105.

35. Rescorla FJ. 2001. Surgical emergencies in the newborn. In *Workbook in Practical Neonatology,* 3rd ed., Polin RA, Yoder MC, and Burg FD, eds. Philadelphia: Saunders, 423–459.

36. Gilchrist BF, and Lessin MS. 2005. Lesions of the stomach. In *Pediatric Surgery,* 4th ed., Ashcraft KW, Holcomb GW, and Murphy JP, eds. Philadelphia: Saunders, 405–415.

37. Mitchell LE, and Risch N. 1993. The genetics of infantile hypertrophic pyloric stenosis: A reanalysis. *American Journal of Diseases of Children* 147(11): 1203–1211.

38. Kobayashi H, Wester T, and Puri P. 1997. Age related changes in innervation in hypertrophic pyloric stenosis. *Journal of Pediatric Surgery* 32(12): 704–707.

39. Dillon PW, and Cilley RE. 1993. Newborn surgical emergencies: Gastrointestinal anomalies, abdominal wall defects. *Pediatric Clinics of North America* 40(6): 1289–1314.

40. Miller AJW, Rode H, and Cywes S. 2005. Intestinal atresia and stenosis. In *Pediatric Surgery,* 4th ed., Ashcraft KW, Holcomb GW, and Murphy JP, eds. Philadelphia: Saunders, 416–434.

41. Gleason PE, Eddleman KA, and Stone JL. 2000. Gastrointestinal disorders of the fetus. *Clinics in Perinatology* 27(4): 901–920.

42. Kays DW. 1996. Surgical conditions of the neonatal intestinal tract. *Clinics in Perinatology* 23(2): 353–375.

43. Aiken JJ, and Oldham KT. 2005. Malrotation. In *Pediatric Surgery,* 4th ed., Ashcraft KW, Holcomb GW, and Murphy JP, eds. Philadelphia: Saunders, 435–447.

44. Cheng W, et al. 2001. Hirshprung's disease: A more generalized neuropathy? *Journal of Pediatric Surgery* 36(2): 296–299.

45. Coit AK. 1999. Necrotizing enterocolitis. *Journal of Perinatal & Neonatal Nursing* 12(4): 53–66.

46. St. Peter SD, and Ostlie DJ. 2005. Necrotizing enterocolitis. In *Pediatric Surgery,* 4th ed., Ashcraft KW, Holcomb GW, and Murphy JP, eds. Philadelphia: Saunders, 461–476.

47. Stoll SJ, and Kliegman RM. 2004. Digestive system disorders. In *Nelson Textbook of Pediatrics,* 17th ed., Behrman RE, Kleigman RM, and Jenson HB, eds. Philadelphia: Saunders, 590–592.

48. Kosloske AM. 1994. Epidemiology of necrotizing enterocolitis. *Acta Paediatrica* 83(supplement 396): S2–S7.

49. Kaul A, and Balistrei WF. 2002. Necrotizing enterocolitis. In *Neonatal-Perinatal Medicine: Diseases of the Fetus and Infant,* 7th ed., Fanaroff RA, and Martin RJ, eds. St. Louis: Mosby, 1299–1307.

50. Ledbetter DJ, and Juul SE. 2000. Necrotizing enterocolitis and hematopoietic cytokines. *Clinics in Perinatology* 27(3): 697–716.

51. Kosloske AM. 1985. Surgery of necrotizing enterocolitis. *World Journal of Surgery* 9(2): 277–284.

52. Pena A, and Levitt MA. 2005. Imperforate anus and cloacal malformations. In *Pediatric Surgery,* 4th ed., Ashcraft KW, Holcomb GW, and Murphy JP, eds. Philadelphia: Saunders, 496–517.

53. Sondheimer JM. 2003. Gastrointesinal tract. In *Current Pediatric Diagnosis and Treatment,* 16th ed., Hay WW, et al., eds. New York: Lange Medical Books/McGraw-Hill, 614-646.

54. Kiely EM, and Pena A. 1998. Anorectal malformations. In *Pediatric Surgery,* 5th ed., O'Neill JA, et al., eds. St. Louis: Mosby, 1425–1439.

55. Pena A. 2004. Surgical conditions of the anus, rectum, and colon. In *Nelson Textbook of Pediatrics,* 17th ed., Behrman RE, Kliegman RM, and Jenson HB, eds. Philadelphia: Saunders, 1285–1288.

56. Rothenberg SS. 2001. Minimally invasive surgery in neonates: A revolution in surgical approach. Lecture at American Academy of Pediatrics Section on Perinatal Pediatrics. Keystone, Colorado.

57. Levitt MA, et al. 1997. The tethered spinal cord in patients with anorectal malformations. *Journal of Pediatric Surgery* 32(3): 462–468.

58. Pena A, and Hong A. 2000. Advances in the management of anorectal malformations. *American Journal of Surgery* 180(5): 370–376.

59. Thomas KS. 2003. Assessment and management of the genitourinary system. In *Comprehensive Neonatal Nursing: A Physiologic Perspective,* 3rd ed., Kenner C, and Lott JW, eds. Philadelphia: Saunders, 673–699.

60. Weber TR, Tracy TF, and Keller MS. 2005. Groin hernias and hydroceles. In *Pediatric Surgery,* 4th ed., Ashcraft KW, Holcomb GW, and Murphy JP, eds. Philadelphia: Saunders, 697–705.

61. Kapur P, Caty MG, and Glick, PL. 1998. Pediatric hernias and hydroceles. *Pediatric Clinics of North America* 45(4): 773–789.

62. Aiken JJ. 2004. Inguinal hernias. In *Nelson Textbook of Pediatrics,* 17th ed., Behrman RE, Kliegman RM, and Jenson HB, eds. Phildelphia: Saunders, 1293–1297.

63. Berseth CL, and Poenaru D. 2005. Abdominal wall problems. In *Avery's Diseases of the Newborn,* 8th ed., Taeusch HW, Ballard RA, and Gleason CA, eds. Philadelphia: Saunders, 1113–1122.

64. DeCou JM, and Gauderer MW. 2000. Inguinal hernia in infants with very low birth weight. *Seminars in Pediatric Surgery* 9(2): 84–87.

65. Raffensperger JG. 1990. Inguinal hernia. In *Swenson's Pediatric Surgery,* 5th ed., Raffensperger JG, ed. Norwalk, Connecticut: Appleton & Lange, 121–133.

66. Misra D. 2001. Inguinal hernias in premature babies: Wait or operate? *Acta Paediatrica* 90(4): 370–371.

Notes

Surgical Conditions of the Liver, Gallbladder, and Biliary Apparatus

Alison Kirse Coit, MN, ARNP

The liver is a complex organ that has several functions. Its principal function is metabolism. It regulates and metabolizes substances absorbed by the intestines and the hormones produced in the gastrointestinal (GI) tract, and it converts glucose to glycogen. It stores and filters blood and excretes bilirubin and other substances into the GI tract. The liver has a double blood supply. It receives the majority of its blood from the portal vein and a smaller portion from the hepatic artery.

Biliary atresia is a rare but potentially fatal disorder of the development of the liver in which the bile ducts fail to form. Biliary atresia begins in early infancy when the incompletely formed bile ducts fail to drain bile into the GI tract. The infant presents with conjugated hyperbilirubinemia, and the liver suffers chronic injury that can lead to cirrhosis and liver failure. Early diagnosis improves prognosis. Biliary atresia is the most serious digestive disease affecting infants. There is obliteration or hypoplasia of part or all of the biliary system (extrahepatic and intrahepatic), resulting in the obstruction of bile flow, causing neonatal jaundice. It is the most common cause of cholestasis in infants and children. Untreated, the cholestasis leads to progressive conjugated hyperbilirubinemia, fibrosis, cirrhosis, and hepatic failure.[1-4]

Neuroblastoma is the most common malignant tumor in neonates. It is the most variable in its clinical presentation and its response to therapy, though it often presents as an abdominal mass with hepatomegaly. Neuroblastoma originates in the neural crest cells, which are located in nearly all viscera and the skin. Tumors can develop anywhere there is neural crest tissue, but are most common in the abdomen or pelvis. Treatment options depend on the staging of the tumor. Therapy can range from no treatment, to surgical excision, to a combination of chemotherapy and surgical removal of the tumor. The prognosis is inversely correlated to the age of the child at diagnosis and the extent of the disease. In the early stages of the disease, surgical treatment is usually curative.

Embryology

See Chapter 4: Neonatal Gastrointestinal Surgical Conditions, FOREGUT.

Biliary Atresia

DEFINITION

Part or all of the biliary system (extrahepatic and intrahepatic) is obliterated, resulting in the obstruction of bile flow. Because bile cannot leave the liver, it accumulates, causing it progressive damage.[1,5–7]

PATHOPHYSIOLOGY

A. Biliary atresia has perplexed physicians since the early 1800s. In 1817, Burns made the earliest report of a case of it, describing early jaundice and acholic stools.[8,9] In 1892, Thomson published a list of all reported cases in which the diagnosis of malformation, obliteration, or absence of the biliary tree was confirmed on postmortem examination.[10] Holmes, a pathologist, described a variety of forms of the disease in a review of 82 autopsies. He noted that approximately 16 percent of these children had patent proximal ducts or bile cysts that were potentially surgically correctable by removal of the obliterated segment.[11] Ladd reported a few surgical successes in removing the obstruction, although, in most cases, unfavorable anatomy made such cases irreparable.[12] Despite over a century of investigation, the pathophysiology of biliary atresia remains uncertain.

B. Bile is characterized by the following.
  1. It is a yellowish-green fluid made in the liver and stored in the gallbladder.
  2. It is made up of bile salts, cholesterol, and waste products (including bilirubin).
  3. It flows through the common bile ducts to the small intestine, where it aids in absorption and digestion of dietary fats and fat-soluble vitamins.[13,14]

C. The degree or extent of the obliteration of the biliary tree is variable (Figure 5-1).
  1. There are several classifications of biliary atresia.
     a. Complete intrahepatic biliary atresia
     b. Complete extrahepatic biliary atresia
     c. Hypoplasia of the extrahepatic biliary trees[13]

D. The most common type of biliary atresia is complete obliteration of the extrahepatic ducts (the delicate ducts outside the liver), patency of the distal biliary tree (gallbladder, cystic duct, and common duct), with proximal obliteration, and proximal hilar bile cysts.[3,15]

E. The extrahepatic bile ducts often have a residual patency into the porta hepatis. These structures communicate through a network with the intrahepatic ducts. The distal portions of the common duct are destroyed and are replaced by thick fibrous tissue. One or two functional bile ducts are seen with tiny functional biliary glands or collecting ducts. Proximally, the bile duct is surrounded by various degrees of fibrosis.[3,15]

F. The degree of fibrous obliteration of the extrahepatic ducts increases with the age of the patient.[3,15] In the first several months of life, there is a variable number

FIGURE 5-1 ■ **Morphologic classification of biliary atresia based on macroscopic and cholangiographic findings.**

Type I, occlusion of common bile duct; **Type IIa,** obliteration of common hepatic duct; **Type IIb,** obliteration of common bile duct, hepatic and cystic ducts, with cystic dilation of ducts at the porta hepatis, and no gallbladder involvement; **Type III,** obliteration of common, hepatic, and cystic ducts without anastomosable ducts at porta hepatic.

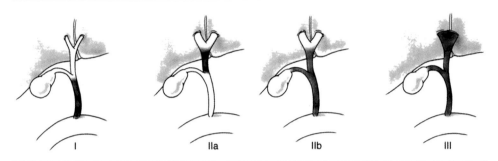

From: Lefkowitch JH, et al. 1998. Biliary atresia. *Mayo Clinic Proceedings* 73(1): 90. Reprinted by permission.

of patent intrahepatic ducts. The obstruction of extrahepatic ducts and fibrosis begin to destroy the intrahepatic ducts, which leads to hepatic fibrosis.[3,15]

G. The obstruction of the common bile ducts prevents bile from entering the duodenum. As a result, there is malabsorption of fats, leading to deficiencies in the fat-soluble vitamins, including vitamin K. Vitamin K deficiency increases the infant's risk of spontaneous bleeding, the most critical type being intracranial hemorrhage.[1,14]

H. The obstruction of the common bile ducts causes bile to accumulate in the ducts and gallbladder, resulting in distention. This atresia progresses to the intra-hepatic ducts, causing biliary cirrhosis and eventually death if bile flow is not established.[1,14]

ETIOLOGY

A. Originally, biliary atresia was thought to be a congenital malformation of the bile ducts.[2,3,16]

B. Some theorize the following.
1. The obstruction is caused by bile ducts that have been injured and become atretic.[4]
2. Biliary atresia occurs in two clinical forms.[9,17]
   a. The embryonic or fetal type (35 percent)
   b. The perinatal type (65 percent)
3. In both subtypes, the ongoing inflammatory process produces complete or partial sclerosis of the bile ducts.[4]

C. Others describe the disease as an inflammatory process.[15,16,18–20]

D. Many attribute the cause of biliary atresia to intrauterine or perinatal viral infections (Table 5-1).[15,16,18–20]
1. Serologic and immunohistochemical studies supported the concept of reovirus Type 3 as a viral causative agent for biliary atresia.[16,21]
2. Other investigations have examined the role of cytomegalovirus (CMV) and Group C rotavirus associated with biliary atresia.[22,23] Tarr and colleagues, in 1996, conducted a retrospective review and noted a 24 percent prevalence

TABLE 5-1 ■ Causes of Biliary Atresia[3,7,33]

Hematologic
Hemolytic disease
Neonatal hemochromatosis

Infectious

Viral
  Cytomegalovirus
  Rubella
  Hepatitis A and B
  Non-A, non-B hepatitis
  Herpes
  Reovirus Type III
  Coxsackie B
  HIV
  Echovirus, also known as enteric cytopathic human orphan (ECHO) virus
  Varicella
  Tuberculosis

Bacterial
  Listeriosis
  Toxoplasmosis
  Syphilis
  Tuberculosis

Metabolic

Disorders of amino acid metabolism
  Tyrosinemia
  Hypermethioninemia
Disorders of lipid metabolism
  Wolman's disease
  Niemann-Pick disease
  Gaucher's disease
Disorders of carbohydrate metabolism
  Galactosemia
  Fructosemia
  Glycogenosis IV

Metabolic disease in which the disease is uncharacterized
  α_1-antitrypsin deficiency
  Cystic fibrosis
  Hypopituitarism
  Hypothyroidism
  Neonatal iron storage disease
  Infantile copper overload
  Multiple acyl-CoA dehydrogenation deficiency (glutaric acid type II)
  Familial erythrophagocytic lymphohistiocytosis

Anatomic abnormalities

Extrahepatic
  Biliary atresia
  Biliary hypoplasia
  Bile duct stenosis
  Choledochal-pancreatic ductal junction anomaly
  Spontaneous perforation of bile duct
  Mass (neoplasia, stone)
  Bile/mucus plug

Intrahepatic
  Idiopathic neonatal hepatitis
  Intrahepatic cholestasis, persistent
    Nonsyndromic paucity of intrahepatic ducts
    Alagille syndrome (arteriohepatic dysplasia)
    Byler disease (severe intrahepatic cholestasis with progressive hepatocellular disease)
    Trihydroxycoprostanic acidemia (defective bile acid metabolism and cholestasis)
    Zellweger syndrome (cerebrohepatorenal syndrome)
  Intrahepatic cholestasis, recurrent
    Familial benign recurrent cholestasis
    Hereditary cholestasis with lymphedema (Aagenaes)
  Congenital cystic fibrosis
  Caroli's disease (cystic dilation of the hepatic ducts)

Systemic
Postnecrotizing enterocolitis intestinal obstruction
Congestive heart failure
Left hypoplastic heart syndrome
Sepsis
Shock/hypoperfusion
Drug induced
Cholestasis associated with parenteral nutrition

Miscellaneous
Histiocytosis X
Polysplenia syndrome
Trisomy 17, 18, 21
Turner's syndrome (XO)

of CMV in patients with biliary atresia. This compared to the typical 1–2.4 percent prevalence of CMV in newborns in the U.S.[24]

E. Some reports note an increased incidence of biliary atresia in infants born August to March.[25,26] Other studies found no such clustering.[27,28]

INCIDENCE

A. The disease is ubiquitous, affecting approximately 1/10,000–15,000 live births.[1,5–7] In the U.S., there are 400–600 cases of biliary atresia annually.[1,5–7]

B. There is a slight predominance of occurrence in females.

C. The incidence of biliary atresia in African-American infants is approximately twice that of Caucasian infants. It is also seen with increased frequency in Japanese and Chinese infants when compared to Caucasian infants.[1,25,29]

D. Biliary atresia has been reported to recur in families, including in twins, but there does not appear to be an increased incidence in families.[22,30–32]

E. Biliary atresia is more common in low birth weight infants, especially those born at term; however, it is rarely seen in stillborns or premature infants.[1]

F. Yoon found no relation between the incidence of biliary atresia and maternal age or parity.[25]

CLINICAL PRESENTATION

A. The history is usually a full-term infant who appeared normal at birth. The primary sign of biliary atresia is increasing, persistent jaundice that develops between two and six weeks of life.

B. Often, the clinical signs are insidious and caused by decreasing bile flow.

C. The direct bilirubin rises, causing a greenish-bronze appearance of the skin, a result of bilirubin mixed with greenish discoloration from biliverdin.[1,3,4,7,14,15]

D. Acholic stools (clay or lightly colored), are caused by the absence of bile in the stool.
  1. In many cases, the infant will pass the clay-colored stools from the fourth or fifth day of life.
  2. Sometimes the stools do not become clay colored for several weeks or months.
    a. This can be attributed to heavily jaundiced epithelial cells that are sloughed off and incorporated into the bulk of the stools.[1,3,14,15,33]
  3. Acholic stools can also be associated with severe neonatal hepatitis.[33]

E. Dark brown urine, resulting from a high bile content

F. Hepatosplenomegaly or distended abdomen[1,3,14,15,33,34]
  1. The liver is enlarged and firm, and there is an appreciable spleen.
  2. Venous dilation appears over the surface of the protuberant abdomen, and ascites develop.
  3. In many cases, this is a reflection of the underlying portal fibrosis.
  4. Liver damage, which can interfere with normal blood flow in the liver
  5. Children who have more progressive liver disease develop malnutrition and clinical findings that indicate portal hypertension.[1]
    a. Portal hypertension is the increase in blood pressure in the veins of the portal system (between the intestines and the spleen to the liver).
    b. This increased pressure may make the veins become enlarged and begin to leak, causing internal bleeding.[1]

    c. Weight loss and malnutrition[1,3,14,15,33]
      1) Adequate bile flow is necessary to aid in the digestion and absorption of dietary fats and fat-soluble vitamins (A, D, E, and K).
      2) When there is a decrease in bile flow, poor growth and malnutrition may result.

ASSOCIATIONS

A. Developmental abnormalities of the heart, digestive tract, or spleen (polysplenia syndrome) and anomalies such as situs inversus, malrotation, preduodenal portal vein, and absent inferior vena cava occur in syndromic (embryonic) biliary atresia (10–20 percent of cases).[2,3,7]

B. Other congenital defects, including small bowel atresia, bronchobiliary atresia, and trisomies 17 and 18, occur in approximately 15 percent of reported cases.[14]

C. There is no difference in histologic features of the liver between infants with and without congenital anomalies.

DIFFERENTIAL DIAGNOSIS

A. The inherited metabolic abnormality α_1-antitrypsin deficiency often presents clinically as neonatal jaundice and can imitate biliary atresia. These patients most commonly have jaundice in the first eight weeks of life.[6] This disorder occurs in approximately 5–10 percent of infants with cholestasis and can be ruled out with an α_1-antitrypsin level.[6]

B. Neonates with cystic fibrosis (CF) may develop cholestasis. A liver biopsy demonstrates inspissated bile and mucus in the intrahepatic bile ducts. A sweat chloride test confirms the CF diagnosis. These infants often resolve their jaundice.[6]

C. Another potentially devastating but treatable metabolic illness presenting with cholestasis is galactosemia. The incidence is 1/100,000. These infants present with early onset cholestasis, hepatomegaly, and often have associated emesis, growth failure, acidosis, or Gram-negative sepsis. While these patients are on lactose-containing feedings, galactose will spill into the urine, producing a positive urine for reducing sugars and a negative urine for glucose. The initiation of a galactose- and lactose-free diet may prevent further damage.[6,7,35]

D. Other diagnoses to consider include these.[6,7,35]
    1. Alagille syndrome
    2. Caroli disease
    3. Cholestasis
    4. Cytomegalovirus infection
    5. Neonatal hemochromatosis
    6. Herpes simplex virus infection
    7. Lipid storage disorders
    8. Rubella
    9. Syphilis
  10. Toxoplasmosis
  11. Byler disease
  12. Idiopathic neonatal hepatitis
  13. Inborn errors of bile acid synthesis
  14. Nonsyndromic intrahepatic bile duct hypoplasia

DIAGNOSIS

A. Maternal blood tests
  1. TORCH (an acronym for **t**oxoplasmosis, **o**ther viruses, **r**ubella virus, **c**ytomegalovirus, and **h**erpes simplex virus)
  2. VDRL (Venereal Disease Research Laboratories) titers
  3. Hepatitis profile
B. Neonatal blood tests (Table 5-2)
  1. Total and direct bilirubin serum levels (a direct bilirubin elevated more than 2 mg/dl (34 μmol/liter) or 20 percent of the total bilirubin level)
  2. Rh, type, Coombs test
  3. Complete blood count (CBC)
    a. The red and white blood cell counts are within the normal range.
    b. The hemoglobin level is normal.
    c. There is no excess of nucleated erythrocytes or reticulocytes.
  4. Peripheral smear
    a. Blood counts are normal in the neonatal period.
    b. By four to six weeks of age, many infants are anemic, with increases in their reticulocyte count.[3,7,14,35]
  5. Viral and bacterial cultures of blood, urine, and spinal fluid[3,7,14,35]
  6. A metabolic screen that includes urine and serum amino acids and urine-reducing substances
    a. This will identify treatable metabolic causes of biliary atresia, including the following.
      1) α_1-antitrypsin deficiency
      2) Cystic fibrosis
      3) Galactosemia
    b. Early detection of any of these metabolic or endocrine disorders aids in evaluating neonatal jaundice.[3,7,14,35]
  7. Liver function tests
    a. These usually are abnormal once cirrhotic changes have started.
    b. Blood cholesterol levels tend to rise as liver damage increases.[3,7,14,24,35]
  8. Other laboratory tests
    a. Vitamin deficiency may exist.[3,7,14,24,35]
      1) The absence of bile salts in the intestine leads to poorly absorbed fat-soluble vitamins.
      2) The deficiencies of vitamins A, D, and K do not manifest themselves until after the neonatal period because hepatocellular damage is not immediately present.
      3) Vitamin E deficiency may be demonstrated by laboratory tests.

TABLE 5-2 ■ Evaluation of Infant with Jaundice

Recognize the infant with prolonged jaundice, including evaluation of stool color

Review family history, prenatal course, postnatal course

Laboratory work:
• TORCH, VDRL, hepatitis profile to rule out perinatal infections
• Total and direct bilirubin
• Type and blood group
• Coombs test
• CBC, including:
  Reticulocyte count
  Peripheral smear
  Prothrombin time
• Viral and bacterial cultures (blood, urine, and spinal fluid)
• α_1-antitrypsin phenotype
• Metabolic screen (urine/serum amino acids, urine reducing substances)
• Thyroxine and thyroid stimulating hormone
• Sweat chloride test

Diagnostic studies:
• Abdominal ultrasound to exclude structural abnormalities of the biliary tree
• Hepatobiliary scintigraphy or duodenal intubation for bilirubin content
• Liver biopsy to differentiate biliary atresia from other forms of intrahepatic cholestasis

    4) Vitamin K deficiency results in a prolonged prothrombin time (PT).

    5) These children are at risk for developing a coagulopathy due to vitamin K deficiency and subsequently are at risk for developing spontaneous hemorrhage.

  b. Serum levels of γ-glutamyl transpeptidase are elevated.

  c. Successive measures of serum alkaline phosphatase, transaminases, or total bilirubin do not distinguish between biliary atresia and other forms of cholestasis. However, these tests help the clinician to recognize infants who need further evaluation.[1,14]

C. Ultrasonography

  1. This is an expeditious, noninvasive tool with real-time imaging.[1,6,14,36,37]

  2. Ultrasound can illustrate the hepatobiliary tree structure for the following.[1,38]

    a. The presence and size of the gallbladder

    b. Choledochal cysts

    c. Cholelithiasis

    d. Perforation of the bile duct

    e. Polysplenia

    f. Vascular anomalies

  3. The abdominal ultrasound will show the following.[1,3,7,37]

    a. No dilation of the biliary ducts

    b. A small, shrunken, noncontractile gallbladder

      1) The gallbladder of normal neonates increases in size during feeding and contracts after feeding.

      2) This process does not occur with biliary atresia because of the obstruction of the biliary tree.[37]

      3) Infants with intrahepatic cholestasis caused by neonatal hepatitis, cystic fibrosis, and total parenteral nutrition (TPN) liver disease may have similar ultrasound findings.[1]

    c. Increased echogenicity of the liver

D. Computed tomography (CT) and magnetic resonance imaging (MRI)

  1. These provide information similar to that obtained from an abdominal ultrasound.

  2. Heavy sedation is needed for best results.[13]

E. Hepatobiliary scintigraphy or hepatobiliary iminodiacetic acid (HIDA) scan

  1. Hepatobiliary scintigraphy with technetium-99-IDM (TC-99) has been the "gold standard" in the evaluation of infants with hyperbilirubinemia. TC-99, a radioactive dye, is injected intravenously into the infant. In the normal physiologic state, hepatocytes remove this compound from the blood, secrete it into the bile canaliculi, to the bile ducts, and eventually into the intestinal lumen. The dye goes everywhere the bile goes. In biliary atresia, this dye fails to clear the liver and biliary tree.[38]

  2. Hepatobiliary scintigraphy is not specific to biliary atresia because patients with cystic fibrosis and severe neonatal hepatitis also fail to excrete the isotope into the gut.[1] Pretreatment with phenobarbital for three to five days will maximize bile excretion, presumably by relieving cholestasis, and enhance the accuracy of hepatobiliary imaging.[15,37] Although cholescintigraphy is a sensitive diagnostic tool, it will not identify other structural or vascular anomalies.[1]

F. Endoscopic retrograde cholangiopancreatography (ERCP)[1,39]
  1. Clinicians who support the use of ERCP contend that its use will prevent unnecessary laparotomy if the endoscopist finds patent bile ducts.
  2. The procedure is expensive, requires significant endoscopic skill, and is not widely available.
G. Liver biopsy
  1. If laboratory tests, ultrasound, HIDA scan, and perhaps other tests suggest biliary atresia, a percutaneous liver biopsy should be done.
  2. This is the most specific and valuable method of diagnosis.
  3. It can be performed on the smallest infants using sedation and local anesthesia.
  4. If an adequate sample is obtained, with five to seven portal spaces, the diagnostic accuracy is 95 percent.[40]
  5. The diagnosis of biliary atresia is confirmed when the gallbladder is replaced by a fibrous remnant with a proliferation of the bile ducts, demonstrating bile duct obliteration.[5,6,41] The amount of fibrosis or cirrhosis correlates with the infant's age. The older the infant, the greater the amount of fibrosis or cirrhosis seen.[42]
  6. If the diagnosis is verified, hepatic portoenterostomy is recommended as soon as possible. Evaluation and therapeutic intervention among the primary care provider, pediatric gastroenterologist, and pediatric surgeon should be completed within approximately one week of identification of an infant with biliary atresia.

TREATMENT OPTIONS AND NURSING CARE

A. In 1959, Kasai and Suzuki described hepatic portoenterostomy, a new procedure that transformed the management of biliary atresia. Improved diagnostic technology and the portoenterostomy procedure have become the standards for diagnosis and treatment of extrahepatic biliary atresia. Liver transplantation is used when intrahepatic disease or damage is severe.[43]
B. Nurses are instrumental in assisting with the task of evaluation, diagnosis, and treatment of biliary atresia. The age at surgery is critical in both short-term and long-term outcomes. Long-term survival decreases with increasing age at surgery.[44]
C. Many skills the nurse will utilize preoperatively involve obtaining necessary blood and urine samples and assisting with procedures. Daily laboratory blood work results of electrolyte levels, total and direct bilirubin, clotting time, and CBC with differential will be monitored. If the infant is anemic, blood transfusions are imperative.[45-47]
D. Hypoprothrombinemia is a typical complication in untreated patients with biliary atresia. If the PT is elevated, daily administration of 10 mg of vitamin K_1 usually improves serum thrombin time in five to seven days. If the patient's prothrombin level is within normal limits, 1–2 mg of vitamin K_1 is indicated.
E. The bowel is prepared for surgery by the administration of antibiotics. Kanamycin (Neomycin), 50 mg by mouth every 8 hours, is given approximately 24–36 hours prior to surgery.[45,46]
F. The bedside nurse remains critical in providing support to parents and family members. Included is the challenging task of helping the parents to cope. The diagnosis of biliary atresia and its consequences can be overwhelming to a

family, who for the first several weeks of their infant's life thought they had a normal child.

SURGICAL MANAGEMENT

A. Kasai portoenterostomy
1. This procedure consists of removal of the obliterated extrahepatic ducts and anastomosis of an intestinal conduit to the transected ducts at the liver hilum. This permits bile drainage from the liver surface to the GI tract. Its success is based on the residual patency of the tiny bile ducts in the fibrous cone at the porta hepatis.[48,49]
2. In an effort to reduce postoperative cholangitis, improve bile drainage, and lengthen survival, portoenterostomy has been altered by many surgeons. Several use a temporary exteriorization of the conduit, thinking this will decrease the gradient the hepatic secretory pressure has to overcome. In addition, exteriorization allows monitoring of bile output and bilirubin clearance. Commonly used exteriorization techniques are double-Y anastomosis of Kasai, Sawaguchi's total exteriorization of the conduit, and a double-barreled exteriorization of the midportion of the Roux-en-Y.[3] If a stoma is used, it should be closed as soon as the bile flow reaches a steady state to avoid complications such as variceal hemorrhage.[3] Using a valve in the conduit also appears to lessen the susceptibility to cholangitis, presumably by decreasing the bacteria count above the valve.[3]
3. Following these procedures, it is difficult to predict when sufficient bile drainage will be established and when jaundice will clear. Serum bilirubin may fall to normal anytime between three weeks and six months later.[47] Bile ducts in the porta hepatis lined with columnar epithelium correlate with favorable prognosis.[50]
4. Since the introduction of the Kasai portoenterostomy, the results of operative treatment have continuously improved. Many children grow well and lead normal lives of good quality. In all forms of biliary atresia, success depends on timely recognition of signs and symptoms and expeditious facilitation before the obstruction leads to biliary cirrhosis.

B. Liver transplantation
1. In children, biliary atresia is the most common indication for a liver transplant. However, primary transplantation is not recommended and may not significantly alter survival.[1,2,40,51]
2. There are advantages to using a Kasai portoenterostomy prior to transplantation.[1,52]
   a. Allowing the patient to grow and gain weight
   b. Allowing time for immunizations to be given prior to transplantation and subsequent immunosuppression
   c. Improved donor availability
   d. Decreased allograft complications
   e. More time for the family to plan for living-related donor options
3. Approximately 50–65 percent of infants who have undergone a portoenterostomy will require liver transplantation.[40,43,53]
   a. The most important prognostic factor in pediatric liver transplantation is the age and size of the recipient. Children weighing less than 10–12 kg had a lower survival rate, and hepatic artery thrombosis was a frequent complication.[4,13,40]

    b. If a graft is too large, it impinges on breathing and can prevent closure of the abdomen.

    c. If the donor organ is too small, its function may not be adequate for survival.[51]

    d. Most biliary atresia recipients need transplantation within the first two years of life.[4,13,40]

    e. Children older than two years who receive a transplant are at decreased risk of developing a posttransplant lymphoproliferative disease.[13,40,52]

4. When the Kasai portoenterostomy is unsuccessful or the signs and symptoms of end-stage liver disease appear, which may be 9–18 months after a failed portoenterostomy, transplantation is the last option and can be a lifesaving alternative.[1,2,40]

5. Signs and symptoms of end-stage liver disease include the following.[40]

    a. Recurrent cholangitis

    b. Progressive jaundice

    c. Portal hypertension

    d. Ascites

    e. Decreased liver function

    f. Malnutrition and growth failure

6. The length of time waiting for a donor organ is critical to children with biliary atresia because they can develop complications of cirrhosis and portal hypertension by 12 months of age. It is crucial to identify children who did not benefit from portoenterostomy because their disease will rapidly progress, and their need for a liver transplant becomes vitally important.[1,40]

7. Since the mid-1980s, liver transplantation has been increasingly successful. However, the availability of donor organs does not meet the demand. This remains a critical obstacle for a successful outcome. This incongruity has led to the development of several surgical procedures to increase the donor organ pool. These include reduced-size liver transplantation, living-related donor transplantation, and donor livers with ABO blood types mismatched with the recipient's blood type. These factors have increased the donor pool size and allowed for better patient preparation and timing of the procedure.[38,52,54]

8. Many centers now report a one-year survival rate of approximately 90 percent.[43,53] Efforts to improve organ donor resources will allow more timely transplantation, which will decrease morbidity and improve the long-term survival of children with this devastating disease.

COMPLICATIONS

A. Complications associated with Kasai portoenterostomy are cholangitis, decreased bile flow, portal hypertension, metabolic dysfunction, pruritus, ascites, and surgical failure.

1. Cholangitis

    a. This is the most frequent and severe complication after surgery, occurring in up to 50 percent of survivors.[1,45]

    b. The bile ducts become inflamed.

    c. The primary cause is reflux of intestinal contents into the bile duct and stenosis of the anastomosis. Because the bowel is colonized by bacteria, this reflux of organisms results in edema of the bile duct, which disturbs bile flow. The bile flow is inhibited secondary to a narrowing of the anastomosis, and infection can develop.[45] Repetitive attacks of cholangitis are serious because permanent hepatic damage can result from each attack.[7,47] For this reason, routine antibiotics, choleretics, and steroids are used as postoperative medications.[55]

1) Broad-spectrum antibiotics, including a cephalosporin at 50–80 mg/kg/day and gentamicin at 2–4 mg/kg/day, are administered for several weeks after the surgery. Then oral antibiotics are given for several months. Long-term prophylactic antibiotics may reduce the incidence of cholangitis.[47,55]

2) For choleretics, an intravenous injection of 3 ml of 10 percent dehydrocholic acid, diluted with 7 ml of 5 percent glucose, is started on the day of surgery and administered every 12 hours for several months until the serum bilirubin is less than 2 mg/dl. Ursodeoxycholic acid, 15–40 mg/kg/day divided every 6–8 hours, is given orally.[40,55] These bile salts may decrease the rate and pace of occlusion of the draining bile duct and promote bile flow.[40]

3) In the immediate postoperative period, steroids are started: Methylprednisolone, 1.6–2 mg/kg/day, divided four times a day, is administered intravenously.[55] Corticosteroids are a potent anti-inflammatory agent that may stimulate bile salt flow. Some centers have found that high-dose, short-term therapy may improve the likelihood of achieving adequate bile drainage.[55]

   d. These measures have succeeded in reducing the frequency and severity of biliary infection, but they have not eliminated the problem.

2. Portal hypertension
   a. Elevated portal pressure is present in the majority of infants and remains a major complication after surgery.[3,47]
   b. It results from an increased resistance of venous flow to the liver[3,47]
   c. Postoperative cholangitis prevents the portal pressure from decreasing, and it aggravates the portal hypertension.[56]
   d. Postoperatively, portal hypertension can progress despite adequate bile flow.[3,47]
   e. Clinical manifestations include enlargement of the esophageal, umbilical, and rectal veins, which appear as splenomegaly, hemorrhoids, enlarged abdominal veins, ascites, and blood in the stool.[3,14]
   f. The complications associated with portal hypertension, particularly esophageal variceal hemorrhage and, less frequently, hepatopulmonary syndrome, occur in greater than 60 percent of long-term survivors.[1]

      1) GI bleeding from esophageal varices can suddenly occur in patients up to three to five years after surgery. Over time, the severity and frequency of variceal bleeding diminish in some patients. This may be due to the improved portosystemic shunts.[3,57] Others require endoscopic sclerotherapy to effectively treat esophageal varices.[5]

B. Complications of liver transplant include the following.[1,40,52]
   1. Biliary anastomotic leaks (Most can be repaired surgically.)
   2. Biliary strictures (repaired surgically)
   3. Hepatic artery thrombosis
   4. Portal vein thrombosis
   5. Venous outflow obstruction (present with graft dysfunction)
   6. Infection

7. Rejection (Some are treated with cyclosporin therapy; others with chronic rejection need to be retransplanted.)
8. Bowel perforation, both small and large bowel (surgically treated)
9. Lymphoproliferative disease

POSTOPERATIVE NURSING CARE

A. Post-Kasai portoenterostomy
  1. Immediate postoperative care
     a. Monitor vital signs. Monitor for signs and symptoms of infection (fever, tachycardia, increased work of breathing). Rule out cholangitis.
     b. Decompress the GI tract. Accurately record intake and output. Note color and amount of GI secretions. Decreasing bile secretion postoperatively could indicate cholangitis. If there is bloody drainage, suspect GI bleeding.
     c. Intravenous fluid is the source of hydration until feedings are established. Accurately infuse a volume sufficient to avoid electrolyte imbalances. Monitor daily electrolyte blood levels. If the infant has ascites, restrict fluids and sodium.
     d. Evaluate lab values.
        1) Leukocytosis
        2) Shift in white blood cell differential
        3) Increasing bilirubin
        4) Worsening liver function
        5) Positive blood cultures (Notify the attending physician when positive blood cultures are reported.)
        6) Worsening PT or partial thromboplastin time (PTT)
     e. Liver biopsy is performed if a failed procedure is suspected.
        1) Signs and symptoms of liver failure (as noted above)
     f. Administer postoperative medications.
        1) Antibiotics to decrease the rate of infection
        2) Choleretics to improve drainage of the bile ducts
        3) Steroids to decrease edema of the bile ducts
  2. Bile flow
     a. Infants who excrete large quantities of bile after surgery have improved survival rates. Poor bile flow is associated with cholangitis, and the operation is unsuccessful unless bile flow is reestablished. Monitoring serum bilirubin concentrations is of critical importance postoperatively.[1,3]
     b. Corticosteroids are started to augment bile flow and to reduce inflammation. If bile flow is not reestablished, reoperation may be indicated.[1,3]
  3. Pruritus
     a. Pruritus is difficult to manage and appears more frequently when there is more fibrosis.[58] Improve patient comfort as much as possible.
     b. To decrease itching, there needs to be an increase in the conversion of cholesterol to bile acids, and the elimination of retained bile acids must increase.[33] If biliary drainage is poor, this is difficult to achieve.
     c. Medications used to help with pruritus include antihistamines, cholestyramine, phenobarbital, and rifampin. Antihistamines provide a tranquilizing effect, cholestyramine reduces enterohepatic circulation of bile acids, and phenobarbital increases biliary flow.[7] Phenobarbital and

cholestyramine will be effective only if there is adequate bile drainage to allow bile acids to reach the GI lumen.[33]

4. Skin care/ascites

   a. Limit handling, turning the infant approximately every three hours.

   b. Ascitic fluid develops when lymph formation exceeds the limits of lymph absorption. If ascites and liver failure develop, the infant should be placed on restricted sodium intake (1–2 mEq/kg/day).[3,6]

   c. If the fluid management does not decrease the ascites, then the use of diuretics should be considered. Acute diuresis can be managed with furosemide. Spironolactone is preferred over furosemide for chronic diuretic therapy.[3,6]

   d. Dressing changes.

      1) A dressing will cover the wound.

      2) Monitor it for drainage (both color and quantity).

      3) A thin, soft rubber drain may have been inserted below the incision to allow excess fluid to drain.[3,6]

   e. Once the incision has healed, the sutures will be removed, usually about two weeks after surgery.[3,6]

5. Nutrition

   a. Intravenous fluids and nasogastric decompression are continued until bowel activity returns. This usually happens within three to five days after surgery.[55]

   b. Optimizing nutritional intake reduces malnutrition. TPN minimizes these effects and provides adequate vitamins, minerals, and calories. But metabolic problems associated with the absorption of vitamins, minerals, and the metabolism of fats and proteins can still occur.[55]

   c. Meeting nutritional requirements is challenging because hepatic dysfunction results in poor weight gain. Poor nutritional support can result in diminished linear growth, decreased weight gain, decreased fat stores, and increased muscle wasting.[1]

      1) Protein/calorie malnutrition results from low caloric intake, fat malabsorption caused by cholestasis, insensitivity to growth hormone, and increased energy expenditure.

      2) The sequelae of fat-soluble vitamin deficiencies are rickets (vitamin D), ataxic neuropathy (vitamin E), coagulopathy (vitamin K), and keratopathy (vitamin A). Essential fatty acid deficiency is also a major problem of malabsorption. Because of impaired absorption, phenobarbital, cholestyramine, and vitamins A, D, E, and K are given for at least one year after surgery.[47,55]

      3) Intraluminal bile salts are essential for enteral absorption of fat. Abnormalities in the metabolism of fat, protein, water, fat-soluble vitamins, iron, calcium, zinc, and copper have been described in children with liver disease both pre- and postoperatively.[59]

   d. Careful monitoring of the clinical symptoms of nutritional deficiencies and serum vitamin levels is needed long after surgery.

   e. Feeding proceeds as follows.

      1) It is started after five to six postoperative days to allow adequate bowel rest.[14,55]

      2) Once the child is ready to eat, the pressure on the stomach contributes to the difficulty with managing feedings.[14]

3) Until normal bile drainage is achieved, formulas should contain medium-chain triglycerides (MCTs) for easier absorption.[14]

4) Breastfed infants should be given MCT supplements.[14]

5) Monitor the following.
  a) Daily weights, to evaluate fluid retention
  b) Weekly head circumferences, to track growth
  c) Nutritional deficiencies

6) Consider the following in regard to discharge.
  a) If there are no complications following surgery, discharge home can occur within two weeks.
  b) Discharge criteria include the following.[14,55]
    • Having no fever or signs of infection
    • Tolerating feedings
    • Gaining weight

OUTCOMES

A. Untreated, biliary atresia will have a survival time of less than two years, with a median survival of eight months.

B. Kasai's portoenterostomy has positively affected the outcome of biliary atresia, but its long-term impact is controversial. One study from Japan concluded that biliary atresia patients had a 10-year survival rate of 70 percent if surgery occurred before 60 days.[1,60] Ten-year survival rates of 73 percent and 92 percent have been reported for infants in whom jaundice has cleared.[55,60,61] For those patients who remain jaundiced with inadequate bile flow, the 3-year survival rate decreased to 20 percent. However, a nationwide study of the surgical section of the American Academy of Pediatrics found that long-term survival rate was only 25 percent.[42] The overall survival rate 5 years after the initial Kasai portoenterostomy ranges from 40 to 62 percent, decreasing to 25 to 33 percent at 10 years and 10 to 20 percent by 20 years.[40]

C. The portoenterostomy may allow children with only partially sufficient drainage time to grow before consideration of a liver transplant.

D. Long-term prognosis after surgery depends on several factors.[40,44,47,62,63]
  1. Age at surgery
  2. Histology of tissue resected from the porta hepatis
  3. Incidence of cholangitis
  4. Severity of portal hypertension
  5. Progress of intrahepatic inflammatory disease
  6. Technical aspects of Kasai's operation
  7. Presence of ducts in the extrahepatic biliary remnant (Histologic studies show that this is time related. By four months of age, there remains only fibrous tissue in the hilum.)[3]

Neuroblastoma

DEFINITION

Neuroblastoma is the most common extracranial malignant tumor in infancy. It originates from the neural crest cells that normally give rise to the adrenal medulla and sympathetic ganglia.

Pathophysiology

A. It arises from primitive, pluripotent, sympathetic cells (sympathogonia), which are derived from the neural crest and normally form the tissues and the different organs of the sympathetic nervous system.

   1. May arise anywhere along the sympathetic ganglia or within the adrenal medulla[64–66]

B. Neuroblastoma is a lobular, fleshy tumor, most commonly found in the abdominal cavity (adrenals, paraspinal ganglia).

   1. Other presenting sites include the following.

      a. Thorax

      b. Pelvis

      c. Neck

   2. It has poorly defined margins.

   3. Infants present with more cervical and thoracic tumors, and older children present with abdominal tumors.[64-66]

C. Seen under a light microscope, the tumor is composed of uniform small round blue cells in a fibrovascular matrix.

   1. The typical tumor shows small uniform cells with scant cytoplasm and hyperchromatic nuclei.

   2. Fifty percent of tumors have microcalcification and form Homer-Wright pseudorosettes with eosinophilic fibrillar material in the interstitial space.[64,66,67]

D. Electron microscopy reveals these subcellular features.[65,67,68]

   1. Dense core

   2. Membrane-bound neurosecretory granules

   3. Microfilaments

   4. Parallel arrays of microtubules

E. There are three histopathologic patterns of neurocrest tumors. These represent a variety of maturation, differentiation, and clinical behavior:[67,68]

   1. Neuroblastoma

   2. Ganglioneuroblastoma

   3. Ganglioneuroma

Etiology

A. This is unknown in most cases.

B. Environmental factors may increase the risk in offspring. However, most studies suggesting this are not confirmed.[69–76]

   1. Prenatal exposure to hydantoin, phenobarbital, or alcohol

   2. Maternal exposure to diuretics, tranquilizers, prescription pain medications, or hair coloring

   3. Paternal occupational exposure to electromagnetic fields

Incidence

A. Neuroblastoma accounts for 8–10 percent of all childhood cancers.[77]

   1. There are approximately 650 newly diagnosed cases in the U.S. each year.

   2. This corresponds to an incidence of 9.5 million cases/year.[77–81]

B. Neuroblastoma is slightly more common in boys than girls, with a male to female ratio of 1.2:1.[77–81]

C. A subset of patients may develop this disease with an autosomal dominant pattern of inheritance. Median age at diagnosis is 9 months versus 22 months in nonfamilial-related neuroblastomas.[82–84]
   1. Twenty-two percent may be the result of germinal mutation.[85]
   2. Twenty percent with familial neuroblastoma have bilateral adrenal or multifocal primary tumors.[86]
D. There is no consistent pattern of chromosomal abnormalities. Approximately 70 percent have a deleted or rearranged short arm of chromosome 1.[87–92]

CLINICAL PRESENTATION

A. Neuroblastomas can arise from anywhere along the sympathetic nervous system. The locations of the primary tumors are varied and change with the age of the child at the time of diagnosis. The signs and symptoms reflect the location of the primary, regional, and metastatic tumors.
   1. Abdominal mass, the most common clinical presentation, occurs in 65 percent.[93–98]
      a. Abdominal distention secondary to abdominal mass[93–98]
      b. Anorexia secondary to abdominal mass[96]
      c. Weight loss secondary to abdominal mass[96]
   2. Subcutaneous masses occur in approximately 32 percent.[93,94,99]
   3. Primary tumors cannot be located in 1 percent of patients.[93,99,100]
   4. Thoracic neuroblastomas also occur.
      a. Respiratory distress secondary to thoracic neuroblastomas that develop in the posterior mediastinum[93–98]
      b. Dyspnea secondary to thoracic tumors
   5. Paraspinal tumors may invade the intravertebral foramina, causing cord compression and "dumbbell-shaped tumors" that result in bladder and bowel dysfunction.[77]
      a. Bladder dysfunction secondary to cord compression from a paraspinal tumor[97,98]
      b. Bowel/anal sphincter dysfunction secondary to spinal cord compression from a paraspinal tumor[97,98]
      c. Gait disturbances secondary to a spinal column tumor (i.e., dumbbell-shaped tumors) and bone pain[77,93–98,101]
      d. Paraplegia secondary to a spinal column tumor (This represents a medical emergency because of the possibility of spinal cord compression and the long-term effects of paraplegia.)[77]
   6. Other presentations include the following.
      a. Abdominal pain may be secondary to a hemorrhage within the lesion.[97,98]
      b. Anemia may be secondary to a hemorrhage and bone marrow involvement.[94,96]
      c. Hypertension may be secondary to catecholamine production or renal vascular compression.[96]
      d. Cervical masses are usually fixed and hard to locate. They may be associated with Horner's syndrome and tracheal compression.[93–98]
      e. "Raccoon eyes" occur when there is a periorbital hemorrhage secondary to a metastatic tumor.[82,100,102–105]
      f. Bluish subcutaneous nodules are present in 30 percent.[65,95,101]

    g. Kerner-Morrison syndrome consists of intractable diarrhea, an unusual presentation, and is related to the release of vasoactive intestinal peptide. Symptoms resolve when the tumor is removed.[105,106–108]

    h. Scrotal and lower extremity edema may be secondary to abdominal tumors that compress venous and lymphatic drainage.[97,98]

    i. Horner's syndrome, which consists of unilateral eyelid drooping, sinking in of the eyeball, constriction of the pupil, narrowing of the palpebral fissure, and anhidrosis, is associated with thoracic and cervical tumors. Symptoms do not resolve with tumor removal.[82,100,102–105]

    j. Hutchinson syndrome involves metastasis to the bone marrow and causes bone pain and limping in older children.[82,100,102–105,109–111]

    k. Lung, bone, brain, skull, and orbit metastasis is rare in the newborn.[99,112] The tendency is to metastasize to cortical bone, skull and facial bones, pelvis, and proximal long bones.[77,96]

    l. Pepper syndrome consists of massive involvement of the liver with metastatic disease with or without respiratory distress.[82,100,102–105]

    m. Opsoclonus-myoclonus ataxia syndrome (dancing eyes and dancing feet syndrome) is associated with a small, slow-growing tumor primarily located in the chest. Involuntary random movement of the eyes (opsoclonus) and muscle jerking (myoclonus) may or may not resolve after the tumor is removed.[82,100,102–105]

DIFFERENTIAL DIAGNOSIS

A. The differential diagnosis includes a variety of neoplastic and nonneoplastic conditions and varies according to tumor location.

    1. Tumors that arise in the suprarenal location (Wilms' tumor and hepatoblastoma) should be considered.[93,96,98]

    2. In thoracic and retroperitoneal locations, lymphoma, germ cell tumors, and infection should be considered.[96,98,100,102]

B. Metastatic involvement of the bone marrow should be distinguished from lymphoma, small cell osteosarcoma, mesenchymal chondrosarcoma, the Ewing's sarcoma family of tumors, primitive neuroectodermal tumors, and undifferentiated soft tissue sarcomas such as rhabdomyosarcoma and leukemia, particularly megakaryoblastic leukemia.[96,98,100,102]

C. Opsoclonus-myoclonus syndrome occurs in 1–3 percent of cases with neuroblastoma. Twenty to 50 percent of children with opsoclonus-myoclonus syndrome have an underlying neuroblastoma.[100,102]

D. Skin nodules may be dermoid and other cysts, subcutaneous fat necrosis, benign tumors (e.g., infantile myofibromatosis, congential self-healing reticulohistiocytosis), or malignant tumors (e.g., infantile fibrosarcoma, rhabdomyosarcoma, and congential leukemia).[100,102]

DIAGNOSIS

A. Median age at diagnosis: 22 months

    1. Thirty-five percent of cases occur before the age of one year.[77]

    2. Seventy-nine percent occur before age four.[82]

    3. Ninety-seven percent are diagnosed before age ten.[113]

    4. Some studies have shown a biphasic peak before the first year and again between 2 and 4 years of age.[82,113]

B. Laboratory tests
1. Urine screening
   a. Test for the urinary catecholamine metabolites: Homovanillic acid (HVA) and vanillylmandelic acid (VMA). With neuroblastoma, 90–95 percent of children will have elevated levels.[114,115] An increased catecholamine level is considered to be 3 standard deviations above the age-appropriate mean.[77,79,112,115,116]
   b. Perform a urine/serum dopamine screening. Dopamine is converted primarily to HVA, and norepinephrine is converted primarily to VMA. Neuroblastomas lack the enzyme that converts dopamine to HVA and norepinephrine to VMA.[74,79,112,115,116]
2. Blood tests
   a. A CBC is done to identify anemia or thrombocytopenia. The presence of either of these could suggest bone marrow involvement.[77]
   b. Dopa, dopamine, or norepinephrine levels will be elevated because neuroblastomas lack the enzyme that converts dopamine to HVA and norepinephrine to VMA (see DIAGNOSIS, B. 1. b., above).[77,79,112,115,116]
   c. Biochemical markers associated with a poor prognosis include elevated levels of the following.[117,118]
      1) Ferritin
      2) Serum lactate dehydrogenase (LDH)
      3) Serum neuron-specific enolase (NSE)
   d. Molecular markers have been identified in neuroblastomas. These assist in determining the prognosis.
      1) Deletion of the short arm of chromosome 1 is the most common abnormality and, if present, represents a poor prognosis. It correlates with increased ferritin and LDH levels.[3]
      2) N-myc is the most important biologic marker. It is a proto-oncogene expressed in the distal arm of chromosome 2. This gene is amplified in approximately 25 percent of new diagnoses and is more common in patients with advanced stage disease. Patients who have N-myc amplification tend to have rapid tumor progression and a poorer prognosis.
   e. Serum markers are elevated in patients with advanced neuroblastoma.[117,119]
      1) NSE
      2) Lactic dehydrogenase
      3) GD2
      4) Ganglioside
      5) Chromogranin
      6) N-myc oncogene
   f. Other lab tests should include the following.
      1) Liver function tests
         a) Alanine transferase
         b) Aspartate aminotransferase
      2) Total bilirubin
      3) Alkaline phosphatase level
      4) Electrolytes
      5) Creatinine
      6) Calcium
      7) Magnesium

C. Imaging studies
1. Chest and abdominal radiographs, anterior, posterior, and lateral views, can initially help the clinician evaluate primary tumors located in the chest and abdomen. If the radiograph confirms a mass, follow-up chest CT or MRI should be done.[77,115,120]
2. CT scan is a standard test that provides three-dimensional information about abdominal metastases, including lymph node enlargement and liver disease. It can define metastases to the skull, orbit, mandible, or brain.[113,121–124]
3. MRI is another standard test useful in evaluation of soft tissue disease and skull, orbit, mandible, or brain metastases. It provides accurate three-dimensional measurements of the involved tumor.[113,121–124]
4. Ultrasound is useful in providing information about abdominal disease, including lymph node enlargement and liver metastases.[122]
5. Methyliodobenzylguanadine (MIBG) scintiscan distinguishes between bone and soft tissue involvement and between active tumors and scar tissue. MIBG is a norepinephrine-iodine analog that is absorbed by most neuroblastomas.[77,113,125]
6. Technetium-99m bone scan is a standard test for detecting bone disease.[120] It is less reliable in children under one year of age because of the increased activity of the bone marrow.[77]

D. Biopsy
1. Bone marrow aspirates and biopsy from both posterior iliac crests are recommended. Two separate sites are assayed, resulting in four samples (two aspirations, two biopsies).
   a. A positive marrow from any site and elevated urine or serum catecholamines confirm the diagnosis of neuroblastoma.[126]
2. A biopsy or resection of the tumor is performed to assign the patient to the appropriate risk category.
3. Tissue diagnosis is essential.[3] Tissue samples from a primary or metastatic tumor may be undifferentiated and confused with other small, round, blue cell tumors of childhood. The pathologist must evaluate the tumor thoroughly because regions with different gross appearances may exhibit different histology.[3]

E. Baseline tests to obtain prior to beginning therapy
1. Electrocardiogram
2. Echocardiogram
3. Hearing
4. Creatinine clearance

F. Staging
1. The revised International Neuroblastoma Staging System is based on clinical, radiographic, and surgical evaluation of children suspected to have neuroblastoma (Table 5-3).[127]

TREATMENT OPTIONS AND NURSING CARE

A. The type and intensity of treatment are based on the age of the patient and the staging of the neuroblastoma.
1. Patients with localized tumors have an excellent outcome.
B. Treatment modalities include the following.
1. Surgery
2. Chemotherapy
3. Radiation therapy

TABLE 5-3 ■ International Neuroblastoma Staging System Criteria

Stage	Definition
1	Localized tumor with complete gross excision, with or without microscopic residual disease; representative ipsilateral lymph nodes negative for tumor microscopically (nodes attached to and removed with the primary tumor may be positive)
2A	Localized tumor with incomplete gross excision; representative ipsilateral nonadherent lymph nodes negative for tumor microscopically
2B	Localized tumor with or without complete gross excision, with ipsilateral nonadherent lymph nodes positive for tumor. Enlarged contralateral lymph nodes must be negative microscopically
3	Unresectable unilateral tumor infiltrating across the midline,* with or without regional lymph node involvement
	or
	Localized unilateral tumor with contralateral regional lymph node involvement
	or
	Midline tumor with bilateral extension by infiltration (unresectable) or by lymph node involvement
4	Any primary tumor with dissemination to distant lymph nodes, bone, bone marrow, liver, skin, or other organs (except as defined for Stage 4S)
4S	Localized primary tumor (as defined for Stage 1, 2A, or 2B), with dissemination limited to skin, liver, and bone marrow† (limited to infants under one year)

* The midline is defined as the vertebral column. Tumors originating on one side and crossing the midline must infiltrate to or beyond the opposite side of the vertebral column.

† Marrow involvement in Stage 4S should be minimal (i.e., <10 percent of total nucleated cells identified as malignant on bone marrow biopsy or on marrow aspirate). More extensive marrow involvement would be considered to be Stage 4. The metaiodobenzylguanidine scan (if performed) should be negative in the marrow.

From: Kiely EM. 2005. Neuroblastoma. In *Pediatric Surgery*, 4th ed., Ashcraft KW, Holder TM, and Murphy JP, eds. Philadelphia: Saunders, 936. Reprinted by permission.

SURGICAL MANAGEMENT

A. Stage 1. Surgery to completely excise the tumor; no benefits from radiation or chemotherapy[128–130]

B. Stage 2A. Surgery to completely excise the tumor; no benefits from radiation or chemotherapy[128–130]

C. Stage 2B. Surgery to completely excise the tumor; no benefits from radiation or chemotherapy[128–130]

D. Stage 3. Combination of chemotherapy, local surgery, and radiation therapy
   1. If tumor cannot be removed completely, radiation and chemotherapy are recommended.
   2. Chemotherapy agents include the following.[131–138]
      a. Cisplatin
      b. Cyclophosphamide
      c. Dacarbazine
      d. Etoposide
      e. Ifosfamide
      f. Vincristine
      g. Doxorubicin
      h. Carboplatin
   3. These chemotherapy agents are almost always given in combinations. Commonly used combinations include the following.
      a. Vincristine, cyclophosphamide, doxorubicin
      b. Carboplatin and etoposide
      c. Cisplatin and etoposide
      d. Ifosfamide and etoposide

E. Stage 4. Combination of chemotherapy, local surgery, and radiation therapy
   1. Combinations of the chemotherapy agents administered for six months to one year yield a survival rate of 50 percent in infants younger than one year.
   2. Chemotherapy agents include the following.[131–138]
      a. Cisplatin
      b. Cyclophosphamide
      c. Dacarbazine
      d. Etoposide
      e. Ifosfamide
      f. Nitrogen mustard
      g. Vincristine
      h. Doxorubicin
F. Stage 4S
   1. Most of these patients will have spontaneous regression.[138,139]
   2. In this stage, the primary tumor is localized, with any dissemination limited to the skin, liver, and bone marrow.

COMPLICATIONS

A. Spinal cord compression
   1. Cord compression can develop from a paraspinal tumor.[93–98]
   2. Evaluation by a neurosurgeon and radiologist oncologist is important.
B. Hypertension or renal insufficiency, which can delay the start of chemotherapy[96]
C. Immunosuppression and myelosuppression
   1. These increase the infant's risk of bleeding and infection.[131,132]
      a. If the infant's temperature increases, immediate medical attention is necessary to start broad-spectrum antibiotics.[131,132]
      b. Monitor CBC and platelets at least twice weekly.
   2. Impaired renal function, hearing loss, and abnormal lab values (e.g., low hematocrit, low platelet count, and abnormal electrolyte levels) may develop in patients after several cycles of therapy.[118,119,127,131,140]
D. Central line complications
   1. Infection
E. Renal function
   1. Some medications can affect renal function (e.g., cisplatin, carboplatin, ifosfamide).[131,132,140]
   2. Monitor serum electrolyte levels closely and provide supplements as needed.
F. Bleeding[94,96]
   1. Blood products should be provided if:
      a. Hemoglobin is <8 gm/dl (80 gm/liter)
      b. Platelet count is <10,000/mm^3
      c. Bleeding is present
G. Diarrhea[103,105]
   1. Intractable diarrhea is a rare paraneoplastic symptom that resolves after the tumor is removed.
      a. The diarrhea is caused by the secretion of a vasoactive intestinal peptide by the tumor and is rarely associated with neuroblastomas.
      b. It is more often a result of the less aggressive ganglioneuroblastomas and ganglioneuromas.

Postoperative Nursing Care

A. Care of the postoperative patient

B. Care of the patient receiving chemotherapy and radiation therapy

Outcomes

A. The outcome is based on the stage of the disease, the age of the patient at diagnosis, and the site of the primary tumor.[141–146]

1. Stage 1

   a. Survival is 75–90 percent.[82,147,148]

   b. If the patient has a localized tumor, negative Ipsilateral lymph nodes, and there is no amplification of N-myc, there is a 90–100 percent survival rate with surgery alone, independent of age.[66,138,140]

2. Stage 2

   a. Stage 2A. If the patient has a localized tumor and negative ipsilateral nonadherent lymph nodes without amplification of N-myc, there is a 90–100 percent survival with surgery alone, independent of age.[66,138,140]

   b. Stage 2B. If there is a localized tumor and/or complete gross excision with ipsilateral nonadherent lymph nodes positive for tumor, survival is 75–90 percent.[82,147,148]

   c. If the patient has Stage 2A/2B disease, is older than one year, has amplified N-myc, and the histology of the tumor is unfavorable, this infant is considered high risk. The survival rate is 20 percent.

3. Stage 3

   a. This stage involves an unresectable unilateral tumor infiltrating across the midline and/or regional lymph node involvement or localized unilateral tumor with contralateral regional lymph node involvement.[66,147,148]

   b. Survival rate is 90 percent for children less than one year with localized disease.

   c. Survival rate is 50 percent for children greater than one year with advanced Stage 3.[66,138,140]

4. Stage 4

   a. This stage includes any primary tumor with dissemination to distant lymph nodes, bone, bone marrow, liver, skin, and/or other organs.

   b. Survival for children less than one year of age with nonamplified N-myc and with favorable histology is 60–75 percent. In those over one year of age with amplified N-myc and unfavorable histology, survival is 20 percent.[82,147,148]

   c. For children less than one year of age with disseminated disease, survival is 90 percent. For infants greater than one year, survival rates range between 10 and 30 percent.[66,138,140]

5. Stage 4S

   a. This state involves a localized primary tumor (as defined for Stages 1, 2A, or 2B) with dissemination limited to skin, liver, and/or bone marrow (less than 10 percent involvement).

   b. For children less than one year of age with nonamplified N-myc and favorable histology, the survival rate is 75–90 percent.[82,147,148]

   c. For children with amplified N-myc and unfavorable histology, survival is 20 percent.[66,138,140]

B. Patients with primary tumors that present in the adrenal glands have poorer outcomes.[82]

C. Infants younger than one year of age have a good prognosis, even if there is metastatic disease present. Children over one year fare poorly—even with aggressive therapy.

D. Follow-up care includes the following.

1. Close surveillance of the patient
2. Monitoring of urinary catecholamines
3. Physical examinations
4. Diagnostic imagining

E. Most recurrences happen within the first two years following treatment.

REFERENCES

1. Bates MD, et al. 1998. Biliary atresia: Pathogenesis and treatment. *Seminars in Liver Disease* 18(3): 281–293.

2. Lefkowitch JH. 1998. Biliary atresia. *Mayo Clinic Proceedings* 73(1): 90–95.

3. Miyano T. 2005. Biliary tract disorders and portal hypertension. In *Pediatric Surgery*, 4th ed., Ashcraft KW, Holder TM, and Murphy JP, eds. Philadelphia: Saunders, 586–608.

4. Balistreri W, et al. 1996. Biliary atresia: Current concepts and research directions. Summary of a symposium. *Hepatology* 23(6): 1682–1692.

5. Knisely AS. 1990. Biliary atresia and its complications. *Annals of Clinical and Laboratory Science* 20(2): 113–118.

6. Haber BA, and Lake AM. 1990. Cholestatic jaundice in the newborn. *Clinics in Perinatology* 17(2): 483–506.

7. Vicente HL. 1995. Biliary atresia: An overview. *Boletin-Asosiacion Medica de Puerto Rico* 87(7-9): 147–153.

8. Burns J. 1817. *Principles of Midwifery, Including the Diseases of Woman and Children*. London: Longman, 601.

9. Mowat AP. 1996. Biliary atresia into the 21st century: A historical perspective. *Hepatology* 23(6): 1693–1695.

10. Thomson J. 1892. On congenial obliteration of the bile ducts. *Edinburgh Medical Journal* 37: 604–616.

11. Holmes JB. 1916. Congenital obliteration of the bile ducts. *American Journal of Diseases of Children* 11: 405–431.

12. Ladd WE. 1928. Congenital atresia and stenosis of the bile ducts. *JAMA* 91: 1082–1085.

13. MacMahon JR, Stevenson DK, and Oski FA. 1998. Obstructive jaundice due to biliary atresia and neonatal hepatitis. In *Avery's Diseases of the Newborn*, 7th ed., Taeusch HW, and Ballard RA, eds. Philadelphia: Saunders, 1021–1029.

14. Thigpen J, and Kenner C. 2003. Assessment and management of the GI system. In *Comprehensive Neonatal Nursing: A Physiologic Perspective*, 3rd ed., Kenner C, and Lott JW, eds. Philadelphia: Saunders, 448–485.

15. Altman RP. 1991. Infantile obstructive jaundice. In *Pediatric Surgery of the Liver, Pancreas, and Spleen*, Schiller M, ed. Philadelphia: Saunders, 59–75.

16. Morecki R, et al. 1982. Biliary atresia and reovirus type 3 infection. *New England Journal of Medicine* 307(8): 481–484.

17. Desmet VJ. 1992. Congenital diseases of intrahepatic bile ducts: Variation on the theme "ductal plate malformation." *Hepatology* 16(4): 1069–1083.

18. Strauss L, and Bernstein J. 1968. Neonatal hepatitis in congenital rubella: A histopathological study. *Archives of Pathology* 86(3): 317–327.

19. Gautier M, Jehan P, and Odievre M. 1976. Histologic study of biliary fibrous remnants in 48 cases of extrahepatic biliary atresia: Correlation with postoperative bile flow restoration. *Journal of Pediatrics* 89(5): 704–709.

20. Witzleben CL, et al. 1978. Studies on the pathogenesis of biliary atresia. *Laboratory Investigation* 38(5): 525–532.

21. Brown WR, et al. 1988. Lack of correlation between infection with reovirus 3 and extrahepatic biliary atresia or neonatal hepatitis. *Journal of Pediatrics* 113(4): 670–676.

22. Jevon GP, and Dimmick JE. 1999. Biliary atresia and cytomegalovirus infection: A DNA study. *Pediatric and Developmental Pathology* 2(1): 11–14.

23. Riepenhoff-Talty M, et al. 1996. Detection of group C rotavirus in infants with extrahepatic biliary atresia. *Journal of Infectious Diseases* 174(1): 8–15.

24. Tarr PI, Haas JE, and Christie DL. 1996. Biliary atresia, cytomegalovirus, and age at referral. *Pediatrics* 97(6 part 1): 828–831.

25. Yoon PW, et al. 1997. Epidemiology of biliary atresia: A population-based study. *Pediatrics* 99(3): 376–382.

26. Strickland AD, and Shannon K. 1982. Studies in the etiology of extrahepatic biliary atresia: Time spacing clustering. *Journal of Pediatrics* 100(5): 749–753.

27. Ayas MF, Hillemeier AC, and Olson AD. 1996. Lack of evidence for seasonal variation in extrahepatic biliary atresia during infancy. *Journal of Clinical Gastroenterology* 22(4): 292–294.

28. Davenport M, and Dhawan A. 1998. Epidemiologic study of infants with biliary atresia. *Pediatrics* 101(4): 729–730.

29. Shim WK, Kasai M, and Spence MA. 1974. Racial influence on the incidence of biliary atresia. *Progress in Pediatric Surgery* 6: 53–62.

30. Sweet LK. 1932. Congenital malformation of the bile ducts. *Journal of Pediatrics* 1: 496–501.

31. Werlin SL. 1981. Extrahepatic biliary atresia in one of twins. *Acta Paediatrica Scandinavica* 70(6): 943–944.

32. Smith BM, et al. 1991. Familial biliary atresia in three siblings including twins. *Journal of Pediatric Surgery* 26(11): 1331–1333.

33. Balistreri WF. 1985. Neonatal cholestasis. *Journal of Pediatrics* 106(2): 171–184.

34. Glassman JA. 1989. *Biliary Tract Surgery*. New York: Macmillan, 58–68.

35. Balistreri WF. 1987. Neonatal cholestasis: Lessons from the past, issues for the future (foreword). *Seminars in Liver Disease* 7(2): 61–66.

36. Hernandez-Cano AM, et al. 1987. Portal vein dynamics in biliary atresia. *Journal of Pediatric Surgery* 22(6): 519–521.

37. Choi SO, Park WH, and Lee HJ. 1998. Ultrasonographic "triangular cord": The most definitive finding for non-invasive diagnosis of extrahepatic biliary atresia. *European Journal of Pediatric Surgery* 8(1): 12–16.

38. Cox KL, et al. 1987. Hepatobiliary scintigraphy with technetium-99m disofenin in the evaluation of neonatal cholestasis. *Journal of Pediatric Gastroenterology and Nutrition* 6(6): 885–891.

39. Wilkinson M. 1996. The art of diagnostic imaging: The biliary tree. *Journal of Hepatology* 25(1): 5–19.

40. Ryckman FC, et al. 1998. Biliary atresia—Surgical management and treatment options as they relate to outcome. *Liver Transplantation and Surgery* 4(5 supplement 1): S24–S33.

41. Middlesworth W, and Altman RP. 1997. Biliary atresia. *Current Opinions in Pediatrics* 9(3): 265–269.

42. Karrer FM, et al. 1990. Biliary atresia registry, 1976–1989. *Journal of Pediatric Surgery* 25(10): 1076–1081.

43. Ryckman F, et al. 1993. Improved survival in biliary atresia patients in the present era of liver transplantation. *Journal of Pediatric Surgery* 28(3): 382–386.

44. Mieli-Vergani G, et al. 1989. Late referral for biliary atresia—Missed opportunities for effective surgery. *Lancet* 1(8635): 421–423.

45. Kasai M. 1974. Treatment of biliary atresia with special reference to hepatic porto-enterostomy and its modifications. *Progress in Pediatric Surgery* 6: 5–52.

46. Ohi R, and Ibrahim M. 1992. Biliary atresia. *Seminars in Pediatric Surgery* 1(2): 115–124.

47. Kasai M, et al. 1968. Surgical treatment of biliary atresia. *Journal of Pediatric Surgery* 3(6): 665–675.

48. Kasai M, and Suzuki S. 1959. A new operation for non-correctable biliary atresia: Hepatic portoenterostomy. *Shujutsu* 13: 733–739.

49. Azarow KS, et al. 1997. Biliary atresia: Should all patients undergo a portoenterostomy? *Journal of Pediatric Surgery* 32(2): 168–172.

50. Schweizer P. 1986. Treatment of extrahepatic bile duct atresia: Results and long-term prognosis after hepatic portoenterostomy. *Pediatric Surgery International* 1(1): 30–36.

51. Whitington PF, Alonso EM, and Piper JB. 1994. Pediatric liver transplantation. *Seminars in Liver Disease* 14(3): 303–317.

52. Nagral S, et al. 1997. Liver transplantation for extra hepatic biliary atresia. *Tohoku Journal of Experimental Medicine* 181(1): 117–127.

53. Otte JB, et al. 1994. Sequential treatment of biliary atresia with Kasai portoenterostomy and liver transplantation: A review. *Hepatology* 20(1 part 2): S41–S48.

54. Broelsch CE, et al. 1990. Application of reduced-size liver transplants as split grafts, auxiliary orthotopic grafts, and living related segmental transplants. *Annals of Surgery* 212(3): 368–377.

55. Ohi R. 1998. Surgical treatment of biliary atresia in the liver transplantation era. *Surgery Today* 28(12): 1229–1232.

56. Kasai M. 1982. Double-Y hepatic porto-jejunostomy for biliary atresia. In *Liver Surgery*, Calne RY, ed. Philadelphia: Saunders, 75–88.

57. Hasegawa T, et al. 1998. Portal hypertension enteropathy in biliary atresia. *Pediatric Surgery International* 13(8): 602–604.

58. Schweizer P, and Lunzmann K. 1998. Extrahepatic bile duct atresia: How efficient is the hepatoportoenterostomy? *European Journal of Pediatric Surgery* 8(3): 150–154.

59. Merritt RJ. 1986. Cholestasis associated with total parenteral nutrition. *Journal of Pediatric Gastroenterology and Nutrition* 5(1): 9–22.

60. Kasai M, et al. 1989. Surgical limitation for biliary atresia: Indication for liver transplantation. *Journal of Pediatric Surgery* 24(9): 851–854.

61. Laurent J, et al. 1990. Long-term outcome after surgery for biliary atresia: Study of forty patients surviving for more than 10 years. *Gastroenterology* 99(6): 1793–1797.

62. Lopez-Santamaria M, et al. 1998. Long-term follow-up of patients with biliary atresia successfully treated with hepatic portoenterostomy. The importance of sequential treatment. *Pediatric Surgery International* 13(5-6): 327–330.

63. Grosfeld JL, et al. 1974. The efficacy of hepatoportoenterostomy in biliary atresia. *Surgery* 106(4): 692–701.

64. Beckwith JB, and Perrin EV. 1963. In situ neuroblastomas: A contribution to the natural history of neural crest tumors. *American Journal of Pathology* 43: 1089–1104.

65. Shimada H. 1982. Transmission and scanning electron microscopic studies on the tumors of neuroblastoma group. *Acta Pathologica Japanica* 32(3): 415–426.

66. Kaneko M, et al. 1998. Complete resection is not required in patients with neuroblastoma under 1 year of age. *Journal of Pediatric Surgery* 33(11): 1690–1694.

67. Shimada H, and Brodeur G. 1998. Tumors of the peripheral neuroblasts and ganglion cells. In *Russell and Rubinstein's Pathology of Tumors of the Central Nervous System*, 6th ed., Bigner DD, McLendon RF, and Bruner JM, eds. New York: Oxford University Press, 493–533.

68. Shimada H, et al. 1999. The International Neuroblastoma Pathology Classification (the Shimada system). *Cancer* 86(2): 364–372.

69. Allen RW, et al. 1980. Fetal hydantoin syndrome, neuroblastoma, and hemorrhagic disease in a neonate. *JAMA* 244(13): 1464–1465.

70. Kinney H, Faix R, and Brazy J. 1980. The fetal alcohol syndrome and neuroblastoma. *Pediatrics* 66(1): 130–132.

71. Schwartzbaum JA. 1992. Influence of the mother's prenatal drug consumption on risk of neuroblastoma in the child. *American Journal of Epidemiology* 135(12): 1358–1367.

72. Seeler RA, et al. 1979. Ganglioneuroblastoma and fetal hydantoin-alcohol syndromes. *Pediatrics* 63(4): 524–527.

73. Spitz MR, and Johnson CC. 1985. Neuroblastoma and paternal occupation. A case control analysis. *American Journal of Epidemiology* 121(6): 924–929.

74. Wilkins JRI, and Hundley VD. 1990. Paternal occupational exposure to electromagnetic fields and neuroblastoma in offspring. *American Journal of Epidemiology* 131(6): 995–1008.

75. Bunin GR, et al. 1990. Neuroblastoma and parental occupation. *American Journal of Epidemiology* 131(5): 776–780.

76. Kramer S, et al. 1987. Medical and drug risk factors associated with neuroblastomas: A case control study. *Journal of the National Cancer Institute* 78(5): 797–804.

77. Alexander F. 2000. Neuroblastoma. *Urologic Clinics of North America* 27(3): 383–392.

78. Miller RW, Young JL Jr, and Novakovic B. 1995. Childhood cancer. *Cancer* 75(1 supplement): S395–S405.

79. Gurney JG, et al. 1995. Incidence of cancer in children in the United States. *Cancer* 75(8): 2186–2195.

80. Campbell AN, et al. 1987. Malignant tumors in the neonate. *Archives of Disease in Childhood* 62(1): 19–23.

81. Gale GB, et al. 1982. Cancer in the neonate: The experience of the Children's Hospital in Philadelphia. *Pediatrics* 70(3): 409–413.

82. Brodeur GM, and Castleberry RP. 2001. Neuroblastoma. In *Principles and Practice of Pediatric Oncology*, 4th ed., Pizzo PA, and Poplack DG, eds. Philadelphia: Lippincott Williams & Wilkins, 895–938.

83. Chatten J, and Voorhess M. 1967. Report of a kindred with multiple disorders, including neuroblastomas in four siblings. *New England Journal of Medicine* 277(23): 1230–1236.

84. Kushner BH, Gilbert F, and Helson L. 1986. Familial neuroblastoma: Case reports, literature review, and etiologic considerations. *Cancer* 57(9): 1887–1893.

85. Knudson AGJ, and Strong LC. 1972. Mutation and cancer: Neuroblastoma and pheochromocytoma. *American Journal of Human Genetics* 24(5): 514–532.

86. Kushner BH, and Helson L. 1985. Monozygotic siblings discordant for neuroblastoma: Etiologic implications. *Journal of Pediatrics* 107(3): 405–409.

87. Mead RS, and Cowell JK. 1995. Molecular characterization of a(1;10)(p22;q21) constitutional translocation from a patient with neuroblastoma. *Cancer Genetics and Cytogenetics* 81(2): 151–157.

88. Laureys G, et al. 1990. Constitutional translocation t(1;17)(p36;q12-21). *Genes, Chromosomes & Cancer* 2(3): 252–254.

89. Biegel JA, et al. 1993. Constitutional 1p36 deletion in a child with neuroblastoma. *American Journal of Human Genetics* 52(1): 176–182.

90. Brodeur GM, and Sekhon GS. 1977. Chromosomal aberrations in human neuroblastomas. *Cancer* 40(5): 2256–2263.

91. Hayashi Y, et al. 1987. Chromosome findings and prognosis in neuroblastoma. *Cancer Genetics and Cytogenetics* 29(1): 175–177.

92. Gilbert F, et al. 1984. Human neuroblastomas and abnormalities of chromosome 1 and 17. *Cancer Research* 44(11): 5444–5449.

93. Rosen EM, et al. 1984. Neuroblastoma: The Joint Center for Radiation Therapy/Dana-Farber Cancer Institute/Children's Hospital experience. *Journal of Clinical Oncology* 2(7): 719–732.

94. Voute PA Jr, Wadman SK, and van Putten WJ. 1970. Congenital neuroblastoma. Symptoms in the mother during pregnancy. *Clinical Pediatrics* 9(4): 206–207.

95. Schneider KM, Becker JM, and Krasna IH. 1965. Neonatal neuroblastoma. *Pediatrics* 36(3): 359–366.

96. McGahren ED, Rodgers BM, and Waldron PE. 1998. Successful management of stage 4S neuroblastoma and severe hepatomegaly using absorbable mesh in an infant. *Journal of Pediatric Surgery* 33(10): 1554–1557.

97. Kedar A, et al. 1981. Severe hypertension in a child with ganglioneuroblastoma. *Cancer* 47(8): 2077–2080.

98. Weinblatt ME, Heisel MA, and Siegel SE. 1983. Hypertension in children with neurogenic tumors. *Pediatrics* 71(6): 947–951.

99. Kellie SJ, et al. 1991. Primary extracranial neuroblastoma with central nervous system metastases characterization by clinicopathologic findings and neuroimaging. *Cancer* 68(9): 1999–2006.

100. Pranzatelli MR. 1992. The neurobiology of the opsoclonus-myoclonus syndrome. *Clinical Neuropharmacology* 15(3): 186–228.

101. Evans AE, D'Angio GJ, and Randolph JA. 1971. A proposed staging for children with neuroblastoma. Children's Cancer Study Group A. *Cancer* 27(2): 374–378.

102. Altman AJ, and Baehner RL. 1976. Favorable prognosis for survival in children with coincident opsomyoclonus and neuroblastoma. *Cancer* 37(2): 846–852.

103. El Shafie M, et al. 1983. Intractable diarrhea in children with VIP-secreting ganglioneuroblastomas. *Journal of Pediatric Surgery* 18(1): 34–36.

104. Roberts KB, and Freeman JM. 1975. Cerebellar ataxia and "occult neuroblastoma" without opsoclonus. *Pediatrics* 56(3): 464–465.

105. Scheibel E, et al. 1982. Vasoactive intestinal polypeptide (VIP) in children with neural crest tumors. *Acta Paediatrica Scandinavica* 71(5): 721–725.

106. Iida Y, et al. 1980. Watery diarrhoea with vasoactive intestinal peptide-producing ganglioneuroblastoma. *Archives of Disease in Childhood* 55(12): 929–936.

107. Delalieux C, et al. 1975. Myoclonic encephalopathy and neuroblastoma. *New England Journal of Medicine* 292(1): 46–47.

108. Swift PGF, Bloom SR, and Harris F. 1975. Watery diarrhoea and ganglioneuroma with secretion of vasoactive intestinal peptide. *Archives of Disease in Childhood* 50(11): 896–899.

109. Scott JP, and Morgan ER. 1983. Coagulopathy of disseminated neuroblastoma. *Journal of Pediatrics* 103(2): 219–222.

110. Labotka RJ, and Morgan ER. 1982. Myelofibrosis in neuroblastoma. *Medical and Pediatric Oncology* 10(1): 21–26.

111. Quinn JJ, and Altman AJ. 1979. The multiple hematologic manifestations of neuroblastoma. *American Journal of Pediatric Hematology/Oncology* 1(3): 201–205.

112. Shaw PJ, and Eden T. 1992. Neuroblastoma with intracranial involvement: An ENSG study. *Medical and Pediatric Oncology* 20(2): 149–155.

113. Voute PA, et al. 1985. Detection of neuroblastoma with 131I-meta-iodobenzylguanidine. *Progress in Clinical and Biological Research* 175: 389–398.

114. Laug W, et al. 1978. Initial urinary catecholamine metabolite concentrations and prognosis in neuroblastoma. *Pediatrics* 62(1): 77–83.

115. LaBrosse EH, et al. 1980. Urinary excretion of 3-methoxy-4-hydroxymandelic acid and 3-methoxy-4-hydroxyphenylacetic acid by 288 patients with neuroblastoma and related neural crest tumors. *Cancer Research* 40(6): 1995–2001.

116. Graham-Pole J, et al. 1983. Tumor and urine catecholamines (CATS) in neurogenic tumors: Correlations with other prognostic factors and survival. *Cancer* 51(5): 834–839.

117. Hann HWL, et al. 1981. Biologic differences between neuroblastoma stages IV-S and IV. Measurement of serum ferritin and E-rosette inhibition in 30 children. *New England Journal of Medicine* 305(8): 425–429.

118. Hann HW, Stahlhut MW, and Evans AE. 1985. Serum ferritin as a prognostic indicator in neuroblastoma: Biological effects of isoferritins. *Progress in Clinical and Biological Research* 175: 331–345.

119. Matthay KK, et al. 1998. Successful treatment of stage III neuroblastoma based on prospective biologic staging: A Children's Cancer Group study. *Journal of Clinical Oncology* 16(4): 1256–1264.

120. Heisel MA, et al. 1983. Radionuclide bone scan in neuroblastoma. *Pediatrics* 71(2): 206–209.

121. Daubenton JD, et al. 1987. The relationship between prognosis and scintigraphic evidence of bone metastases in neuroblastoma. *Cancer* 59(9): 1586–1589.

122. White SJ, et al. 1983. Sonography of neuroblastoma. *American Journal of Roentgenology* 141(3): 465–468.

123. Golding SJ, McElwain TJ, and Husband JE. 1984. The role of computed tomography in the management of children with advanced neuroblastoma. *British Journal of Radiology* 57(680): 661–666.

124. Fletcher BD, et al. 1985. Abdominal neuroblastoma: Magnetic resonance imaging and tissue characterization. *Radiology* 155(3): 699–703.

125. Feine U, et al. 1987. Metaiodobenzylguanidine (MIBG) labeled with 123I/131I in neuroblastoma diagnosis and follow-up treatment with a review of the diagnostic results of the International Workshop of Pediatric Oncology held in Rome, September 1986. *Medical and Pediatric Oncology* 15(4): 181–187.

126. Moss TJ, et al. 1991. Prognostic value of immunocytologic detection of bone marrow metastases in neuroblastoma. *New England Journal of Medicine* 324(4): 219–226.

127. Brodeur GM, et al. 1993. Revisions of the international criteria for neuroblastoma diagnosis, staging, and response to treatment. *Journal of Clinical Oncology* 11(8): 1466–1477.

128. Evans AE, Baum E, and Chard R. 1981. Do infants with stage IV-S neuroblastoma need treatment? *Archives of Disease in Childhood* 56(4): 271–274.

129. Nickerson HJ, et al. 1985. Comparison of stage IV and IV-S neuroblastoma in the first year of life. *Medical and Pediatric Oncology* 13(5): 261–268.

130. Stephenson SR, et al. 1986. The prognostic significance of age and pattern of metastases in stage IV-S neuroblastoma. *Cancer* 58(2): 372–375.

131. Starling KA, et al. 1974. Drug trials in neuroblastoma: Cyclophosphamide (NSC-26271) alone; vincristine (NSC-67574) plus cyclophosphamide; 6-mercaptopurine (NSC-755) plus 6-methylmercaptopurine riboside (NSC-40774); and cytosine arabinoside (NSC-63878) alone. *Cancer Chemotherapy Reports* 58(5 part 1): 683–688.

132. Thurman WG, Fernbach DJ, and Sullivan MP. 1964. Cyclophosphamide therapy in childhood neuroblastoma. *New England Journal of Medicine* 270(25): 1336–1340.

133. Kamalakar P, et l. 1977. Clinical response and toxicity with cis-dichlorodiammineplatinum(II) in children. *Cancer Treatment Reports* 61(5): 835–839.

134. Wang JJ, et al. 1971. Therapeutic effect and toxicity of adriamycin in patients with neoplastic disease. *Cancer* 28(4): 837–843.

135. Campbell RP, et al. 1993. Escalating dose of continuous infusion combination chemotherapy for refractory neuroblastoma. *Journal of Clinical Oncology* 11(4): 623–629.

136. Rubie H, et al. 1998. Unresectable localized neuroblastoma: Improved survival after primary chemotherapy including carboplatin-etoposide. Neuroblastoma Study Group of the Societe Francaise d'Oncologie Pediatrique (SFOP). *British Journal of Cancer* 77(12): 2310–2317.

137. Cheung NK, and Heller G. 1991. Chemotherapy dose intensity correlates strongly with response, median survival, and median progression-free survival in metastatic neuroblastoma. *Journal of Clinical Oncology* 9(6): 1050–1058.

138. Castleberry RP, et al. 1991. Radiotherapy improves the outlook for patients older than 1 year with Pediatric Oncology Group stage C neuroblastoma. *Journal of Clinical Oncology* 9(5): 789–795.

139. Guglielmi M, et al. 1996. Resection of primary tumor at diagnosis in stage IV-S neuroblastoma: Does it affect the clinical course? *Journal of Clinical Oncology* 14(5): 1537–1544.

140. Katzenstein HM, et al. 1998. Prognostic significance of age, MYCN oncogene amplification, tumor cell ploidy, and histology in 110 infants with stage D(S) neuroblastoma: The pediatric oncology group experience—a pediatric oncology group study. *Journal of Clinical Oncology* 16(6): 2007–2017.

141. Oppedal BR, et al. 1988. Prognostic factors in neuroblastoma. Clinical, histopathologic, and immunohistochemical features and DNA ploidy in relation to prognosis. *Cancer* 62(4): 772–780.

142. Hassenbusch S, Kaizer H, and White JJ. 1976. Prognostic factors in neuroblastic tumors. *Journal of Pediatric Surgery* 11(3): 287–297.

143. Evans AE, et al. 1987. Prognostic factors in neuroblastoma. *Cancer* 59(11): 1853–1859.

144. Coldman AJ, et al. 1980. Neuroblastoma: Influence of age at diagnosis, stage, tumor site and sex on prognosis. *Cancer* 46(8): 1896–1901.

145. Grosfeld JL, et al. 1978. Metastatic neuroblastoma: Factors influencing survival. *Journal of Pediatric Surgery* 13(1): 59–65.

146. Jereb B, et al. 1984. Age and prognosis in neuroblastoma. Review of 112 patients younger than 2 years. *American Journal of Pediatric Hematology/Oncology* 6(3): 233–243.

147. Evans AE, D'Angio GJ, and Koop CE. 1984. The role of multimodal therapy in patients with local and regional neuroblastoma. *Journal of Pediatric Surgery* 19(1): 77–80.

148. Matthay KK, et al. 1989. Excellent outcome of Stage II neuroblastoma is independent of residual disease and radiation therapy. *Journal of Clinical Oncology* 7(2): 236–244.

Notes

Notes

6

Genitourinary
Surgical Conditions

Donna L. Buchanan, APRN, MS, NNP
Terese M. Donovan, RNC, MS

This chapter provides the clinician with information to care for infants with conditions leading to genitourinary surgery. Diagnostic testing measures are included. An understanding of testing methods and the timing of testing is critical to effective education of the family. The infant often needs ongoing testing after he leaves the hospital.

Specific surgical procedures that range from circumcision, performed daily in hospital nurseries and the most commonly performed genitourinary procedure, to surgery for cloacal exstrophy, a condition that may not have been seen by even the most experienced neonatal nurses, are addressed. For some of the disorders presented, surgery may not occur in the immediate neonatal period; however, family education about follow-up, ongoing care, and prophylaxis against urinary tract infection is the priority of the clinician in the neonatal intensive care unit. Nursing care practices such as measurement of intake and output, which are considered routine, must be attended to with scrupulous attention for infants with anomalies of the kidney, bladder, or collecting system.

The routine use of prenatal ultrasound has changed our understanding of the pathophysiologic processes associated with many conditions of the genitourinary system. Many infants are now diagnosed before the onset of clinical symptoms. Surgical outcomes reported in the literature may predate antenatal diagnosis, and our understanding of the impact of early diagnosis on the progression of renal injury is evolving.

Embryology

RENAL SYSTEM[1-9]

A. The renal system emerges from three separate embryonic excretory systems. These form from a ridge of mesodermal tissue that lies along the posterior wall of the abdominal cavity on each side of the aorta. Two of these systems, the pronephros and mesonephros, will regress by the fourth to fifth week of

FIGURE 6-1 ■ The three sets of excretory system in an embryo during the fifth week.

A. Lateral view. **B.** Ventral view. The mesonephric tubules have been pulled laterally; their normal position is shown in A.

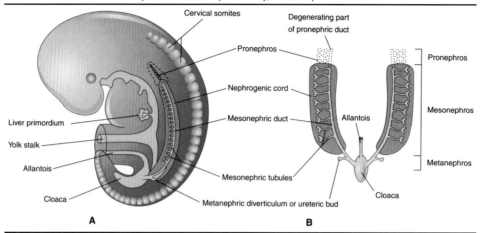

From: Moore KL, and Persaud TVN. 2003. *The Developing Human: Clinically Oriented Embryology,* 7th ed. Philadelphia: Saunders, 290. Reprinted by permission.

gestation, leaving the third system, the metanephros, to differentiate into the renal and urinary structures (Figures 6-1 and 6-2).[3]

1. Pronephros[1,3,10–14]
   a. This is nonfunctional and will degenerate by the fourth week.
2. Mesonephros[1,3,10–14]
   a. The ureteral bud arises from the mesonephric duct at four to five weeks gestatation.[4]

FIGURE 6-2 ■ Positional changes of the kidneys.

A–D. Ventral views of the abdominopelvic region of embryos and fetuses (sixth to ninth weeks) showing medial rotation and "ascent" of the kidneys from the pelvis to the abdomen. **A and B.** Observe also the size regression of the mesonephric. **C and D.** Note that, as the kidneys "ascend," they are supplied by arteries at successively higher levels and that the hilum of the kidney (where the vessels and nerves enter) is eventually directed anteromedially.

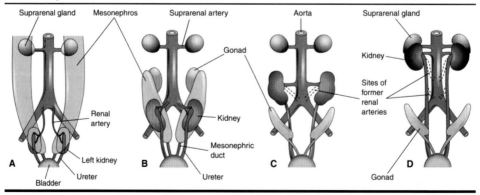

From: Moore KL, and Persaud TVN. 2003. *The Developing Human: Clinically Oriented Embryology,* 7th ed. Philadelphia: Saunders, 295. Reprinted by permission.

FIGURE 6-3 ■ **Development of the permanent kidney.**

A. Lateral view of a five-week embryo showing the primordium of the metanephros. B–E. Successive stages in the development of the metanephric diverticulum or ureteric bud (fifth to eighth weeks). Observe the development of the ureter, renal pelvis, calices, and collecting tubules.

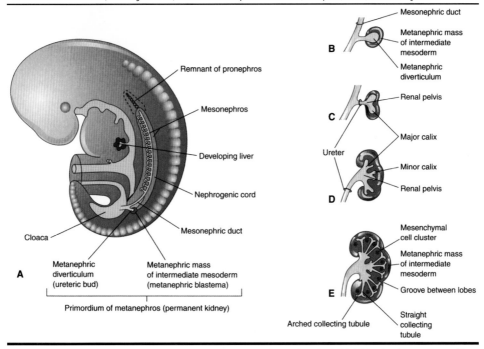

From: Moore KL, and Persaud TVN. 2003. *The Developing Human: Clinically Oriented Embryology,* 7th ed. Philadelphia: Saunders, 293. Reprinted by permission.

    b. At four weeks, the mesonephric nephrons form cranially and develop in a caudal direction along the nephrogenic cord. These nephrons will degenerate in a reverse direction, leaving the tubules and duct system.[4]

    c. The genital duct contributes to the further differentiation of the male internal sexual structures.

    d. Duplication of the renal system may result if the mesonephros does not degenerate.

  3. Metanephros[1,3,10–14]

    a. Developed by the fifth week of gestation, this will ultimately differentiate into the kidneys and ureters.

    b. The metanephros arises from two separate tissue sources.

      1) Ureteric bud[5,7,10,14,15]

        a) The ureteric bud induces nephron formation within the metanephric blastema. When these cells meet the ureteric bud, they differentiate to form the following.[10]

         • Glomerulus

         • Proximal convoluted tubule

         • Loop of Henle

         • Distal convoluted tubule

        b) The ureteric bud further differentiates into the following.[10]

         • Ureter

- Renal pelvis
- Major and minor calyces
- Collecting tubules
  c) As the ureteric bud grows, it meets the metanephric mass.[10,13–15]
  2) Metanephric mass[10]
    a) The metanephric mass forms a cap over the ureteric bud.
    b) Differential development of the kidney occurs in a centrifugal pattern beginning in the center of the kidney mass, progressing to the periphery.[10,13,14]
      - This forms the tissue mass into which the tubules develop through a staged sequence of branching (Figure 6-3).[13,14]

B. The allantois is a small outpouch that develops at 16 days gestation.[16]
  1. It extends from the caudal wall of the yolk sac, then joins with the urogenital sinus.
  2. It contributes to early blood formation.
  4. It is continuous with the urogenital sinus from which the bladder forms.
  5. It develops into a patent structure between the bladder and the umbilicus that ultimately constricts to form a thick, fibrous cord, the median umbilical ligament, extending from the bladder apex to the umbilicus.

C. The kidney develops.[2,4,10]
  1. Primitive kidney
    a. This is functional by 8 weeks gestation, with further differentiation complete by 14 weeks.
    b. This kidney produces urine by 12 weeks gestation.[3,14,15,17]
    c. The kidneys initially develop in the pelvis, then migrate to the abdomen.
      1) This movement is primarily the result of fetal growth caudal to the kidneys.
      2) This migration results in rotation of the kidneys into their final position and the development of new arterial support.[11,13,14]
      3) Failure of this migration may result in the development of a horseshoe kidney.
  2. Nephrons[1,4,5–7]
    a. Each nephron consists of a renal corpuscle (composed of the glomerulus and Bowman's capsule) and a uriniferous tubule containing the following.[3,11,13]
      1) Proximal tubule
      2) Loop of Henle
      3) Distal tubule
      4) Collecting tubule
    b. The full complement of approximately one million nephrons is developed by 35 weeks gestation.[3,5,10,14,17]
    c. Further growth of the existing nephrons will occur in the third trimester.[10,17]
    d. Following birth, nephron growth continues.
      1) Glomeruli are formed in the nephrogenic zone of the kidney and migrate into deeper zones of the cortex during maturation of the kidney.
      2) More mature glomeruli formed earlier in gestation will migrate to the juxtamedullary cortex.
      3) More immature nephrons formed later in gestation remain in the cortex and contribute little to filtration in the fetus until 35 weeks gestation.

    4) Increasing numbers of nephrons combined with a growing proportion of juxtamedullary glomeruli will improve the infant's ability to concentrate urine.[10,14,15]

  e. The nephron has a complex vascular network that develops from the efferent arteriole of the nephron, forming peritubular capillaries. These capillaries surround the primary as well as the adjacent nephrons. In deeper juxtamedullary nephrons, the peritubular capillaries extend into the medulla as a complex of vascular loops known as the *vasa recta,* which further develops to form a capillary network surrounding the ascending limbs of the loop of Henle and the collecting ducts. This structure of vascular support serves the following functions.[5]

    1) Delivery of oxygen and nutrients to the nephron

    2) Delivery of substances for nephron secretion

    3) A pathway for reabsorbed water and solutes into the circulatory system

    4) Concentration and dilution of urine

3. Collecting tubules[4,5,14,15]

  a. During the second trimester, growth of the medulla supports the developing system of collecting tubules.

  b. The tubules of the developing nephron join with the collecting tubules.

  c. Together they form the proximal tubule, the loop of Henle, and the distal tubule.

D. The urinary system develops.[4–6,8,14,18,19]

1. The dilated end of the hindgut, known as the cloaca, divides to form the following.[11]

  a. Urinary system

  b. Anorectal canal

  c. Urogenital sinus

2. The urinary bladder and ureters are formed.[4–6,14]

  a. The bladder epithelium develops from the urogenital sinus.[4,12]

  b. The muscles and serosa develop from the adjacent splanchnic mesenchyme.[12]

  c. As the bladder grows, the dorsal wall meets and incorporates itself into the caudal aspect of the mesonephric ducts.

    1) In the male, the metanephric duct forms the appendix of the epididymis, vas deferens, and ejaculatory duct.

    2) In the female, mesonephric duct development is suppressed.

  d. The mesonephric ducts are absorbed, and urinary drainage into the bladder is replaced by exclusive flow through the ureters, which are patent around the 11th week of gestation.[20]

  e. The bladder can be easily identified by ultrasound at 16 weeks gestation.[13]

3. The urachus develops.[4,5,11,14]

  a. Failure of the urachus to fibrose into the median umbilical ligament will result in a patent fistula known as a patent urachus. This allows drainage of urine into the umbilical orifice directly from the bladder.

    1) Partial patency remains at the level of the bladder in 50 percent of infants.[19]

    2) Complete patency is rare.[19]

  b. The urachus eventually becomes the median umbilical ligament.

4. The urethra develops.[4,5,14,18,21]
  a. The prostatic urethra of the male and the entire urethra of the female develop from the vesicourethral canal of the urogenital sinus.
  b. In the male, the glandular portion of the penile urethra develops from a cluster of ectodermal cells that canalize the glans from the tip (Figure 6-4).[4]

REPRODUCTIVE SYSTEM

A. The strict sequence of differentiation in the sexual development of the human fetus.[1,4,6,8,9,11,22–25]
  1. This process occurs early in pregnancy, with sexual organ and internal structure differentiation complete by 7 to 8 weeks gestation.
  2. The development of external genitalia is complete by 16 weeks.
  3. Sexual differentiation begins with the presence of X or Y chromosomes and completes under the influence of testosterone.[25]
    a. The short arm of the Y chromosome contains the gene responsible for the differentiation of the primitive gonad into a testis.
    b. Although genes regulate differentiation of gonads, hormones mediate phenotype.
B. Internal sexual organs and structures[4,11,23,24]
  1. Gonadal development[4,11]
    a. The development of male or female gonads is dependent on chromosomal influence and is separate from the development of internal and external sexual structures.
    b. Undifferentiated gonads are present by 5 weeks gestation.
    c. Ovaries develop as follows.
      1) In the presence of XX (lack of Y), primordial germ cells migrate to the cortical region of the urogenital ridge. As the medulla regresses, ovaries develop from the cortex.
      2) Ovaries are identifiable by 10 weeks gestation (Figure 6-5).

FIGURE 6-4 ■ Schematic longitudinal sections of the distal part of the developing penis illustrating development of the prepuce (foreskin) and the distal part of the spongy urethra.

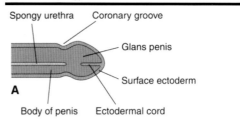

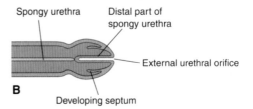

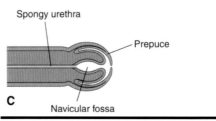

From: Moore KL, and Persaud TVN. 2003. *The Developing Human: Clinically Oriented Embryology,* 7th ed. Philadelphia: Saunders, 306. Reprinted by permission.

FIGURE 6-5 ■ Differentiation of the indifferent gonads of a five-week embryo (top) into ovaries or testes.

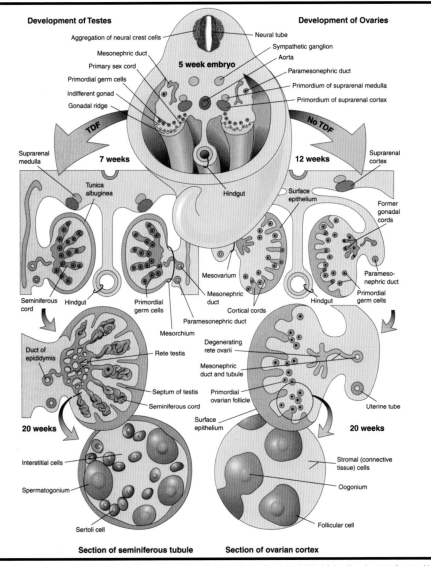

From: Moore KL, and Persaud TVN. 2003. *The Developing Human: Clinically Oriented Embryology,* 7th ed. Philadelphia: Saunders, 310. Reprinted by permission.

3) The ovary descends to its final position in the pelvis by 12 weeks gestation.

   a) It is secured by the development of the round and ovarian ligaments.[23]

d. Testes develop as follows.[25–29]

   1) In the presence of XY, primordial germ cells migrate to the medulla, with subsequent regression of the cortex. This results in the development of testes (see Figure 6-5).[4,23]

   2) Migration or descent of the testes through the inguinal canals into the scrotum is complete by 32–34 weeks gestation.

e. Primordial germ cells are located in the wall of the yolk sac.

FIGURE 6-6 ■ **Internal genital duct development.**

A. Indifferent stage showing large mesonephric body. **B.** Female ducts. Remnants of the mesonephros and wolffian ducts are now termed the epoophoron, paroophoron, and Gartner's duct. **C.** Male ducts before descent into the scrotum. The only müllerian remnant is the testicular appendix. The prostatic utricle (vaginal masculina) is derived from the urogenital sinus.

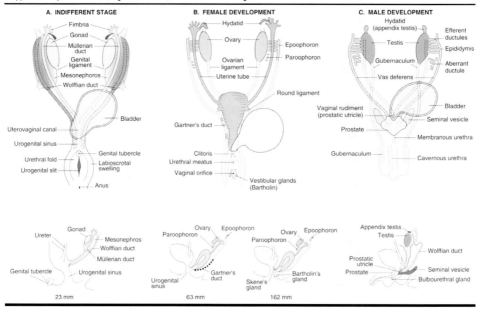

From: Grumbach MM, and Conte FA. 1985. Disorders of sexual differentiation. In *William's Textbook of Endocrinology*, 7th ed., Wilson JD, and Foster DW, eds. Philadelphia: Saunders, 329. Reprinted by permission.

     1) These cells migrate to the gonads to develop as oogonia and spermatogonia.

     2) This migration occurs by the sixth week of gestation.[23]

     3) The full complement of oogonia is developed prior to birth.[23]

  2. Internal sexual structures[4,11,23]

    a. Internal sexual structures differentiate under the influence of the presence or absence of testosterone produced by the testes.

    b. In the female, following the regression of the medullary region of the urogenital ridge, the paramesonephric (Müllerian) ducts of the primitive genital ducts differentiate into internal female structures in the absence of Müllerian-inhibiting substance (MIS) (Figure 6-6).[25]

      1) Fallopian tubes

      2) Uterus

      3) Cervix

      4) Upper vagina

    c. In the male, cortical regression supports the differentiation of the mesonephric genital ducts.[25]

      1) Under the influence of testosterone and MIS, these ducts subsequently develop as male internal structures (see Figure 6-6).[25]

        a) Epididymis

        b) Vas deferens

        c) Seminal vesicles

        d) Ejaculatory ducts

C. External genitalia (Figure 6-7)[4,23]

1. In the male, testosterone produced from the testes supports the differentiation into male external genitalia. This occurs between 9 and 12 weeks gestation.[25]

   a. The genital tubercle differentiates into the external male sexual structures and prostate.

      1) The enlargement and elongation of this tissue results in the development of a penis.

   b. As the genital tubercle elongates, the urogenital folds form the lateral walls of the urethral groove.

      1) This forms the under surface of the penis.

      2) The fusion of the urogenital folds form the penile urethra.

   c. The glandular plate on the tip of the penis splits to form a groove on the ventral side of the glans.

      1) As this groove meets the urethral groove, the external urethral orifice moves to the tip of the glans (Figure 6-8).

   d. During the 12th week of gestation, the foreskin begins to form from a fold of skin at the distal margin of the penis.

      1) The glans is completely covered by the foreskin at 14 weeks gestation.

   e. The scrotum forms from a pouch of tissue in the inguinal area that migrates to each side of the urogenital folds anterior to the perineum.[30]

   f. Testes descend into the scrotum during the third trimester.[25]

   g. The inguinal canals remain patent between the peritoneal cavity and the scrotum until anatomic closure several months following birth.[31]

   h. The prostate differentiates from the urogenital sinus in response to testosterone stimulation. Testosterone production begins at 8 weeks and peaks at 12–18 weeks.[32]

      1) Multiple endodermal outgrowths from the prostatic portion of the urethra grow into the surrounding tissue forming the prostate.

         a) Ductal budding begins at 10 weeks gestation.[33]

         b) Prostatic bud development is complete by 20–23 weeks gestation; bud tubule development by 30–31 weeks, and acinotubular development by 37–42 weeks.[32,34]

         c) Further differentiation occurs up to one year of age.[32]

FIGURE 6-7 ■ **Differentiation of the external genitalia in the male and female fetus from the common primordia.**

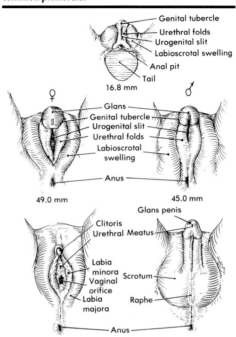

From: Grumbach MM, et al. 1992. Disorders of sexual differentiation. In *William's Textbook of Endocrinology*, 8th ed., Wilson JD, and Foster DW., eds. Philadelphia: Saunders, 853. Reprinted by permission.

FIGURE 6-8 ■ **Development of the external genitalia.**

A and B. Diagrams illustrating the appearance of the genitalia during the indifferent stage (fourth to seventh weeks). **C, E, and G.** Stages in the development of male external genitalia at 9, 11, and 12 weeks, respectively. To the left are schematic transverse sections of the developing penis, illustrating formation of the spongy urethra. **D, F, and H.** Stages in the development of female external genitalia at 9, 11, and 12 weeks, respectively.

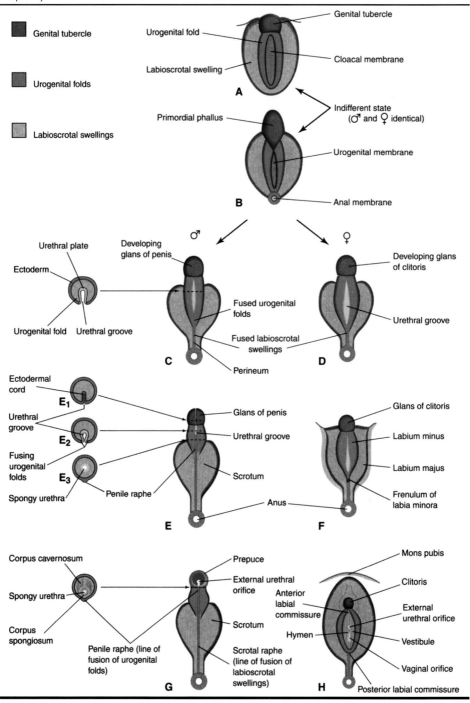

From: Moore KL, and Persaud TVN. 2003. *The Developing Human: Clinically Oriented Embryology,* 7th ed. Philadelphia: Saunders, 316. Reprinted by permission.

2. In the female, the absence of testosterone supports the differentiation into female external genitalia (see Figure 6-7).[25]

   a. The genital swellings differentiate as the labia majora and labia minora.

   b. The anterior aspect of the labioscrotal folds fuse to form the mons pubis.

   c. The posterior aspect of the labioscrotal folds fuse to form the posterior labial commissure.

   d. The unfused portion of the labioscrotal folds form the labia majora.

   e. The lower vagina develops from the urogenital sinus.

      1) It develops inward to meet the upper vagina, which is developing as part of the internal sexual structures.

      2) The urogenital folds fail to fuse, forming the labia minora.

      3) The vagina initially develops as a solid cord of tissue. The central epithelial cells break down to form the lumen of the vagina. The peripheral cells remain as the vaginal epithelium.

      4) The hymen separates the cavity of the urogenital sinus from the vaginal lumen. It usually ruptures during the perinatal period.[35]

Physiology

RENAL SYSTEM

A. Effects of normal renal function *in utero*[10,36]

   1. Normal growth

   2. Lung development

   3. Protective autoregulation of fetal vascular volume

B. The kidney regulates[10,17,36,37]

   1. Fluids and electrolytes

   2. Excretion of toxins

   3. Arterial blood pressure

   4. Activation of erythropoietin (for production of red blood cells) and vitamin D

C. Primary renal functions[5,11]

   1. Ultrafiltration of plasma by the glomerulus

   2. Reabsorption of water and solutes from the ultrafiltrate

   3. Secretion of solutes into the tubular fluid

D. Determinants of renal clearance[5,17,20]

   1. Glomerular filtration

   2. Reabsorption of substances from tubular fluid into blood

   3. Secretion of substances from blood into tubular fluid

   4. Total balance of input from the renal arteries combined with the output from the renal veins and ureters

      a. *In utero*[37]

         1) The fetus relies primarily on the placenta for homeostatic function.

            a) The placenta is the primary excretory organ of the fetus.[3,10]

            b) Renal function is diminished and not necessary for homeostasis.

      b. At birth[2,3,17,37,38]

         1) Cardiac output and the relationship between peripheral vascular resistance (PVR) and renal vascular resistance (RVR) determine renal blood flow (RBF).[10,18]

         2) The increase in RBF is primarily a result of the simultaneous increase in PVR and decrease in RVR combined with the rise in cardiac output and

mean arterial pressure that occurs at the time of birth.[10,25] RVR continues to fall throughout the first year of life.[39]

3) Cardiac output received by the fetal kidney increases from approximately 5 percent of cardiac output in the previable infant to approximately 9 percent by one week of age in the term infant.[10]

4) After birth, the glomerular filtration rate (GFR) doubles in the first two weeks, primarily in response to the increase in RBF.[20]

c. Glomerular filtration rate[3,11,16,37,39,40]

1) GFR represents the rate at which fluid is filtered by the glomerulus. It is affected by any process that induces a change in filtration surface or tubular permeability, including the following.[5,36]

a) Hydration

b) Arterial blood pressure

c) Physiologic maturity

d) Anatomic maturity

e) Drugs

f) Vascular resistance

g) Plasma protein concentration

h) Glomerular capillary permeability

2) GFR reflects renal function.[11]

3) Serum creatine levels are a direct reflection of GFR.[5]

4) A progressive and proportional increase in GFR and urine output volumes begins upon development of the first nephrons and continues as the fetus grows to term.[20] This increase is primarily the result of the following.[5,17,36,38,41]

a) Decrease in RVR

b) Increase in RBF

c) Increase in glomerular surface area

5) A functional GFR develops between 9 and 12 weeks simultaneous to the first ultraurine production, which occurs between 8 and 10 weeks.[5,10,11]

6) GFR increases after birth in both the preterm and the term neonate.[5,10,36,38,41]

a) In the preterm neonate, the increase in GFR at birth is slightly less than that of the term infant and remains lower throughout the first month of life.[42]

b) In term infants, serum creatinine levels will steadily decrease over the first several days to approximately 0.6–1 mg/dl and will continue to drop to normal levels of 0.2–0.3 mg/dl by 6 months of age.[43]

d. Tubular function[1,3,5,10,37,44,45]

1) The nephron is a complex functional unit consisting, in part, of an elongated tubular segment. Function along the tubule assures a balance of filtration and reabsorption effecting homeostasis.

2) Tubular reabsorption is a process of both active and passive transport as well as diffusion across a semipermeable membrane. Sodium is a primary ion involved in many of the known transporters.

3) Proximal tubule[10,45]

a) Transport proteins facilitate the reabsorption of 70 to 80 percent of water and elements in the proximal tubule.[10]

b) Although tubular function regulating the reabsorption of sodium is present in the fetus by 24 weeks gestation, sodium and calcium reabsorption is limited in the proximal tubule prior to 34 weeks gestation.[5,10]

      c) The proximal tubule is short and immature in the very low birth weight infant, limiting excretion of organic acids.

      d) The proximal tubule has a lower renal threshold for bicarbonate.[46]

   4) Loop of Henle[10,45]

      a) In the neonate, only long-looped nephrons extend into the medulla. Short-looped nephrons remain superficial to the cortex.

      b) Short-looped nephrons are critical to the recycling of urea, on which the concentrating process is dependent.[47]

      c) The loop of Henle provides passive transport of calcium.[48]

      d) It demonstrates significant ability for reabsorption of potassium.[49]

   5) Distal tubule/collecting duct[10,45]

      a) Factors affecting function of the distal tubule are responsible for the changes in the handling of sodium by the nephron.[46]

      b) These remain impermeable to water except under the influence of antidiuretic hormone (ADH) secreted by the posterior pituitary.[50]

      c) The distal tubules are critical to the maintenance of homeostasis through the control of water and solute concentrations.[5,10]
- Sodium, phosphate, bicarbonate, and amino acids are absorbed.
- Hydrogen ions are secreted.
- Potassium and organic acids are absorbed and secreted.
- There is active transport of calcium.[49]

      d) Sodium delivery to the distal tubule is greater and sodium reabsorption is less in the premature than in the term infant.[46]

      e) In the distal tubule, the following are diminished.[5]
- Levels of aldosterone
- Sensitivity to aldosterone

F. Renal autoregulation[5,11,38]

   1. GFR and RBF are maintained in a constant state by a pressure-sensitive myogenic mechanism.

G. Regulation of fluid and electrolytes[5,51]

   1. The processes of fluid and electrolyte balance are dependent on tubular:

     a. Secretion

     b. Reabsorption

     c. Excretion

   2. Water balance[3,5,42,52]

     a. The ability to concentrate urine correlates to the length of the long loops of Henle. As the loops elongate into the medulla, the ability to concentrate urine improves.[47]

     b. The shorter loops of Henle allow the accumulation of urea, thereby maintaining a physiologic gradient.[47]

     c. There is limited water reabsorption in the thin ascending limbs of the loops of Henle.[47]

     d. The immature kidney maintains sodium and water homeostasis through the following.[33]

       1) Diminished glomerular filtration

       2) Diminished maximum sodium reabsorption

       3) Diminished renal capacity for dilution and concentration of urine

       4) Diminished bicarbonate reabsorption parallel to potassium and hydrogen ion secretion

  e. The diffusion of water is primarily a passive process related to osmotically active sodium and chloride concentrations.[53]

     1) Osmosis

       a) Is the primary means of water transport. It is regulated by osmotic pressure, which is determined exclusively by the concentration of solute particles.[39]

     2) Hydrostatic pressure[5,52]

       a) This is the primary regulator of GFR and is directly affected by any fluctuation in RBF.[11]

       b) Obstruction results in increased hydrostatic pressure.[37]

H. Factors affecting renal hemodynamics

  1. Renin production[5,10,54,55]

    a. Renin, angiotensinogen, and angiotensin converting enzyme are detectable in the metanephros at six weeks gestation.[10]

    b. Juxtamedullary cells produce increasing amounts of renin beginning at three months gestation.[2,10,53]

    c. Renin is produced, stored, and released from the smooth muscle cells of the nephron.

    d. When RBF decreases, the renin-angiotensin cycle is activated at the level of the kidney; renin secretion results in an increase in RBF and GFR.[2,10,56]

  2. Angiotensin, aldosterone, and catecholamines[55]

    a. The fetal response to angiotensin is vital to the control of the following.

     1) Placental blood flow to the fetus

     2) Fetal blood pressure

     3) Renal blood flow and pressure in the fetus and newborn[10,14,53]

    b. Angiotensin II levels increase as a result of elevated renin, stimulating water and sodium chloride (NaCl) reabsorption in the proximal tubule.[5]

    c. Aldosterone is secreted from the adrenal cortex in response to increased serum levels of potassium and angiotensin II. It promotes NaCl reabsorption from the thick ascending limb of Henle's loop, the distal tubule, and the collecting duct and stimulates potassium secretion from the distal tubule and the collecting duct.[5] Fetal response to aldosterone is decreased, resulting in diminished sodium reabsorption.[10,17,37,53]

    d. Catecholamines (norepinephrine and epinephrine) do the following.[5,10]

     1) They increase RVR.

     2) They increase efferent arteriolar tone.

     3) They increase renin release.

     4) They increase angiotensin II release.

     5) They affect the distribution of potassium across cell membranes.[5]

     6) They promote water and NaCl reabsorption.

     7) Epinephrine, norepinephrine, and angiotensin II cause vasoconstriction, resulting in increased vascular resistance. This decreases both RBF and GFR.[2,10,37,50,56]

  3. ADH[5]

    a. Is the primary regulatory hormone of water balance

    b. Increases water reabsorption in the collecting duct

4. Prostaglandin production
    a. Prostaglandins are antagonistic to angiotensin II.[11]
    b. Prostaglandins PGE_2 and PGI_2 cause vasodilation, inducing a decrease in vascular resistance.[2,10,37,39,53]
5. Kallikrein-kinin system
    a. This system is activated at birth and is involved in the regulation of sodium and water by influencing renal hemodynamics.[10,37,53,56]
    b. Kallikrein is a proteolytic enzyme produced in the kidneys. It cleaves kininogen to bradykinin.
    c. Bradykinin is a diuretic and vasodilator peptide that stimulates the release of nitric oxide and prostaglandins.[5,7,10]
        1) It increases GFR and RBF.[5]
6. Nitric oxide (NO)
    a. NO is produced by the renal vascular endothelium.[10,37,56]
    b. It is a vasodilator in the developing kidney.[10,37,56]
    c. It counteracts the vasoconstrictive effects of angiotensin II and catecholamines.[5]
    d. It induces vasodilation of the afferent and efferent arterioles in the kidneys.[5]
7. Atrial natriuretic factor[37,50,55,56]
    a. Hormone secreted in the heart by cardiac myocytes
    b. A potent vasodilator, diuretic, and natriuretic[7]
    c. Increases GFR with little change in RBF through vasodilation of the afferent arteriole and vasoconstriction of the efferent arteriole[5]
    d. Inhibits renin and aldosterone release
    e. Increases vascular permeability
    f. Decreases both arterial pressure and blood volume by reducing peripheral vascular resistance and enhancing sodium and water excretion[6,7]
    g. Produces renal vasodilation in the renal splanchnic bed[7]
8. Urodilatin[5]
    a. Hormone secreted in the distal tubule and the collecting duct that inhibits sodium and water reabsorption across the medullary portion of the collecting duct
9. Endothelin B
    a. A potent vasoconstrictor that increases fetal urine flow and electrolyte excretion and decreases GFR and RBF[5,37]
10. Dopamine and dopamine receptors[5]
    a. Dopamine is a vasodilator hormone.
    b. Secretion is stimulated by an increase in extracellular fluid volume.
    c. Dopamine increases RBF.
    d. It inhibits renin secretion.
    e. It inhibits NaCl and water reabsorption in the proximal tubule.
11. Arginine vasopressin (AVP)[10,55]
    a. This is a potent intrarenal vasoconstrictor.
    b. In response to stress, AVP may induce a decrease in RBF and a secondary increase in RVR.
I. Electrolyte balance[51,55,57,58]
    1. In general, the functional transport of ions in the immature kidney is diminished when compared to the mature kidney, with the exception of phosphate, which is more active in the immature nephron.[45]

2. Sodium (Figure 6-9)[1,5,10,17,37,45,52,53,59]
   a. The sodium-hydrogen exchanger is responsible for the majority of sodium bicarbonate and NaCl reabsorption. It maintains intracellular pH and regulates cell growth.[45]
   b. The highest concentration of sodium is found in extracellular fluid.
   c. Positive sodium balance is required for growth.
   d. The ability to reabsorb sodium is present by 24 weeks gestation.
   e. In the immature infant, a partial compensatory increase in sodium reabsorption occurs in the distal tubule in response to limited reabsorption in the proximal tubule. This mechanism is responsive to the increased circulating levels of renin, angiotensin, and aldosterone. The compensation cannot fully accommodate the increased sodium delivery to the distal tubule. Therefore, the overall net effect is a persistent state of salt wasting.[36]
   f. Renal tubular maturation will result in increased sodium reabsorption in the proximal tubules. This will precipitate a gradual decrease in renin, angiotensin, and aldosterone levels.[36]
   g. Total body sodium and chloride are higher per kilogram in the premature infant than in the term infant.[55]
   h. In the term infant, a diminished fractional excretion of sodium (FENa) results in an improved ability to preserve sodium and maintain a positive sodium balance.
   i. Conversely, the decrease in FENa and low GFR limit the infant's ability to excrete a sodium load.[3,36]
   j. FENa may be increased with the following.[17]
      1) Hypoxia
      2) Respiratory distress
      3) Hyperbilirubinemia
      4) Acute tubular necrosis
      5) Polycythemia
      6) Drugs such as
         a) Diuretics
         b) Theophylline
         c) Caffeine
   k. Cortisol has been shown to decrease sodium reabsorption.
3. Potassium[1,3,10,17,37,49,60]
   a. Potassium regulation is achieved through the balance of potassium reabsorption in the proximal tubule and loop of Henle with the secretion of potassium in the distal tubule and the collecting duct.[5]
   b. Potassium excretion in the neonate is diminished. This results in a serum potassium level that is higher in the neonate than in the adult.[36]
   c. Potassium and hydrogen are present in the distal tubule as a process of tubular secretion.
      1) Hydrogen ion concentration directly impacts potassium excretion into urine.
      2) Serum potassium levels are increased in the presence of metabolic acidosis; alkalosis results in decreased serum potassium levels.
   d. Fractional reabsorption of potassium is decreased in the loop of Henle.[45]
   e. Approximately 50–65 percent of filtered potassium is reabsorbed in the proximal tubule.[10,49] Reabsorption closely follows water reabsorption.[49]

4. Chloride[5]
   a. Chloride reabsorption in the proximal tubule is both passive and active and is closely linked to sodium transport.[45]
   b. Chloride transport is indirectly linked to hydrogen ion transport.[45]
   c. Fractional reabsorption of chloride is decreased in the loop of Henle.[5,45]
5. Calcium[5,10,19,48,61–63]
   a. The kidney is a primary organ regulating extracellular calcium concentration.[62]
   b. Calcium homeostasis is regulated by parathyroid hormone (PTH).[5]

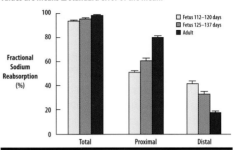

FIGURE 6-9 ■ Fractional sodium reabsorption in different renal tubular segments in two groups of fetal sheep and in nonpregnant ewes.

Values are means ± standard error of the mean.

From: Lumbers ER, Hill KJ, and Bennett VJ. 1988. Proximal and distal tubular activity in chronically catheterized fetal sheep compared with the adult. *Canadian Journal of Physiology and Pharmacology* 66(6): 697–702. Reprinted by permission.

   1) Increased production of PTH in response to decreased plasma calcium levels will do the following.
      a) It increases calcium resorption from bone, thereby raising calcium concentrations in the extracellular fluid.
      b) It increases calcium reabsorption in the proximal tubule, thereby decreasing calcium excretion.[64]
      c) It increases absorption of calcium from the small intestine.
   2) There is diminished response to PTH in the ascending limb of the loop of Henle.[50]
   c. Calcitonin produced by the thyroid gland inhibits the release of calcium from bone and increases renal tubular excretion of calcium.[55,62,64]
   d. There is increased calcium excretion with decreasing gestational age.[17,64]
   e. Fractional reabsorption of calcium is decreased in the loop of Henle.[10]
   f. Altered renal regulation most commonly results in hypercalcemia as a result of a decrease in calcium excretion.[62]
   g. Most renal calcium reabsorption occurs in the proximal tubule.
   h. Renal tubular excretion of calcium and sodium are normally parallel; however, their reabsorption may be independent.[5]
   i. Acid-base balance impacts the plasma concentration of ionized calcium (iCa) by altering calcium binding in competition with hydrogen ions. Total calcium levels are not impacted.[5]
   j. Ionized calcium levels are decreased in the first 48 hours of life.
   k. The following factors affect ionized levels.[62]
      1) The total serum calcium level.
      2) Elevated serum albumin decreases serum iCa.
      3) Elevated serum phosphate decreases serum iCa.
      4) Elevated bicarbonate decreases serum iCa.
      5) Elevated levels of heparin in the blood will decrease serum iCa.
      6) Serum iCa is inversely related to blood pH.
      7) Elevated serum magnesium will increase serum iCa.

6. Magnesium[5,10,62,63,65]
   a. Most magnesium is in bone and is not exchanged with extracellular magnesium. Therefore, the serum magnesium levels cannot be utilized to evaluate total body magnesium. Decreased levels at birth will rise over the first week of life.[64]
   b. Contrary to calcium and phosphorus, magnesium homeostasis is not hormonally regulated. The dominant regulation of magnesium is through the balance of magnesium concentrations in the intestine, kidney, and intracellular fluid.[62,64]
   c. The kidney is the primary regulatory organ for total body serum magnesium concentrations.
   d. Reabsorption of magnesium in the renal tubule is stimulated by the following.[10]
      1) PTH
      2) Calcitonin
      3) Glucagon
      4) AVP
   e. Increased excretion of magnesium occurs as a result of the following.[64,65]
      1) Hypercalcemia
      2) Hypermagnesemia
      3) Expansion of the extracellular fluid compartment
      4) Decreased PTH levels
      5) Acidosis
      6) Estrogen
      7) Thyroxine
      8) Aldosterone
   f. Decreased excretion of magnesium occurs as a result of the following.[64,65]
      1) Hypocalcemia
      2) Hypomagnesemia
      3) Contraction of the extracellular fluid compartment
      4) Increased PTH levels
      5) Alkalosis
      6) Epinephrine
      7) Glucocorticoids
      8) Progesterone
7. Phosphate[2,37,45,63,64]
   a. Phosphorus exists as either organic or inorganic forms in the plasma. Only the inorganic form is measured in the clinical setting. Approximately 10–15 percent of total plasma inorganic phosphorus is protein bound. The remaining 85 to 90 percent is filtered by the renal glomerulus as phosphate ions. Phosphate measurements are expressed as the amount of elemental phosphorus, therefore, the terms phosphorus concentration and phosphate concentration are used interchangeably in the clinical setting.[60]
   b. Phosphorus is an important buffer affecting acid-base balance.
   c. Homeostasis is controlled by total body phosphorus and the distribution between intracellular and extracellular fluid compartments.[5]
      1) Total phosphate is regulated by the following.[10]
         a) PTH
         b) Dietary intake
         c) Growth hormone

d) Insulin-like growth factors

e) Glucocorticoids

2) PTH has the greatest effect on homeostasis of serum phosphorus through its response to serum calcium levels. The result is the increase in ionized phosphorus excretion.

d. Excretion is affected by the following.[5]

1) Changes in the extracellular fluid (ECF) volume

2) Acid-base imbalance

3) Glucocorticoids (increase phosphorus excretion by inhibiting calcium reabsorption in the proximal tubule)

4) Growth hormone (decreases phosphorus excretion)

5) Calcitrol induced by hypophosphatemia (decreases ionized phosphorus and calcium)

e. Phosphorus tubular reabsorption is increased by the following.[5,10,61]

1) Growth hormone

2) $1,25(OH)_2D$

3) Insulin

4) Somatomedins

f. Even in the preterm neonate, the kidney has a high reabsorptive capacity for phosphate.

g. Reabsorptive ability increases to 85–99 percent between 28 weeks gestation and term.[10,17]

J. Acid-base balance[5,58,66–68]

1. Acid-base homeostasis is maintained through the excretion of acid from the body at a rate equal to the addition of acid products. The parallel reabsorption of filtered bicarbonate together with acid excretion is defined as net acid excretion. Net acid excretion in balance with acid production maintains serum pH at 7.35–7.45.

2. To maintain acid-base balance, the following occurs.

a. Renal response to acid-base disturbance is slow and gradual.[60]

b. Kidneys cannot excrete free acids. They must excrete sodium salts and conserve bicarbonate. This is done by the reabsorption of excreted hydrogen ions as bicarbonate (HCO_3), therefore producing acid urine.[5]

3. Acid-base balance is affected by the following.

a. Mineralocorticoids increase net acid excretion. They stimulate renal tubular acidification, increasing ammonium production.[60]

b. Hypercalcemia and excess vitamin D increase tubular reabsorption of bicarbonate leading to metabolic acidosis, nephrocalcinosis, and renal insufficiency.[60]

c. PTH inhibits tubular reabsorption of bicarbonate and increases net acid excretion. Combined with the resulting increase in plasma bicarbonate, a metabolic alkalosis results.[60]

4. Bicarbonate is a major buffer in both plasma and erythrocytes.[1,3,37,60]

a. Bicarbonate is produced by the metabolism of amino acids, aspartate, glutamate, and organic anions.[5,60]

b. Under normal conditions, the majority of tubular bicarbonate is reabsorbed in the proximal tubule. Therefore, very little is actually excreted in the urine.[5,66]

c. Within the cell, hydrogen ion and bicarbonate are produced. Hydrogen ion is secreted into the tubule, whereas bicarbonate passively exits the cell coupled with other ions, of which sodium is dominant.[5,66] The bicarbonate and hydrogen ion within the tubule are easily uncoupled, creating CO_2 and water, which are rapidly reabsorbed.[5,66]

    d. Bicarbonate homeostasis is altered by factors affecting hydrogen ion secretion.[5]

    e. PTH inhibits bicarbonate reabsorption in the proximal tubule.[5]

    f. In the term infant and even more so in the preterm infant, the proximal tubule has a low threshold for bicarbonate.

    g. This inability to preserve bicarbonate combined with the limited ability to excrete an acid load results in the susceptibility of the preterm infant to the development of metabolic acidosis.[10,17]

    h. The bicarbonate threshold increases with gestational age.[10]

5. Hydrogen ion effects are as follows.

    a. Tubular excretion of hydrogen ions is insufficient to maintain homeostasis.[5]

    b. Hydrogen ions are vital to the synthesis of ammonium, which is then excreted in the urine, which in turn results in the reabsorption of bicarbonate.[5]

    c. Hydrogen ions are excreted with urinary buffers such as phosphate to form titratable acids.[5]

    d. Hypokalemia stimulates the secretion of hydrogen by the proximal tubule. Conversely, hyperkalemia will inhibit hydrogen secretion.[5]

    e. Decreased ECF will increase hydrogen ion secretion.

    f. Increased ECF will decrease hydrogen ion secretion.

    g. Aldosterone will stimulate sodium reabsorption in the collecting tubule, resulting in increased hydrogen ion secretion.[5]

    h. At birth, there is diminished ability of the collecting duct to secrete hydrogen ion.

        1) This ability improves by two weeks of age, increasing the infant's ability to acidify urine to a pH of ≤5.[10]

    i. At maturity, secretion of hydrogen ion is limited only by the availability of urinary buffers.[17,60]

6. Urinary buffers are necessary to the control of renal acidification.[10,60,69]

    a. Reabsorption of bicarbonate is not enough to maintain homeostasis. New bicarbonate must be produced.[5]

    b. There is limited ability in the neonate for renal acidification as a result of decreased excretion of urinary buffers such as phosphates and ammonia.[10]

    c. Distal urine acidification is critical to the reabsorption of filtered bicarbonate, titration of phosphorus, and excretion of ammonium.[66] It is dependent on mineralocorticoids, sodium transport, presence of urinary buffers, tubular fluid pH, and systemic pH and CO_2 content.[66]

    d. Because bicarbonate is reabsorbed at and above the level of Henle's loop, hydrogen ions in the fluid of the collecting duct combine with urinary buffers.

    e. The most active urinary buffer is phosphorus. Once combined, it is excreted, leaving bicarbonate to be reabsorbed back into the bloodstream.[5]

    f. Ammonium is produced in the proximal tubule through the metabolism of glutamate. The excretion of ammonium and acid salts produces new sodium bicarbonate ($NaHCO_3$), which is reabsorbed into the plasma. This process is dependent on the excretion of ammonium into tubular fluid.

1) If ammonium reenters the circulation without excretion into tubular fluid, it will be converted to urea. The hydrogen ions produced are buffered by bicarbonate. This process will result in the consumption of bicarbonate by the metabolism of ammonium. This pathway will negate the contribution of ammonium as a major buffer responsible for the production of new bicarbonate.[5]

2) Ammonium regulation is affected by the following.

    a) Acidosis increases production of the enzymes necessary for glutamine metabolism in the proximal tubule.[5]

    b) Alkalosis will inversely increase ammonium production.

    c) Hyperkalemia inhibits ammonium production, and hypokalemia stimulates increased production.[5]

K. Organic components of urine

  1. Glucose[1,10,37,70,71]

    a. Premature infants have higher fractional glucose excretion and lower glucose reabsorption.

      1) This results in a higher urine glucose concentration.

      2) This limitation is caused by the following.[45]

        a) Limitation of the number of glucose transporters

        b) Increased extracellular fluid volume

        c) Diminished GFR

        d) Increased intracellular sodium

        e) Diminished electrical potential across the tubular epithelium

    b. All newborns have a lower renal threshold for glucose.

      1) The threshold increases with gestational age.

      2) At term, the infant has the capacity for maximum reabsorption of glucose.[17]

      3) Transport is sodium dependent.[45]

    c. Increased reabsorptive ability is primarily supported by the following.[45]

      1) Development of new nephrons

      2) Increase in cell membrane surface

      3) Changes in expression and density of transporter proteins

      4) Changes in membrane permeability to sodium affecting membrane potential

  2. Amino acids[3,10,17,45,72]

    a. Renal reabsorption of many amino acids is low in the neonate resulting in higher urinary amino acid levels. Mild proteinuria in the first week is normal.[36]

    b. Transport is sodium dependent.

    c. Acidic amino acids require potassium for transport.

    d. Limited reabsorptive ability in the immature infant results in diminished ability to adapt to states of amino acid deficiency.

    e. Peptides (angiotensin II, bradykinin, and glucagons) are filtered freely at the glomerulus. They are reabsorbed in the proximal tubule after being hydrolyzed by peptidases.

    f. Proteins are filtrated by the glomerulus, dependent on their molecular size.

  3. Organic acids[3,10,45,73]

    a. Renal clearance of organic acids is low in the neonate.[17]

    b. Organic acids are divided into anions and cations. Many are end products of metabolism that are eliminated both by filtration and secretion in the proximal tubule.[45]

        1) Cations include the following.

            a) Creatinine

            b) Dopamine

            c) Epinephrine

            d) Norepinephrine

            e) Atropine

            f) Morphine

        2) Anions include the following.

            a) Prostaglandins

            b) Bile salts

            c) Oxalate

            d) Urate

            e) Furosemide

            e) Chlorothiazides

            f) Penicillin

    c. Uric acid is filtered at the glomerulus and transported by the proximal tubule in exchange for chloride.[45]

        1) Decreased solubility in alkaline urine results in the uric acid crystals commonly seen in normal infants.[36]

        2) Decreases in the fractional excretion of urate is thought to be secondary to maturation of the superficial renal cortex, resulting in increased reabsorptive capacity.[45]

L. Urine output[1,3,62]

    1. Urine concentration[17,37,47,53,62]

        a. The final concentration of urine occurs in the renal collecting ducts, primarily as a result of ADH.[10,42]

        b. Both preterm and term infants have a limited ability to concentrate urine.[10]

            1) This ability improves after 35 weeks of gestation.

            2) Normal concentrating ability occurs by one year of life.[11,12]

            3) In contrast, the ability to dilute urine is fairly efficient.

                a) Both premature and term infants can produce urine with an osmolarity as low as 50 mOsm/liter.[55]

                b) The resulting clinical impact is the limited ability to handle high osmotic and fluid volume loads.[17]

        c. The neonate has diminished responsiveness to ADH.[10,42]

        d. Anatomic immaturity of the neonatal kidney results in a low medullary gradient.[10]

        e. Both term and preterm infants have the ability to produce highly dilute urine. However, a low GFR limits the ability of newborns to excrete a hypotonic load.[10]

            1) This may be related to the enhanced ability of the distal tubule to reabsorb sodium, resulting in a high urine sodium content.[36,42]

    2. Volume

        a. Urine production begins at 10 weeks gestation.[10]

        b. Fetal urine is a primary contributor to amniotic fluid volume after 16 weeks gestation; therefore, oligohydramnios may be present in the absence of adequate fetal urine output.[10,13,17,20]

    c. Urine output at 20 weeks gestation is approximately 5 ml/hour. At 30 weeks gestation it is 10 ml/hour, increasing to 50 ml/hour by 40 weeks gestation.[10]

    d. Contraction of the large extracellular fluid volume will result in a steady diuresis in the first week of life.[36]

    e. The neonate has limited ability to suddenly increase GFR, therefore cannot excrete a large fluid volume rapidly.[36]

  3. Voiding

    a. Initial voiding occurs in 50 percent of healthy infants by 12 hours.[36] It occurs by 24 hours in 92 percent of all infants. Ninety-eight percent of infants will void by 48 hours of life.[33]

    b. A smaller group of approximately 8 percent of the normal population may not void until 48 hours of life. Approximately 17 percent of all infants void in the delivery room.[36]

    c. Voiding prior to birth may play a role in the timing of the first documented void.

    d. Delays in voiding may be associated with the following.

      1) Genitourinary anomalies

      2) Perinatal drugs such as magnesium sulfate

      3) Perinatal-neonatal events impacting fluid volume and renal perfusion

M. Body composition[1,55,74]

  1. Total body water includes both intracellular and extracellular volumes.

  2. The fetus and newborn have a higher total body water composition than the adult.

  3. As the fetus develops, extracellular volumes decrease and intracellular volumes increase.

  4. The increase in intracellular volume reflects the growth of organs and body cell proliferation during gestational growth and development.

  5. With the shift in the ratio of extracellular to intracellular water volume, total body electrolyte concentrations change as well. Intracellular electrolytes increase as extracellular electrolytes decrease.

  6. Fetal growth produces an increase in total body protein, carbohydrate, fat, and cellular tissue. This results in a diminished percentage of total body water.

  7. After birth, there is a responsive increase in extracellular fluid consistent with the shift of fluid out of the interstitial compartment. The initial 5–10 percent of weight loss after birth is a reflection of the diuresis resulting from these fluid shifts. The obligatory fluid and sodium losses associated with these compartment shifts are a normal and vital part of transition. In the normal infant, this period usually lasts for approximately three days.

REPRODUCTIVE SYSTEM

A. There is a highly interdependent physiologic relationship between the fetus and the placenta.

B. The functioning of the fetal reproductive system is dependent on the competency of the following.

  1. Pituitary gland[1,25,75]

    a. Gonadotropin-releasing hormone (GnRH) stimulates the anterior pituitary to produce luteinizing hormone (LH) and follicle-stimulating hormone (FSH). These glycoproteins influence the differentiation of fetal gonads and phenotypic development of both male and female.[75]

    b. LH and FSH are detectable in the fetus by 10 weeks gestation.[75]

    c. Plasma concentrations of LH and FSH increase slowly to physiologic levels by 20 weeks gestation, at which time they become regulated by the process of negative feedback.[75]

    d. LH and FSH reach peak levels by 25–29 weeks gestation in the female and 35–40 weeks in the male.[75]

        1) Both LH and FSH contribute to penile lengthening in later gestation.[24]

        2) FSH stimulates the development of ovarian follicles in the female and seminiferous tubules in the male.

        3) LH enhances the production of testosterone from the testes and steroid synthesis from ovarian cells.

    e. The development of functional negative feedback is important to the regulation of LH and FSH, which are released in response to GnRH.[25,75]

        1) Testosterone inhibits the release of GnRH.

        2) Inhibin, which is produced by both fetal testes and ovaries, inhibits FSH but not LH and is present by midgestation. It is higher in females and premature infants.

    f. Both LH and FSH decline with advancing gestational age.

  2. Adrenal glands[1]

    a. Adrenocorticotropic hormone (ACTH), a releasing hormone produced in the anterior pituitary, is produced by the fetal pituitary by eight weeks gestation. ACTH acts on the fetal adrenal glands, stimulating their growth.[25]

    b. The fetal adrenal glands produce the following.

        1) Glucocorticoids

        2) Adrenal androgens

        3) Precursors to the production of estrone and estradiol-17β in the placenta

    c. The fetus cannot convert pregnenolone to progesterone.

        1) The placenta provides a source of progesterone to the fetal adrenal gland; it is then converted by the fetus to corticosteroids.[12]

    d. The corticosteroids produced by the fetal adrenal glands are used by the placenta to produce estrogen.[12]

  3. Gonads[1]

    a. Testosterone can be detected from the fetal testes by eight weeks gestation.

    b. The rise in testosterone secretion may be affected by the levels of human chorionic gonadotropin (hCG) produced by the placenta.

C. The normal development of the human genitalia is dependent on the following.[1,11,24,76]

    a. Genetic integrity

    b. Fetal endocrine function

    c. Fetal hormonal exposure

    d. Teratogenic events

Posterior Urethral Valves

DEFINITION

Posterior urethral valves (PUVs) are not a part of normal urethral development. They are mucosal folds that can obstruct the urethra and cause obstructive uropathy.

PATHOPHYSIOLOGY

A. Three different types of valves have been classified.[77–81]

    1. Type I

        a. This is the most common (about 95 percent of cases).

        b. It consists of a pair of tissue folds or leaflets that extend down and laterally from the lower border of the verumontanum.

        c. The membranous tissue may be thin and transparent or thick and rigid.

        d. The fusion of the valve leaflets may be complete, or there may be a slitlike opening separating them.

        e. The leaflets act as a one-way valve, creating variable degrees of urine flow obstruction.

        f. Antegrade flow is impaired; easy retrograde flow is possible.

    2. Type II

        a. This was originally described as nonpathologic hypertrophy of the posterior urethral folds that did not produce obstruction.

        b. It is currently accepted that Type II valves do not exist.[82,83]

    3. Type III

        a. This type occurs infrequently (in 5 percent of infants who present with PUVs).

        b. It consists of a transverse membrane crossing the urethra.

        c. A pinhole-sized perforation allows the passage of some urine.

        d. There is resistance to urine flow in both directions.

        e. It is associated with greater obstruction and a worse long-term prognosis than Type I valves.

B. The degree of urethral obstruction affects the developing urinary tract by increasing voiding pressure and urine storage.

C. Because the urinary system matures in an environment of elevated intraluminal pressures, consequences may be seen in the proximal urethra, bladder, ureters, and kidneys.[78]

    1. High pressures can cause hypertrophy of the proximal urethra and the bladder neck. The distal urethra may be of normal size.[83]

    2. Bladder changes may be caused by increased collagen deposition and include the following.[78,84,85]

        a. Thickening

        b. Increased connective tissue

        c. Decreased elasticity and compliance

        d. Trabeculation

        e. Diverticula

        f. Hyperplasia of the detrusor muscle

    3. Increased resting pressures in the bladder produce the following.[85]

        a. Vesicoureteral reflux

        b. Ureteral dilation

        c. Hydronephrosis

        d. Renal injury

    4. Polyuria can alter bladder function.[83]

    5. Renal injury may occur because of obstruction or dysplasia.[78,86]

        a. Obstructive uropathy has been observed in nearly all cases.[78]

            1) Increased intraluminal pressure interferes with the following renal processes.

      a) Perfusion

      b) Filtration

      c) Tubular function

    2) The infant may be unable to concentrate and acidify the urine; polyuria is the result.

  b. Dysplasia represents a significant injury. It can be caused by pressure elevations early in fetal life or abnormal embryologic development of the ureteral bud.

    1) Some degree of dysplasia is present in nearly all cases.[78]

      a) The degree of dysplasia cannot be predicted by renal ultrasound.[87]

      2) The renal architecture is disordered; cysts, ectopic tissue, and primitive ductules may be present. Glomeruli are immature.[88]

6. Hydronephrosis may be caused by obstruction or vesicoureteral reflux.[78,84]

  a. The hypertrophied bladder may distort the ureterovesical junction and interfere with urine drainage from the upper tracts.[85]

  b. Reflux may be caused by increased bladder pressure or ectopy of the ureteral orifice.

7. Compensatory processes may develop to protect renal function.[78,80] The following mechanisms provide a "pop off" for the high pressure and may preserve the function of at least one kidney and improve later bladder function.[89]

  a. Development of urinary ascites

  b. Creation of large bladder diverticuli

  c. Urachal patency

  d. Massive unilateral reflux into a single ureter

ETIOLOGY

A. The embryologic derivation of PUVs has not been determined.[78,80] Current theories include the following.

  1. Type I valves are thought to derive from:

    a. An aberrant insertion of the mesonephric duct into the fetal cloaca

    b. Failure of the ventrolateral folds of the urogenital sinus to regress

  2. Type III valves are thought to be caused by incomplete regression of the urogenital membrane.[78,82]

B. Because posterior urethral valves develop early in embryonic life, the developmental impact on the kidney, ureter, and bladder are permanent.

INCIDENCE

A. This condition occurs exclusively in males

B. Most commonly seen form of congenital urethral obstruction

C. 1/4,000 live male births[89]

D. 1/5,000–8,000 male births[77]

E. 1/8,000–25,000 live births[90]

CLINICAL PRESENTATION

A. Clinical presentation depends on the severity of the obstruction and the extent of the involvement of the urinary tract. The spectrum of findings may range from abnormal voiding patterns to advanced renal failure.

  1. The most severely affected infants are usually diagnosed in the neonatal period.

a. These infants may present with severe respiratory distress, urinary ascites, and renal failure.

b. Progressive respiratory failure may result from pulmonary hypoplasia.

2. In the fetus, obstruction changes the amniotic fluid dynamics and can result in the oligohydramnios sequence with the following.

   a. Uterine compression

   b. Potter facies

   c. Limb deformations

   d. Pulmonary hypoplasia

3. A pneumothorax in the newborn period may be the initial finding and can occur across the entire spectrum of presenting acuity.[90]

4. Less severely affected infants may appear asymptomatic in the neonatal period.

5. Other clinical findings include these.

   a. Lethargy, pallor, poor muscle tone, and other signs of systemic illness[78,80,83,84,91]

   b. Palpable mass or masses in the abdomen and/or flanks (distended bladder, ureters, kidneys)

   c. Abdominal distention due to urinary ascites (The abdomen may feel tense, and respirations may be compromised.)

   d. Delayed voiding with dribbling or a poor urinary stream due to "overflow" voiding (Delayed voiding results in incomplete emptying of the bladder.)

   e. Nonspecific signs of sepsis with concurrent urosepsis

B. Laboratory findings include the following.

1. Acidosis

2. Azotemia/uremia

3. Electrolyte abnormalities

Associations

A. Male gender

B. Oligohydramnios sequence

C. VURD syndrome[78,80] (an acronym for valves; unilateral reflux; dysplasia)

Differential Diagnosis[78]

A. Prune belly syndrome

B. Bilateral ureteropelvic junction obstruction

C. Severe vesicoureteral reflux

D. Bilateral ureterovesical junction obstruction

E. Congenital urethral atresia

F. Anterior urethral valves

Diagnosis

A. Most infants are now diagnosed by prenatal ultrasound.[87]

1. PUVs are the third most common prenatally made genitourinary diagnosis after ureteropelvic junction obstruction and megaureter.[78,80]

   a. When diagnosed before 24 weeks gestation, a poor outcome (death or chronic renal failure) is more likely.[92]

   b. Respiratory distress at birth is a predictor of poor outcome.[92]

2. The following are characteristic ultrasound findings.[78]

   a. Hydroureteronephrosis

   b. Dilated bladder neck with a thickened bladder wall

c. Dilated posterior urethra
3. Oligohydramnios and poor uterine growth may be seen.
B. The extent of bladder dysfunction cannot be predicted on the basis of diagnosis alone. Urodynamic studies of the bladder are needed.[83]
C. Imaging studies include the following.
   1. Abdominal and renal ultrasound studies are done when posterior urethral valves are suspected. All infants with a prenatal diagnosis of hydronephrosis should have a repeat ultrasound following normalization of total body water and vascular volume.
   2. A voiding cystourethrogram (VCUG) provides confirmatory evidence of urethral obstruction and reflux (Figure 6-10).[78,93]
      a. Classic findings
         1) Bladder trabeculation
         2) Enlarged bladder capacity
         3) Elongated and dilated posterior urethra
         4) Presence of residual urine after voiding
   3. Radionuclide scanning to assess renal function is ordered when the infant stabilizes.
   4. Renal ultrasound, computed tomography (CT) scan, and intravenous pyelography are not diagnostic for posterior urethral valves.
D. A urine specimen for culture, urinalysis, and electrolytes is obtained to assess for renal tubular dysfunction and infection.
E. Serial measures of serum electrolytes, blood urea nitrogen (BUN), and creatinine are needed over the first several days of life to assess renal function and to distinguish between newborn and maternal regulation.

FIGURE 6-10 ■ Voiding cystourethrogram.

A. Classic dilated posterior urethral and "pop-off" bladder diverticulum.
B. Classic dilated posterior urethral and "pop-off" unilateral vesicoureteral reflux. C. CT scan of the abdomen: Massive urinary ascites secondary to a renal sinus leak from posterior urethral valves. Note that the kidneys are well preserved.

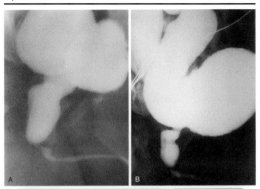

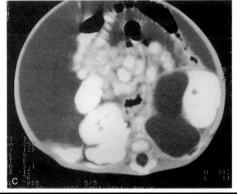

From: Baskin LS, and Kogan BA. 1998. Urethral anomalies and obstruction. In *Urologic Surgery in Infants and Children*, King LR, ed. Philadelphia: Saunders, 211. Reprinted by permission.

TREATMENT OPTIONS AND NURSING CARE

A. The following are management priorities.
   1. Provide cardiopulmonary and hemodynamic support.
      a. Extracorporeal membrane oxygenation has been used successfully to treat associated pulmonary hypertension.[94]
   2. Restore acid-base balance.
   3. Maintain fluid and electrolyte balance.

FIGURE 6-11 ■ Algorithm for treatment of PUV.

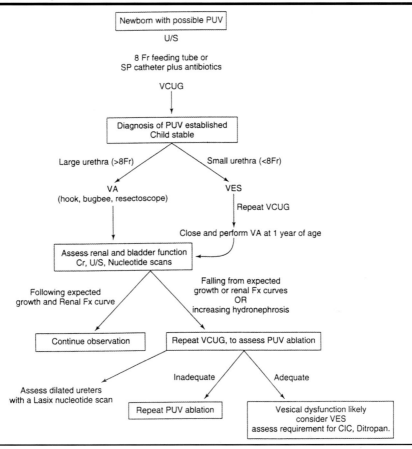

PUV = posterior urethral valves; U/S = ultrasound; SP = suprapubic; Fr = French; VCUG = voiding cystourethrogram; VA = valve ablation; VES = vesicostomy; Cr = creatinine; Fx = function; CIC = clean intermittent catheterization.

From: Smith GH, and Duckett JW. 1996. *Adult and Pediatric Urology,* 3rd ed., Gillenwater JY, ed. St. Louis: Mosby. Reprinted by permission of the author.

    4. Prevent infection.
    5. Facilitate drainage of the bladder.
B. Figure 6-11 provides an algorithm for treatment of PUV.
C. A urethral catheter is placed. Urinary drainage is particularly critical when diagnostic evaluation must be deferred because of respiratory distress, sepsis, or other conditions.[78,95]
    1. A straight catheter (size 5.0 French to 8.0 French) is recommended. A balloon catheter has a smaller internal lumen. The balloon occupies space within the bladder and can obstruct urine flow. The balloon may stimulate bladder fullness or spasms, which can also impede drainage of urine from the upper tracts.[8,83,95]
    2. A urine culture is obtained at the time of catheter placement.
    3. It may be difficult to direct the catheter through the dilated posterior urethra and the bladder neck.[80]

FIGURE 6-12 ■ Ablation.

Type I posterior urethral valves demonstrating ablation with a stylet and ureteral catheter.

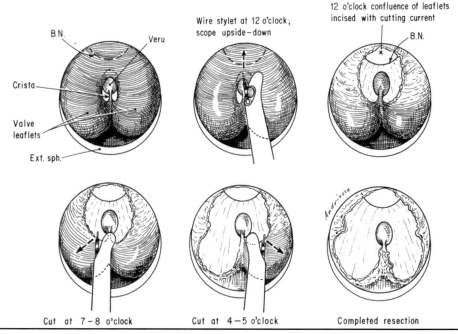

B.N. = bladder neck; Ext. sph. = external sphincter.

From: Hendren WH. 1993. Urethral valves. In *Pediatric Surgery,* 2nd ed., Ashcraft KW, and Holder TM, eds. Philadelphia: Saunders. 210. Reprinted by permission.

4. Various practices for catheter insertion depth exist. Preliminary guidelines for balloon catheter placement in children (not newborns) with normal urinary tracts have been proposed.[96]

5. The catheter is secured to avoid tension or excess play. Securing the catheter to the lower abdomen of male infants may reduce later stricture formation.[91]

6. Catheter care is performed at regular intervals with soap-and-water cleansing of the urinary meatus.

7. Symptoms of a urinary tract infection (UTI) and voiding around the catheter may indicate ineffective bladder drainage.

D. Percutaneously placed suprapubic catheters may be used.

1. Conditions for their use include the following.

   a. The urethra cannot be catheterized.

   b. A urethral catheter drains ineffectively.[80]

   c. The physician prefers this approach, with the intent of preventing injury to the urethra.[95]

2. A suprapubic catheter may be placed in critically ill newborns who cannot be catheterized. This procedure may be done in the NICU.

   a. A local anesthetic is used.

   b. The thick-walled, spastic bladder makes catheter positioning difficult.[80]

3. Suprapubic catheter care proceeds as follows.

      a. Until healed, the catheter site is cleaned at regular intervals with sterile water. Half-strength hydrogen peroxide may be used to remove crusts after healing has occurred.

      b. The insertion site is assessed for healing, catheter security, and signs of inflammation and infection.

      c. If the catheter stops draining, it may need irrigation with sterile saline. Aseptic technique is necessary.

    4. Complications include the following.[85,97]

      a. Infection

      b. Spasm

      c. Stone formation

      d. Deterioration of the upper urinary tract.

E. Assess fluid and electrolyte balance and renal function on a regular basis.

    1. With renal failure, hyperkalemia may be life threatening.

F. Anticholinergics may be used to alleviate bladder spasm.[80,85]

SURGICAL MANAGEMENT

A. The following are the goals of surgical treatment.

    1. Relieve the obstruction.

    2. Prevent further injury to the kidneys.

B. Endoscopic valve ablation is the primary treatment procedure.

C. Urethral valve ablation (Figure 6-12) may be done.

    1. The primary surgical technique used is endoscopic valve ablation. Open procedures may be complicated by injury to the urethra or the bladder.

      a. The endoscopic procedure is intended to "disrupt the ability of the valves to obstruct the flow of urine from the bladder" (p. 231).[78]

        1) An antegrade approach to valve ablation may be successful in preterm infants.[98]

    2. Valve *resection* is not needed and may result in urethral damage and stricture formation.

    3. A number of instruments and differing surgical approaches may be used, including the following.

      a. Infant resectoscope with hook or flattened loop

      b. Bugbee electrode using cystoscopic guidance

      c. Laser techniques

D. Urethral valve ablation may be deferred for these patients.[80]

    1. Preterm infants (The urethra may be too small for the surgical instruments.)

    2. Infants with sepsis

    3. Infants with severe respiratory illness

E. There are differing opinions about whether primary urethral valve ablation or temporary diversion is the preferred initial surgical procedure. There are no random, controlled, clinical trials.[99]

F. Infants with renal dysfunction and creatinine levels >1 mg/dl after several days of effective bladder drainage with an indwelling urethral catheter may need some type of operative urinary diversion.[85,100,101]

    1. The abnormal dynamics of the "valve bladder" with high resting pressures and detrusor instability that persist after valve ablation may contribute to the development of renal failure.

    2. Percutaneous nephrostomy drainage may be used in some circumstances.[83] **(See Megaureter later in this chapter.)**

3. Surgical techniques for diversion are performed to avoid the complications associated with extended use of suprapubic or urethral catheters.
    a. Vesicostomy is preferred when there is free vesicoureteral reflux; high diversion is preferred when there is no reflux.[85]
    b. Upper urinary tract diversion is needed after failure of valve ablation or vesicostomy to adequately drain the upper urinary tract.
    c. Other indications for diversion at the time of or shortly after valve ablation are as follows.[99]
        1) Severe hydronephrosis
        2) Severe infection with hydronephrosis
        3) Persistent septicemia
        4) Persistent poor renal function in spite of adequate bladder drainage
        5) Urinary ascites
4. High diversion techniques include the following.[84,85,101–104]
    a. Cutaneous pyelostomy
    b. Cutaneous ureterostomy
    c. Cutaneous loop ureterostomy
5. High diversion proceeds as follows.
    a. The renal pelvis or upper ureter is mobilized to the skin, and a stoma is created.
    b. The stoma may be on the abdomen or on the flank.[102,103]
    c. Urine flows freely into the infant's diaper.
6. High diversion procedures are not done by some surgeons for these reasons.
    a. Later ureteral surgery may be needed to correct vesicoureteral reflux.[80]
    b. Effects on bladder compliance and capacity if it is not filled may result.

FIGURE 6-13 ■ Vesicostomy.

A. Vesicostomy incision and identification of urachal remnant to confirm location of bladder dome. **B.** Properly placed functional vesicostomy.

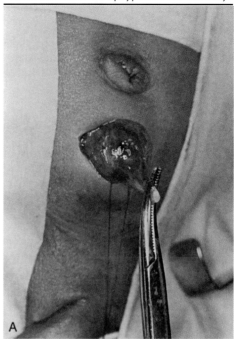

A

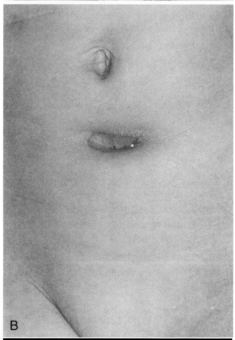

B

From: Baskin LS, and Kogan BA. 1998. Urethral anomalies and obstruction. In *Urologic Surgery in Infants and Children,* King LR, ed. Philadelphia: Saunders, 215. Reprinted by permission.

7. The Sober-type diversion procedure allows urine to flow into the bladder without adversely affecting bladder outcome.[105]

G. Vesicostomy (Figure 6-13) is a safe and efficient procedure for temporary decompression and drainage of the urinary tract.[84,106]

1. It allows normal cycling of urine through the bladder.

2. It proceeds as follows.

a. The vesicostomy is created by a transverse incision halfway between the umbilicus and the symphysis pubis.

b. A triangle of anterior rectus fascia is removed, and the bladder dome is mobilized into the incision, secured, and incised.[80,97]

c. Urine drains into the diaper without a need for any collection appliance.

3. Vesicostomy may not always provide effective drainage of the upper urinary tracts for the following reasons.[77,79,101,107]

a. Altered bladder structure and function

b. Associated ureterovesical junction obstruction

H. Nephroureterectomy for nonfunctioning hydronephrotic kidneys will need to be done at some point.[84]

I. Circumcision may be recommended to further reduce the risk of UTI.

COMPLICATIONS

A. Complications of valve ablation are rare and include the following.[98]

1. Leakage of urine at the site of valve disruption caused by perforation of the urethra

2. Stricture

3. Bleeding

B. Even after successful valve ablation, there may be poor drainage through the ureterovesical junction, and renal function may not improve.[78,80,83,85,101]

C. Reflux may spontaneously correct after valve ablation, or ureteral reimplantation may be needed for surgical repair of reflux.

1. This surgery can be technically difficult because of the abnormal bladder structure.

D. Repeat ablation may be needed with increasing hydronephrosis or with failure to meet expected growth or renal function norms.

E. The primary complication of vesicostomy is severe urinary infection.[78] Other complications include the following.

1. Prolapse

2. Stenosis

F. Stenosis of high diversion stomas is possible; revision may be necessary.[105]

G. Bladder function must be carefully assessed when vesicoureteral reflux or recurrent infections occur.

1. Potential serious consequences of reflux[101]

a. Altered bladder dynamics

b. Increased risk of renal scarring

c. Obstruction of urine flow

d. Hydronephrosis

e. Irreversible renal damage

POSTOPERATIVE NURSING CARE

A. High diversion procedure
1. In the immediate postoperative period, the stoma may be covered with a petrolatum gauze dressing or a dressing with antibiotic ointment.
   a. The dressings are changed when saturated with urine.
2. A petrolatum ointment will protect the surrounding skin from draining urine.
3. The stoma is assessed with diaper changes for the following.
   a. Color
   b. Drainage
   c. Bleeding
   d. Irritation
   e. Odor due to wound infection or UTI
   f. Skin breakdown
   g. Edema
   h. Prolapse
   i. Stenosis
4. The urine will initially be blood tinged and will clear in a few days.
5. If a unilateral procedure was done, urine output from the stoma and from the bladder need to be monitored separately.
B. Vesicostomy
1. The vesicostomy initially appears red and "angry" looking; this color will gradually fade.
2. Dressings may be used initially to cover the stoma.
   a. Change dressings frequently to prevent maceration of the surrounding skin.
3. Triple antibiotic ointment may be applied several times daily to the wound edges until healing has occurred.[102]
4. Dermatitis around the stoma has not been considered a significant problem.[106]
   a. Petrolatum ointment application to the skin can help protect it.
C. Valve ablation
1. The urinary catheter remains indwelling for about 24 hours postoperatively unless there is increased bleeding during surgery.
2. Therapeutic antibiotics are administered for several days, and then prophylactic antibiotics are given until reflux is no longer a problem.
3. Pain is assessed at regular intervals and analgesics administered to relieve pain.
4. Circumcision care is provided according to unit-specific protocols.
5. Periodic checks of serum creatinine levels and follow-up imaging studies are needed to evaluate the following.
   a. Urine drainage through the upper tracts
   b. Renal function
D. Important points in family education[78,101]
1. The types of care needed with urinary diversion procedures
   a. Hygiene
   b. Skin assessment
   c. Site care
2. Protection from UTI
   a. Importance of taking prescribed antimicrobials as ordered
   b. Rationale for medication and expected effects and side effects of medication

    c. Signs of UTI that must be reported
      1) Fever
      2) Irritability or inconsolability
      3) Poor feeding
      4) Failure to gain weight
      5) Vomiting or diarrhea
      6) Change in the odor of the urine
  3. Susceptibility to dehydration during the following as a result of the decreased ability to concentrate urine
    a. Illness
    b. Hot weather
    c. Periods of activity
  4. Referrals and support
    a. Exploring available support systems
    b. Evaluating community resources
    c. Providing assistance to the parents in navigating the health care system
    d. Teaching and reinforcing findings so that parents are realistic about their infant's prognosis

OUTCOMES

A. Respiratory failure accounts for nearly all mortality; only a 1–2 percent mortality rate is reported in neonatal patients.[78,85] Improvements in neonatal intensive care and the treatment of pulmonary hypoplasia have contributed to these outcomes.

B. Long-term issues depend on the severity of the initial presentation and the degree of renal dysplasia.
  1. Dysplasia is not reversible after effective drainage is established.
  2. Poor prognostic factors include the following.[101]
    a. Neonatal azotemia
    b. Severe bilateral reflux

C. Later bladder problems are common.[80,108,109]
  1. Delayed continence caused by poor bladder compliance
  2. Decreased bladder capacity
  3. Instability of the detrusor muscle
  4. Polyuria that may exceed the capacity of the bladder
    a. Later bladder problems were more common in infants receiving high loop ureterostomy than those receiving vesicostomy and primary valve ablation.[109]
    b. Bladder function is improved when there is a pressure pop-off.[89]

D. Abnormal urodynamic patterns are commonly found.[85]
  1. A similar frequency of bladder dysfunction was seen in infants treated with primary ablation and those with persistent elevated creatinine and hydroureteronephrosis who were treated with temporary pyeloureterostomy.[100]

E. Poor growth patterns may be evident.
  1. Necessitate careful attention to nutrition and diet[101]
  2. Are present whether valves are treated with primary ablation or vesicostomy[99]

F. End-stage renal disease—renal dysfunction that necessitates dialysis or transplant or causes death from renal failure—occurs frequently.[78,101,108–110]
  1. The highest rates are during the first year of life and late adolescence.[108]

2. The age at initial presentation of posterior urethral valves does not influence the likelihood of renal failure.[109,110]
3. UTI contributes to deteriorating renal function.[85]

G. A preliminary report suggests that plasma renin activity may be an early marker for renal damage.[111]

Torsion of the Testicle

DEFINITION

Twisting or torsion of a testis or spermatic cord

PATHOPHYSIOLOGY

A. During testicular descent, there is free rotation of the testis and spermatic cord within the inguinal canal and the scrotum.
   1. This ability to freely rotate lasts for about seven to ten days after birth.[112]
B. Clinical features and consequences of torsion are caused by interruption of the arterial blood supply (internal spermatic artery) and venous congestion.[113]
   1. Torsion may be incomplete or intermittent with sporadic ischemia.
   2. Necrosis and atrophy follow without prompt spontaneous correction by surgical intervention.
      a. Irreparable testicular damage may occur within a matter of hours.
   3. In experimental models of testicular ischemia, there is loss of spermatogenesis after six hours and elimination of Leydig cells with loss of hormonal function after ten hours.[114]
C. Torsion is classified as one of the following.[112,113,115]
   1. Extravaginal (extratunical): Torsion of the spermatic cord above the level of the tunica vaginalis (Most cases of newborn torsion are extravaginal.)[116,117]
   2. Intravaginal: Torsion of the spermatic cord within the tunica vaginalis

ETIOLOGY

A. The cause of testicular torsion has not been determined.
B. It is thought that elevated hormone levels may play a role because testosterone levels are high at the times of peak incidence.[91]
   1. Perinatal period
   2. Peripubertal period
C. Trauma to the scrotum may be contributory.[91]

INCIDENCE

A. Peak incidence occurs during the following periods.[91,118]
   1. Early neonatal period
   2. Adolescence
B. Torsion can occur *in utero.*
C. Torsion has been reported in preterm infants.[117,119]
D. Torsion can be unilateral or bilateral.[91,113,116]
   1. When it is unilateral, the left side is two times more likely to be affected because there is a longer spermatic cord on the left.
E. One series describing extravaginal torsion reported these rates of occurrence.[120]
   1. Prenatally: 72 percent
   2. Postnatally: 28 percent
   3. Bilateral: 21 percent

CLINICAL PRESENTATION

A. Signs of torsion may be present at delivery or early in the neonatal period.
   1. This palpable, firm, solid, painless mass in the scrotum does not transilluminate.
   2. A unilateral, nonpalpable testis may represent *in utero* extravaginal torsion.[91]
B. The infant with postnatal torsion has a normal scrotal exam initially, with later scrotal swelling and discoloration.
   1. The scrotum is plethoric or discolored, with a bluish or bruised appearance.
      a. This discoloration may be sporadic.
   2. Scrotal edema may occur, or the skin can become fixed to the necrotic testis.
C. The cremasteric reflex may be absent.[113]
D. Pain may occur as ischemia is progressing.[112]

ASSOCIATIONS

A. Factors that seem to be associated with this condition:
   1. Average birth weight
   2. Stress of labor and delivery
      a. Intrapartum stress has not been implicated in all studies.[80]
   3. Breech presentation
   4. Overactive cremasteric reflex.[112,121]

DIFFERENTIAL DIAGNOSIS

A. Many of these conditions are rarely seen in newborns. Rule out the following.
   1. Hydrocele
   2. Hematocele
   3. Incarcerated inguinal hernia
   4. Hematoma due to birth trauma
   5. Meconium peritonitis
   6. Benign or malignant tumor
   7. Scrotal abscess
   8. Ectopic adrenal or splenic tissue
   9. Idiopathic testicular infarction
   10. Epidymo-orchitis
   11. Torsion of the appendix testis or epididymis[112,116]

DIAGNOSIS

A. Clinical examination
B. Adjunctive studies[91,117]
   1. Doppler stethoscope examination to assess arterial flow
   2. Doppler ultrasound studies
      a. Flow may be seen on Doppler ultrasound when torsion is present.[122]
   3. Radionuclide scanning to assess testicular blood flow
   4. The accuracy of all results depends on the experience of the clinician.
      a. Complete accuracy never attainable
C. Surgical exploration to confirm the diagnosis of torsion
   1. Testing performed to support a clinical diagnosis may only delay surgery and increase the duration of ischemia.[112,113]
   2. The duration of ischemia is the most important factor affecting the ability to salvage the testicle.[120]

Treatment Options and Nursing Care

A. Controversies in management include the following.
1. The need for emergent surgical intervention
   a. Emergency surgery should be performed if testicular salvage is believed possible.
   b. Infants with *in utero* torsion and symptoms suggesting a chronic process are unlikely to benefit from immediate surgery; testicular function is not likely to improve.
      1) Of 23 newborns with abnormal scrotal exams at birth, 17 were surgically explored before 24 hours of age, and no viable testes were found.[116]
      2) Six newborns had testes surgically replaced within the scrotum; all were atrophied at later follow-up.[116]
2. How to manage the contralateral testicle when unilateral torsion is suspected
3. How to treat testicles that are found to be necrotic at operation
B. Because incarcerated inguinal hernia is a differential diagnosis, careful abdominal assessment is needed.

Surgical Management

A. Surgical approaches
1. Inguinal (especially if an incarcerated hernia is a likely differential diagnosis)
2. Transscrotal[112,116,123]
B. Consider the following if the infant is preterm.
1. Concurrent disease processes
2. The risks of general anesthesia (Regional anesthesia is an alternative.)
   a. One case report has described the use of local anesthesia in a preterm infant with respiratory distress after external manipulation and fixation of a torsed testis was attempted.[117]
C. Many practitioners advocate contralateral exploration and orchiopexy with the goal of preserving the function of the remaining testicle.[113,117,119,121]
1. Their viewpoints are based on experience and reports of asynchronous bilateral torsion.[117,121]
2. Proponents of this approach feel that there are no harmful effects of this surgery.[116,119,121]
3. Failure to explore and perform contralateral orchiopexy has resulted in infants becoming anorchid.[121]
D. Other practitioners feel that because neonatal torsion is nearly always extravaginal and adhesions develop to "fix" the testicle in the scrotum, surgery is not necessary.[112,116,119]
E. Early orchiectomy is recommended to remove a nonviable testis and for surgical exploration to establish the diagnosis.[112,113,116,123]
1. It was previously recommended that detorsion and orchiopexy be done even when the testicle was necrotic in the hopes of preserving some endocrine function.[112,118,121]
2. Data from animal studies suggest that the nonviable testis may induce the production of autoantibodies that affect the functioning of the remaining testicle and, later, fertility.[112,116,121,124]
3. No evidence of autoimmunization was found in humans who were evaluated between two and ten years after torsion.[125]

COMPLICATIONS

A. No immediate surgical complications are expected.

POSTOPERATIVE NURSING CARE

A. Care of the scrotum
  1. Assess the scrotum for the following.
    a. Swelling
    b. Discoloration
    c. Warmth
  2. Position the infant to avoid pressure on the scrotum and to be comfortable.
  3. Apply the diaper so that excessive scrotal pressure is avoided.
  4. Administer analgesics based on assessment of pain.
B. Care of the incision
  1. A transparent semipermeable dressing is usually applied to the incision.
  2. Evaluate the incision for the following.
    a. Healing
    b. Signs of infection
    c. Effects of urine contact on the healing process
  3. Gently clean the scrotum and the perineum during diaper changes.
C. Postoperative maintenance of intravenous (IV) fluids until bowel function resumes and the infant shows signs of hunger and readiness to take a feeding
D. Teaching
  1. Teach the family about the signs of torsion if contralateral orchiopexy was not performed.
  2. Explain that their physician must be called immediately if the scrotum changes color or swelling is seen.

OUTCOMES

A. Long-term care issues[123]
  1. Hormone replacement therapy if the torsion was bilateral and the infant is anorchid
  2. Psychological issues related to
    a. Body image
    b. Gender identity
    c. Potential effects on fertility.

Patent Urachus (of Any Degree)

DEFINITION

The urachus is a tubular structure that extends from the allantoic duct to the dome of the bladder.[4,126,127] The urachus may provide a route for drainage of the bladder during early fetal life while the urethra and urinary sphincter are maturing.[128,129]

PATHOPHYSIOLOGY

A. Embryology
  1. The allantois is a small outpouching that develops from the caudal wall of the embryo during the third week of gestation.
    a. The allantois grows into the body stalk from which the urogenital sinus is derived.[4]
    b. During early gestation, blood formation occurs within its walls; its vessels evolve into the umbilical vessels.

2. The inferior portion of the urogenital sinus develops into the urethra.
3. The bladder forms from the superior portion of the urogenital sinus and remains connected to the allantois.
    a. As the bladder grows and enlarges, the allantois involutes, forming a tubular structure called the urachus.
        1) Because the bladder is continuous with the allantois, both structures are involved in the derivation of the urachus.[127,128]
        2) The lumen of the urachus normally obliterates during the fourth or fifth month of gestation, forming the median umbilical ligament that extends from the umbilicus to the bladder.
            a) The urachus is obstructed by desquamated epithelium.[128]
4. Urachal anomalies occur when the urachus fails to obliterate.[127,128,130,131]
    a. Patent urachus: There is an open tract from the bladder to the umbilicus.
    b. Urachal sinus: The proximal urachus (closest to the bladder) is obliterated, and the distal urachus is patent.[127,130]
    c. Urachal cyst: Both the proximal and the distal ends of the urachus are obliterated, and there is an intervening segment that is patent.[127,131]
    d. Urachal diverticulum: This is a cyst-like structure that communicates with the bladder.[128] This condition is very uncommon and is not discussed in this chapter.

ETIOLOGY

A. The etiology of patent urachus is not known.
B. It has been proposed that bladder outlet obstruction and subsequent elevated intravesical pressure inhibit the obliteration of the urachus.[127]

INCIDENCE

A. Incidence figures are difficult to obtain because urachal anomalies are uncommon and are often asymptomatic.
B. Patent urachus was noted in 2 percent of adult autopsy specimens.[132]
C. One series reported a clinical diagnosis of patent urachus in 3 of 200,000 admissions to a children's hospital.[133]
D. Over a 20-year period, only 3 cases of patent urachus were diagnosed in over 1 million hospital admissions.[134]
E. Young adults are most commonly affected because symptoms occur in response to infection.[128,135]
F. Distribution of anomalies (infancy to age 20) is as follows.[128,132,136]
    1. Patent urachus: 10–15 percent
    2. Urachal cysts: 30–43 percent
    3. Urachal sinus: 43–59 percent
    4. Urachal diverticulum: 4–6 percent. (See earlier comment under PATHOPHYSIOLOGY.)
G. The male to female ratio is about 3:1.[134]

CLINICAL PRESENTATION

A. Patent urachus (Figure 6-14)
    1. The umbilicus is wet from urine leakage.
        a. A skin rash similar to diaper dermatitis may be seen.[127,130]
        b. The urine leak may be minimal or intermittent.[128,137]
        c. The urine leak may be increased with crying, straining, or voiding.[127]

2. The following may be present.
   a. Umbilical hernia
   b. Mass protruding from the umbilicus
   c. Large, tense umbilical cord caused by the reflux of urine[126]

B. Urachal sinus (Figure 6-14)[126,128,131]
   1. Umbilical inflammation
      a. Tenderness
      b. Redness
      c. Excoriation of the periumbilical area or lower abdomen in the midline
   2. Umbilical drainage (may be intermittent or persistent)
   3. Possible pain and fever

C. Urachal cyst (Figure 6-14)[131,138]
   1. Most are asymptomatic unless infected.
      a. Infection may be due to seeding from the bloodstream or lymphatics or by direct extension from the bladder.[126]
      b. Most infections are caused by *Staphylococcus aureus*.[128,138]
      c. Umbilical drainage is an unusual finding.
      d. The following may occur.
         1) Suprapubic or flank pain
         2) Fever
         3) Dysuria
         4) Palpable midline suprapubic mass
         5) Mild periumbilical erythema
      e. Complications of urachal cysts, which are rare, may include the following.[138]
         1) Stone formation within the cyst
         2) Hemorrhage into the cyst
         3) Intra-abdominal rupture, which can cause peritonitis
         4) Intestinal obstruction
         5) Urinary tract obstruction
         6) Extra-abdominal rupture with fasciitis and/or myonecrosis of the abdominal wall

FIGURE 6-14 ■ Urachal anomalies.

A. Urachal cysts. The most common site is the superior end of the urachus just inferior to the umbilicus. B. Two types of urachal sinus. One opens into the bladder; the other opens at the umbilicus. C. Patent urachus or urachal fistula connecting the bladder and the umbilicus.

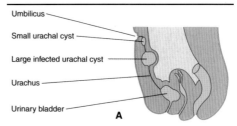

Umbilicus
Small urachal cyst
Large infected urachal cyst
Urachus
Urinary bladder
A

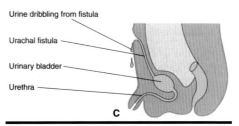

Umbilicus
Discharge from sinus
Urachal sinus
Urachus
Urinary bladder
B

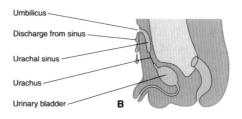

Urine dribbling from fistula
Urachal fistula
Urinary bladder
Urethra
C

From: Moore KL, and Persaud TVN. 2003. *The Developing Human: Clinically Oriented Embryology,* 7th ed. Philadelphia: Saunders, 303. Reprinted by permission.

ASSOCIATIONS

A. Urachal anomalies are usually isolated.[128]
B. Urachal patency has been associated with the following.[128,139]
   1. Posterior urethral valves
   2. Prune belly syndrome

C. Urachal patency may provide a pressure "pop-off" to protect the kidney; however, most infants with a bladder outlet obstruction do not have a patent urachus. Other pressure pop-offs may be present. **(See Posterior Urethral Valves earlier in this chapter.)**

DIFFERENTIAL DIAGNOSIS

A. Differential diagnoses for patent urachus and urachal sinus are similar and include the following.[127,128]
   1. Omphalitis
   2. Patent omphalomesenteric duct cyst
   3. Granuloma of the umbilical stump
   4. Infected umbilical vessels
   5. Various types of urachal patency
   6. Omphalocele
B. The following are differential diagnoses for urachal cysts.[131,138]
   1. Severe cystitis
   2. Pelvic inflammatory disease
   3. Appendicitis (with or without abscess)
   4. Inflammatory bowel disease
   5. Intra-abdominal or pelvic abscess
   6. Perforated viscus
   7. Strangulated umbilical hernia
   8. Meckel's diverticulum

DIAGNOSIS

A. Patent urachus
   1. Diagnosis is made by the observation of urine leaking from the umbilicus; this may be noted during umbilical vessel cannulation.[126,130]
   2. Ultrasound detects the following.
      a. A patent urachal channel
      b. Other abnormalities of the urinary tract or bladder
   3. Sinogram is an injection of the tract with contrast material under fluoroscopy.
      a. When there is umbilical drainage, this permits the differentiation of urachal anomalies from an omphalomesenteric defect. This may be the preferred early study.[132]
B. Urachal sinus[138]
   1. Diagnosis is made by abdominal ultrasound or sinogram.
C. Urachal cyst
   1. Diagnosis is made by abdominal ultrasound.
   2. CT scan is used if ultrasound is not diagnostic.
      a. CT scan can show whether there is involvement of the bowel or other structures.[128]
D. VCUG is used as an adjunct in the identification of the following.[126,127,130]
   1. Vesicoureteral reflux
   2. Urethral and bladder anomalies
E. Prenatal diagnosis case reports
   1. Umbilical cord edema[140]
   2. Cysts in communication with the fetal bladder, later noted to be ruptured[141]

TREATMENT OPTIONS AND NURSING CARE

A. Patent urachus

1. This urachal condition is the most likely to require surgery in the neonatal period.

2. Preoperative nursing care includes the following.

   a. The goals of treatment of the wet umbilicus

      1) Maintain skin integrity.

         a) The periumbilical area is kept dry by folding diapers below the umbilicus.

            • Dressings used to absorb urine must be changed frequently.

            • Wet or saturated dressings can cause maceration of the skin.

         b) A thin layer of petrolatum jelly may be applied to the skin as protection against the effects of urine.

         c) The use of tape or transparent dressings around the umbilicus is discouraged.

            • Their removal can produce skin abrasions in close proximity to the surgical incision.

      2) Prevent infection.

         a) Assessment focuses on the identification of signs suggesting local or systemic infection.

B. Urachal sinus

1. Surgery is delayed until acute infection and inflammation have subsided.[126,127]

SURGICAL MANAGEMENT

A. Patent urachus

1. Excision of the urachus with a cuff of bladder. This is done through a small subumbilical incision.[126,130]

2. The umbilicus is left intact.

3. Early surgical correction is performed to avoid associated problems of these.[126]

   a. Umbilical excoriation

   b. Recurrent UTI

   c. Sepsis

   d. Stone formation within the urachus or bladder

B. Urachal sinus

1. An infraumbilical surgical approach is used unless extensive inflammation due to infection necessitates a midline incision.

2. With extensive inflammation (unusual), it may be necessary to excise remnants of the umbilicus or the omphalomesenteric duct.

C. Urachal cyst

1. Surgical treatment is excision and drainage of the cyst.

2. Complete excision is needed to prevent recurrence and reinfection.

3. A laparoscopic approach to urachal cyst removal has been described in children and adults.[137,138]

   a. Care must be taken to avoid vascular or bowel injury.

COMPLICATIONS

A. Surgical correction of patent urachus is generally accomplished without complications.

POSTOPERATIVE NURSING CARE

A. An indwelling urinary catheter may be placed to promote drainage of the bladder. **(See Posterior Urethral Valves earlier in this chapter.)**

B. Assess the incision for drainage, signs of bleeding and infection, and evidence of healing.

C. IV fluids will be continued until resumption of bowel function suggests that enteral feedings may be initiated.

D. If the peritoneum was entered during surgery, there may be a longer period of postoperative ileus. Nasogastric drainage may be needed. Perform abdominal assessments initially every four hours.

E. If enteral feedings are delayed due to prolonged ileus, parenteral nutritional support should be provided to supply essential nutrients for wound healing.

F. Perform pain assessment at regular intervals; administer analgesics for pain relief.

G. The duration of postoperative antibiotics (if used) will depend on whether the urachal anomaly was associated with infection.

OUTCOMES

A. Complete resolution is anticipated for isolated urachal anomalies.

B. Urachal cysts that are drained only may recur and become reinfected.

C. When patent urachus accompanies other anomalies, overall outcome depends on the infant's primary diagnosis.

D. Removal of all urachal remnants is recommended because of the possible later development of neoplasms, including the following.
   1. Adenocarcinoma[127,131,135,138]
   2. Other cell types[130]
      a. Transitional cell carcinoma
      b. Neuroblastoma
      c. Rhabdomyosarcoma
      d. Teratoma
      e. Yolk sac carcinoma

Bladder Exstrophy (Classic)

DEFINITION

A. The exstrophy-epispadius complex comprises a wide spectrum of defects including classic bladder exstrophy and cloacal exstrophy.

B. "Classic" or "typical" bladder exstrophy is characterized by the following.
   1. Exposed bladder plate
   2. Epispadius
   3. Pelvic bony defects
   4. Defects of the genitalia
   5. Other anatomic defects **(See PATHOPHYSIOLOGY below.)**

C. Cloacal exstrophy is a more severe condition associated with multiple anomalies. **(See Cloacal Exstrophy later in this chapter.)**

D. The omphalocele-exstrophy-imperforate anus-spinal (OEIS) complex has been conceptualized as a more severe condition than cloacal exstrophy.[142] **(See Cloacal Exstrophy later in this chapter.)**

PATHOPHYSIOLOGY

A. The spectrum of these anomalies has deficient development of the dorsal wall of the urethra as the common denominator.[143]

   1. Earlier failure of migration of mesenchymal cells results in a more severe defect.[144]

B. Isolated epispadias involves only the urethra and not the bladder

   1. Variations include the following.

     a. Continent epispadias

     b. Incontinent epispadias

     c. Pubovesical cleft

   2. The position of the urinary meatus varies.[143,144]

ETIOLOGY

A. The etiology of exstrophy of the bladder has not been determined.

   1. Abnormal development of the cloacal membrane and failure of migration of mesenchymal cells have been implicated.[143–145] Failure of mesenchymal migration results in instability of the cloacal membrane.

   2. Abnormal placement of the paired primordia of the genital tubercle may cause the cloacal membrane to rupture on the anterior abdominal wall.[146]

   3. Premature rupture of the cloacal membrane after separation of the genitourinary tract by descent of the urorectal septum results in classic bladder exstrophy.

B. Although genetic inheritance has not been determined, a genetic predisposition is presumed because there is a recurrence risk within a family of 1/275 live births.[147]

   1. The likelihood of a parent with bladder exstrophy having a child with bladder exstrophy is estimated to be 1/70 live births.[147]

INCIDENCE

A. The incidence ranges from 1/10,000 to 1/100,000 live births.[144,145,148,149]

   1. One study reported a prevalence rate of classic bladder exstrophy of 3.3/100,000 live births.[150]

     a. In that report, the average prevalence of epispadias was 2.4/100,000 live births, with a higher rate (8.1/100,000) in the U.S.

     b. Epispadias almost always occurred in boys.[150]

   2. The Healthcare Cost and Utilization Project Nationwide Inpatient Sample (NIS) reported an overall weighted incidence of exstrophy at 2.15/100,000 live births.[151]

     a. Cases of cloacal exstrophy may be included in these numbers.

     b. The incidence was stable over the years 1988 to 2000.

     c. The incidence was greater in the following.

       1) Whites

       2) Infants born in the South and Midwest

       3) Infants born of parents of middle socioeconomic status

B. Bladder exstrophy is more likely to occur in males than in females, with reported ratios of 1.5:1 to 5:1.[144,145,148,149]

   1. The NIS reported the ratio of males to females to be almost equal.[151]

C. In all cases of exstrophy, about 50–60 percent are classic bladder exstrophy.[144,145,152]

   1. Classic bladder exstrophy usually occurs in full-term infants who have no other associated anomalies.

D. Other variants of bladder exstrophy occur infrequently.[145]

CLINICAL PRESENTATION[143–145,152,153]

A. See **DIFFERENTIAL DIAGNOSIS: B below.**

   1. Exposed bladder through open lower abdominal defect

   2. Widely spaced pubic bones

   3. Thighs widely separated by a broad perineum with external rotation of the hips

   4. Low insertion of the umbilical cord

   5. Inguinal hernias possible

   6. Anus apparently displaced anteriorly; normal sphincter development

   7. Males

      a. Short, wide penis with dorsal curvature

      b. Flat and wide scrotum

   8. Females

      a. The mons pubis is separated by the opening of the bladder neck.

      b. The labia do not meet.

      c. The clitoris is bifid.

      d. The vagina is displaced anteriorly.

ASSOCIATIONS

A. Bladder exstrophy typically occurs in full-term infants with no other anomalies.[143,153]

B. The NIS reported associations with the following.[151] Infants with cloacal exstrophy may have been included in this sample.

   1. Spina bifida

   2. Cleft palate

   3. Preterm birth

   4. Gastrointestinal anomalies

DIFFERENTIAL DIAGNOSIS

A. Rare variants of bladder exstrophy are:[145,154]

   1. Covered exstrophy

   2. Duplicate exstrophy

   3. Superior vesical fissure

   4. Pseudoexstrophy

B. Cloacal exstrophy is characterized by:[144,148,154]

   1. Exstrophy of the bladder—appears as two hemibladders

   2. Gastrointestinal (GI) anomalies, including omphalocele

   3. Central nervous system (CNS) anomalies

   4. Upper urinary tract anomalies

   5. Musculoskeletal anomalies, including a greater degree of pelvic deformity than classic bladder exstrophy

   6. Rudimentary penis in males

   7. Vaginal agenesis or duplication anomalies in females

   8. **See Cloacal Exstrophy later in this chapter.**

DIAGNOSIS

A. Prenatal diagnosis may be made.
   1. Prenatal ultrasound diagnostic criteria are as follows.[144,148,149]
      a. Bladder never seen
      b. Bulge on the lower abdomen
      c. Small penis with an anterior scrotum
      d. Low-set insertion of the umbilical cord
      e. Wide iliac crests
   2. Bladder exstrophy is not always diagnosed prenatally by ultrasound even though the fetal bladder can be seen at about 14 weeks gestation.
   3. A three-dimensional ultrasound may confirm the diagnosis of bladder exstrophy prenatally.[155]
B. Clinical diagnosis results from an abnormal physical examination.
   1. This is made at birth by observation of the exposed bladder.[143–145,152,154]
      a. Usually appears small and hypoplastic
      b. May be asymmetric in shape
      c. Sometimes appears quite large
      d. Can have a smooth or irregular surface
      e. May contain polyps
      f. May show congestion of the mucosa at birth
         1) Edema and thickening of the mucosa typically increase during the first few days after birth.
      g. Appears to have the openings of the ureters widely gaping or small and difficult to visualize[143,145]
   2. The pubic bones are widely spaced, and the pelvis has an open, C-shaped position.
   3. The thighs are widely separated by a broad perineum, and there is external rotation of the hips.[143,145,153,154]
   4. The umbilical cord often has a low insertion just above the edge of the bladder plate.
      a. Three vessels are usual.
      b. Remnants of the urachus may be present.
      c. Small umbilical hernias or small omphaloceles may be seen.
      d. Large omphaloceles are more typically associated with cloacal exstrophy.[144,145]
   5. Inguinal hernias may be apparent; more than 80 percent of affected males have inguinal hernias.[143–145,154]
   6. The rectum and anus seem to be displaced anteriorly because of the deficient development of the anterior structures.
      a. The anal sphincter is usually normal, but it may be stenotic and need dilation.
      b. Rectal prolapse is common due to weakness of the perineal floor.
         1) There may be rectal prolapse through the abdominal wall defect.[145,152,154]
   7. The following occurs in males.[143–145]
      a. The urethra is a short mucosal strip (one-quarter to one-third the usual length).
      b. The penis is short and wide with a dorsal curvature.
         1) The glans may appear bifid and flattened.
         2) The bases of the penis and scrotum are widely separated.

       3) There is a congenital deficiency of anterior corporal tissue.[154]

       4) The dorsal foreskin is deficient or absent.[143]

    c. The scrotum is flat and wide.

       1) The testes may be retractile or undescended.

  8. The following occurs in females.

    a. The labia do not meet because the mons pubis is separated by the opening of the bladder neck.

    b. The urethral strip passes between two halves of a bifid clitoris.

    c. The urethra and the vagina are short, and the vaginal orifice is anteriorly displaced and may be stenotic.

    d. The uterus, fallopian tubes, and ovaries are usually normal, but there may be duplications.

C. Renal ultrasound is done to assess the kidneys and ureters.[145,153]

TREATMENT OPTIONS AND NURSING CARE

A. One goal of preoperative treatment is to protect the exposed bladder from trauma and injury.

  1. Minimize handling of the exposed bladder mucosa.

  2. Recommended coverings include the following.

    a. Damp Teflon or Silastic sheeting[145]

    b. Plastic wrap[149]

    c. Petrolatum dressing and gauze[11]

    d. Hydrated gel dressing, such as Vigilon[156]

  3. Any wrap that is applied should not be too tight and constricting.

  4. Change plastic wrap or gel dressings daily.

  5. Fold diapers below the defect.

  6. Avoid the following, which may injure the bladder if efforts are made to remove them.[153]

    a. Ointments

    b. Powders

    c. Cornstarch

  7. Ligate the umbilical cord with a suture to keep the cord clamp from damaging the bladder.[144,145,149,152,153]

B. The bladder mucosal surface may be gently irrigated with warm saline to remove old urine and mucus from the bladder and the surrounding skin.[149,153]

  1. This will hydrate the bladder.[156]

  2. Irrigation should be performed after each void/diaper change.[156,157]

C. Initiate latex precautions.[157]

D. Assess cardiopulmonary function carefully; the infant will require extensive surgery under general anesthesia.[149,153]

E. Examine the infant closely for spinal abnormalities or altered innervation to the lower extremities.[148]

F. Begin broad-spectrum antibiotics as ordered, and continue for seven to ten days postoperatively.[145,149]

G. Some infants may not be candidates for early surgical closure of the bladder because of the following.[154,158]

  1. The bladder diameter is <3 cm.

  2. There are multiple polyps on the bladder surface.

  3. The bladder is not elastic.

4. Other variants such as ectopic bowel within the bladder or significant hydronephrosis are present.
  a. These infants may be maintained with open bladder drainage.
  b. The bladder tissue is protected with plastic and irrigated frequently with sterile saline.
  c. Trauma to the tissue by constrictive dressings or clothing is avoided.
  d. Skin irritation or candidal rash may occur despite scrupulous skin care.

SURGICAL MANAGEMENT

A. The following are the goals of surgery.[144,148,152,153,159]
  1. Closure of these structures.
    a. Bladder
    b. Abdominal wall
    c. Pelvis
  2. Preservation of function of the upper urinary tract and the kidneys
  3. Urinary continence
  4. Satisfactory appearance and function of the external genitalia
B. A staged approach is often used, or total reconstruction may be performed in the neonatal period.
  1. The initial operation in the immediate newborn period involves the following.
    a. Closing the bladder
    b. Placing the bladder within the pelvis
    c. Approximating the symphysis pubis
    d. Establishing urethral drainage
  2. The immediate newborn period is the best time for surgery because during the first 72 hours of life the pelvic ring is cartilaginous and flexible due to the effects of the maternal hormone relaxin.[143,145,148,154,156]
    a. Early repair reduces injury and scarring of the bladder plate.
    b. The infection risk is less.
    c. The bladder is easier to handle when there is less mucosal swelling.
    d. Successful early closure of the pelvic ring accomplishes the following.
      1) Reduces postoperative complications such as incisional breakdown and dehiscence (from tension on the incision)
      2) Increases the likelihood of adequate bladder capacity and urinary continence[148]
  3. The epispadius repair is performed between three months and one year of age.[143,145,148,154]
  4. Bladder neck reconstruction is delayed until four to five years of age. The goals of this surgery are voluntary voiding and urinary continence.[143,145,148,154]
    a. It is expected that 75–85 percent of infants will achieve urinary continence without compromise of renal function.[148,149]
C. Staged repair proceeds as follows.
  1. The bladder is examined under anesthesia to estimate its capacity.
    a. Visual estimation alone cannot predict the capacity of the bladder, and polyps may interfere with the assessment.
    b. An estimated bladder capacity of 5 ml or greater after closure is believed to be adequate.[149]
  2. The umbilicus may be excised and the vessels ligated.
    a. The umbilical vessels may interfere with the ability to place the bladder deep into the pelvis.

FIGURE 6-15 ■ The combined anterior innominate and posterior vertical osteotomies for closure of bladder exstrophy.

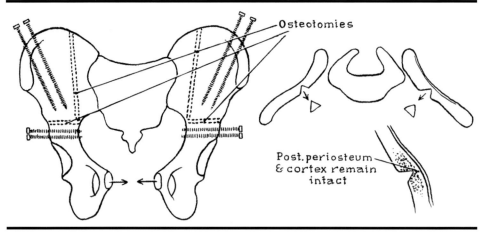

Osteotomies

Post. periosteum & cortex remain intact

From: Baskin LS, and Kogan BA. 1998. Urethral anomalies and obstruction. In *Urologic Surgery in Infants and Children*, King LR, ed. Philadelphia: Saunders, 109. Reprinted by permission.

    b. The umbilicus is a potential source of wound infection.[143,145,149]

3. A patent urachus is repaired.

4. The bladder muscle is gently freed from the surrounding rectus muscle and positioned in the pelvis.[144,149]

5. The posterior urethra (especially in males) may be lengthened using paraexstrophy flaps.

    a. This technique, however, may increase the likelihood of later stricture or fistula formation.[145,149]

6. The bladder is closed in the midline after placement of a suprapubic (Malecot) cystostomy tube and bilateral ureteral stents. These are brought out through the bladder wall and the neoumbilicus.[145,149]

    a. The ureteral catheters (size 3.5 French or 5.0 French), acting as stents, are passed nearly to the level of the kidney.

        1) They allow direct kidney drainage in the immediate postoperative period.

        2) They are left in place for 10 to 14 days (longer if still draining).[143,148]

    b. The suprapubic catheter remains in place for four to six weeks postoperatively until the following occur.[145,148]

        1) The lumen of the bladder outlet and urethra are adequate.

        2) There are low residual urine volumes.

    c. The suprapubic catheter is left in place for three weeks after complete primary repair of exstrophy.[160]

7. The inguinal areas are explored and hernias repaired.

    a. Some surgeons delay repair until hernias are clinically evident.[144,148,149]

8. Steps are taken to accomplish the following.[148,149]

    a. Allow the penis to increase in length

    b. Allow the penis to become more dependent

    c. Correct chordee

9. The posterior urethra is closed so that it is not obstructed, but with enough resistance to stimulate bladder growth and prevent prolapse.[149]

   a. Urine flow is diverted.
    1) Promotes healing
    2) Ensures integrity of the suture line
    3) Decreases infection
   b. Urethral catheters are avoided.[145,148,149,152]
    1) Potential pressure necrosis
    2) Possible accumulation of secretions that can lead to infection and wound disruption
  10. The pelvis is closed by rotation of the greater trochanters, and the pubis is approximated.
   a. Closure of the pelvic ring is critical to achieving successful repair, reducing incisional tension, and decreasing the likelihood of later uterine and rectal prolapse.
    1) Later continence may be influenced by the early approach used.[143,148,149]
    2) The pubic suture knot is kept away from the location of urethral closure.[148]
   b. Osteotomy may be done to restore pelvic anatomy and to ensure a secure closure of the abdomen (Figure 6-15).[149]
    1) After the first few days of life or if there is wide separation of the pubic bones, some form of osteotomy is needed to achieve pelvic closure.
    2) Osteotomy makes the pelvic ring unstable; an internal or external fixation device is needed.[152,156,161]
     a) Osteotomy with external fixation devices may be used with infants under six months of age because intrafragmentary pins do not hold as well.[149,161]
    3) Osteotomy is the preferred approach if it is believed that external closure will not be effective and following failure of an earlier closure.[148,159,162] The pelvis is closed before the final suturing of the outer layers of the abdominal wall.
  11. The abdominal wall is closed.
   a. A nonlatex drain is placed in the prevesical space and exits the skin at the neoumbilicus.
    1) This area is covered with a gauze dressing.[149]
D. The following is the procedure for complete primary repair of bladder exstrophy and epispadius.[156]
 1. It may be performed in the neonatal period.
 2. It incorporates many of the same steps as staged repair.
 3. The bladder, bladder neck, and urethra are moved posteriorly within the pelvis so the urethra is in a position that is anatomically normal.
 4. In males, the penis is totally disassembled.
  a. The reconstructed urethra may not be long enough to reach the penile glans.
   1) A hypospadias that can be repaired later may be created.
   2) In one series, newborns undergoing complete primary repair did not need to have a hypospadias created.[163]
  b. Ureteral stents exit from the reconstructed urethra.
 5. Osteotomy is not necessary if the surgery is done within 72 hours of birth.
 6. When an initial staged closure of bladder exstrophy has been unsuccessful and complicated by wound dehiscence, the complete primary repair procedure may be done.[154]

      a. A theoretical advantage of this approach is that early cycling of urine through the bladder will promote normal bladder development and improved urinary continence.[156]

      b. Posterior positioning of the bladder may facilitate closure of the symphysis pubis.

E. One surgical approach in females is total urogenital complex mobilization.[164]

   1. The pelvic floor anterior to the rectum is completely disassembled.

   2. The urethra and anterior vagina are placed in a normal anatomic position, eliminating the need for later surgery.

   3. The goals are as follows.

      a. Improved bladder function

      b. Continence

      c. Cosmetic appearance

F. The following factors are associated with successful surgical outcomes.[149,156,165]

   1. Pelvic immobilization and fixation

   2. Appropriate use of osteotomies

   3. Use of postoperative antibiotics

   4. Effective pain relief measures

   5. Effective control of movement and straining

   6. Relief of bladder spasms

   7. Avoidance of abdominal distention

   8. Adequate nutritional support

   9. Secure fixation of urinary drainage catheters

COMPLICATIONS

A. Wound dehiscence with bladder extrusion is the most serious early complication and may be caused by inadequate fixation of the pelvis.[145,148,149,154] Conditions that may contribute to wound dehiscence include the following.

   1. Abdominal distention

   2. Bladder prolapse

   3. Use of urethral catheters

   4. Early loss of a suprapubic catheter within six days of closure

      a. Attempt to reclose is delayed for four to six months to permit healing and renewed tissue strength.[148,149,159] Too long a delay and exposure of bladder mucosa may produce inflammation, decreased elasticity, and reduced potential for bladder growth.[159]

   5. Wound infection[143,145]

B. UTI may occur despite antimicrobial therapy.[143,166]

C. Urethral stricture is associated with the use of paraexstrophy flaps.

D. Calculi in the bladder or the urethra have been associated with use of the following.[143,145]

   1. Nonabsorbable sutures

   2. Infection

   3. Abnormal mucosa

   4. Urinary retention

E. Suprapubic leak is common.

   1. This may be a protective mechanism when urethral edema increases pressure within the bladder.[143]

   2. Leakage may be seen after removal of the suprapubic catheter.[162]

F. The nylon suture approximating the pubis may produce the following.[148]
   1. Stitch abscess
   2. Urethral polyp
   3. Erosion into the urethra
G. Penile ischemia can occur due to compromise of the blood supply and may be evidenced by the following.
   1. Small areas of skin loss
   2. Delayed healing
   3. Minor wound separation
H. Complications of early primary repair and staged repair are similar.[165]

Postoperative Nursing Care

A. Different techniques of ensuring continued closure of the pelvic ring may be used.
   1. Spica cast[152,156,157,167]
      a. Assess circulation to ensure that there is no interference with the arterial or venous blood supply as indicated by the following.
         1) Pallor
         2) Cyanosis
         3) Prolonged capillary refill
         4) Cool temperature
         5) Reduced pulses
         6) Edema
         7) Pain
      b. Cleanse the skin of any cast residue.
      c. Pad the cast edges with moleskin to prevent irritation.
      d. Inspect the skin at the cast edges to locate any pressure points.
      e. Tuck a disposable diaper into the cast edges with the absorbent side showing to keep the cast from coming into contact with stool.
      f. Perform meticulous skin hygiene after bowel movements.
   2. Modified Buck's traction or Bryant's traction
      a. The traction is held in place by elastic bandages wrapped around the legs.[145,148,149,152,153]
      b. Traction may be needed for four weeks.
      c. Maintenance of proper alignment is crucial. The hips are kept elevated 1–2 inches off the mattress.[153,167]
      d. Nursing interventions include these.[167–169]
         1) Maintain the desired weights.
            a) Do not remove or add weights.
         2) Ensure that the weights hang freely.
            a) Avoid bumping or jarring the weights.
         3) Ensure that all knots are intact and that the ropes are not frayed.
         4) Thoroughly wash and dry the infant's skin daily.
         5) Use a pressure relief mattress.
         6) Assess pressure points and wraps to maintain skin integrity.
         7) Alter weight-bearing areas within the limitations of the traction setup.
         8) Assess circulation as outlined in Spica cast above.
   3. External fixation devices in conjunction with traction[148]
   4. "Mummy wrapping" or "mermaid wrapping" of the lower extremities (not recommended because pelvic closure is not secure)[145,148]

B. Assess pain at regular intervals.
  1. Medicate to keep the infant comfortable and relaxed.[148]
    a. Crying, straining, and twisting movements are to be avoided.
  2. Morphine or fentanyl infusions are used in the immediate postoperative period.
  3. A midazolam infusion for sedation may be used as adjunctive therapy.
  4. Muscle relaxants such as pancuronium bromide may be used initially to reduce muscle movements that may put strain on the closure.
C. Antispasmodics may also be needed to relieve painful bladder spasms.[148,159]
  1. Oxybutynin chloride (Ditropan) may be administered directly into the bladder.
D. IV antibiotics are given for seven to ten days.
  1. Oral antimicrobials are then given until reflux is managed.
E. Insert a nasogastric tube to prevent abdominal distention, which can cause the pubic closure sutures to cut through soft tissue.[148,154]
  1. A nasogastric tube may not be routinely needed.[156]
F. Every two to four hours, assess urine output from both stents and suprapubic catheter.
  1. Initially, a large amount of urine output is expected from the stents.
    a. Postoperative swelling may keep urine from reaching the bladder.[153]
    b. Reduced drainage from the stents without a corresponding increase in suprapubic output may indicate obstruction and the need for irrigation.
  2. The suprapubic drainage is bloody.
    a. The suprapubic catheter may become obstructed with blood or mucus and need to be irrigated with sterile saline at regular intervals.
    b. Obstruction to urine flow may result in pain.
  3. As bladder and ureteral swelling decreases, suprapubic output increases, and the urine gradually becomes less bloody and more yellow/amber in appearance.
    a. This may take seven to ten days.[153]
    b. After the urine clears, the reappearance of blood may indicate spasm.
    c. Persistence of bloody urine is not normal.
  4. Aseptic technique is used when handling these devices.[149,153]
    a. Tubings are secured to the abdomen and the bed so that the urine drains freely.
    b. The urine drainage bag is kept below the level of the kidneys at the mattress level.
      1) If the bag is too low, changes in pressure may stimulate bladder spasms.
    c. Cleanse the skin around the stents and suprapubic catheter with half-strength hydrogen peroxide if crusts form; otherwise, sterile water may be used for cleansing.
G. Support of the family
  1. Reinforce what the surgery was to achieve.
    a. Explain the equipment the infant has.
    b. Educate the family to be alert to a lack of urine output and changes in the color of the urine.
      1) These can indicate an outlet obstruction and must be reported immediately.[149]
  2. Talk with the family about the anticipated length of hospitalization.[156,170]
    a. Four weeks or more with traction
    b. Approximately three weeks with an uncomplicated complete primary repair

3. Teach the family about the following.
   a. Site care of the suprapubic catheter that is necessary if the catheter is still in place at discharge
   b. To be alert for bloody drainage, which indicates possible bladder spasm
   c. Signs of UTI and the importance of adhering to the prescribed medication regimen
4. Because casts, traction, and fixation devices limit holding, creativity is needed in facilitating the following.
   a. Parent-infant bonding
   b. Parental performance of caregiving tasks

OUTCOMES

A. Long-term issues
   1. The ability to gain urinary continence is influenced by the following.[159]
      a. Initial postoperative course
      b. Frequency of infections
      c. Presence of stones
      d. Gender (Females have a greater likelihood of achieving continence than males.)[171]
   2. The "waddling gait" usually resolves; there may be some restriction of internal rotation of the hips.[145]
   3. Psychological issues are related to the inability to achieve continence and the need for multiple surgical procedures. These patients are at high risk for emotional and psychological issues involving self-image.[170,171]
   4. Opinions and evolving evidence regarding gender reassignment are changing to favor preservation of genetic gender. Multiple-stage reconstruction of the phallus may be needed for adequate function in males.
   5. Adult females born with bladder exstrophy require caesarean delivery to avoid possible disruption of urinary continence by vaginal delivery. Uterine prolapse is common during pregnancy due to abnormal pelvic support.[145]
B. Early complete primary repair
   1. Early reimplantation of the ureters may be needed after complete primary repair.[162,165]
   2. The effect of an early primary repair on the patient's ability to achieve continence is not yet known because there has not yet been any long-term follow-up.[156,165]
   3. Vesicoureteral reflux may occur after complete primary repair.[162]
C. Adenocarcinoma
   1. Has been related to exposure of the bladder with either delayed repair or failed initial closure[145,166]
   2. May also be a consequence of bladder augmentation procedures that use GI mucosa[145]

Cloacal Exstrophy

DEFINITION

A. Cloacal exstrophy is the most severe defect of the exstrophy-epispadius complex.
   1. It is characterized by a severe defect in the formation of the abdominal wall.
   2. Cloacal exstrophy includes a number of defects involving the unseparated urogenital and gastrointestinal tracts.

B. Cloacal exstrophy is also known as the following.[148,172]
1. Vesicointestinal fistula or fissure
2. Ileovesical fissure
3. Splanchnic exstrophy
4. OEIS complex

Pathophysiology[148,173,174]

A. Cloacal exstrophy is characterized by exstrophy of both the bladder and the bowel. Variable pathology and presentation may be due to different levels of descent of the urorectal septum during development. The urorectal septum separates the urogenital sinus and the hindgut.
1. The exstrophied bladder typically takes the form of two hemibladders that are separated by exstrophied bowel.
2. There is abnormality of the hindgut with imperforate anus.
3. A short, blind-ending distal colon is believed to be persistent tail gut.
4. The exstrophied bowel is from the ileocecal segment; multiple orifices may be visible.

B. Abnormalities of the genitalia are more severe than with classic bladder exstrophy.

C. Associated anomalies are very common.

D. Extensive reconstruction of the genitourinary and intestinal tracts is needed, with effects on later bladder, bowel, and sexual function

Etiology

A. The pattern of inheritance is unknown because of the rarity and the apparent sporadic incidence of cloacal exstrophy.

B. Cloacal exstrophy has been observed in both monozygotic twins (with only one or both twins affected) and in dizygotic twins.[175–178]

C. Recurrence in siblings has been reported.[176]

D. The embryology is as follows.[144,148,154,172]
1. Overdevelopment of the cloacal membrane prevents normal migration of mesenchyme.
2. In contrast to classic bladder exstrophy, the unstable cloacal membrane ruptures *before* the urorectal septum has descended caudally, separating the hindgut from the anterior structures.
3. The end result is extrusion of both the bladder and the bowel.
4. It is generally believed that the cloacal membrane rupture occurs between weeks 4 and 8 of gestation.[144,148,172,179]
   a. Prenatal ultrasound reports, however, have demonstrated rupture of the cloacal membrane sometime between 18 and 24 weeks gestation.[176,180]
   b. Variability in the timing of rupture may explain differing presentations.[180]

Incidence

A. This is a rare anomaly.
1. It occurs in 1/200,000–400,000 live births.[144,154,181]

B. The male to female ratio is 2:1.[144,148,154,172]
1. Earlier reports suggested equal distribution between males and females.[148,171]

Clinical Presentation

A. Infants with cloacal exstrophy are often preterm and/or small for gestational age (SGA) and so may require management of conditions typically associated with prematurity.[148,172,173,177]

B. Cloacal exstrophy is a complex set of anomalies. Use of the term *OEIS complex* perhaps allows for the easiest explanation of its presentation.
1.   Omphalocele
   a. GI anomalies are a typical feature of cloacal exstrophy.[148,154,172,178,181,182]
   b. Omphalocele is present in 85–100 percent of cases.
     1) Omphaloceles may be ruptured.[181,182]
   c. The extruded intestinal mucosa consists of the ileocecal region of the bowel or the foreshortened hindgut.
     1) The terminal ileum is often prolapsed, presenting as the "elephant trunk deformity."[173,183]
     2) Multiple orifices may be observed in the terminal ileum and the hindgut.
     3) A single appendix or paired appendices may be seen on the surface of the everted cecum.
2.   Exstrophy of the cloaca[144,148,172,174,176,181,184]
   a. Through the defect in the abdominal wall, the exstrophied bladder and urethra are evident.
     1) The bladder is divided into two "hemibladders," which are separated by a strip of intestinal mucosa.
       a) These hemibladders may be of different sizes.
3.   Imperforate or absent anus
4.   Spinal anomalies, such as tethered cord (in up to 80 percent of cases)
5.   Frequent lower limb anomalies[148,172,173,177,183]
   a. Clubfoot
   b. Congenital hip dislocation
   c. Agenesis
   d. Severe deformities of the foot and leg
C. In male infants, the phallus is usually diminutive in size and is widely separated into right and left halves that may be attached to each hemibladder.[144,148,173,181]
1.   Occasionally, the penis is together in the midline.
2.   It may be difficult to determine gender because of the absence of external genitalia.
3.   The testes are usually undescended.
D. In female infants, the clitoris is widely separated.[144,148,154,181]
1.   Commonly observed anomalies
   a. Duplication anomalies of the uterus and vagina (These may be partial or complete.)
   b. Bifid uterus
   c. Vaginal agenesis
   d. Vaginal atresia
E. Life-threatening anomalies of the cardiopulmonary system are unusual, although the following have been described.[148]
1.   Cyanotic heart disease
2.   Aortic duplications
3.   Duplications of the vena cava
F. Rare anomalies have been reported involving the following.[179]
1.   Lung
2.   Liver
3.   Brain
4.   Spleen
5.   Other structures

ASSOCIATIONS

A. Unlike classic bladder exstrophy, associated anomalies are common. **(See CLINICAL PRESENTATION above.)**[144,148,154,172,173,177]

  1. The bony pelvis contains a widened symphysis pubis with an enlarged pubic diastasis, and the hips are externally rotated and abducted.[148]
  2. Various forms of myelodysplasia may be evident and range from lipomeningocele to severe spinal dysraphism.[148,154,172]
     a. The reported incidence varies from 29 to 86 percent.[148,173]
     b. There may be associated hydrocephalus.
  3. Upper urinary tract anomalies are common, occurring in as many as two-thirds of the affected infants. These may include the following.[148,154,172,177]
     a. Renal agenesis
     b. Multicystic kidney disease
     c. Pelvic kidney
     d. Fused kidneys
     e. Ureteral duplication
     f. Ectopic ureteral drainage into the uterus, vagina, or fallopian tubes
     g. Hydronephrosis
     h. Hydroureter
  4. Deficiencies of the musculature of the abdominal wall and the pelvic floor may be seen.
  5. Inguinal hernias may be present.
  6. Short-bowel syndrome occurs in 25–50 percent of cases and has been reported even when the bowel is of normal length.[177,181,182]
  7. Additional GI malformations may occur.[173,184]
     a. Omphalocele
     b. Malrotation
     c. Bowel duplication
     d. Duodenal atresia or web
     e. Meckel's diverticulum
     f. Hypoplasia of the colon
     g. Imperforate anus
     h. Double or absent appendix
  8. There may be large ovarian cysts.[185]

DIFFERENTIAL DIAGNOSIS

See Bladder Exstrophy (Classic) earlier in this chapter.

A. Gastroschisis

B. Omphalocele

DIAGNOSIS

A. Alpha-fetoprotein analysis may allow prenatal detection of a large percentage of affected fetuses.

B. The following prenatal ultrasound findings suggest cloacal exstrophy.
  1. Midline abdominal wall defect
  2. Large cystic mass below the umbilicus
  3. Sacral myelomeningocele
  4. Splaying of the pubic rami[154]
  5. "Rocker bottom" deformity[180]

C. Most infants with cloacal exstrophy are identified at delivery; definitive diagnosis by antenatal ultrasound may not be possible.

D. Renal ultrasound is done to identify renal parenchymal disease or urinary tract abnormalities.[144]

E. Radiographs of the spine and lower extremities are done to evaluate the integrity of the spine, pelvis, and lower limbs.

F. Magnetic resonance imaging (MRI) is done to assess for skeletal and CNS abnormalities, including tethered cord.

G. Laboratory analysis of serum electrolytes, BUN, and creatinine levels is done to evaluate renal function.

H. Chromosomal analysis is done to determine if the infant is genetically male or female.[172]

TREATMENT OPTIONS AND NURSING CARE

A. Because of the rarity of this anomaly, newborns with cloacal exstrophy should be transferred to a center with surgeons who are experienced in its management.
   1. Not all Level III NICUs have experience with this complex malformation.

B. If the infant is premature and has respiratory distress syndrome and other complications of prematurity, manage these while assessing the overall gravity of the infant's condition.

C. Position the infant.
   1. Do this to avoid damage to susceptible tissue (especially when a myelomeningocele is present).
   2. A supported, side-lying position is helpful to use if there is a myelomeningocele or large omphalocele because venous return may be reduced with supine positioning.

D. Protect the exposed tissue.
   1. Use gentle handling, and avoid contamination of exposed viscera from stool.
   2. If moist saline dressings are used on the omphalocele or myelomeningocele, keep them moist so that they do not adhere to the mucosa.[144]
   3. Moist, nonadherent dressings may be applied to a myelomeningocele as an alternative to saline and gauze dressings.
   4. A bowel bag is another alternative to protect the exposed abdominal viscera.

E. For treatment options for bladder exstrophy, **see Bladder Exstrophy (Classic) earlier in this chapter.**

F. Treat omphalocele as follows.
   1. Use aseptic technique, especially if ruptured.
   2. Avoid constrictive dressing.
   3. Remove the cord clamp and ligate the cord with a suture.
   4. **See Omphalocele in Chapter 4: Neonatal Gastrointestinal Surgical Conditions; and Bladder Exstrophy (Classic) earlier in this chapter.**

G. Treat myelomeningocele as follows.
   1. Use strict asepsis, especially if the sac is ruptured. **(See Myelomeningocele in Chapter 7: Neurosurgical Conditions.)**

H. Initiate latex precautions.

I. Carefully assess the infant to determine the extent and severity of the associated anomalies.
   1. This is important for managing the infant and for counseling the family about the infant's condition and expected outcome.

    2. Gender identification may need to be deferred pending chromosomal analysis.

J. Carefully assess respiratory and cardiovascular function.

    1. Even in the absence of respiratory distress, an extended duration of general anesthesia will be needed, so knowledge of respiratory and cardiovascular function is important.

K. Initiate IV fluids.

    1. Assess intake hourly and output every two to four hours.

    2. There is increased potential for insensible water loss because there is not a protective skin covering over the defects.

    3. Central venous access will be needed for optimal, long-term, parenteral nutrition.

L. Maintain a neutral thermal environment; deficits of skin integrity increase the potential for evaporative water loss.

M. Place a nasogastric tube to low intermittent suction for gastric decompression to prevent abdominal distention while the extent of GI abnormalities is being determined.

N. Administer broad-spectrum IV antibiotics as ordered for seven to ten days.

    1. Oral prophylaxis will be initiated because of the risk of UTI.

O. Provide support to the family, who may be overwhelmed by the extent and severity of the anomalies.

    1. The potential need for gender reassignment for male infants may be especially distressing, particularly if prenatal evaluation predicted male gender.

SURGICAL MANAGEMENT

A. Previously, surgery for cloacal exstrophy was believed to be futile, and death occurred from the following.

    1. Sepsis

    2. Prematurity

    3. Short-bowel syndrome

    4. Renal disease

    5. CNS disease

B. The first report of successful surgical repair of cloacal exstrophy was published in 1960.[184]

    1. Survival rates are now >90 percent and are attributed to the following.[175,177,186]

        a. Improved NICU care and monitoring

        b. More refined surgical techniques and anesthesia management

        c. Improvements in parenteral nutrition and nutritional support

        d. Antibiotic therapy

    2. Mortality is associated with lethal anomalies or extreme prematurity.[172,182]

    3. Efforts are now directed at improving the quality of life for children with this anomaly.[148,173,174,177,184]

C. Multiple surgical procedures are needed to achieve these goals.[175,181]

    1. Protecting the upper urinary tract and preserving renal function

    2. Maximizing the length of the intestine for optimal growth and development

    3. Making the child appear as normal as possible

    4. Maximizing genital structure and function

    5. Promoting later continence reconstructive procedures so that stomas and appliances are eliminated whenever possible

      6. Achieving social continence

      7. Promoting self-esteem

D. A coordinated effort is required of all neonatal and surgical providers.[148,172,183]

   1. The surgical team consists of the following.

      a. General surgeons

      b. Pediatric urologists

      c. Neurosurgeons

      d. Orthopedic surgeons

   2. Genetic evaluation and karyotyping are done immediately so that gender assignment issues can be discussed with the family.[172]

E. Procedure options are as follows.

   1. A single-stage (primary) closure procedure is preferred when there are few associated anomalies.[148,177,181,182]

      a. Prolonged exposure of the bladder plate may cause thickening of the mucosa and inflammatory changes.[144]

   2. A staged approach is recommended in the following cases.[148]

      a. Preterm infant

      b. SGA infant

      c. Severe associated anomalies

   3. As with classic bladder exstrophy, early surgery when the pelvis is still flexible may contribute to improved surgical outcome.

   4. Closure of the myelomeningocele may need to be the first priority if there is spinal fluid leakage or concern about rupture of the covering membrane.

      a. If myelomeningocele closure is deferred, scrupulous attention to protection of the spinal cord defect is imperative.[172]

F. These are the steps in surgical management.[148,172,177,182]

   1. Closure of the omphalocele

      a. Primary closure is possible unless the omphalocele and exstrophy involve most of the anterior abdominal wall or if a large omphalocele contains the liver.

      b. If surgery is delayed, the omphalocele needs to be protected from rupture.

   2. Separation of the bowel from the bladder halves (Caution is needed.)

      a. Proper management of the bowel is crucial to later success.[148,172,177,181,182,186]

      b. All bowel segments should be saved for use in later urinary tract and other reconstructive procedures.

      c. Short-bowel syndrome may be life threatening.

   3. Closure of the lateral vesicointestinal fistula

   4. Creation of a short colostomy or ileostomy

      a. The bowel is brought through the abdomen rather than through the perineum in most cases.

      b. The hindgut has been found to increase in length during infancy.[148,172,173,177]

      c. The colostomy or ileostomy should be placed lateral to the site of abdominal wall closure (to avoid contamination) and where it can easily be managed with an appliance.[172]

   5. Reapproximation of the hemibladders into the midline to create a single exstrophied bladder

      a. The lower urinary tract is reconstructed as in classic bladder exstrophy.[148,172]

      b. It may be necessary to approximate the hemibladders and leave the bladder exposed for later closure.[172]

6. Possible anoplasty when there is an intact colon and anterior placement of the anus[172]
   a. With severe spinal dysraphism, a very short residual colon, and inadequate pelvic musculature, it is unlikely that bowel continence will be achieved.[175,177,181]
7. Stabilization of the pelvis
   a. The pelvis is stabilized as with classic bladder exstrophy.[148]
   b. Osteotomy may be necessary for stability of the pelvic closure. (**See Bladder Exstrophy [Classic] earlier in this chapter.**)
8. Gender assignment
   a. In females, the clitoris may be brought together at the time of bladder closure; other reconstruction is done later.[175]
   b. Sexual conversion of genotypic males to females is advocated by some.[148,172,173,175]
      1) Given the diminutive size of the penis and current surgical techniques, creating a penis that is functional and cosmetically acceptable may not be possible.[172,173]
      2) Orchiectomy may be performed at the time of initial surgery in order to decrease the infant's exposure to testosterone.[172,173,181]
9. Possible casts or splints for the treatment of limb anomalies. (**See Chapter 8: Surgical Repair of Defects and Injuries of the Extremities in the Neonatal Period.**)

COMPLICATIONS

A. Similar to those for classic bladder exstrophy (**See COMPLICATIONS in Bladder Exstrophy [Classic] earlier in this chapter.**)

POSTOPERATIVE NURSING CARE

A. General care and management are similar to bladder exstrophy. (**See Bladder Exstrophy [Classic] earlier in this chapter.**)
B. The order in which surgical procedures are done will alter postoperative priorities.
C. Use of aseptic technique is imperative because there are multiple surgical sites and incisions.
   1. Use care while working from clean areas to dirty areas.
D. Myelomeningocele requires the following. (**See Myelomeningocele in Chapter 7: Neurosurgical Conditions.**)
   1. Pelvic immobilization makes access to the myelomeningocele repair site difficult.
   2. Monitor head circumference, and assess for signs of increased intracranial pressure that may be associated with developing hydrocephalus.
   3. Consult with occupational therapy/physical therapy to manage the following.
      a. Musculoskeletal conditions
      b. Splints
      c. Positioning
E. For care of omphalocele, **see Omphalocele in Chapter 4: Neonatal Gastrointestinal Surgical Conditions.**
F. Avoid contamination of multiple healing surgical sites of ostomy. (**See OSTOMY CARE IN THE NEWBORN in Chapter 11: Skin Care after Surgical Intervention.**)
G. Nutrition care includes the following.
   1. Total parenteral nutrition for approximately four weeks
      a. Central access

2. An in-bed scale for evaluating weight
3. Generally, feedings delayed until two weeks postoperatively
4. Possibly a calorically dense, predigested formula at discharge[177]

OUTCOMES

A. Slow weight gain is anticipated.
   1. This is especially so when an end ileostomy has been performed.
   2. Children with ileostomies may have frequent hospitalizations for the following.[182]
      a. Diarrhea
      b. Dehydration
      c. Metabolic acidosis
   3. Short-bowel syndrome occasionally requires long-term parenteral nutrition, which may contribute to hepatic failure and death.[177]
B. Multiple surgical procedures are needed for urinary tract reconstruction, intestinal tract continuity, and genital reconstruction.
   1. Many children later require the following.
      a. Bladder augmentation
      b. Continence diversion procedures
      c. Bowel management programs
   2. A permanent colostomy is often needed when there are severe spinal defects or a muscular deficiency of the pelvis.[172]
   3. Vesicoureteral reflux is expected in all; later ureteral reimplantation may be needed.[175] **(See Megaureter later in this chapter.)**
C. A waddling gait is common; there may never be complete approximation of the pelvis.
D. Genetic boys who are raised as girls may demonstrate male-type behavior despite early removal of the gonads.[175]
E. Genetic females have successfully conceived.[172]
F. Normal intellectual function is expected.[182]

Megaureter

DEFINITION

A. A wide or dilated ureter[187,188]
   1. The ureter may be very elongated and tortuous.
   2. Many different terms have been used to describe ureteral dilation.[188,189]

PATHOPHYSIOLOGY

A. Ureteral dilation
   1. The normal ureter is a muscular tube that is consistent in size throughout.
      a. In children, the diameter is no greater than 7 mm.
   2. The ureter functions to transfer a urine bolus from the renal pelvis to the bladder.[188]
   3. Dilation is usually seen in the distal one-half or one-third of the ureter.[189]
   4. Ureteral dilation may be caused by the following.[103,187,188]
      a. Obstruction
      b. Vesicoureteral reflux
      c. Elevated intravesical pressure (posterior urethral valves or neurogenic bladder)

TABLE 6-1 ■ Classification of Megaureter

Refluxing		Obstructed		Nonrefluxing and Nonobstructed	
Primary	**Secondary**	**Primary**	**Secondary**	**Primary**	**Secondary**
Primary reflux	Neuropathic bladder	Intrinsic (primary obstructed megaureter)	Neuropathic bladder	Nonrefluxing, nonobstructive	Diabetes insipidus
Megacystic-megaureter syndrome	Hinman syndrome		Hinman syndrome		Infection
	Posterior urethral valves	Ureteral valve	Posterior urethral valves		Persistent after relief of obstruction
Ectopic ureter	Bladder diverticulum	Ectopic ureter	Ureteral calculus		
Prune belly syndrome	Postoperative	Ectopic uretocele	Extrinsic		
			Postoperative		

From: Elder JS. 2004. Urologic disorders in infants and children: Obstructions of the urinary tract. In *Nelson Textbook of Pediatrics*, 17th ed., Berhman RE, Kliegman RM, and Jenson HB, eds. Philadelphia: Saunders, 1800. Reprinted by permission.

    d. High urinary flow rates (diabetes insipidus)

    5. The neonatal ureter can dilate without loss of peristaltic function.

B. Megaureter

    1. Megaureter has been classified according to the presence of reflux and/or obstruction and whether the condition is primary or secondary (Table 6-1).[103,188–190]

    2. Primary defects have their origin in the ureter.

    3. Secondary defects originate outside the ureter.

      a. Bladder outlet obstruction

      b. Neurogenic bladder

      c. Polyuria

C. Primary obstructive megaureter

    1. A narrow distal segment of ureter is present approximately 1 cm above the ureteral-vesical junction.[191]

      a. This segment is 0.5–4 cm in length.[188,189]

      b. It is adynamic and does not effectively transmit the peristaltic wave necessary to propel urine to the bladder.[189]

    2. This narrow, distal segment can produce retrograde peristaltic waves.[191]

    3. This narrowing is not considered to be a true stricture or stenosis and will permit retrograde passage of a catheter.[189–191]

    4. Obstruction may be unilateral or bilateral. When it is unilateral, the unaffected ureter may be completely normal.[187–189,191]

      a. Histologic analysis of the abnormal ureteral segment shows deviations from the typical muscle pattern: There is increased deposition of collagen within the adynamic segment.[187,188]

      b. The fibrous terminal has been described as an "inelastic collar" that interferes with the normal transmission of the urinary bolus.

    5. The bladder and ureteral orifices appear normal.

    6. Although this condition may seem to be comparable to Hirschsprung's disease, an abnormal nerve supply has not been demonstrated.

      a. The normal ureter does not contain neural ganglia within its walls.[187–189]

    7. The following are consequences of untreated primary obstructive megaureter.[192,193]

      a. Urinary stasis

      b. Dilation of the upper urinary tract

      c. Recurrent infections

   d. Calculi
   e. Irreversible deterioration of renal function

ETIOLOGY

A. Congenital megaureter can be caused by the following.
   1. Vesicoureteral reflux
   2. Abnormal development of the ureteral musculature
   3. Obstructive pathology
   4. High urine flow rates when the kidney is unable to concentrate urine or with diabetes insipidus
      a. The ability of the ureter to transport urine is overtaxed.
B. Ureterocele is a common cause of megaureter, especially in females with a duplex collecting system.[187]

INCIDENCE

A. Primary obstructive megaureter occurs with greater frequency in males than in females.
   1. The estimated male to female ratio varies from 2:1 to 4:1.[103,188,189,192]
B. Obstruction occurs more often on the left side and is bilateral in about 20 percent of infants with primary obstructed megaureter.[102,191,192]

CLINICAL PRESENTATION

A. Postnatal symptoms that often appear during the first year of life:[103,190,191]
   1. UTI
   2. Flank pain or cystic abdominal pain
   3. Abdominal mass
   4. Asymmetric or generalized fullness of the abdomen or flank(s)
   5. Hematuria (after minor trauma or due to stones in the distal ureter)

ASSOCIATIONS

A. Obstructive megaureter has been reported in association with contralateral renal agenesis.[188,189]

DIFFERENTIAL DIAGNOSIS

A. Other primary ureteral anomalies may affect the flow of urine.[187,188]
   1. Ureteral valves are most often in the upper ureter; they are persistent transverse folds of tissue that cause obstruction.
   2. True congenital strictures of the ureter may be present; they are associated with abnormal muscularization.
   3. Ectopic implantation of the ureters into the bladder neck or the urethra will produce obstruction.

DIAGNOSIS

A. Diagnosis can frequently be made by prenatal ultrasound.
   1. The prenatal ultrasound finding that suggests primary obstructive megaureter is a dilated ureter(s) with a normal bladder.[191]
      a. Additional investigation is needed to determine if:[187,190]
         1) There is a primary or secondary problem.
         2) Obstruction is present.
         3) There is a potential for renal deterioration.
B. Ureteral dilation may not be seen on prenatal ultrasound; hydronephrosis may be the finding that prompts further evaluation after delivery.[192]

C. Postnatal abdominal ultrasound may be done.
  1. Delay this procedure for at least 48 hours after birth because low urine volumes during the first day of life may minimize existing dilation and lead to an inaccurate diagnosis.[188,190]
    a. Delay may not be possible in these circumstances.
      1) A life-threatening condition is suspected.
      2) There is concern for deterioration of renal function.
  2. Ultrasound and other diagnostic procedures should be done immediately under the following conditions.[190,191]
    a. There is bilateral disease.
    b. Posterior urethral valves are suspected.
    c. There is concern for obstruction in a solitary kidney.
D. A VCUG may be necessary to determine if vesicoureteral reflux is responsible for the megaureter.
  1. A VCUG will also identify other conditions that can occur with megaureter such as:[188]
    a. Posterior urethral valves
    b. Bladder diverticula or trabeculation
    c. Neurogenic bladder
    d. Ureterocele
    e. Ectopic refluxing ureters
E. Diuretic renal scan may be done.
  1. It is used to assess the following.[188]
    a. Differential renal function
      1) When megaureter is not caused by obstruction, differential renal function should be 50 percent in each kidney.
    b. Transit time of the tracer material through the urinary tract
      1) When megaureter is not caused by obstruction, the isotope should promptly wash out of the renal pelvis and ureter.
      2) With obstruction, the isotope is delayed proximal to the obstruction.
      3) Good hydration is essential because dehydration prolongs transit time.
      4) Poor renal function will be identified by delayed washout of the isotope through the kidney.
  2. If possible, renal scan is delayed for two to four weeks after birth to allow some maturation of the kidneys.
F. Diagnostic measures may not distinguish those cases that will require surgery from those that will spontaneously resolve or those in which ureteral dilation will stabilize without loss of renal function.[192,193]
  1. Urinary tract dilation does not always mean obstruction, and expectant management may be appropriate.
  2. Even with ureteral dilation, the kidneys may grow and develop normally.

TREATMENT OPTIONS AND NURSING CARE

A. Medical management
  1. With prenatal diagnosis, it is likely that cases are now being identified that previously would have resolved prior to the appearance of symptoms.[191]
    a. Spontaneous resolution may occur in mild, moderate, and even severe cases of hydronephrosis.
  2. Antimicrobial prophylaxis is needed to protect against UTI until spontaneous resolution occurs or until corrective surgery is performed.

3. With nonsurgical management, regular screening ultrasounds and diuretic renal scans are necessary.[193]
4. The following appeared in a published series of 53 infants (67 megaureters) with primary obstructive megaureter.[192]
   a. Only 17 percent of the cases required surgery because of breakthrough infections or deteriorating renal function.
   b. In 34 percent of the cases, dilation resolved spontaneously.
   c. The time to resolution varied between three months and four years.
   d. In 49 percent of the infants, persistent dilation of the ureter was observed.
   e. Infants with ureters >10 mm in diameter and whose kidneys were noted on renal scan to drain poorly were more likely to need surgery.
5. The effect of the condition on renal function is taken into account when determining the timing of surgery.
   a. Normally, renal function improves during the first year of life so that adult renal function is achieved by one year of age.
      1) Because of this, delay of needed surgical repair may interfere with the achievement of the infant's full potential of renal function.[187]

B. Placement of nephrostomy tubes
   1. Nephrostomy tubes are infrequently used in current practice to promote urinary drainage and to protect the kidneys.[77,191] However, they may be needed for temporary relief of obstruction.
   2. Technical considerations for nephrostomy tube placement in newborns have been described.[194]
   3. Nursing considerations postplacement include the following.
      a. Bleeding is a potentially serious complication following nephrostomy tube placement.
         1) Vital signs are closely monitored after the procedure because bleeding may not always be obvious.
         2) The dressing is assessed for excessive bleeding and drainage.
         3) The urine may be pink tinged or streaked with blood for a day or two following tube placement. Assess urine for the following.
            a) Amount
            b) Color
            c) Clarity
            d) Odor
         4) If clots are present, the tubes may not drain effectively.[11,195,196]
            a) Irrigation of obstructed tubes is not generally a nursing intervention. Unit protocols may vary.[11,195,196]
      b. The site of insertion is assessed two to three times daily for skin breakdown or infection.
      c. To promote urine flow, do the following.
         1) Maintain drainage tubing without kinks or tension.
         2) Keep the drainage bag below the level of the kidney.[195–197]
         3) Check the tube site for urine leakage, which may indicate obstruction.
      d. Aseptic technique is used for all aspects of care, including site care and dressing changes.
         1) The drainage system is maintained as a closed system.
      e. The infant is assessed for local and systemic signs of infection.[11,195–197]
         1) Prophylactic IV antibiotics may be ordered.
      f. Analgesics are administered to treat pain associated with the puncture and tube placement.

  g. Chronic infection and stone formation may be associated with long-term nephrostomy tube use.[77]

  h. Leakage of urine from the site is normal for about 24 hours after tube removal.[11]

SURGICAL MANAGEMENT

A. Surgical correction is recommended when any of the following is present.[188,191,193,198]

  1. Evidence of impaired renal function on renal scan

  2. Marked hydroureteronephrosis with thinning of the renal parenchyma

  3. Hypertension

  4. Hematuria

  5. Pyelonephritis

  6. Renal calculi

  7. Recurrent pain

  8. Signs of disease progression during a period of observation

B. A urinary diversion procedure is needed if the infant is too small for surgery.

  1. Proximal ureterostomy is preferred over distal ureterostomy to eliminate the potential compromise of the distal ureteral blood supply.

  2. See Posterior Urethral Valves earlier in this chapter.

C. The following are the goals of surgery.[188,190]

  1. Removal of the abnormal obstructing segment

  2. Tapering and reimplantation of the ureter

D. The following procedure is used in ureteral reimplantation—intravesical approach.

  1. The urine should be sterile at the time of surgery.[191]

  2. Antibiotics are given intraoperatively and for 10–14 days postoperatively.[103]

  3. Caution is needed during surgery to ensure that the ureteral blood supply is preserved.[188,190,193]

   a. This reduces the likelihood of later obstruction from fibrosis and stricture.

  4. The caliber of the distal ureter is tapered to achieve more effective peristalsis.

   a. The tortuous upper ureter often straightens spontaneously after the obstruction is removed.

  5. The distal ureter must be tunneled into the bladder at an optimal ratio.

   a. The ratio of diameter to submucosal tunnel length is 1:5 to prevent postoperative reflux.[188,190,193]

   d. The ureter must be reimplanted in such a way that angulation and hooking are avoided—these can create later obstruction.[192,194]

  6. The ureter may be stented with a 5.0 French or 8.0 French feeding tube to eliminate leakage prior to complete healing.

   a. The stent also accomplishes the following.

    1) Supports the ureter as it is healing

    2) May lessen the potential for later kinking of the ureter

   b. The stents are left in place from 3 to 12 days, depending on the surgical technique.[187,188,191,199]

   c. A shorter duration of stenting is needed when the ureter is plicated rather than tapered.[190,199]

   d. Stents may not be necessary in all cases.[199]

7. A urethral catheter is inserted to keep the bladder empty.
    a. Balloon catheters are avoided because they may compress the site of ureteral repair.[187]
8. A Penrose drain may be placed in the paravesical area.
    a. Urine leakage from this site must be reported.

E. The following procedure is used in ureteral reimplantation—extravesical approach.[188,198]
  1. The bladder mucosa remains intact.
  2. The ureter is detached from the ureterovesical junction and tapered.
  3. The ureter is reanchored, and the bladder muscle is reapproximated over the ureter to create a submucosal tunnel.
  4. Internal catheters are used to stent the repair; they remain in place for four to six weeks.

F. Bilateral megaureters are repaired simultaneously, necessitating a lengthy operation and an extended duration of anesthesia.[187]

COMPLICATIONS

A. The complication rate is higher for newborns than for older children because of the technical challenge of reimplanting a dilated ureter into a small bladder.[193,198]
B. The following are the most common complications.
  1. Reflux caused by an inadequate ratio of ureteral diameter to submucosal tunnel length or abnormal bladder function
  2. Obstruction
    a. Causes[187,188,191,199]
      1) Angulation at the ureterovesical junction
      2) Ischemia and later fibrosis at the tapered segment of the ureter
      3) Postoperative edema that persists after stent removal
  3. Anastomosis leaks[188]
  4. Urosepsis, which may occur even after postoperative and prophylactic antibiotics[199]

POSTOPERATIVE NURSING CARE[199,200]

A. Document the quality and amount of urine output from all sources (stents and urinary catheter) every two to four hours.
  1. Assess adequacy of urine output.
  2. Note any changes in the amount of urine output from any site.
    a. A decrease in output may indicate obstruction of a stent.
  3. Urine that is initially blood tinged should clear.
    a. Blood-tinged drainage may continue for as long as two to three weeks after surgery.
B. A straight indwelling urinary catheter is placed to keep the bladder empty. (**See Posterior Urethral Valves, TREATMENT OPTIONS, earlier in this chapter for catheter care.**)
  1. The urinary catheter will remain in place until after stent removal so that the effect of removal of the stents on urine output can be evaluated.
  2. If a bilateral repair is done, the stents are removed one at a time so that each ureter can be evaluated separately.
C. Maintain ordered IV fluids.
  1. Feedings will be resumed when bowel function is assured and the infant demonstrates an interest in feeding.

D. Assess for pain on a regular basis.
   1. Administer IV analgesics initially for pain relief.
   2. Caudal or epidural nerve blocks can be administered by an anesthesiologist to provide postoperative pain relief.
   3. Bladder spasms may be a source of pain for some infants.
      a. Oxybutynin (Ditropan) may be prescribed to alleviate bladder spasms.
      b. Sitting the infant in a shallow tub of warm water (taking care not to immerse the incision) may be comforting.
E. Administer IV antibiotics as ordered.
   1. Oral antibiotics will be continued following discharge until it has been determined that there is no vesicoureteral reflux.
F. Assess the surgical incision, drain sites, and stent sites for signs of infection, bleeding, urine leakage, and evidence of healing.
   1. Cleanse drain and stent sites two to three times daily with sterile water. Half-strength hydrogen peroxide may be used if there is crusted drainage at the sites after healing has occurred.
   2. The frequency of site care will vary, depending on the type of dressing used.
      a. The dressing over the Penrose drain will need more frequent changing if there is considerable urine drainage.
         1) Avoid skin maceration from a wet dressing.
         2) Wash the skin around the drain to remove all urine.
         3) Dry the skin before applying a new dressing.
G. Measure abdominal girth—initially, every four hours, then every eight hours.
H. Teach the parents the following.
   1. To encourage fluids so that the infant is able to maintain an adequate output of dilute urine
   2. That changes in the amount, color, or odor of the urine may indicate dehydration or malfunction of stents
   3. That the physician should be notified if there is a reduction in urine output because edema in the ureter can continue for four to five weeks
   4. How to manage drains, stents, and catheters that are still in place
   5. What to do if drains, stents, or catheters become dislodged
   6. The importance of continuing to administer antibiotics until they have been discontinued by the physician
   7. The signs of a UTI and the importance of reporting them to the health care provider
   8. The importance of keeping follow-up medical appointments
      a. If the extravesical surgical approach was used, the internal stents will be removed at about four to six weeks postoperatively.
         1) Removal of the stents will require administration of anesthesia.
      b. Diagnostic studies will be done to evaluate renal function and to look for vesicoureteral reflux.

OUTCOMES

A. A postoperative success rate of 95 percent is expected for primary obstructed megaureter.[191]
   1. Infants with abnormal bladders will not have the same success rate.[187]
B. When postoperative success was defined as improved hydroureteronephrosis and no vesicoureteral reflux, the following occurred.[198]
   1. Overall success was comparable for intravesical and extravesical techniques.

2. The extravesical technique was less successful in children with obstructive megaureter and voiding dysfunction.
3. The incidence in of UTI and stone formation was similar.
4. The average length of hospital stay was significantly less in children having extravesical surgery (4.7 days compared to 6.8 days).

Prune Belly Syndrome

DEFINITION

A. This condition is characterized by abnormal musculature of the abdominal wall, undescended testicles, and urinary tract abnormalities.
B. Sir William Osler first used the term *prune belly* in 1901 to describe the wrinkled, prunelike appearance of the abdominal wall.[104,187,201]
C. It is also known as the following.[104,201,202]
   1. Triad syndrome
   2. Eagle-Barrett syndrome
   3. Urethral obstruction malformation complex
   4. Abdominal muscular deficiency syndrome

PATHOPHYSIOLOGY

A. Abdominal wall
   1. The rectus abdominis and the transversus abdominis muscles are the most affected. They may do the following.
      a. Be absent
      b. Be hypoplastic
      c. Show patchy, asymmetric defects
   2. With severe abdominal wall atrophy, muscle may be replaced with collagen.[139]
   3. The rectus muscle may be more poorly developed in the lower abdomen.
      a. Normal abdominal musculature may be necessary for testicular descent.[139,201]
B. Ureters and bladder
   1. The ureters are typically dilated, elongated, and tortuous, with thickened walls.
      a. Megaureter is a universal finding.
         1) The upper portions of the ureters have a normal appearance and histology.[187,203]
         2) The lower, distal ureter is abnormal, with diminished smooth muscle, blood supply, and nerve plexus.[187]
      b. Ureteral muscle is replaced by fibrous tissue and collagen, resulting in ineffective peristalsis and stasis of urine.[104,187,202,203]
      c. Kinking and folding of the ureter creates secondary obstruction.[104]
      d. The ureteropelvic junction may be either of the following.[187]
         1) Obstructed
         2) Very tortuous and not obstructed
   2. There are pseudodiverticula in the bladder dome.
      a. They affect the bladder as follows.
         1) It is very large.

 2) It is thick walled.
   a) The wall is thickened from the deposition of collagen and fibrous tissue.
   b) Ureteral orifices are positioned laterally and may be widely dilated.
   c) Vesicoureteral reflux is common.
 3) It may be irregular in shape.
 b. Unlike with PUVs, the bladder is not usually trabeculated.[104,187,202,203]
3. The dilated ureters and distended bladder may interfere with testicular descent.[201,202]
4. The bladder neck and prostatic urethra are usually dilated; a lack of muscular support has been hypothesized.[202]
 a. There may be an abrupt junction between the prostatic and membranous urethra that gives the appearance of obstruction.[104]
 b. Congenital urethral stenosis or posterior urethral valves occasionally may be present.[187]
5. Hypoplasia of the prostate is common and may contribute to functional obstruction.[86,104,203–205]
 a. The hypoplasia is caused by a decrease in smooth muscle or an increase in connective tissue.
 b. It has been suggested that an obstructing lesion may rupture during development and not be visible at birth.
 c. Delay in canalization of the glandular urethra between gestational weeks 11 and 16 may cause a temporary obstruction.[104]
C. Possible renal dysplasia in variable degrees
1. Severe dysplasia may be associated with the oligohydramnios sequence with characteristic Potter's facies and pulmonary hypoplasia.[86]
2. The most severely affected infants may die from respiratory failure shortly after birth.
 a. In a study reported in 1995, data from the Congenital Malformations Registry of New York State for 1983–1989 indicated a mortality rate of 60 percent.[206]
   1) Nearly half of the deaths were *in utero* or during the first 24 hours of life.
   2) Two-thirds of the deaths occurred during the first week of life.
 b. The current mortality rate is reported as 20 percent.[207]
3. Later mortality is usually due to renal failure.[187]

ETIOLOGY

A. The underlying cause of prune belly syndrome has not been determined.
B. Two primary theories of origin have been proposed.[104,202]
1. Urethral obstruction blocks the flow of urine, contributing to distended bladder, megaureter, hydronephrosis, and renal dysplasia.
 a. Bladder distention and urinary ascites produce degeneration of the muscle of the abdominal wall.[104]
 b. Prune belly syndrome has been induced in an experimental model of complete urethral obstruction in a fetal lamb.[208]
2. A primary embryologic defect of mesenchyme development affects muscle development in the abdominal wall and urinary tract.[209] This mesodermal arrest may occur at 6–10 weeks gestation, perhaps even earlier.[187]
C. Neither theory completely explains all of the findings or the preponderance in males.

D. Comparable abdominal wall changes are not seen with obstruction associated with posterior urethral valves.

E. Most cases are sporadic.

  1. Occurrence in twin gestation and association with autosomal trisomies have been reported.[104,202,204,210]

  2. No specific teratogenic agent has been identified.

INCIDENCE

A. This condition is rare.

  1. It has been reported to occur with a frequency of 1/29,000–50,000 live births.[104,201,202]

  2. The Congenital Malformations Registry of New York State reported an incidence of 3.2/100,000 live births.[206]

  3. The true incidence may be higher because the characteristic abdominal wall appearance may not always be present.[202]

B. Its prevalence was higher in African-Americans than in Caucasians.[206]

C. Its prevalence was higher in twin pregnancies than in singletons.[206]

D. Prune belly syndrome appears in boys 95 percent of the time.[104]

E. Similar findings, without cryptorchidism, have been described in females.[139,211]

  1. Affected females present with genitourinary anomalies such as the following.

    a. Urethral atresia

    b. Vaginal atresia

    c. Uterine agenesis

    d. Uterine duplication

    e. Bicornuate uterus

    f. Fistulae formation

    g. Anorectal anomalies

  2. These findings may or may not represent true prune belly syndrome.[104,201]

  3. Affected females are more likely than males to have severe anomalies or syndromes than are males.[206]

CLINICAL PRESENTATION

A. Abdominal wall

  1. Coarse

  2. Wrinkled

  3. Lax appearance

  4. Often protuberant with bulging flanks

  5. Provides the first clue to the diagnosis

B. Abdominal skin

  1. It may be very thin, allowing visualization of the dilated ureters and the intestines.[187]

  2. Abdominal organs are easily palpated.

  3. Peristalsis may be visible.

C. Flaring of the rib margins and depression of the lower sternum.

D. Universal cryptorchidism, usually bilateral

  1. The testes are usually:

    a. Small

    b. Intra-abdominally located

    c. Histologically abnormal with decreased numbers of spermatogonial cells[104,139,202]

E. Possibly a patent urachus
F. Dimpling of the outer aspect of the knees and elbows (possibly caused by fetal compression)
G. Likely immediate respiratory distress requiring oxygen and assisted ventilation in the newborn with maternal oligohydramnios
 1. There may be concurrent renal failure because of severe dysplasia.[104]

ASSOCIATIONS

A. The high incidence of orthopedic problems favors the mesenchymal deficiency theory of pathogenesis.
B. Musculoskeletal anomalies are common, with an incidence ranging from 45 to 63 percent.[139,212,213] These may be a consequence of oligohydramnios and fetal compression.[214]
 1. The following are the most common.
  a. Clubfoot
  b. Hip abnormalities (congenital subluxation or dislocation)
  c. Thoracic abnormalities (such as pectus excavatum)
 2. Vertebral anomalies and limb defects have been reported.
 3. Associated congenital hip dislocation is more severe and more complex than isolated hip dislocation and is thought to reflect a teratogenic process.
C. Observed cardiac anomalies include the following.[104,139]
 1. Patent ductus arteriosus
 2. Septal defects
 3. Tetralogy of Fallot
D. The following GI malformations have been reported.[104,139,187,201,202,210]
 1. Gastroschisis
 2. Atresias/stenoses
 3. Malrotation/volvulus
 4. Omphalocele
 5. Anorectal anomalies
E. Isolated cases of a variety of malformations have been observed.[206,215]
F. There are reported associations with trisomies 13, 18, and 21.[104,202,204]

DIFFERENTIAL DIAGNOSIS

A. Posterior urethral valves
B. Massive primary vesicoureteral reflux
C. Megacystis-megaureter syndrome
D. Potter syndrome
E. Polycystic kidney disease

DIAGNOSIS

A. Antenatal diagnosis
 1. Many infants with prune belly syndrome are now identified by antenatal ultrasound.[202]
  a. Ultrasound findings that suggest prune belly syndrome
   1) Hydronephrosis
   2) Hydroureter
   3) Enlarged bladder
 2. A lax abdominal wall and fetal ascites may be seen.
 3. Oligohydramnios may be present.

B. Postnatal diagnosis
  1. Chest x-rays are done to assess for the following.
    a. Pulmonary hypoplasia
    b. Pneumothorax
    c. Pneumomediastinum
    d. Other air leaks
  2. Abdominal and renal ultrasounds are done to evaluate the following.
    a. Extent of bladder and ureteral dilation
    b. Extent of hydronephrosis
    c. Amount of renal parenchyma
    d. Presence of a patent urachus **(See Patent Urachus [of Any Degree] earlier in this chapter.)**
    e. Renal parenchyma for cystic changes and other findings associated with dysplasia
  3. A VCUG is done to determine the presence and degree of vesicoureteral reflux.
  4. Routine ultrasound of the hips has been recommended even if signs of subluxation or dislocation are not evident on exam.[213]
    a. Ongoing evaluation by an orthopedic specialist is necessary as the child grows.
    b. Traditional orthopedic treatments such as casting for hip dislocation must be carefully evaluated before use.
  5. Radionuclide renal scan is done once the infant stabilizes so that renal function can be evaluated.
  6. An echocardiogram is done.[202]
  7. Other diagnostic studies are performed as dictated by physical findings or as recommended by consulting specialists.

TREATMENT OPTIONS AND NURSING CARE

A. In the immediate newborn period, attention is directed toward the following.
  1. Supporting cardiopulmonary function
  2. Promoting effective urine drainage
  3. Determining the extent of urinary and other malformations and their impact on renal function
  4. Initiating prophylaxis against UTI
  5. Supporting the family
    a. Even with anticipatory guidance following an antenatal diagnosis, support of the family is a priority.
    b. They may be shocked, disturbed, and fearful because of their infant's appearance.
  6. Evaluating serum electrolytes, BUN, and creatinine regularly
    a. Pulmonary manifestations of fluid overload such as crackles heard on auscultation are worrisome because of:
      1) The mechanical restriction to lung inflation
      2) Possible associated pulmonary pathology
  7. Evaluating the caliber of the urinary stream
    a. Dribbling or poor caliber may mean urethral obstruction.
B. The infant must be protected against upper respiratory infection.
  1. The lack of abdominal musculature contributes to weakened pulmonary defenses because of an ineffective cough.[213]

C. Vesicoureteral reflux is common. Antimicrobial treatment is recommended because of presumed reflux and the urinary stasis associated with impaired ureteral peristalsis.[104,216]

   1. Urinary catheters are avoided unless absolutely necessary.

     a. When catheters are used, strict asepsis is mandatory.

     b. The massively dilated urinary system is extremely susceptible to bacteriuria, and the infection is difficult to clear once it is established.[104,201–203]

   2. A program of clean, intermittent catheterization is not recommended.

     a. These infants have normal penile and urethral sensation and experience discomfort during catheterization.[202]

D. Constipation is a problem because of the lack of abdominal wall musculature for effective bowel movements.[103,212]

   1. Adequate fluid intake is essential.

   2. The addition of dilute prune juice or the use of glycerin suppositories may be necessary.

SURGICAL MANAGEMENT

A. Management issues

   1. There is no consensus regarding the optimal timing of surgery.

     a. The timing of surgery depends on the severity of the anomalies and the adequacy of renal function.

   2. Surgery is contemplated under the following conditions.[201,203]

     a. Deteriorating renal function

     b. Increasing serum creatinine

     c. Instability of serum creatinine level

     d. Increasing obstruction

     e. Recurrent UTIs

   3. Surgery may be advantageous to those who exhibit improved renal function following decompression of the urinary tract.[104]

   4. Proponents of an aggressive approach to surgery are concerned about the following.[201]

     a. The long-term effects of urinary stasis

     b. The effects of recurrent UTIs on later renal function

   5. Chronic renal failure and renal transplantation are potential long-term consequences of prune belly syndrome.

B. Potential surgical procedures

   1. Urinary diversion procedures may include the following.

     a. Vesicostomy

       1) Vesicostomy may be less effective in infants with prune belly syndrome because of the tortuous nature of the ureters.[201]

       2) Bladder prolapse due to straining at stool with concurrent constipation may complicate vesicostomy.[202]

     b. Upper tract diversion procedures **(See Posterior Urethral Valves earlier in this chapter.)**

       1) Ureterostomies are directed laterally, away from the abdominal wall, so they are removed from the future site of peritoneal dialysis catheters.[202]

       2) Low distal cutaneous ureterostomies may be used with the proximal ureter left intact.[104]

   2. A patent urachus may be surgically expanded to permit more effective drainage.[103]

3. Urethrotomy may be advantageous to those who have some degree of urethral obstruction or poor bladder emptying.[202,203]
4. Reconstruction of the abnormal urinary tract may be done in the neonatal period or later, either as primary or staged procedures.[203]
   a. The following are the goals of reconstruction.
      1) Better ureteral peristalsis
      2) More effective urine drainage
      3) Elimination of reflux (See Megaureter earlier in this chapter.)
   b. The distal tortuous ureters are excised, and the proximal ureters are tapered and reimplanted into the bladder.
   c. Bladder reconstruction involves the excision of the dome of the bladder and reduction cystoplasty.[203]
   d. Orchidopexy, placement of the testes in the scrotum, will be done at the time of reconstructive surgery.
      1) This surgery is easier in young infants because of the length of the spermatic cord.[202]
   e. Abdominal wall reconstruction can be done at the same time as urinary tract reconstruction or with other procedures.
      1) This surgery is important for the later self-image of the child.[104]
      2) There may be improved ability to generate intra-abdominal pressure, resulting in more effective bladder emptying.[202,217]
      3) The abdominal wall may still be lax after the excess skin is removed.

COMPLICATIONS

A. Continued urinary stasis due to poor bladder emptying and/or vesicoureteral reflux[203]
B. UTI[203]
C. Wound dehiscence
D. Fascial defect or abdominal wall laxity after abdominoplasty

POSTOPERATIVE NURSING CARE

A. The needs of the infant following surgery are dictated by the surgical procedures performed.
B. Postoperative pulmonary complications such as atelectasis and pneumonia are of concern.[202,203]
   1. Postoperative respiratory distress has been observed in infants and children with prune belly syndrome even when there has been no prior history of pulmonary problems.[212]
   2. The onset of respiratory distress may be unpredictable.[203]
C. Following reconstructive surgery, the bladder may enlarge, with loss of tone and inadequate emptying.
   1. Follow-up evaluation for residual urine is necessary.
D. Avoid abdominal distention and tension on the suture line after abdominoplasty.[218]
   1. Nasogastric tube drainage will be needed when other intra-abdominal procedures are done or if an intraperitoneal incision is made.
   2. An abdominal binder or wrap is used for eight to ten weeks to eliminate tension on the incision.

E. With or without surgery, infants with prune belly syndrome have unique discharge planning issues.
  1. Pulmonary complications are a concern, and upper respiratory infection may progress to lower tract disease.
     a. The family needs to be vigilant about protecting their infant from respiratory infection and reporting any infection to their pediatric care provider.
     b. The infant may benefit from respiratory syncytial virus prophylaxis.
  2. Management of constipation may be problematic, requiring the following.
     a. Dietary modification
     b. Evaluation of output and stooling
  3. Referral to an early intervention program is recommended.
     a. Deficiencies of the abdominal wall musculature make it difficult to change from supine to sitting positions.
     b. Delayed ambulation may occur.[104]
     c. Ongoing orthopedic evaluation is needed.
  4. As the infant grows and becomes more active, protection of the abdomen is needed.
     a. The abdominal organs, including the bladder and the kidneys, are susceptible to trauma.

OUTCOMES

A. The prognosis for the infant with prune belly syndrome is worse when this condition is associated with posterior urethral valves, urethral atresia, or urethral stenosis.[86]
B. Ongoing surveillance of the status of the urinary tract is essential.
  1. This includes frequent urine culture and aggressive treatment of UTI.[219]
  2. Despite antibiotic therapy, UTIs related to urine stasis may lead to eventual renal failure.
  3. Instrumentation of the urinary tract is to be avoided.
C. Renal failure develops in 25 to 30 percent of patients with prune belly syndrome. The following factors correlate with renal failure.[219]
  1. Nadir creatinine (lowest creatinine level after day 5 of life) >0.7mg/dl
  2. Pyelonephritis
  3. Urosepsis (defined as positive blood culture and symptoms of pyelonephritis)
  4. Bilateral kidney abnormalities
D. Renal transplantation may be required because of progressive renal failure. The success of renal transplantation in children with prune belly syndrome is comparable to that of children with malformations of the upper urinary tract.
E. Developmental abnormalities such as scoliosis are seen on later follow-up.
F. Adult males are sterile.[104,201]

Ureteropelvic Junction Obstruction

DEFINITION

Obstruction to urine flow can occur at any location within the urinary system, but it most often occurs at the meeting of two structures such as the pyeloureteral junction or the ureterovesical junction.[220]

PATHOPHYSIOLOGY

A. The renal pelvis exits the kidney at the renal hilum, posterior to the renal vein and artery.

B. Normally, "pacemaker" sites located in the proximal collecting system regulate the frequency of muscle contractions within the renal calyces, pelvis, and ureter. These contractions propel urine from the renal pelvis through the ureter.

    a. The ureteropelvic junction closes during ureteral peristalsis to prevent retrograde flow of urine from the ureter to the renal pelvis.

C. Three types of ureteropelvic junction anomalies have been described.

    1. Extraparietal (extraluminal)

        a. This obstruction is external or mechanical.[220–223]

           1) It may be the result of aberrant vessels that cross the ureteropelvic junction, resulting in kinking or compression and interruption of urine flow.

               a) It has been suggested that a dilated renal pelvis associated with intrinsic obstruction becomes draped over a branch of the renal artery, giving the impression that the vessel causes obstruction.[224]

           2) The following are other potential sources of extrinsic obstruction.

               a) Kinking of the ureter

               b) Bands

               c) Adhesions

               d) Inflammation

               e) Tumors

               f) Arteriovenous malformations

    2. Parietal (luminal)

        a. This is the most common obstruction and is associated with an abnormal distribution of muscle and collagen fibers at the level of the ureteropelvic junction.[220–223]

           1) A segment of the ureter may be narrowed or/and aperistaltic.

           2) This obstruction is similar to that seen in primary obstructed megaureter.[220] **(See Megaureter earlier in this chapter.)**

    3. Intraparietal (intraluminal)

        a. This obstruction is a rare finding and occurs when true ureteral strictures, valvelike folds, or polyps are present.

D. Different types of obstruction are associated with differing patterns of urine flow across the ureteropelvic junction.[222]

    1. Extraparietal and parietal obstruction may be seen simultaneously.[220]

    2. Variable histologic findings have been observed, including hypertrophic smooth muscle growth and muscle deficiency at the level of the ureteropelvic junction.[223]

E. Obstruction at the ureteropelvic junction initially produces distention of the renal pelvis and the calyces (hydronephrosis) due to elevated pressure from the increased urine volume.[220,221]

    1. Complete obstruction of the upper urinary tract is rare.[225]

    2. Hydronephrosis alone does not signify obstruction, and renal function may be maintained.[221,226,227]

    3. Significant or long-standing distention can produce changes in the renal parenchyma and alter renal function.[220,221]

  a. Total obstruction can produce cystic dysplasia and complete loss of function.[225]

  b. Increased pelvic pressure stimulates the release of vasoactive mediators such as the following.[220,223]

   1) Angiotensin II

   2) Thromboxane A_2

   3) Prostaglandins

  c. In experimental models, there is an initial increased renal blood flow and later decreased renal blood flow and glomerular filtration rate.[220]

  d. Renal blood flow and glomerular filtration rate are also mediated by the activity of the renin-angiotensin-aldosterone system.

 4. Upward transmission of ureteral pressure alters tubular pressure and tubular function.[221,223]

  a. Impaired tubular function results in the following.

   1) Excess sodium loss

   2) Reduced ability to acidify and concentrate the urine

  b. Consequences of urinary obstruction that result in a decreased glomerular filtration rate include the following.[223]

   1) Inflammation

   2) Fibrosis

   3) Glomerulosclerosis

  c. Increased tubular pressure opposes glomerular filtration.[221]

 5. It is theorized by some that hydronephrosis is a compensatory mechanism that protects the kidneys by preventing the transmission of pressure to the nephrons.[221-223] Others do not support this theory.[219,227]

  a. A kidney of larger than normal size has been found opposite a hydronephrotic kidney that required surgery.[228]

ETIOLOGY

A. It has been theorized that parietal ureteropelvic junction obstruction is caused by the failure of recanalization of the ureter during embryonic development.[77,223,225]

 1. As the ureter normally develops from the ureteral bud, it undergoes a process of obstruction and recanalization.

  a. Recanalization through apoptosis begins in the middle of the ureter and extends equally toward the kidneys and the bladder. The final areas to cannulate are the junctions between the ureter and the renal pelvis and the ureter and the bladder.[225]

  b. This process is completed by about six weeks gestation.

B. A familial tendency has been noted.[220]

INCIDENCE

A. Ureteropelvic junction obstruction is the most common congenital anomaly of the urinary tract.

B. Ureteropelvic junction obstruction occurs with greater frequency in males than females (65 percent males).[221,229]

C. Unilateral obstruction is more often on the left side.[221,223]

D. Obstruction is bilateral in 5 to 30 percent of cases.[221,223]

CLINICAL PRESENTATION

A. Many infants have no clinical findings in the newborn period, especially when hydronephrosis is unilateral.[229] Other infants may have significant impairment of renal function.

B. Clinical findings include the following.[220,221,223]
1. Recurrent UTIs or urosepsis
2. Abdominal or flank mass (Ureteropelvic junction obstruction is the most common cause of abdominal mass in the newborn.)[220]
3. Variable size of the kidney on palpation (It may be absent, small, or enlarged.)
4. Failure to thrive
5. GI discomfort or loin pain

ASSOCIATIONS

A. Renal and urologic anomalies
1. Ureteral hypoplasia
2. Partial or complete ureteral duplication
3. Horseshoe and ectopic kidney
4. Multicystic dysplastic kidney
5. Vesicoureteral reflux[220,221,223]
   a. The presence of reflux may complicate management further.
   b. Vesicoureteral reflux may produce secondary ureteropelvic junction obstruction if the reflux impairs urine flow at that level.
   c. When reflux and obstruction are both present, correction of reflux may not correct the obstruction.

B. Nonurologic anomalies[221,223,226,230]
1. VACTERL (an acronym for **v**ertebral anomalies; **a**nal atresia; **c**ardiac abnormalities; **t**racheo**e**sophageal abnormalities; **r**enal abnormalities; and **l**imb anomalies) association
2. Imperforate anus
3. Congenital heart disease
4. Pyloric stenosis
5. Esophageal atresia

DIFFERENTIAL DIAGNOSIS

A. Other pathologic causes of dilation seen on prenatal ultrasound include:[87,220,221,223,224]
1. Vesicoureteral reflux
2. Obstructed or nonobstructed megaureter
3. Neurogenic bladder
4. Prune belly syndrome
5. Posterior urethral valves
6. Ureterocele
7. Renal cysts
8. Multicystic dysplastic kidneys
9. Duplication anomalies
10. Ovarian cyst
11. Neoplasms

DIAGNOSIS

A. Prior to the use of routine prenatal ultrasound, only 25 percent of cases were diagnosed during the first year of life.[223] The following clinical and laboratory findings were observed.[77,220,221,224]

   1. Recurrent UTIs or urosepsis (most common)

   2. Abdominal or flank mass

   3. Failure to thrive

   4. GI discomfort or loin pain (may be due to intermittent distention of the renal pelvis or renal ischemia)

   5. Hypertension (rare)

   6. Hematuria with mild trauma (especially in older children or adolescents)

   7. Pelvic and calyceal lithiasis

   8. Mild anemia, polycythemia, and renal tubular acidosis (possible but not usual)

   9. Systemic or pulmonary compromise not anticipated

B. Most infants are now diagnosed by prenatal ultrasound.

   1. Dilation of the fetal renal pelvis does not always indicate pathology.

     a. Most hydronephrosis that is detected prenatally is physiologic and resolves spontaneously; it is difficult to distinguish physiologic from pathologic dilation.[88,225]

   2. Transient physiologic dilation of the ureteropelvic junction may occur because of the following.[220]

     a. High fetal urine flow rate

     b. Delayed canalization of the urinary system

     c. Slow maturation of the urinary system

   3. Hydronephrosis is the most common congenital condition seen on prenatal ultrasound, and ureteropelvic junction obstruction is the most common cause of hydronephrosis.[77,220,221,224]

   4. Ureteropelvic junction obstruction is suspected when the ureters cannot be seen and the dilated pelvis communicates with the dilated calyces.[87,221]

     a. Lack of communication suggests multicystic kidney disease.

   5. A grading system for consistency in evaluating hydronephrosis has been developed.[231]

     a. Grade 0

       1) Intact central renal complex

       2) Normal renal parenchymal thickness

     b. Grade 1

       1) Slight splitting of the central renal complex

       2) Normal renal parenchymal thickness

     c. Grade 2

       1) Evident splitting of the central renal complex

       2) Complex confined within the renal border

       3) Normal renal parenchymal thickness

       4) Grade 2 or less demonstrated by 95 percent of children with nonobstructed hydronephrosis[231]

     d. Grade 3

       1) Wide splitting of the central renal complex

       2) Renal pelvis dilated outside renal border

       3) Calices uniformly dilated

       4) Normal renal parenchymal thickness

       5) Grade 3 or higher demonstrated by 89 percent of children with obstructed hydronephrosis[231]

    e. Grade 4

       1) Further dilation of the renal pelvis and calices (The calices may appear convex.)

       2) Thin renal parenchymal thickness

  6. Significant pathology is suspected when the following occurs.[220]

    a. There are changes in the renal parenchyma.

    b. Oligohydramnios is present.

    c. The anomaly is bilateral.

  7. Dilation of the ureter usually means a more distal condition.

    a. A dilated ureter may look like bowel on ultrasound.[87]

  8. The timing of the prenatal ultrasound is important.

    a. Studies performed before 24 weeks gestation are difficult to interpret.

    b. Beyond 24 weeks gestation, renal pelvic diameter exceeding 10 mm is well correlated with significant postnatal dilation.[88,223,232]

C. A prenatal diagnosis of hydronephrosis is not always confirmed by a postnatal ultrasound.[88]

  1. Unless a diagnosis of posterior urethral valves is suspected, ultrasounds should be delayed for 48 to 72 hours after birth.[88,232]

    a. The newborn typically has a decreased intake and oliguria during the first days after birth, and hydronephrosis may be missed.[88,232]

  2. Even if the initial postnatal ultrasound is normal, it should be repeated.

    a. The recommended interval for retesting ranges from five to ten days to two to three months.[77,222,225]

D. If dilation persists on postnatal ultrasound, a radionuclide scan will be necessary.

  1. This is usually delayed for several weeks to allow the kidneys some time to mature.[220,221]

  2. Nuclear scanning will show the differential function of each kidney and the presence of obstruction.

E. A VCUG is done to evaluate reflux, which is present in 10 to 18 percent of infants.[77,221,223,225,233]

  1. A VCUG is recommended even if the postnatal ultrasound is normal.[88,232]

F. Angiography is reliable for the detection of vascular conditions associated with ureteropelvic junction obstruction.

G. MRI offers no advantage in diagnosis.

H. No tests are able to show definitively which kidneys are obstructed enough to need surgery.[223,228]

I. Diagnostic studies are more difficult to interpret when bilateral disease is present.[220]

TREATMENT OPTIONS AND NURSING CARE

A. There is no consistently recommended approach to management. Options for management include these.

  1. Observation and conservative management

    a. Conservative management approaches are based on the premise that most cases of hydronephrosis will improve or spontaneously resolve over time.[88,227]

        1) Most infants with unilateral obstruction can be observed for several months if under the following conditions.

           a) They remain asymptomatic.

           b) Pelvic dilation is stable or decreasing.

           c) Relative renal function is stable or improved.

        2) Children with unilateral obstruction monitored regularly for up to three years demonstrated no loss of renal function.[234]

        3) An interval of no longer than three months between evaluations has been recommended.[227]

    b. Prophylactic antimicrobials are given to protect against UTIs.

    c. Circumcision may be recommended to reduce the likelihood of UTI.[232]

2. Temporary diversion

    a. Temporary diversion may be recommended when there is bilateral disease or severe unilateral disease with relatively poor function.[220]

        1) Unilateral nephrostomy drainage may improve the drainage in both kidneys.

        2) Percutaneous nephrostomy drainage may be needed when there is complete obstruction or oligohydramnios with pulmonary compromise.

3. Surgical management

    a. Advocates of early surgery are concerned about early loss of renal function.[235]

    b. Controversy exists because there is no clear-cut definition of significant obstruction.[225]

    c. There have also been concerns that unnecessary operations have been performed since the advent of prenatal diagnosis.[88]

SURGICAL MANAGEMENT

A. The following are indications for surgery.[220,225,227,235]

  1. The presence of symptoms

  2. Worsening function of the dilated kidney

  3. Moderate to severe bilateral pelvic dilation

  4. Advancing hydronephrosis/obstruction

  5. Unilateral pelvic dilation (There is no agreement on what extent of this warrants surgery.)[220,225,227]

B. The goals of surgery are as follows.[220]

  1. Improve the flow of urine

  2. Prevent renal parenchymal injury

  3. Relieve symptoms

C. Dismembered pyeloplasty is the procedure of choice for most cases.

  1. Other procedures may be needed under these conditions.[220,221,223]

    a. There are renal abnormalities (horseshoe kidney).

    b. Abnormal insertion of the ureter exists.

    c. There are changes in the renal parenchyma.

    d. Pyeloplasty has previously failed.

  2. Laparoscopic techniques are successful.

  3. Balloon techniques have been attempted in children and have been less successful than in adults.[223]

D. Surgery proceeds as follows.[220,221,223,234]

  1. The renal pelvis is opened and emptied.

  2. The pyeloureteral junction is excised; no abnormal ureteral segments should remain.

3. A feeding tube is passed to the bladder to check for other ureteral abnormalities.
4. Excess renal pelvic tissue may be excised.
5. The proximal end of the ureter is spatulated and anastomosed to the renal pelvis.
   a. It is important to ensure that the ureter is long enough to reach the pelvis without tension.
   b. Interrupted, rather than continuous, sutures are used to avoid later narrowing at the anastomosis.
6. Ureteral stents may or may not be placed. These can drain internally or externally.
7. Penrose drains are placed through two separate incisions.[220]
   a. A single drain may not sufficiently drain the retroperitoneum, and urinoma may develop.
   b. The drains are usually removed after a week.
   c. Little drainage is expected at the time of discharge, and a gauze dressing is all that is needed.
   d. These drains may help prevent ileus from urine extravasation.[234]
8. A bladder catheter may be placed for one or two days postoperatively; this depends on the preference of the surgeon.
9. Some surgeons prefer to avoid nephrostomy tubes because they keep the anastomosis dry.[220] Others have reported successful results with nephrostomy tube drainage and pyeloplasty.[234]
10. A nasogastric tube is passed to the stomach when a transperitoneal incision has been made for simultaneous bilateral repair because postoperative bowel obstruction is possible.

COMPLICATIONS

A. Recurrent stenosis
   1. There is a 2 to 5 percent rate of reoperation.[88]
B. Leakage across the anastomosis[220]
C. Bleeding and infection (uncommon)
D. Manifestations of a failed repair
   1. Prolonged drainage
   2. UTI requiring hospitalization
   3. Need for temporary internal stenting for pain or hydronephrosis several weeks postoperatively[235]

POSTOPERATIVE NURSING CARE[221,236]

A. Postoperative nursing care is similar to that for described for ureteral reimplantation surgery. **(See Megaureter earlier in this chapter.)**
B. Assess and document urine output from all sites: Urethral catheter **(see Posterior Urethral Valves earlier in this chapter)**, ureteral stents, and/or nephrostomy tubes **(see Megaureter earlier in this chapter)**.
C. A nasogastric tube for decompression is placed when postoperative ileus is a concern.
   1. This is typically removed in one to two days when there are signs of bowel function.
   2. Feedings can then be resumed.

D. Pain must be managed.
  1. A caudal block may be administered in the operating room, to be followed by IV narcotics.
  2. An epidural catheter may be placed for delivery of postoperative analgesics for one to two days after surgery.
  3. The infant will be given oral analgesics when pain scores are decreasing.
  4. Oxybutynin (Ditropan) may need to be ordered for bladder spasms.
E. Antibiotics
  1. IV antibiotics will be administered in the immediate postoperative period.
  2. Oral antibiotics and UTI prophylaxis will be given until relief of obstruction is ensured.
F. Discharge teaching includes the following.
  1. The Penrose drain may be left in place until after discharge and removed in the urologist's office.
     a. Explain to the family that local redness and a small amount of drainage are to be expected.
     b. Teach family members how to clean the site and apply a dry gauze dressing.
  2. If the infant is discharged with stents or nephrostomy tubes, care of these devices must be explained to the primary caregiver and other family members/support persons.
  3. Instruct families to encourage sufficient fluid intake to ensure an adequate volume of dilute urine.
  4. The urologist must be informed about the following.
     a. Fever
     b. Bleeding
     c. Vomiting
     d. Deceased urine output
     e. Irritability or inconsolability
  5. Emphasize the importance of follow-up visits.
     a. Removal of drain and other drainage devices seven to ten days following surgery
     b. Renal ultrasound at one to two months to see if there is relief from obstruction or evidence of blockage
     c. Renal scan to evaluate renal function

OUTCOMES

A. Excellent surgical results are expected, with success rates exceeding 90–95 percent for open procedures.[221,223,232,234]
  1. Successful surgical repair does not always produce improved differential renal function.[222,223]
B. Newborns have a higher rate of complications than older children.[223]
C. A poorer prognosis is expected when the following exist.[226,232]
  1. Nonrenal anomalies
  2. Oligohydramnios
  3. Urethral atresia
  4. Infravesical obstruction
D. Pyeloplasty at less than six months did not produce greater improvement in renal function when compared to infants with delayed surgery.[227]
  1. Maximal ultrasound improvement occurred within the first year after pyeloplasty.

Ovarian Cysts

DEFINITION
A sac containing fluid that develops within the ovary

PATHOPHYSIOLOGY[237–242]
A. Large cysts may cause compression of the following.
   1. Abdominal organs
   2. Urinary tract structures
   3. Thorax, thereby producing pulmonary hypoplasia
B. The ovary can be lost due to the following.
   1. Torsion
   2. Autoamputation
C. The ovary can become incarcerated within an inguinal hernia.
D. The cyst can rupture, with resultant hemorrhage into the pelvic cavity.
E. Maternal polyhydramnios may be seen; it is caused by compression of the fetal small bowel or umbilical cord.[237]
F. Intestinal perforation may occur; this is caused by mechanical obstruction or may follow torsion and the development of adhesive bands from the necrotic ovary to the bowel.

ETIOLOGY
A. Ovarian cysts develop from ovarian follicles; their etiology is not clear.[237,239]
   1. The ovary is a functional organ during fetal life. Follicular growth and maturation are ongoing processes that begin in the fetus and continue through childhood and into adulthood.[237,240,242]
      a. Neonatal ovaries have a structure and function similar to pubertal and adult ovaries and contain both differentiating and maturing follicles and oocytes.[237]
      b. Primary follicles can be seen in the fetus as early as 20 weeks gestation.[239]
      c. *In utero*, follicular growth is influenced by the following.[237,240–244]
         1) FSH
            a) FSH from the fetal pituitary is the primary stimulus to follicular growth, increasing both the size and number of follicles.[237,239]
         2) Maternal estrogens
         3) hCG produced by the placenta
   2. After delivery and separation of the placenta, the hormonal milieu changes with the loss of maternal estrogen and hCG.[237,239]
      a. FSH levels drop in response to low levels of estrogen.[239]
   3. This removal of hormonal stimulation may explain the spontaneous regression of many ovarian cysts, especially those that are small in size.[237,239,243,245]
B. Theories on the origins of ovarian cysts include the following.
   1. Excessive stimulation of the fetal ovary by placental and maternal hormones[237,243]
   2. Disordered folliculogenesis in the fetal ovary[237]
   3. Disordered enzyme activity[243]
   4. Increased responsiveness of the ovaries to gonadotropins[246]

INCIDENCE

A. Ovarian cysts are being observed with increasing frequency because of the routine use of antenatal ultrasound. Most are diagnosed in the third trimester.[242,247]

  1. On ultrasound, small, follicular cysts (<7 mm) are common and are considered a normal finding.[237,243–245]

    a. Cyst size may be a factor in the determination of whether a cyst is pathologic or physiologic. There usually is no change in cyst size from the time of diagnosis until the fetus is delivered.[242]

  2. The traditional view held that ovarian cysts were uncommon in children younger than age six, with most cysts being seen after puberty.[237,244]

  3. Ovarian cysts are the most common intra-abdominal cysts seen antenatally.[243]

B. The incidence of symptomatic or pathologic cysts has been estimated to be about 1/2,600 live births.[242]

  1. Cysts may persist into the neonatal period and beyond.[237,243]

C. Ovarian cysts are the most commonly diagnosed abdominal masses originating in the female genital tract during the neonatal period.[240,248]

CLINICAL PRESENTATION

A. Clinical findings depend on the size and nature of the cyst and whether complications are present.

  1. Ovarian cysts are typically isolated occurrences without associated anomalies or genetic factors.[242,247]

B. Potential physical examination findings include a palpable abdominal mass.[245,249]

  1. Size varies; the mass can fill the entire abdomen.

  2. It is usually asymptomatic unless torsion is present.[245]

C. Abdominal distention, which can be caused by the presence of a large cyst or ascites[249–251]

  1. Ascites can be the result of cyst rupture or peritonitis.

  2. Marked abdominal distention may be associated with one or more of the following.

    a. Large cysts

    b. Ascites

    c. Dilated bowel

D. Bilious vomiting, ileus, and gasless abdomen on x-ray, possibly with bowel obstruction with distention

  1. Caused by:

    a. Mechanical obstruction created by the ovarian cyst[237,239,240,251–254]

    b. Development of adhesive bands following torsion and inflammatory reaction[239,252,253]

    c. Cecal perforation, reported in conjunction with ovarian cyst and torsion[252]

E. Pain, emesis, fever, distention, leukocytosis, and signs of peritonitis are signs associated with torsion.

  1. Torsion may be asymptomatic. When torsion occurs antenatally, surgery to salvage the ovary is futile.[239]

  2. Torsion is one of the most common complications of ovarian cyst and can occur antenatally.[237,239,241,250,251,254,255]

    a. Long fallopian pedicles may anchor the cyst; these are easily twisted.

    b. Torsion can produce adhesion of the necrotic ovary to the bowel or other viscera. Intestinal perforation may be the result.[241]

3. Torsion is more likely to occur in large cysts, but the likelihood of torsion cannot be directly correlated to the size of the cyst.[237,239,242,250,251]

F. Respiratory distress may be evident.[241,249,250,255]

1. Large cysts can contribute to thoracic compression with resulting pulmonary hypoplasia.[237,240,242]

G. Hemorrhage may occur with or without torsion.[237,248]

1. It can manifest as progressive abdominal distention with a decreasing hematocrit.[250]

2. Mechanical stress during delivery may contribute to bleeding.[237]

Associations

A. The following conditions have been associated with ovarian cysts.[237,240,242,243,248,256]

1. Maternal diabetes

2. Maternal toxemia

3. Rh isoimmunization

4. Maternal and congenital hypothyroidism

a. Nonspecific stimulation of the synthesis of pituitary glycoprotein may explain the association with congenital hypothyroidism.[256]

B. It has been hypothesized that there may be increased secretion of hCG due to an enlarged placenta or other factors or increased placental permeability to hCG.

Differential Diagnosis

A. There are many differential diagnoses that can be considered for intra-abdominal cystic masses. Ultrasound can differentiate many of them.[237,240,243,248,256]

1. Ovarian cysts are usually seen in the lower abdomen or pelvis, but large cysts may be seen high in the abdomen.

2. It is crucial to distinguish the cyst from the kidneys and the urinary collecting system.

B. Possible differential diagnoses include the following.[237,239,240,243,248,256]

1. Mesenteric cysts

2. Enteric duplication cysts

3. Hydrometrocolpos

4. Urachal cysts

5. Cystic meconium peritonitis

6. Distended bladder

7. Anterior myelomeningocele

8. Bowel atresia or obstruction

9. Lymphangioma

10. Renal cysts

11. Hydronephrosis

C. Cysts of the omentum, pancreas, spleen, adrenals, and choledochal cysts have been reported as confounding diagnoses.

D. Complex cysts may be indistinguishable from neoplasms.

1. Ovarian neoplasms, however, are rare in the newborn.[237,240,248,256]

2. Solid or complex abdominal masses may be the following.[247]

a. Teratomas

b. Nephroblastomas

c. Neuroblastomas

d. Hemangiomas

e. Lymphangiomas

DIAGNOSIS

A. Ovarian cysts are typically diagnosed by ultrasound.
    1. They are variable in size and may be small or large enough to occupy nearly the entire abdomen.[237,239,243,248–250]
    2. Most are unilateral.[242]

B. Ovarian cysts are generally classified as follows.
    1. Simple (uncomplicated)
        a. On ultrasound, simple cysts are anechoic with a thin or imperceptible wall and "through transmission."[237,248,250,257]
        b. Simple cysts are usually <2.5 cm in diameter.[245]
    2. Complex (complicated)
        a. On ultrasound, complex, or complicated, cysts contain the following.
            1) A fluid-debris level
            2) Retracting clot
            3) Septa
        b. They may be characterized as follows.[237,239,243,250,257]
            1) Completely echogenic or consisting of mixed anechoic and echogenic areas
            2) Solid in appearance
                a) A solid mass is the rarest form of ovarian cyst; only about 1 percent of cysts are completely echodense on ultrasound.[247]
            3) Having echogenic walls because of calcification associated with infarction
        c. The above findings suggest antenatal torsion or hemorrhage, but may be indicative of neoplasia.[237,239,243,250]
        d. A "wandering" cyst may be the consequence of torsion with subsequent necrosis of the pedicle.
            1) The cyst may appear in the midabdomen rather than the lower abdomen or pelvis.[242,243]
        e. Cysts may be adherent to other abdominal structures.[248]

C. The ovarian origin of the cyst may be difficult to determine if it extends into the abdomen or is on a pedicle.[257]

D. Some authors feel that an ultrasound diagnosis of ovarian cyst should always be considered presumptive because the appearance of the cyst on ultrasound is similar to that of other rare lesions.[239,243]
    1. Ultrasound may not be able to distinguish between benign and malignant lesions when a complex cyst is present.[258]

E. Clinical findings that may suggest ovarian cyst are abdominal distention and abdominal mass.
    1. These are not specific for ovarian cyst.

F. A plain film of the abdomen may show displacement of the bowel gas pattern.[240]

TREATMENT OPTIONS AND NURSING CARE

A. Management depends on the following.
    1. The size and nature of the cyst
        a. Many simple cysts will regress spontaneously within three to four months.
            1) Those <4 cm in diameter are most likely to regress.
            2) Observation and follow-up ultrasound are recommended.[237,239,244,259]
        b. Complicated cysts can also involute spontaneously.

> **1)** A conservative approach can be taken when the infant is asymptomatic.[259]

2. The presence of complications
3. Whether there are concerns that the mass may be a tumor[237,239,244]

B. A risk of conservative management is that torsion can occur and can be difficult to diagnose clinically.[239]

C. There is disagreement about *in utero* treatment.
   1. Because of the tendency for many simple cysts to regress, it is believed that *in utero* treatment is not necessary.[243]
      a. Other concerns are that antenatal treatment may not be effective because there will be ongoing hormonal stimulation with possible cyst recurrence.
      b. Lack of correlation between cyst diameter and risk of torsion creates controversy regarding the most efficacious management.[241]
   2. *In utero* cyst decompression has been reported to be beneficial for the following.
      a. Anechoic cysts of 4 cm in diameter or larger
      b. Cysts noted to be "wandering" about the abdomen on serial ultrasounds
      c. Rapidly enlarging cysts (increasing in size >1 cm/week)[240,241]
   3. Antenatal cyst decompression may be the best management strategy for cysts >10 cm in diameter.[247]
   4. Successful decompression may eliminate the need for later surgery for the infant.

D. Postnatally, assess the abdomen for the following.
   1. Signs that indicate the presence of a mass
   2. Signs of obstruction
   3. Signs of torsion

E. Assess respiratory status for signs of distress due to the following.
   1. Lung hypoplasia
   2. Mechanical obstruction of the diaphragm

F. Assess for the adequacy of cardiac output if hemorrhage is a consideration.
   1. Support circulation with the following in the rare event of circulatory collapse.
      a. Volume
      b. Blood components
      c. Inotropic agents

SURGICAL MANAGEMENT

A. A primary goal of surgical management is to preserve as much gonadal tissue as possible.[237,239,242,244]
   1. This necessitates decompression of the cyst before torsion occurs.[241]
   2. Because ovarian cysts often adhere to the ovary or appear to completely replace it, oophorectomy may be necessary.[237,239]

B. Surgery has been recommended under these conditions.[239,240,243,244,247,257]
   1. Symptoms (including a palpable abdominal mass) are present.
   2. The cyst is complex—suggesting torsion.
   3. Neoplasm cannot be ruled out.
   4. A cyst recurs or fails to regress after several months of observation.

C. Cysts >4 cm in diameter have a greater risk of torsion and possible loss of the ovary and are more likely to be surgically removed or aspirated to remove the fluid.[237,239,244,247]

D. These surgical options exist.
1. Open surgery
    a. Open surgery is the most invasive; however, postoperative complications are not likely.
2. Laparoscopic surgery
    a. Advantages[260]
        1) Small scars
        2) Reduced likelihood of adhesion formation
        3) Greater ability to avoid loss of the ovary
3. Needle aspiration
    a. Preservation of the ovary is most likely when ultrasound-guided cyst aspiration is performed; however, cyst recurrence is possible.[237,239,244,261]
        1) Cyst aspiration has been recommended for simple cysts of >4 cm in diameter.[259]
        2) Cyst aspiration may prevent the development of torsion.[238]
        3) Aspiration may not be possible when the contents of the cyst are consolidated.[243]
        4) A disadvantage of this approach is the possible failure to diagnose a neoplasm.[240]
        5) Multiple pericystic adhesions can occur.[243]

COMPLICATIONS

A. Maternal complications are rarely associated with fetal ovarian cyst.
1. Polyhydramnios occurs in about 10 to18 percent of cases and is thought to be caused by partial obstruction of the fetal small bowel or by umbilical cord compression.[237,239–242,248,256]
2. Dystocia is possible with large cysts.[248,251]
    a. Vaginal delivery is generally acceptable.
    b. Cesarean section is recommended in the following cases.[239,242–244,250]
        1) The cyst is very large, and there is a strong likelihood of dystocia.
        2) It is an effort to prevent torsion or cyst rupture.
B. Neonatal complications may occur.
1. Hemorrhagic ascites and/or peritonitis are rare but potentially lethal complications of cyst rupture.[237,239,240,251,254]
    a. Ovarian cyst rupture is a surgical emergency.[255]
2. Urinary tract obstruction may occur.[239,241] Urinary tract obstruction with vesicoureteral reflux and intrarenal reflux has been reported.[254]
3. The cyst may become incarcerated within an inguinal hernia.[237,240,241,243,254]
4. Edema of the labia majora attributed to altered hormone levels may occur.[240]

POSTOPERATIVE NURSING CARE

A. Position the infant to make her comfortable and for ease of respirations.
B. Maintain IV fluids postoperatively until bowel function resumes and the infant shows signs of hunger and readiness to feed.
C. Evaluate the operative site for healing and signs of infection.
D. Address the family's concerns about later development and fertility as needed.

OUTCOMES

A. Many cysts involute spontaneously; surgery is not needed.[242,258,259]

B. Ultrasound-guided cyst aspiration may be associated with cyst reoccurrence.[237,239,244,261]

C. Most infants requiring surgery, even those needing acute surgery for torsion, are expected to recover without complications.[238,242,260]

D. Postoperative adnexal adhesion formation and the removal of functional ovarian tissue might affect later fertility.[242]

E. The outcome of infants with other organ involvement, such as pulmonary hypoplasia or peritonitis, or those with cyst rupture depends on hemodynamic stability and the extent of organ compromise. Some associated conditions may be lethal.[237,240]

Newborn Circumcision

DEFINITION
Removal of the foreskin (prepuce) to a level near the coronal sulcus

INCIDENCE
A. Circumcision is the most commonly performed genitourinary surgery. In most circumstances, it is an elective procedure.

POTENTIAL MEDICAL BENEFITS[113,262–266]
A. Slightly decreased risk of UTI
   1. The estimated risk of UTI in uncircumcised males during the first year of life is 7–14/1,000. For a circumcised infant, that risk is about 1–2/1,000.[259]
B. Lower risk of cancer of the penis (This is a very rare condition. The estimated risk in uncircumcised males is 1/600 men in the U.S.)[267]
C. Possible lower risk of sexually transmitted diseases[262]

POSSIBLE INDICATIONS FOR CIRCUMCISION[113,264–266]
A. The presence of urinary tract anomalies or vesicoureteral reflux when there is an increased risk of UTI.
B. Phimosis—narrowing of the preputial ring resulting in the inability to retract the foreskin when it should be fully retractable (In newborn infants, the foreskin is normally not retractable. In most children, the foreskin should be fully retractable by age five.)
   1. Pathologic phimosis occurs under these conditions.
      a. The foreskin cannot be retracted after it has been retractable.
      b. Retraction of the foreskin after completion of puberty is not possible.[265,266]
   2. The following are possible causes of phimosis.
      a. Inflammation or trauma that produces an inelastic scar
      b. Forceful disruption of "physiologic adhesions" in infants
      c. Recurrent posthitis that produces scarring[113]
   3. Phimosis or recurrent episodes of balanoposthitis (inflammation of both the glans [balanitis] and the foreskin [posthitis]) are reasons for circumcision, but these conditions rarely exist in the newborn period.[266]
C. Paraphimosis—retention of the preputial ring proximal to the coronal sulcus
   1. Paraphimosis produces tension and elevated lymphatic pressure resulting in edema of the prepuce and glans.
      a. This may be caused by forcible retraction of the foreskin.

CONTRAINDICATIONS TO CIRCUMCISION[91,113,263–265]

A. Presence of the following.
   1. Hypospadias
      a. About 5 percent of newborns with hypospadias have a completely formed prepuce that masks the hypospadias.
         1) It is essential to locate the urinary meatus prior to circumcision.[145]
   2. Ambiguous genitalia
   3. Structural abnormalities of the external genitalia (e.g., chordee or a small unusual appearing penis)
B. Clinically unstable infant
C. Evidence of bleeding tendencies (e.g., oozing from puncture sites or slow clotting after punctures)
   1. Family history of a bleeding disorder may be a relative contraindication, pending evaluation of the infant.

PREPROCEDURAL ASSESSMENT

A. Determine the family's understanding of the procedure, including the rationale and the expected risks and benefits.
B. Ascertain whether there is any family history of bleeding or any bleeding tendencies in the infant.
   1. Confirm that vitamin K has been administered.
C. Discuss the use of anesthesia/analgesia/pain relief measures.
D. Inspect the penis, checking for the following.
   1. Abnormalities in the position of the meatus
   2. Any other visual abnormality
E. Identify whether the infant has been voiding normally.
F. Examine the equipment to be used prior to the procedure for the following.[268]
   1. Appropriate fit of all parts
   2. Signs of wear or corrosion
   3. Inadequate closure of the clamp
   4. Matching of all marks on the components of the device
   5. Defects, which may injure the penis
G. The three most common devices used are these:
   1. Gomco clamp
   2. Mogen clamp
   3. Plastibell device
H. Electrocautery should not be used with metal clamps; burns can result.[269]

SURGICAL MANAGEMENT[262,263,266,269–271]

A. Secure and position the infant for the procedure.
   1. The infant is provided with supportive interventions during the procedure.
   2. Swaddling the upper body, padding the immobilization device, and dimming the lights may ameliorate the infant's distress.
B. Cleanse the genital area.
C. Administer an anesthetic agent.
   1. Acetaminophen given prior to circumcision may help to reduce postcircumcision pain.[271]
   2. Oral sucrose administered on a pacifier or into the mouth decreases pain behaviors during local anesthetic administration and the circumcision procedure.

3. Dorsal penile nerve block and ring block both provide effective local anesthesia.
   a. Using buffered lidocaine reduces the pain of injection.
   b. Discomfort caused by administration of lidocaine can be alleviated by the following.
      1) Warming the lidocaine
      2) Injecting the drug slowly
      3) Using a small-gauge needle
4. If EMLA (eutectic mixture of local anesthetics) cream is used, apply it at least 60 minutes prior to the procedure.
   a. EMLA may provide some anesthetic benefit when no other agents are used.
D. Dilate the preputial ring.
E. Visualize the glans.
F. Release the inner preputial epithelium from the epithelium of the glans (also referred to as lysing the adhesions).
   1. There is a common epithelium between the inner surface of the prepuce and the glans; these are not true adhesions.[269]
G. Estimate the amount of foreskin to be removed.
H. Apply the device, and leave it in place to achieve hemostasis.
   1. Applying a hemostat to the prepuce and dorsal slit may precede application of the device.
   2. Use of a Mogen clamp in combination with a dorsal penile nerve block (DPNB) was more effective than Gomco clamp plus DPNB in decreasing pain and distress of newborns undergoing circumcision.[272]
I. Excise the foreskin.
J. Remove the device and assess for immediate complications.

COMPLICATIONS[91,263–266,269,270,273–275]

A. The estimated frequency of complications ranges from 0.2 to 5 percent.[262,263]
B. The following are the most common complications.
   1. Bleeding
      a. Bleeding is the most common early complication.[262]
      b. It can be controlled by the application of direct pressure.
      c. An absorbable hemostatic cellulose product (e.g., Surgicel) may be applied.
      d. Occasionally, a suture may be needed.
      e. If a solution such as epinephrine is used to control bleeding, it should be diluted to a concentration of 1/100,000. Otherwise, absorption through the open wound can result in significant cardiovascular effects.[266]
   2. Infection
      a. Infection can be mild or severe.
      b. Severe infection may produce scarring and deformity of the penis.
C. The foreskin may be cut so that it is too short or too long.
D. Injuries to the foreskin, shaft, and glans may include the following.
   1. Degloving injuries to the prepuce and the shaft when too much skin is drawn up through the clamp and excised
   2. Partial amputation of the glans
      a. When this is observed, the infant should be immediately referred to a urologic surgeon for reconstruction of the penis.
E. Side effects associated with the local anesthetic occur rarely.
   1. Hematoma formation at the site of the injections
   2. Local skin necrosis

POSTOPERATIVE NURSING CARE

A. Postcircumcision care is directed toward the following.
1. Assessing for acute complications
   a. Bright red, prolonged bleeding
   b. Urinary retention
   c. Possible effects on feeding and behavior
2. Promoting healing
   a. Following circumcision and inspection of the penis, the site is dressed with an emollient dressing to promote healing and to prevent adherence of the penis to the diaper.
      1) Emollients are not used with the Plastibell device.
      2) Unit protocols will vary according to type of dressing. Recommended dressings include the following.
         a) Petrolatum jelly–impregnated gauze
         b) Petrolatum jelly alone
         c) Aquaphor ointment[276]
      3) The use of antimicrobial ointments is not recommended.
         a) They do not prevent infection.
         b) They do not promote healing.
         c) They may result in bacterial resistance and later induction of allergic contact dermatitis.[276,277]
3. Preventing infection
4. Instructing the family in home care[91,265,278]
   a. Describe the expected appearance of the penis.
      1) The penis may look raw, and a yellowish-white coating may develop on the glans. This does not indicate infection.
      2) This coating should not last for longer than a week.
      3) Full healing will not occur for seven to ten days.
   b. The infant may cry vigorously during the initial voidings following circumcision.
      1) The infant does experience pain, and this may affect feeding and sleeping patterns.
   c. If acetaminophen has been ordered, the parents need to know the correct dose and method of administration.
   d. Change the dressing with each diaper change. If the dressing is adherent, use warm water to soak it and facilitate removal. The recommended duration of dressing use varies from three to four to seven to ten days after circumcision.[91,278]
   e. Avoid tub baths until the site is completely healed. The penis should be nontender and noninflamed, and the yellow-white coating should have disappeared.
B. The infant is assessed periodically for pain; acetaminophen may be ordered for analgesia.
C. If the infant leaves the hospital prior to voiding, the pediatrician should be called if the infant has not voided 8–12 hours after the circumcision.
D. The Plastibell ring is expected to drop off in five to eight days.
E. Call the pediatrician if any of the following occur (the parent should call if the infant has been discharged):
1. Persistent, bright red bleeding

2. Signs of infection
3. Urinary retention

OUTCOMES

A. Later complications may occur outside the nursery setting.[113,263,264,266,269,278]
   1. Meatitis due to exposure to wet diapers
      a. This may lead to meatal stenosis.
   2. Postcircumcision phimosis as the scar contracts
      a. There may be interference with urine flow.
   3. Adhesions
      a. These can appear as skin bridges between the shaft and the glans.
      b. Curvature of the penis can result from the formation of scar tissue.
   4. Urethrocutaneous fistulas
      a. The etiology is thought to be crushing of the urethra with the clamp, with resulting ischemia.
   5. Inclusion cysts along the incision line
   6. Altered pain responses resulting from circumcision performed without adequate anesthesia.[278,279]

Summary

The routine use of prenatal ultrasound has changed our understanding of the pathophysiologic processes associated with many conditions. Many infants are now diagnosed before the onset of symptoms. A genitourinary anomaly is detected in 0.5 percent of all pregnancies assessed.[280]

Urinary tract dilation does not always mean that obstruction is present; there may be spontaneous resolution of dilation. Many anomalies of the genitourinary tract identified in the neonate do not require surgery in the newborn period.

The family needs to understand the long-term implications of their infant's diagnosis. The infant will be followed by the primary pediatric provider in collaboration with specialists, such as a urologist, nephrologist, and others specific to the infant's needs. The importance of seeing these specialists as scheduled cannot be overemphasized. Family members must know the symptoms of a UTI and be able to assess hydration status of the infant. Teaching the parents the special skills they will need will help them to advocate and better care for their infant.

REFERENCES

1. Blackburn ST. 2003. *Maternal, Fetal, and Neonatal Physiology: A Clinical Perspective,* 2nd ed. Philadelphia: Saunders, 19–23, 75–91, 387–411.

2. Fletcher MA. 1998. *Physical Diagnosis in Neonatology.* Philadelphia: Lippincott Williams & Wilkins, 357–387.

3. Kim MS, and Herrin JT. 2004. Renal conditions. In *Manual of Neonatal Care,* 5th ed., Cloherty JP, Eichenwald EC, and Stark AR, eds. Philadelphia: Lippincott Williams & Wilkins, 621–623.

4. Moore KL, and Persaud TVN. 2003. The urogenital system. In *The Developing Human: Clinically Oriented Embryology,* 7th ed. Philadelphia: Saunders, 288–328.

5. Koeppen BM, and Stanton BA. 2001. *Renal Physiology,* 3rd ed. Philadelphia: Mosby, 17–29, 31–47, 49–72, 75–91, 93–114, 117–132, 133–152, 155–167, 181–190.

6. Bolender DL, and Kaplan S. 2004. Basic embryology. In *Fetal and Neonatal Physiology,* 3rd ed., Polin RA, Fox WW, and Abman SH, eds. Philadelphia: Saunders, 25–40.

7. Sweeney WE Jr, and Avner ED. 2004. Embryogenesis and anatomic development of the kidney. In *Fetal and Neonatal Physiology,* 3rd ed., Polin RA, Fox WW, and Abman SH, eds. Philadelphia: Saunders, 1223–1241.

8. Lerman SE, McAleer IM, and Kaplan GW. 2001. Embryology of the genitourinary tract. In *Clinical Pediatric Urology,* 4th ed., Belman AB, King LR, and Kramer SA, eds. London: Martin Dunitz, 1–22.

9. Ritchey M. 2001. Anomalies of the kidney. In *Clinical Pediatric Urology,* 4th ed., Belman AB, King LR, and Kramer SA, eds. London: Martin Dunitz, 537–558.

10. Nafday SM, et al. 2005. Renal disease. In *Avery's Neonatology: Pathophysiology and Management of the Newborn,* 6th ed., MacDonald MG, Mullett MD, and Seshia MMK, eds. Philadelphia: Lippincott Williams & Wilkins, 981–1065.

11. Thomas KS. 2003. Assessment and management of genitourinary system. In *Comprehensive Neonatal Nursing: A Physiologic Perspective,* 3rd ed., Kenner C, and Lott JW, eds. Philadelphia: Saunders, 673–699.

12. Lott JW. 2003. Fetal development: Environmental influences and critical periods. In *Comprehensive Neonatal Nursing: A Physiologic Perspective*, 3rd ed., Kenner C, and Lott JW, eds. Philadelphia: Saunders, 151–172.

13. Silva JM, et al. 1998. Abnormalities of the kidney: Embryogenesis and radiologic appearance. In *Textbook of Neonatal Ultrasound*, Haller JO, ed. New York: Parthenon, 101–116.

14. Woolf AS. 2004. Embryology. In *Pediatric Nephrology*, 5th ed., Avner ED, Harmon WE, and Niaudet P, eds. Philadelphia: Lippincott Williams & Wilkins, 3–24.

15. Hawkins EP. 1999. Morphologic development of the kidney. In *Oski's Pediatrics: Principles and Practice*, 3rd ed., McMillan JA, et al., eds. Philadelphia: Lippincott Williams & Wilkins, 1542–1543.

16. Gallini F, et al. 2000. Progression of renal function in preterm neonates with gestation age ≤32 weeks. *Pediatric Nephrology* 15(1-2): 119–124.

17. Vogt BA, Dell KM, and Davis ID. 2006. The kidney and urinary tract. In *Neonatal-Perinatal Medicine: Diseases of the Fetus and Infant*, 8th ed., Martin RJ, Fanaroff AA, and Walsh MC, eds. St. Louis: Mosby, 1659–1683.

18. Belman AB. 2001. Hypospadias and chordee. In *Clinical Pediatric Urology*, 4th ed. Belman AB, King LR, and Kramer SA, eds. London: Martin Dunitz, 1061–1092.

19. Belman AB. 2002. Hypospadias and chordee. In *Guide to Clinical Pediatric Urology*, Belman AB, King LR, and Kramer SA, eds. London: Martin Dunitz, 299–311.

20. Arant BS. 1999. Renal and genitourinary diseases. In *Oski's Pediatrics: Principles and Practice*, 3rd ed., McMillan JA, et al., eds. Philadelphia: Lippincott Williams & Wilkins, 336–345.

21. Barthold JS, and Kass EJ. 2002. Abnormalities of the penis and scrotum. In *Guide to Clinical Pediatric Urology*, Belman AB, King LR, and Kramer SA, eds. London: Martin Dunitz, 267–298.

22. Aaronson IA. 2001. Sexual differentiation and intersexuality. In *Clinical Pediatric Urology*, 4th ed., Belman AB, King LR, and Kramer SA, eds. London: Martin Dunitz, 995–1060.

23. Palmert MR, and Dahms WT. 2006. Abnormalities of sexual differentiation. In *Neonatal-Perinatal Medicine: Diseases of the Fetus and Infant*, 8th ed., Martin RJ, Fanaroff AA, and Walsh MC, eds. St. Louis: Mosby, 1550–1596.

24. Spack NP, and Scott MD. 2004. Ambiguous genitalia. In *Manual of Neonatal Care*, 5th ed., Cloherty JP, Eichenwald EC, and Stark AR, eds. Philadelphia: Lippincott Williams & Wilkins, 607–619.

25. Porterfield SP. 2001. Male reproductive system. In *Endocrine Physiology*, 2nd ed. Philadelphia: Mosby, 21–47, 49–58, 153–175, 177–199.

26. Husmann DA. 2002. Cryptorchidism. In *Guide to Clinical Pediatric Urology*, Belman AB, King LR, and Kramer SA, eds. London: Martin Dunitz, 313–335.

27. Barthold JS, and Kass EJ. 2001. Abnormalities of the penis and scrotum. In *Clinical Pediatric Urology*, 4th ed., Belman AB, King LR, and Kramer SA, eds. London: Martin Dunitz, 1093–1124.

28. Husmann DA. 2001. Cryptorchidism. In *Clinical Pediatric Urology*, 4th ed., Belman AB, King LR, and Kramer SA, eds. London: Martin Dunitz, 1125–1154.

29. Franco I. 2001. Evaluation and management of impalpable testes. In *Clinical Pediatric Urology*, 4th ed., Belman AB, King LR, and Kramer SA, eds. London: Martin Dunitz, 1155–1172.

30. Rabinowitz R, and Hulbert WC. 1995. Acute scrotal swelling. *Urologic Clinics of North America* 22(1): 101–106.

31. Bloom DA, Wan J, and Kew DW. 1992. Disorders of the male external genitalia and inguinal canal. In *Clinical Pediatric Urology*, vol. 2, 3rd ed., Kelalis PP, King LR, and Belman AB, eds. Philadelphia: Saunders, 1015–1049.

32. Barnett DH, et. al. 2002. The human prostate expresses sonic hedgehog during fetal development. *Journal of Urology* 168(5): 2206–2210.

33. Barratt TM, and Niaudet P. 2004. Clinical evaluation. In *Pediatric Nephrology*, 5th ed., Avner ED, Harmon WE, and Niaudet P, eds. Philadelphia: Lippincott Williams & Wilkins, 387–398.

34. Xia TG, Blackburn WR, and Gardner WA Jr. 1990. Fetal prostate growth and development. *Pediatric Pathology* 10(4): 527–537.

35. Mor N, Merlob P, and Reisner SH. 1986. Types of hymen in the newborn infant. *European Journal of Obstetrics, Gynecology, and Reproductive Biology* 22(4): 225–228.

36. Swinford RD, et al. 2006. Neonatal nephrology. In *Handbook of Neonatal Intensive Care*, 6th ed., Merenstein GB, and Gardner SL, eds. Philadelphia: Mosby, 736–772.

37. Robillard JE, Guillery EN, and Petershack JA. 1999. Renal function during fetal life. In *Pediatric Nephrology*, 4th ed., Barrett TM, Avner ED, and Harmon WE, eds. Philadelphia: Lippincott Williams & Wilkins, 1–20.

38. Solhaug MJ, and Jose PA. 2004. Postnatal maturation of renal blood flow. In *Fetal and Neonatal Physiology*, 3rd ed., Polin RA, Fox WW, and Abman SH, eds. Philadelphia: Saunders, 1242–1249.

39. Yared A, and Ichikawa I. 1999. Glomerular circulation and function. In *Pediatric Nephrology*, 4th ed., Barrett TM, Avner ED, and Harmon WE, eds. Philadelphia: Lippincott Williams & Wilkins, 39–58.

40. Seikaly MG, and Arant BS Jr. 1992. Development of renal hemodynamics: Glomerular filtration and renal blood flow. *Clinics in Perinatology* 19(1): 1–13.

41. Guignard J-P. 2004. Postnatal development of glomerular filtration rate in neonates. In *Fetal and Neonatal Physiology*, 3rd ed., Polin RA, Fox WW, and Abman SH, eds. Philadelphia: Saunders, 1256–1266.

42. Aperia A, and Zetterstrom R. 1982. Renal control of fluid homeostasis in the newborn infant. *Clinics in Perinatology* 9(3): 523–533.

43. Engrum SA, and Rescorda FJ. 1999. Surgical physiology of the neonate. In *Pediatric Urology Practice*, Gonzales ET, and Bauer SB, eds. Philadelphia: Lippincott Williams & Wilkins, 35–51.

44. Jones DP, and Chesney RW. 1992. Development of tubular function. *Clinics in Perinatology* 19(1): 33–57.

45. Jones DP, and Chesney RW. 2004. Tubular function. In *Pediatric Nephrology*, 5th ed., Barrett TM, Avner ED, and Harmon WE, eds. Philadelphia: Lippincott Williams & Wilkins, 45–72.

46. Feld LG, and Corey HE. 2004. Renal transport of sodium during early development. In *Fetal and Neonatal Physiology*, 3rd ed., Polin RA, Fox WW, and Abman SH, eds. Philadelphia: Saunders, 1267–1278.

47. Linshaw MA. 2004. Concentration and dilution of the urine. In *Fetal and Neonatal Physiology*, 3rd ed., Polin RA, Fox WW, and Abman SH, eds. Philadelphia: Saunders, 1303–1327.

48. Woroniecki RP, et al. 2004. Role of the kidney in calcium and phosphorus homeostasis. In *Fetal and Neonatal Physiology*, 3rd ed., Polin RA, Fox WW, and Abman SH, eds. Philadelphia: Saunders, 1286–1294.

49. Benchimol C, and Satlin LM. 2004. Potassium homeostasis in the fetus and neonate. In *Fetal and Neonatal Physiology*, 3rd ed., Polin RA, Fox WW, and Abman SH, eds. Philadelphia: Saunders, 1279–1286.

50. Celsi G, and Aperia A. 1999. Endocrine control. In *Pediatric Nephrology*, 4th ed., Barrett TM, Avner ED, and Harmon WE, eds. Philadelphia: Lippincott Williams & Wilkins, 101–116.

51. Arant BS Jr. 2001. Renal development: Fluid and electrolyte balance in neonates. In *Clinical Pediatric Urology*, 4th ed., Belman AB, King LR, and Kramer SA, eds. London: Martin Dunitz, 23–34.

52. Trachtman H. 2004. Sodium and water. In *Pediatric Nephrology*, 5th ed., Avner ED, Harmon WE, and Niaudet P, eds. Philadelphia: Lippincott Williams & Wilkins, 125–145.

53. Siegel SR. 1982. Hormonal and renal interaction in body regulation in the newborn infant. *Clinics in Perinatology* 9(3): 535–557.

54. Norwood VF, et al. 2004. Development of the renin-angiotensin system. In *Fetal and Neonatal Physiology*, 3rd ed., Polin RA, Fox WW, and Abman SH, eds. Philadelphia: Saunders, 1249–1256.

55. Bell EF, and Oh W. 2005. Fluid and electrolyte management. In *Avery's Neonatology: Pathophysiology and Management of the Newborn*, 6th ed., MacDonald MG, Mullett MD, and Seshia MMK, eds. Philadelphia: Lippincott Williams & Wilkins, 362–379.

56. Gomez RA, El-Dahr S, and Chevalier RL. 1999. Vasoactive hormones. In *Pediatric Nephrology*, 4th ed., Barrett TM, Avner ED, and Harmon WE, eds. Philadelphia: Lippincott Williams & Wilkins, 83–100.

57. Kerr BA, Starbuck A, and Block SM. 2006. Fluid and electrolyte management. In *Handbook of Neonatal Intensive Care*, 6th ed., Merenstein GB, and Gardner SL, eds. Philadelphia: Mosby, 351–367.

58. Dell KM, and Davis ID. 2006. Fluid, electrolyte, and acid-base homeostasis. In *Neonatal-Perinatal Medicine: Diseases of the Fetus and Infant*, 8th ed., Martin RJ, Fanaroff AA, and Walsh MC, eds. St. Louis: Mosby, 695–712.

59. Robilliard JE, et al. 1992. Regulation of sodium metabolism and extracellular fluid volume during development. Clinics in Perinatology 19(1): 15–32.

60. Schwartz GJ. 2004. Potassium. In *Pediatric Nephrology*, 5th ed., Avner ED, Harmon WE, and Niaudet P, eds. Philadelphia: Lippincott Williams & Wilkins, 147–187.

61. Portale AA. 2004. Calcium and phosphorus. In *Pediatric Nephrology*, 5th ed., Avner ED, Harmon WE, and Niaudet P, eds. Philadelphia: Lippincott Williams & Wilkins, 209–236.

62. Koo WWK, and Tsang RC. 2005. Calcium and magnesium homeostasis. In *Avery's Neonatology: Pathophysiology and Management of the Newborn*, 6th ed., MacDonald MG, Mullett MD, and Seshia MMK, eds. Philadelphia: Lippincott Williams & Wilkins, 847–875.

63. Rigo J, and Curtis MD. 2006. Disorders of calcium, phosphorus, and magnesium metabolism. In *Neonatal-Perinatal Medicine: Diseases of the Fetus and Infant*, 8th ed., Martin RJ, Fanaroff AA, and Walsh MC, eds. St. Louis: Mosby, 1491–1523.

64. Namgung R, and Tsang RC. 2004. Neonatal calcium, phosphorus, and magnesium homeostasis. In *Fetal and Neonatal Physiology*, 3rd ed., Polin RA, Fox WW, and Abman SH, eds. Philadelphia: Saunders, 323–341.

65. Koeppen BM, and Stanton BA. 1992. *Renal Physiology*. Philadelphia: Mosby, 140–151.

66. Chan JCM, and Mak RHK. 2004. Acid-base homeostasis. In *Pediatric Nephrology*, 5th ed., Avner ED, Harmon WE, and Niaudet P, eds. Philadelphia: Lippincott Williams & Wilkins, 189–208.

67. Parry WH, and Zimmer J. 2006. Acid-base homeostasis and oxygenation. In *Handbook of Neonatal Intensive Care*, 6th ed., Merenstein GB, and Gardner SL, eds. Philadelphia: Mosby, 210–222.

68. Friedlich PS, and Seri I. 2004. Regulation of acid-base balance in the fetus and neonate. In *Fetal and Neonatal Physiology*, 3rd ed., Polin RA, Fox WW, and Abman SH, eds. Philadelphia: Saunders, 1361–1364.

69. Brewer ED. 2004. Urinary acidification. In *Fetal and Neonatal Physiology*, 3rd ed., Polin RA, Fox WW, and Abman SH, eds. Philadelphia: Saunders, 1327–1330.

70. McGowan JE, Price-Douglas W, and Hay WW Jr. 2006. Glucose homeostasis. In *Handbook of Neonatal Intensive Care*, 6th ed., Merenstein GB, and Gardner SL, eds. Philadelphia: Mosby, 368–390.

71. Kalhan SC. 2004. Metabolism of glucose and methods of investigation in the fetus and newborn. In *Fetal and Neonatal Physiology*, 3rd ed., Polin RA, Fox WW, and Abman SH, eds. Philadelphia: Saunders, 449–464.

72. Friedman AL. 2004. Transport of amino acids during early development. In *Fetal and Neonatal Physiology*, 3rd ed., Polin RA, Fox WW, and Abman SH, eds. Philadelphia: Saunders, 1294–1298.

73. Jones DP, and Stapleton FB. 2004. Developmental aspects of organic acid transport. In *Fetal and Neonatal Physiology*, 3rd ed., Polin RA, Fox WW, and Abman SH, eds. Philadelphia: Saunders, 1299–1302.

74. Vogt BA, Davis ID, and Avner ED. 2001. The kidney. In *Care of the High-Risk Neonate*, 5th ed., Klaus MH, and Fanaroff AA, eds. Philadelphia: Saunders, 425–446.

75. Cuttler L, and Palmert MR. 2004. Luteinizing hormone and follicle-stimulating hormone secretion in the fetus and newborn infant. In *Fetal and Neonatal Physiology*, 3rd ed., Polin RA, Fox WW, and Abman SH, eds. Philadelphia: Saunders, 1896–1906.

76. Donahoe PK, and Hendren WH. 1976. Evaluation of the newborn with ambiguous genitalia. *Pediatric Clinics of North America* 23(2): 361–370.

77. El-Dahr SS, and Lewy JE. 1992. Urinary tract obstruction and infection in the neonate. *Clinics in Perinatology* 19(1): 213–222.

78. Casale AJ. 1999. Posterior urethral valves and other obstructions of the urethra. In *Pediatric Urology Practice*, Gonzales ET, and Bauer SB, eds. Philadelphia: Lippincott Williams & Wilkins, 223–244.

79. Ellis DG, and Mann CM. 1998. Abnormalities of the urethra, penis, and scrotum. In *Pediatric Surgery*, 5th ed., O'Neill JA Jr, et al., eds. St. Louis: Mosby, 1783–1795.

80. Baskin LS, and Kogan BA. 1998. Urethral anomalies and obstruction. In *Urologic Surgery in Infants and Children*, King LR, ed. Philadelphia: Saunders, 209–221.

81. Rink RC, and Mitchell ME. 1990. Physiology of lower urinary tract obstruction. *Urologic Clinics of North America* 17(2): 329–334.

82. Gonzales ET. 2002. Posterior urethral valves and other urethral anomalies. In *Campbell's Urology*, 8th ed., Walsh PC, Retik AB, and Vaughan ED, eds. Philadelphia: Saunders, 2207–2230.

83. Sheldon CA, and Snyder HM. 1998. Structural disorders of the bladder, augmentation. In *Pediatric Surgery*, 5th ed., O'Neill JA Jr, et al., eds. St. Louis: Mosby, 1685–1707.

84. Casale AJ. 1990. Early ureteral surgery for posterior urethral valves. *Urologic Clinics of North America* 17(2): 361–372.

85. Gonzales ET Jr. 1990. Alternatives in the management of posterior urethral valves. *Urologic Clinics of North America* 17(2): 335–342.

86. Kaplan BS, Kaplan P, and Ruchelli E. 1992. Inherited and congenital malformations of the kidneys in the neonatal period. *Clinics in Perinatology* 19(1): 197–211.

87. Reznik VM, and Budorick NE. 1995. Prenatal detection of congenital renal disease. *Urologic Clinics of North America* 22(1): 21–30.

88. Fine RN. 1992. Diagnosis and treatment of fetal urinary tract abnormalities. *Journal of Pediatrics* 121(3): 333–341.

89. Kaefer M, et al. 1995. Posterior urethral valves, pressure pop-offs and bladder function. *Journal of Urology* 154(2 part 2): 708–711.

90. Atwell JD. 1983. Posterior valves in the British Isles: A multicenter B.A.P.S. review. *Journal of Pediatric Surgery* 18(1): 70–74.

91. Sugar EC, and Hoyler-Grant C. 1995. Disorders of the external genitalia in children. In *Urologic Nursing: Principles and Practice*, Karlowicz KA, ed. Philadelphia: Saunders, 498–525.

92. Hutton KAR, et al. 1994. Prenatally detected posterior urethral valves: Is gestational age at detection a predictor of outcome? *Journal of Urology* 152(2): 698–701.

93. Hilton SVW, and Kaplan GW. 1995. Imaging of common problems in pediatric urology. *Urologic Clinics of North America* 22(1): 1–20.

94. Gibbons MD, et al. 1993. Extracorporeal membrane oxygenation: An adjunct in the management of the neonate with severe respiratory distress and congenital urinary tract anomalies. *Journal of Urology* 150(2): 434–437.

95. Jordan GH, and Hoover DL. 1985. Inadequate decompression of the upper tracts using a Foley catheter in the valve bladder. *Journal of Urology* 134(1): 137–138.

96. Smith AB, and Adams LL. 1998. Insertion of indwelling urethral catheters in infants and children: A survey of current nursing practice. *Pediatric Nursing* 24(3): 229–234.

97. Duckett JW Jr. 1974. Cutaneous vesicostomy in childhood: The Blocksom technique. *Urologic Clinics of North America* 1(3): 485–495.

98. Zaontz MR, and Firlit CF. 1985. Percutaneous antegrade ablation of posterior urethral valves in premature or underweight term neonates: An alternative to primary vesicostomy. *Journal of Urology* 134(1): 139–141.

99. Narasimhan KL, et al. 2004. Does mode of treatment affect the outcome of neonatal posterior urethral valves? *Journal of Urology* 171(6 part): 2423–2426.

100. Jaureguizar E, et al. 2000. Does neonatal pyeloureterostomy worsen bladder function in children with posterior urethral valves? *Journal of Urology* 164(3 part 2): 1031–1033.

101. Churchill BM, et al. 1990. Emergency treatment and long-term follow-up of posterior urethral valves. *Urologic Clinics of North America* 17(2): 343–360.

102. Welch VW. 1994. The management of urologic disorders in the neonate. *Journal of Perinatal & Neonatal Nursing* 8(1): 48–58.

103. Montagnino B, Welch VW, and Hoyler-Grant C. 1995. Congenital anomalies that affect the kidney, ureter and bladder. In *Urologic Nursing: Principles and Practice*, Karlowicz KA, ed. Philadelphia: Saunders, 526–564.

104. Joseph DB. 1999. Triad syndrome and other disorders of abnormal detrusor development. In *Pediatric Urology Practice*, Gonzales ET, and Bauer SB, eds. Philadelphia: Lippincott Williams & Wilkins, 323–337.

105. Ghanem MA, and Nijman RJ. 2005. Long-term followup of bilateral high (sober) urinary diversion in patients with posterior urethral valves and its effect on bladder function. *Journal of Urology* 173(5): 1721–1724.

106. Krahn CG, and Johnson HW. 1993. Cutaneous vesicostomy in the young child: Indications and results. *Urology* 41(6): 558–563.

107. Hendren WH. 1998. Diversion and undiversion. In *Pediatric Surgery*, 5th ed., O'Neill JA Jr, et al., eds. St. Louis: Mosby, 1653–1670.

108. Smith GHH, et al. 1996. The long-term outcome of posterior urethral valves treated with primary valve ablation and observation. *Journal of Urology* 155(5): 1730–1734.

109. Ghali AM, et al. 2000. Posterior urethral valves with persistent high serum creatinine: The value of percutaneous nephrostomy. *Journal of Urology* 164(4): 1340–1344.

110. Merguerian PA, et al. 1992. Radiographic and serologic correlates of azotemia in patients with posterior urethral valves. *Journal of Urology* 148(5): 1499–1503.

111. Bajpai M, et al. 2005. Posterior urethral valves: Preliminary observations on the significance of plasma rennin activity as a prognostic marker. *Journal of Urology* 173(2): 592–594.

112. Yerkes EB, and Brock JW III. 1998. Diagnosis and management of testicular torsion. In *Urologic Surgery in Infants and Children*, King LR, ed. Philadelphia: Saunders, 239–245.

113. Bartholomew TH, and McIver B. 1999. Other disorders of the penis and scrotum. In *Pediatric Urology Practice*, Gonzales ET, and Bauer SB, eds. Philadelphia: Lippincott Williams & Wilkins, 533–546.

114. Smith GI. 1955. Cellular changes from graded testicular ischemia. *Journal of Urology* 73(2): 355–362.

115. Sheldon CA. 2001. The pediatric genitourinary examination. *Pediatric Clinics of North America* 48(6): 1339–1380.

116. Brandt MT, et al. 1992. Prenatal testicular torsion: Principles of management. *Journal of Urology* 147(3): 670–672.

117. Ryken TC, Turner JW, and Haynes T. 1990. Bilateral testicular torsion in a pre-term neonate. *Journal of Urology* 143(1): 102–103.

118. Hutson JM. 1998. Undescended testis, torsion and variocele. In *Pediatric Surgery*, 5th ed., O'Neill JA Jr, et al., eds. St. Louis: Mosby, 1087–1109.

119. Kayler L, et al. 1999. Testicular torsion in a pre-term neonate. *Journal of Perinatology* 19(4): 318–319.

120. LaQuaglia MP, et al. 1987. Bilateral neonatal torsion. *Journal of Urology* 138(4): 1051–1054.

121. Steinhardt GF, Boyarsky S, and Mackey R. 1993. Testicular torsion: Pitfalls of color Doppler sonography. *Journal of Urology* 150(2): 461–462.

122. Barada JH, Weingarten JL, and Cromie WJ. 1989. Testicular salvage and age-related delay in the presentation of testicular torsion. *Journal of Urology* 142(30): 746–748.

123. Das S, and Singer A. 1990. Controversies of perinatal torsion of the spermatic cord: A review, survey and recommendations. *Journal of Urology* 143(2): 231–233.

124. Nagler HM, and White RD. 1982. The effect of testicular torsion on the contralateral testis. *Journal of Urology* 128(6): 1343–1348.

125. Fraser I, et al. 1985. Testicular torsion does not cause autoimmunization in man. *British Journal of Surgery* 72(3): 237–238.

126. Bauer SB, and Retik AB. 1978. Urachal anomalies and related umbilical disorders. *Urologic Clinics of North America* 5(1): 195–211.

127. Nasrallah PF, and McMahon DR. 1999. Anatomic abnormalities of the bladder. In *Pediatric Urology Practice*, Gonzales ET, and Bauer SB, eds. Philadelphia: Lippincott Williams & Wilkins, 313–321.

128. Nguyen HT, and Cilento BG Jr. 2001. Bladder diverticula, urachal anomalies, and other uncommon anomalies of the bladder. In *Pediatric Urology*, Gearhart JP, Rink RC, and Mouriquand PDE, eds. Philadelphia: Saunders, 565–576.

129. Gobet R, Bleakley J, and Peters CA. 1998. Premature urachal closure induces hydroureteronephrosis in male fetuses. *Journal of Urology* 160(4): 1463–1467.

130. Cilley RE, and Krummel TM. 1998. Disorders of the umbilicus. In *Pediatric Surgery*, 5th ed., O'Neill JA Jr, et al., eds. St. Louis: Mosby, 1029–1043.

131. Goldman IL, et al. 1988. Infected urachal cysts: A review of 10 cases. *Journal of Urology* 140(2): 375–378.

132. Mesrobian HGO, et al. 1997. Ten years of experience with isolated urachal anomalies in children. *Journal of Urology* 158(3 part 2): 1316–1318.

133. Mahoney PJ, and Ennis D. 1936. Congenital patent urachus. *New England Journal of Medicine* 215(5): 193–195.

134. Nix JT, et al. 1958. Congenital patent urachus. *Journal of Urology* 79(2): 264–273.

135. Cadeddu JA, et al. 2000. Laparoscopic management of urachal cysts in adulthood. *Journal of Urology* 164(5): 1526–1528.

136. Cilento BG, et al. 1998. Urachal anomalies: Defining the best diagnostic modality. *Urology* 52(1): 120–122.

137. Khurana S, and Borzi PA. 2002. Laparoscopic management of complicated urachal disease in children. *Journal of Urology* 168(4 part 1): 1526–1528.

138. Allen JW, Song J, and Velcek FT. 2004. Acute presentation of infected urachal cysts: Case report and review of diagnosis and therapeutic interventions. *Pediatric Emergency Care* 20(2): 108–111.

139. Manivel JC, et al. 1989. Prune belly syndrome: Clinicopathologic study of 29 cases. *Pediatric Pathology* 9(6): 691–711.

140. Scheisser M, et al. 2003. Umbilical cord edema associated with patent urachus. *Ultrasound in Obstetrics & Gynecology* 22(6): 646–647.

141. Van der Bilt JD, et al. 2003. Prenatally diagnosed ruptured vesico-allantoic cyst presenting as patent urachus at birth. *Journal of Urology* 169(4): 1478–1479.

142. Smith NM, et al. 1992. The OEIS complex (omphalocele-exstrophy-imperforate anus-spinal defects): Recurrence in sibs. *Journal of Medical Genetics* 29(10): 730–732.

143. Kelly JH. 1998. Exstrophy and epispadias: Kelly's method of repair. In *Pediatric Surgery*, 5th ed., O'Neill JA Jr, et al., eds. St. Louis: Mosby, 1732–1759.

144. Zaontz MR, and Packer MG. 1997. Abnormalities of the external genitalia. *Pediatric Clinics of North America* 44(5): 1267–1297.

145. Brock JW III, and O'Neill JA Jr. 1998. Bladder exstrophy. In *Pediatric Surgery*, 5th ed., O'Neill JA Jr, et al., eds. St. Louis: Mosby, 1709–1725.

146. Patten BM, and Barry A. 1952. The genesis of exstrophy of the bladder and epispadias. *American Journal of Anatomy* 90(1): 35–57.

147. Shapiro E, Lepor H, and Jeffs RD. 1984. The inheritance of the exstrophy-epispadius complex. *Journal of Urology* 132(2): 308–310.

148. Gearhart JP. 1999. Bladder and cloacal exstrophy. In *Pediatric Urology Practice*, Gonzales ET, and Bauer SB, eds. Philadelphia: Lippincott Williams & Wilkins, 339–363.

149. Gearhart JP, and Ben-Chaim J. 1998. Exstrophy and epispadius. In *Urologic Surgery in Infants and Children*, King LR, ed. Philadelphia: Saunders, 106–118.

150. International Clearinghouse for Birth Defects Monitoring Systems. 1987. Epidemiology of bladder exstrophy and epispadius: A communication from the International Clearinghouse for Birth Defects Monitoring Systems. *Teratology* 36(2): 221–227.

151. Nelson CP, Dunn RL, and Wei JT. 2005. Contemporary epidemiology of bladder exstrophy in the United States. *Journal of Urology* 173(5): 1728–1731.

152. Mollohan J. 1999. Exstrophy of the bladder. *Neonatal Network* 18(2): 17–26.

153. Bowers V, Hannigan KF, and Kushner KL. 1995. Bladder exstrophy and epispadius. In *Urologic Nursing: Principles and Practice*, Karlowicz KA, ed. Philadelphia: Saunders, 565–592.

154. Gearhart JP. 2001. The bladder exstrophy-epispadius-cloacal exstrophy complex. In *Pediatric Urology*, Gearhart JP, Rink RC, and Mouriquand PDE, eds. Philadelphia: Saunders, 511–546.

155. Evangelidis A, Murphy JP, and Gatti JM. 2004. Prenatal diagnosis of bladder exstrophy by 3-dimensional ultrasound. *Journal of Urology* 172(3): 1111.

156. Grady RW, and Mitchell ME. 2000. Complete primary repair of exstrophy. Surgical technique. *Urologic Clinics of North America* 27(3): 569–578.

157. Montagnino BA. 2001. Nursing intervention in pediatric urology. In *Pediatric Urology*, Gearhart JP, Rink RC, and Mouriquand PDE, eds. Philadelphia: Saunders, 259–271.

158. Dodson JL, et al. 2001. The newborn exstrophy bladder inadequate for primary closure: Evaluation, management and outcome. *Journal of Urology* 165(5): 1656–1659.

159. Gearhart JP, et al. 1996. The multiple reoperative bladder exstrophy closure: What affects the potential of the bladder? *Urology* 47(2): 240–243.

160. Allen TD, Husmann DA, and Bucholz RW. 1992. Exstrophy of the bladder: Primary closure after iliac osteotomies without external or internal fixation. *Journal of Urology* 147(2): 438–440.

161. Gearhart JP, et al. 1996. A combined vertical and horizontal pelvic osteotomy approach for primary and secondary repair of bladder exstrophy. *Journal of Urology* 155(2): 689–693.

162. El-Sherbiny MT, Hafez AT, and Ghoneim MA. 2002. Complete repair of exstrophy: Further experience with neonates and children after failed initial closure. *Journal of Urology* 168(4 part 2): 1692–1694.

163. Hafez AT, and El-Sherbiny MT. 2005. Complete repair of bladder exstrophy: Management of resultant hypospadias. *Journal of Urology* 173(3): 958–961.

164. Kropp BP, and Cheng EY. 2000. Total urogenital complex mobilization in female patients with exstrophy. *Journal of Urology* 164(3 part 2): 1035–1039.

165. Gearhart JP. 2001. Complete repair of bladder exstrophy in the newborn: Complications and management. *Journal of Urology* 165(6 part 2): 2431–2433.

166. Mesrobian H-GO, Kelalis PP, and Kramer SA. 1988. Long-term followup of 103 patients with bladder exstrophy. *Journal of Urology* 139(4): 719–722.

167. Redemann S. 2002. Modalities for immobilization. In *Orthopaedic Nursing*, Maher AB, Salmond SW, and Pellino TA, eds. Philadelphia: Saunders, 302–323.

168. Marek JF. 1999. Management of persons with trauma to the musculoskeletal system. In *Medical-Surgical Nursing Concepts and Clinical Practice*, 6th ed., Phipps WJ, Sands JK, and Marek JF, eds. St. Louis: Mosby, 1915–1937.

169. Thompson JM. 1997. Musculoskeletal system. In *Mosby's Clinical Nursing*, Thompson JM, et al., eds. St. Louis: Mosby, 432–448.

170. Mercy N, and Brady-Fryer B. 2004. Bladder exstrophy: A challenge for nursing care. *Journal of Wound, Ostomy, and Continence Nursing* 31(5): 293–298.

171. Capolicchio G, et al. 2001. A population based analysis of continence outcomes and bladder exstrophy. *Journal of Urology* 165(6 part 2): 2418–2421.

172. O'Neill JA Jr. 1998. Cloacal exstrophy. In *Pediatric Surgery*, 5th ed., O'Neill JA Jr, et al., eds. St. Louis: Mosby, 1725–1732.

173. Hurwitz RS, et al. 1987. Cloacal exstrophy: A report of 34 cases. *Journal of Urology* 138(4 part 2): 1060–1064.

174. Manzoni GA, Ransley PG, and Hurwitz RS. 1987. Cloacal exstrophy and cloacal exstrophy variants: A proposed system of classification. *Journal of Urology* 138(4 part 2): 1065–1068.

175. Lund DP, and Hendren WH. 2001. Cloacal exstrophy: A 25-year experience with 50 cases. *Journal of Pediatric Surgery* 36(1): 68–75.

176. Bruch SW, et al. 1996. Challenging the embryogenesis of cloacal exstrophy. *Journal of Pediatric Surgery* 31(6): 768–770.

177. Davidoff AM, et al. 1996. Management of the gastrointestinal tract and nutrition of patients with cloacal exstrophy. *Journal of Pediatric Surgery* 31(6): 771–773.

178. Redman JF, Seibert JJ, and Page BC. 1981 Cloacal exstrophy in identical twins. *Urology* 17(1): 73–74.

179. Fujiyoshi Y, et al. 1987 Exstrophy of the cloacal membrane. A pathologic study of four cases. *Archives of Pathology and Laboratory Medicine* 111(2): 157–160.

180. Langer JC, et al. 1992. Cloacal exstrophy: Prenatal diagnosis before rupture of the cloacal membrane. *Journal of Pediatric Surgery* 27(10): 1352–1355.

181. Tank ES, and Lindenauer SM. 1970. Principles of management of exstrophy of the cloaca. *American Journal of Surgery* 119(1): 95–98.

182. Ricketts RR, et al. 1991. Modern treatment of cloacal exstrophy. *Journal of Pediatric Surgery* 26(4): 444–460.

183. Lund DP, and Hendren WH. 1993. Cloacal exstrophy: Experience with 20 cases. *Journal of Pediatric Surgery* 28(10): 1360–1369.

184. Rickham PP. 1960. Vesico-intestinal fissure. *Archives of Disease in Childhood* 35(179): 97–102.

185. Geiger JD, and Coran AG. 1998. The association of large ovarian cysts with cloacal exstrophy. *Journal of Pediatric Surgery* 33(5): 719–721.

186. Smith EA, et al. 1997. Urologic management of cloacal exstrophy: Experience with 11 patients. *Journal of Pediatric Surgery* 32(2): 256–262.

187. Hendren WH, Carr MC, and Adams MC. 1998. Megaureter and prune-belly syndrome. In *Pediatric Surgery*, 5th ed., O'Neill JA Jr, et al., eds. St. Louis: Mosby, 1631–1651.

188. Massad C, and Smith E. 1999. Megaureter. In *Pediatric Urology Practice*, Gonzales ET, and Bauer SB, eds. Philadelphia: Lippincott Williams & Wilkins, 205–221.

189. Belman AB. 1974. Megaureter. Classification, etiology, and management. *Urologic Clinics of North America* 1(3): 497–513.

190. Keating MA, and Retik AB. 1990. Management of the dilated obstructed ureter. *Urologic Clinics of North America* 17(2): 291–306.

191. Woodard JR. 1998. Megaloureter. In *Urologic Surgery in Infants and Children*, King LR, ed. Philadelphia: Saunders, 67–74.

192. Liu HYA, et al. 1994. Clinical outcome and management of prenatally diagnosed primary megaureters. *Journal of Urology* 152(2): 614–617.

193. Baskin LS, et al. 1994. Primary dilated megaureter: Long term followup. *Journal of Urology* 152(2): 618–621.

194. Douenias R, Smith AD, and Brock WA. 1990. Advances in the percutaneous management of the ureteropelvic junction and other obstructions of the urinary tract in children. *Urologic Clinics of North America* 17(2): 419–428.

195. Carney S, et al. 1995. Urinary tract obstructions. In *Urologic Nursing: Principles and Practice*, Karlowicz KA, ed. Philadelphia: Saunders, 107–140.

196. Bernhardt J. 1986. Percutaneous nephrostomy tubes in the neonate with obstructive uropathy. *Neonatal Network* 4(6): 51–53.

197. Marantides DK, Marek JF, and Moran J. 1999. Management of persons with problems of the kidney and urinary tract. In *Medical Surgical Nursing Concepts and Clinical Practice*, 6th ed., Phipps WJ, Sands JK, and Marek JF, eds. St. Louis: Mosby, 1411–1464.

198. DeFoor W, et al. 2004. Results of tapered ureteral reimplantation for primary megaureter: Extravesical versus intravesical approach *Journal of Urology* 172(4 part 2): 1640–1643.

199. Joseph DB. 2001. Ureterovesical junction anomalies—megaureters. In *Pediatric Urology*, Gearhart JP, Rink RC, and Mouriquand PDE, eds. Philadelphia: Saunders, 347–357.

200. Kogan BA, Baskin LS, and Laedlein MA. 1997. Ureteral reimplant surgery: Frequently asked questions. In *Handbook of Pediatric Urology*, Baskin LS, Kogan BA, and Duckett JW, eds. Philadelphia: Lippincott Williams & Wilkins, 307–310.

201. Greskovich FJ III, and Nyberg LM Jr. 1988. The prune belly syndrome: A review of its etiology, defects, treatment and prognosis. *Journal of Urology* 140(4): 707–712.

202. Mesrobian H-GO. 1998. Prune belly syndrome. In *Urologic Surgery in Infants and Children*, King LR, ed. Philadelphia: Saunders, 182–191.

203. Woodard JR, and Zucker I. 1990. Current management of the dilated urinary tract in prune belly syndrome. *Urologic Clinics of North America* 17(2): 407–418.

204. Hoagland MH, Frank KA, and Hutchins GM. 1988. Prune-belly syndrome with prostatic hypoplasia, bladder wall rupture, and massive ascites in a fetus with trisomy 18. *Archives of Pathology & Laboratory Medicine* 112(11): 1126–1128.

205. Hoagland MH, and Hutchins GM. 1987. Obstructive lesions of the lower urinary tract in the prune belly syndrome. *Archives of Pathology & Laboratory Medicine* 111(1): 154–156.

206. Druschel CM. 1995. A descriptive study of prune belly in New York State, 1983 to 1989. *Archives of Pediatrics & Adolescent Medicine* 149(1): 70–76.

207. Franco I. 2006. Prune belly syndrome. Retrieved May 26, 2006, from www.emedicine.com/med/topic3055.htm.

208. Gonzalez R, et al. 1990. Early bladder outlet obstruction in fetal lambs induces renal dysplasia and the prune-belly syndrome. *Journal of Pediatric Surgery* 25(3): 342–345.

209. Stephens FD, and Gupta D. 1994. Pathogenesis of the prune belly syndrome. *Journal of Urology* 152(6): 2328–2331.

210. Short KL, Groff DB, and Cook L. 1985. The concomitant presence of gastroschisis and prune belly syndrome in a twin. *Journal of Pediatric Surgery* 20(2): 186–187.

211. Reinberg Y, et al. 1991. Prune belly syndrome in females: A triad of abdominal musculature deficiency and anomalies of the urinary and genital systems. *Journal of Pediatrics* 118(3): 395–398.

212. Loder RT, et al. 1992. Musculoskeletal aspects of prune-belly syndrome: Description and pathogenesis. *American Journal of Diseases of Children* 146(10): 1224–1229.

213. Brinker MR, Palutsis RS, and Sarwark JF. 1995. The orthopaedic manifestations of prune-belly (Eagle Barrett) syndrome. *Journal of Bone and Joint Surgery* 77(2): 251–257.

214. Soylu H, et al. 2001. Prune-belly syndrome and pulmonary hypoplasia: A potential cause of death. *Pediatrics International* 43(2): 172–175.

215. Fontaine E, et al. 1997. Long-term results of renal transplantation in children with the prune-belly syndrome. *Journal of Urology* 158(3 part 1): 892–894.

216. Smith EA, and Woodard JR. 2001. Prune-belly syndrome. In *Pediatric Urology*, Gearhart JP, Rink RC, and Mouriquand PDE, eds. Philadelphia: Saunders, 577–592.

217. Woodard JR. 1998. Editorial: Lessons learned in 3 decades of managing the prune-belly syndrome. *Journal of Urology* 159(5): 1680.

218. Furness PD, et al. 1998. The prune-belly syndrome: A new and simplified technique of abdominal wall reconstruction. *Journal of Urology* 160(3 part 2): 1195–1197.

219. Noh PH, et al. 1999. Prognostic factors for long-term renal function in boys with the prune-belly syndrome. *Journal of Urology* 162(4): 1399–1401.

220. Mouriquand P. 1998. Congenital anomalies of the pyeloureteral junction and the ureter. In *Pediatric Surgery*, 5th ed., O'Neill JA Jr, ed. St. Louis: Mosby, 1591–1608.

221. Cilento BG Jr, and Kaplan GW. 1998. Ureteropelvic junction obstruction. In *Urologic Surgery in Infants and Children*, King LR, ed. Philadelphia: Saunders, 18–30.

222. Koff SA. 1990. Pathophysiology of ureteropelvic junction obstruction. Clinical and experimental observations. *Urologic Clinics of North America* 17(2): 263–272.

223. Steinhardt GF. 1999. Ureteropelvic junction obstruction. In *Pediatric Urology Practice*, Gonzales ET, and Bauer SB, eds. Philadelphia: Lippincott Williams & Wilkins, 181–204.

224. Gonzalez R, and Schimke CM. 2001. Ureteropelvic junction obstruction in infants and children. *Pediatric Clinics of North America* 48(6): 1505–1518.

225. Blyth B, Snyder HM, and Duckett JW. 1993. Antenatal diagnosis and subsequent management of hydronephrosis. *Journal of Urology* 149(4): 693–698.

226. Mandell J, Peters CA, and Retik AB. 1990. Current concepts in the perinatal diagnosis and management of hydronephrosis. *Urologic Clinics of North America* 17(2): 247–262.

227. Ulman I, Jayanthi VR, and Koff SA. 2000. The long-term followup of newborns with severe unilateral hydronephrosis initially treated nonoperatively. *Journal of Urology* 164(3 part 2): 1101–1105.

228. Koff SA, et al. 1994. The assessment of obstruction in the newborn with unilateral hydronephrosis by measuring the size of the opposite kidney. *Journal of Urology* 152(2): 596–599.

229. Roth JA, and Diamond DA. 2001. Prenatal hydronephrosis. *Current Opinion in Pediatrics* 13(2): 138–141.

230. Bidair M, Kalota SJ, and Kaplan GW. 1993. Infantile hypertrophic pyloric stenosis and hydronephrosis: Is there an association? *Journal of Urology* 150(1): 153–155.

231. Maizels M, et al. 1992. Grading nephroureteral dilatation detected in the first year of life: Correlation with obstruction. *Journal of Urology* 148(2): 609–614.

232. Elder JS. 1997. Antenatal hydronephrosis. Fetal and neonatal management. *Pediatric Clinics of North America* 44(5): 1299–1321.

233. Bomalski MD, Hirschl RB, and Bloom DA. 1997. Vesicoureteral reflux and ureteropelvic junction obstruction: Association, treatment options and outcome. *Journal of Urology* 157(3): 969–974.

234. Austin PF, Cain MP, and Rink RC. 2000. Nephrostomy tube drainage with pyeloplasty: Is it necessarily a bad choice? *Journal of Urology* 163(5): 1528–1530.

235. MacNulty AE, et al. 1993. Does early pyeloplasty really avert loss of renal function? A retrospective review. *Journal of Urology* 150(2): 769–773.

236. Kogan BA, Baskin LS, and Leadlein. 1997. Pyeloplasty surgery for ureteropelvic junction obstruction: Frequently asked questions. In *Handbook of Pediatric Urology,* Baskin LS, Kogan BA, and Duckett JW, eds. Philadelphia: Lippincott Williams & Wilkins, 311–314.

237. Schmahmann S, and Haller JO. 1998. Sonography of the neonatal ovary. In *Textbook of Neonatal Ultrasound,* Haller JO, ed. New York: Parthenon, 129–136.

238. Strickland JL. 2002. Ovarian cysts in neonates, children and adolescents. *Current Opinion in Obstetrics & Gynecology* 14(5): 459–465.

239. Brandt ML, et al. 1991. Surgical indications in antenatally diagnosed ovarian cysts. *Journal of Pediatric Surgery* 26(3): 276–282.

240. Giacoia GP, and Wood BP. 1987. Radiological case of the month. *American Journal of Diseases of Children* 141(9): 1005–1006.

241. Crombleholme TM, et al. 1997. Fetal ovarian cyst decompression to prevent torsion. *Journal of Pediatric Surgery* 32(10): 1447–1449.

242. Sakala EP, Leon ZA, and Rouse GA. 1991. Management of antenatally diagnosed fetal ovarian cysts. *Obstetrical & Gynecological Survey* 46(7): 407–414.

243. Meizner I, et al. 1991. Fetal ovarian cysts: Prenatal ultrasonographic detection and postnatal evaluation and treatment. *American Journal of Obstetrics and Gynecology* 164(3): 874–878.

244. Kaplan GW, and McAleer IM. 2005. Structural abnormalities of the genitourinary tract. In *Neonatology: Pathophysiology and Management of the Newborn,* 6th ed., MacDonald MG, Seshia MMK, and Mullett MD, eds. Philadelphia: Lippincott Williams & Wilkins, 1092–1093.

245. Kurjak A, et al. 1996. Ultrasound and the ovary. In *Diagnosis and Management of Ovarian Disorders,* Altchek A, and Deligdisch L, eds. New York: Igaku-Shoin, 270–291.

246. Topaloglu AK, Vade A, and Zeller WP. 1997. Congenital adrenal hyperplasia and bilateral ovarian cysts in a neonate. *Clinical Pediatrics* 36(12): 719–720.

247. Katz VL, et al. 1996. Fetal ovarian torsion appearing as a solid abdominal mass. *Journal of Perinatology* 16(4): 302–304.

248. Scully RE, et al. 1995. Case records of the Massachusetts General Hospital. Weekly clinicopathological exercises. Case 6-1995—A one-month-old girl with an intraabdominal mass found on prenatal ultrasonographic examination. *New England Journal of Medicine* 332(8): 522–527.

249. Suita S, et al. 1984. Neonatal ovarian cyst diagnosed antenatally: Report of two patients. *Journal of Clinical Ultrasound* 12(8): 517–519.

250. Nussbaum AR, et al. 1988. Neonatal ovarian cysts: Sonographic-pathologic correlation. *Radiology* 168(3): 817–821.

251. Sandler MA, et al. 1985. Prenatal diagnosis of septated ovarian cysts. *Journal of Clinical Ultrasound* 13(1): 55–57.

252. Scholtz PM, et al. 1982. Large ovarian cyst causing cecal perforation in a newborn infant. *Journal of Pediatric Surgery* 17(1): 91–92.

253. McKeever PA, and Andrews H. 1988. Fetal ovarian cysts: A report of five cases. *Journal of Pediatric Surgery* 23(4): 354–355.

254. Herman TE, and Shackelford GD. 1997. Large torsed neonatal ovarian cysts associated with massive vesicoureteral and intrarenal reflux. *Journal of Perinatology* 17(1): 75–78.

255. Monson R, et al. 1978. Ruptured ovarian cyst in a newborn infant. *Journal of Pediatrics* 93(2): 324–325.

256. Jafri SZH, et al. 1984. Ovarian cysts: Sonographic detection and association with hypothyroidism. *Radiology* 150(3): 809–812.

257. Siegel MJ. 1991. Pediatric gynecologic sonography. *Radiology* 179(3): 593–600.

258. Chiaramonte C, Piscopo A, and Cataliotti F. 2001. Ovarian cysts in newborns. *Pediatric Surgery International* 17(2-3): 171–174.

259. Luzzatto C, et al. 2000. Neonatal ovarian cysts: Management and follow-up. *Pediatric Surgery International* 16(1-2): 56–59.

260. Van der Zee DC, et al. 1995. Laparoscopic approach to surgical management of ovarian cysts in the newborn. *Journal of Pediatric Surgery* 30(1): 42–43.

261. Eggermont E, et al. 1988. Ovarian cysts in newborn infants (letter). *American Journal of Diseases of Children* 142(7): 702.

262. American Academy of Pediatrics Task Force on Circumcision. 1999. Circumcision policy statement. *Pediatrics* 103(3): 686–693.

263. Baskin LS. 1997. Circumcision. In *Handbook of Pediatric Urology,* Baskin LS, Kogan BA, and Duckett JW, eds. Philadelphia: Lippincott Williams & Wilkins, 1–9.

264. Lund MM. 1990. Perspectives on newborn male circumcision. *Neonatal Network* 9(3): 7–12.

265. American Academy of Pediatrics Task force on Circumcision. 1989. Report of the task force on circumcision. *Pediatrics* 84(4): 388–391.

266. Kaplan GW. 1983. Complications of circumcision. *Urologic Clinics of North America* 10(3): 543–549.

267. Kochen M, and McCurdy S. 1980. Circumcision and the risk of cancer of the penis. A life-table analysis. *American Journal of Diseases of Children* 134(5): 484–486.

268. Swayze S. 1999. Clamping down on circumcision. *Nursing* 29(9): 73.

269. Grimes DA. 1978. Routine circumcision of the newborn infant: A reappraisal. *American Journal of Obstetrics and Gynecology* 130(2): 125–129.

270. Alkalay AL, and Sola A. 2000. Analgesia and local anesthesia for non-ritual circumcision in stable healthy newborns. *Neonatal Intensive Care* 13(2): 19–22.

271. Geyer J, et al. 2002. An evidence-based multidisciplinary protocol for neonatal circumcision pain management. *Journal of Obstetric, Gynecologic, and Neonatal Nursing* 31(4): 403–410.

272. Kurtis P, et al. 1999. A comparison of the Mogen and Gomco clamps in combination with dorsal penile nerve block in minimizing the pain of neonatal circumcision. *Pediatrics* 103(2): E23.

273. Patel HI, et al. 2001. Genitourinary injuries in the newborn. *Journal of Pediatric Surgery* 36(1): 235–239.

274. Strimling BS. 1996. Partial amputation of glans penis during Mogen clamp circumcision. *Pediatrics* 97(6): 906–907.

275. Howard CR, Howard FM, and Weitzman ML. 1994. Acetaminophen analgesia in neonatal circumcision: The effect on pain. *Pediatrics* 93(4): 641–646.

276. Lund C, et al. 1999. Neonatal skin care: The scientific basis for practice. *Journal of Obstetric, Gynecologic, and Neonatal Nursing* 28(3): 241–254.

277. Smack DP, et al. 1996. Infection and allergy incidence in ambulatory surgery patients using white petrolatum vs bacitracin ointment. A randomized controlled trial. *JAMA* 276(12): 972–977.

278. Brown MR, Cartwright PC, and Snow BW. 1997. Common office problems in pediatric urology and gynecology. *Pediatric Clinics of North America* 44(5): 1091–1115.

279. Taddio A, et al. 1997. Effect of neonatal circumcision on pain response during subsequent routine vaccination. *Lancet* 349(9052): 599–603.

280. Herndon CD, et al. 2000. Consensus on the management of antenatally detected urological abnormalities. *Journal of Urology* 164(3 part 2): 1052–1056.

Notes

Neurosurgical Conditions

Tracy Karp, RNC, MS, NNP
Julieanne Schiefelbein, RNC, MAppSc, MA(Ed),
RNM, CPNP, CCRN, NNP
Kim Friddle, RNC, BSN, BC
Nancy Shaw, MSN, NNP
Nan Nicholes, RNC, MS
Paula Peterson, MS, CPNP
Laurie Udy, RNC, BSN

General neurosurgical disorders encompass a wide spectrum of problems from congenital anomalies to acquired conditions. The congenital anomalies can range from common, such as spina bifida, to rare, such as arterial venous malformation. Some of the most frequent acquired problems are secondary to other conditions, such as hydrocephalus following intraventricular hemorrhage (IVH). The rate of this disorder is dependent upon the number of at-risk preterm infants seen in one's setting, as well as the incidence of the underlying causal event (IVH). The frequency with which one sees neurosurgical conditions will depend upon the practice setting, services offered, and local custom for care provision. Regardless of the incidences of these conditions or the frequency with which one may see them, the neonatal nurse's responsibility is to be able to provide competent and compassionate care to these patients. For all these conditions, the quality of nursing care may significantly alter the outcome. This chapter presents an overview of some common and not so common neurosurgical conditions in a manner that supplies a framework to provide care across conditions as well as care specific to various ones.

Embryology[1-3]

A. Evolution of the fertilized ovum into the embryo
1. Embryoblasts (cells of the embryo) organize into the two layers of the bilaminar embryo.
   a. The epiblast or primary ectoderm is located at top of the embryonic pole.
   b. The hypoblast or primary endoderm is located directly beneath the ectoderm.

      c. These two layers differentiate during the first week of gestation.
2. Development of the trilaminar embryo occurs during the third week of gestation.
      a. Ectodermal cells migrate through a midline groove in the ectoderm, the primitive streak.
      b. Migrating cells arrange themselves between the two existing layers, the ectoderm and the endoderm.
      c. Creation of this third layer, the mesoderm, is known as gastrulation.
B. Development of the notochord
1. Development of the notochordal process
      a. Mesodermal cells that lie along the midline differentiate into the notochordal process, the precursor of the central nervous system (CNS).
      b. The notochordal process extends along the midline of the embryo from the primitive streak cranially to the primitive mouth.
2. Development of the notochord
      a. Within the notochordal process, a canal that extends caudally from a pit in the primitive streak to the cranial end of the process forms.
      b. The lower portion of the notochordal process fuses with the underlying endoderm and degenerates.
      c. The ends of the remaining U-shaped notochordal process begin to fold in and fuse with each other, eventually creating a solid notochord.
      d. Closure of the U-shaped ends of the notochord also results in fusion and closure of the attached endoderm.
      e. The notochord separates from the endoderm by the fourth week of gestation.
C. Development of the neural tube
1. Neurulation
      a. The notochordal process induces the overlying ectoderm to separate into ectodermal tissue and a specialized neuroectodermal tissue, the neural plate.
      b. The degeneration and subsequent folding of the notochordal process induce similar folding of the neural plate, resulting in the neural tube.
      c. Fusion of the folding neural tube begins in the middle and progresses simultaneously toward both ends.
2. Secondary neurulation
      a. The caudal end completes fusion first in a process known as secondary neurulation.
      b. Specialized mesodermal tissue caudal to the neural tube develops into a structure known as the caudal eminence.
      c. The caudal eminence hollows out and fuses with the neural tube to complete the primitive CNS.
3. Neural crest
      a. A portion of the neuroectodermal tissue extrudes from the developing neural tube to become an independent structure, the neural crest.
      b. Neural crest cells contribute to multiple organ systems, including the peripheral and central nervous systems.
4. Differentiation of the neural tube
      a. The neural tube differentiates early into two portions.
         1) The brain
            a) The primitive brain portion divides into three primary vesicles:

- Prosencephalon (forebrain)
  - Secondary vesicles
    - Telencephalon (cerebral hemispheres)
    - Diencephalon (epithalamus, thalamus, hypothalamus)
  - Mesencephalon (midbrain)
  - Rhombencephalon (hindbrain)
    - Secondary vesicles
      - Metencephalon (cerebellum and pons)
  - Myelencephalon (medulla oblongata)

    2) The spinal cord

5. Flexures
    a. Rapid growth of the cranial portion of the neural tube results in development of flexures.
    b. Three flexures develop at four to eight weeks gestation, allowing the brain to fold as the embryo undergoes craniocaudal folding.
        1) Mesencephalic
            a) The mesencephalic flexure allows the primitive forebrain (telencephalon) to fold ventrally and surround the diencephalon and the mesencephalon, creating the familiar shape of the human brain.
        2) Cervical
            a) The cervical flexure allows ventral folding of the myelencephalon and further definition between the brain and spinal cord.
        3) Pontine
            a) The pontine flexure develops at the level of the metencephalon, promoting reverse dorsal flexion of the portion of the neural tube destined to become the pons.

D. Cytodifferentiation of the brain
    1. Beginning in the rhombencephalon during the fourth week of gestation, cells that line the inner wall of the neural tube proliferate and differentiate.
        a. Ventricular zone
            1) This mitotically active layer surrounds the lumen of the neural canal.
            2) The neuroepithelium initially produces neuroblasts that migrate outward to produce the mantle zone.
                a) Neuronal cells in the mantle develop nerve fibers, eventually becoming the gray matter of the CNS.
                b) Neuronal processes from the mantle zone grow peripherally to form the marginal layer that will become the white matter of the brain.
            3) Completion of neuroblast production prompts the ventricular zone to change to production of glioblasts, cells that provide nutritive and structural support to the brain cells.
            4) After completion of the two outer layers, the neuroepithelial cells of the ventricular zone differentiate into ependymal cells that contribute to the lining of the ventricles and the internal canal of the spinal cord and construction of the choroid plexus, site of cerebrospinal fluid (CSF) production.
    2. The ventricles develop.
        a. Each vesicle retains its inner canal throughout convolution of the developing neural tube.
        b. Ventral folding of the telencephalon results in the creation of two hemispheres with corresponding ventricles, the lateral ventricles.

FIGURE 7-1 ■ CSF flow.

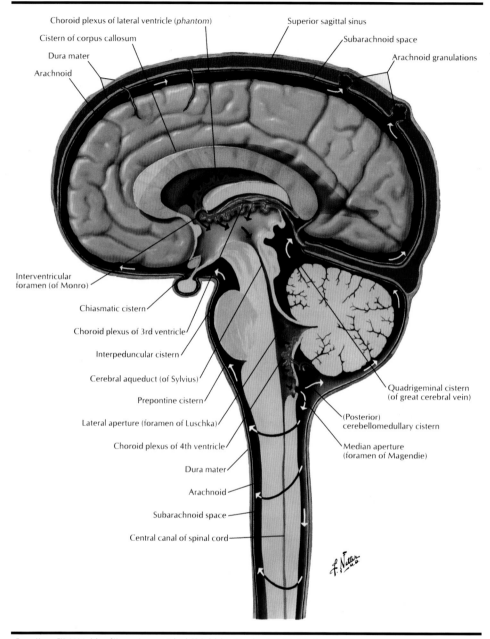

From: Netter FH. 2006. *Atlas of Human Anatomy*, 4th ed. Philadelphia: Saunders, 109. Reprinted by permission.

c. The lateral ventricles join with the third ventricle located in the diencephalon.

d. The cavity of the mesencephalon becomes the aqueduct of Sylvius that connects the third ventricle to the fourth ventricle in the rhombencephalon.

Neurologic Physiology

A. CSF production[4]
1. About 80 percent of the CSF is produced in the choroid plexus of the lateral (most), third, and fourth ventricles.
   a. Adults produce about 504 ml/day,[5] neonates, about 200 ml/day.[6]
2. Turnover is about two to three times per day.
3. CSF functions as a lymphatic system for the brain.

B. CSF flow
1. The basic serial flow scheme is as shown. There is some parallel flow (Figure 7-1).
   a. Lateral ventricles→foramen Monro→third ventricle→foramen Sylvius→fourth ventricle→foramen Luschka and Magendie→subarachnoid space→base of brain→down and around the spinal cord as well as up to be absorbed by archroniod granulations→sagittal sinus

C. CSF control
1. CSF absorption[7]
   a. Absorption occurs mostly by bulk flow mainly through arachnoid villi (or granulations).
   b. Other sites of absorption include the following.
      1) Subarachnoid space
      2) Cranial and spinal nerve roots
   c. Fluid then passes into blood capillaries and the lymphatics.
2. Intracranial pressure (ICP)[7]
   a. ICP is the pressure within the cranial vault.
   b. Neonates are protected to a degree from high ICP by the open fontanel and sutures.
   c. Acute changes are more dependent on cerebral hemodynamics than CSF production.
   d. Removal of large amounts of CSF may reduce ICP only a small amount.
3. Brain blood flow
   a. Cerebral blood flow (CBF)[8]
      1) In preterm infants 25–26 weeks gestational age, CBF is approximately 5–23 ml/kg/minute.
         a) This is about 20–25 percent of CO.
      2) In term infants, CBF is about 22–76 ml/kg/minute.
         a) This is about 20–25 percent of cardiac output.
   b. Pressure autoregulation
      1) Autoregulation keeps CBF constant across changes in pressure.
         a) Alterations in cerebral vascular resistance (CVR) occur in response to changes in mean arterial pressure (MAP) and ICP.
         b) CVR is affected by many things, including the following.
            • Autonomic (sympathetic and parasympathetic) stimulation
            • PCO_2
            • PO_2
            • Local pH
            • Ca
            • K
            • Nitric oxide
   c. Cerebral perfusion pressure (CPP)

1) CPP is defined as MAP minus ICP.
2) The optimum MAP to support CPP is not known for the preterm or term infant.
   a) Some data suggest that a MAP of 24–40 mmHg in preterm infants and 40–50 mmHg in term infants will support CPP.[9]
3) Ischemia may occur when CPP is 20–40 percent of baseline. Ischemia may lead to cell death and brain injury.

  d. Cerebral metabolism
    1) Glucose is the main substrate for energy metabolism.
    2) Other important sources of energy include the following.
     a) Ketones
     b) Lactate
    3) Energy is used for the following.
     a) Synthesis of proteins, lipids, and nucleic acids
     b) Release, synthesis, and uptake of neurotransmitters
     c) Axonal transport
     d) ATPase pumps
     e) Ion channel maintenance and carrier transport

Hydrocephalus and Posthemorrhagic Hydrocephalus (PHH)

DEFINITION

Enlargement of cerebral ventricles or subarachnoid space that causes an increase in the size of the brain[10]

PATHOPHYSIOLOGY

A. Imbalance of CSF production and absorption
  1. Excessive production extremely rare; related to choroid plexus tumors
  2. Impaired or blocked absorption (arachnoid villi)
    a. Obstruction to flow by blood and particulate matter[11]
    b. Obstruction to flow by bone or compression of foramina by displaced tissue
B. Continued imbalance
  1. This leads to accumulation of CSF, which causes changes in the tissue/ pressure relationships.
  2. This leads to the following forces and altered processes being applied to the brain, which may result in further injury.
    a. Compression
    b. Distortion
    c. Stretching
    d. Ischemia
    e. Edema
    f. Demyelination
    g. Gliosis
    h. Breakdown of blood-brain barrier
    i. Bleeding into the underlying brain[12]

ETIOLOGY

A. Intraventricular hemorrhage in the preterm infant
  1. IVH is a major cause of hydrocephalus in the NICU.

     a. IVH is bleeding into the following.
- **1)** The CSF/ventricular system
- **2)** Brain parenchyma surrounding the ventricular system, either as a discrete hemorrhage (most common) or an extension of the ventricular blood

     b. IVH is usually described with a grading system on a scale of I to IV.[13,14]
- **1)** In Grade I, the blood is contained in the subependymal germinal matrix area at the floor of the lateral ventricles.
- **2)** Grade II denotes intraventricular blood without ventricular dilation.
- **3)** Grade III denotes a ventricular clot and ventricular dilation.
- **4)** Grade IV denotes a parenchymal hemorrhage with or without Grade III findings.

     c. Blood causes an acute obstruction in the ventricular drainage system by the following.
- **1)** The presence of a physical clot
- **2)** Obliterative arachnoiditis

     d. Areas of hemorrhage into the brain parenchyma can evolve into cysts.

     e. IVH can occur as a result of the following.
- **1)** Venous congestion
- **2)** Ischemia/reperfusion
- **3)** Acute, rapid increased flow, especially after hypoperfusion

     f. The incidence of IVH is as follows.
- **1)** In general, 32 percent of infants with birth weights of <1,500 gm have a hemorrhage of some grade.[15]
- **2)** Hemorrhages usually occur by day 3 of life, through the first week and into the second week of life. They rarely occur after that time.[16]
- **3)** The incidence of PHH is 20–50 percent of Grade III/IV IVH.[17]

     g. Clinical presentation can vary.
- **1)** There are three types of clinical syndromes.[18]
  - **a)** Catastrophic: Acute cardiopulmonary and neurologic deterioration with anemia
  - **b)** Salutatory: Episodic deteriorations and recoveries in cardiopulmonary and neurologic status as the hemorrhage occurs and progresses
  - **c)** Silent: No obvious clinical signs, but possibly a slowly dropping hematocrit
- **2)** All three types may have concomitant seizures.

B. Other conditions[5]
1. Myelomeningocele
   - **a.** Chiari deformity
     - **1)** This results from downward displacement of the cerebellar vermis and tonsils through the foramen magnum.
     - **2)** There is also downward displacement and folding of the medulla oblongata and fourth ventricle.
     - **3)** This leads to obstruction of the fourth ventricle outlet.
     - **4)** Chiari deformity is found most commonly with spinal cord defects (myelodysplasia).
2. Aqueductal stenosis
   - **a.** The aqueduct of Sylvius is the channel between the third and fourth ventricles.

     b. This channel becomes blocked or narrowed, fully or partially, with bone, with or without other inflammatory signs.

     c. This phenomenon either is developmental or secondary to a viral infection.

  3. Dandy Walker syndrome

     a. Cystic development of the fourth ventricle with

        1) Ballooning into the posterior fossa

        2) Obstruction of the foramina of Magendie and Luschka

     b. Also abnormalities of the cerebellar vermis[5]

  4. Meningitis/ventriculitis

     a. This inflammatory obliteration of the arachnoid villi causes decreased absorption of CSF.

        1) It is usually transient and resolves when the infection resolves.

        2) CSF production may also be temporarily reduced during acute infection.

     b. Inflammatory debris may obstruct various foramina.

  5. Vein of Galen malformation

     a. A dilated vein of Galen compresses the aqueduct of Sylvius and prevents flow from the third to the fourth ventricle.

  6. Choroid plexus papilloma

     a. This very rare tumor causes oversecretion of CSF.

     b. It is treated by removing the tumor.

  7. Holoprosencephaly

     a. A primary failure of neural induction resulting in varying degrees of fusion of the forebrain

  8. Hydranencephaly

     a. Absence of the forebrain secondary to vascular accident or severe infection with accompanying destruction and liquefaction of the cerebral hemispheres

C. Genetic

  1. X-linked hydrocephalus

     a. This is the most common cause of hydrocephalus in related males.

     b. Some are caused by aqueductal stenosis in a sequence with mental retardation, adducted thumbs, shuffling gait, and aphasia.

     c. Gene encoding links the syndrome to L1 located near the telomere of the long arm of chromosome X (Xq28).[19,20]

INCIDENCE

A. For all hydrocephalus: 0.5–0.8/1,000 live births.[1,12]

B. The incidence of PHH is 20–50 percent of those with Grade III/IV IVH.[17]

CLINICAL PRESENTATION

A. The head is macrocephalic for the body size.

B. Head size, as measured by occipitofrontal circumference (OFC), is greater than the 90th percentile for age (Figure 7-2).

C. The rate of head growth is greater than the norm for the age (usually 0.5–1 cm/week).

D. The anterior fontanel is abnormal on exam (bulging, full, tense).

E. Cranial sutures are abnormally separated for age, especially squamosal sutures (part of the temporal bone above the ear).

F. There may be signs of increased intracranial pressure (apnea, hypertension, vomiting, bradycardia, downward deviation of the eyes).

ASSOCIATIONS

A. Over 100 syndromes have hydrocephalus listed as a component.[4,21]

  1. Is frequent in:

    a. Hydrolethalus syndrome (characterized by polydactyly and CNS malformations that include hydrocephalus; mapped to gene 11q23-q25)

    b. Triploidy syndrome

    c. Walker Warburg syndrome

    d. Osteopetrosis: autosomal recessive

    e. X-linked hydrocephalus

  2. Is occasional in more than 50 syndromes and disorders such as:

    a. Apert's syndrome

    b. Trisomy 9 (Mosaic syndrome)

    c. Trisomy 13, 18 syndrome

    d. Vater association

    e. Fetal alcohol syndrome

    f. Hunter's syndrome

    g. Hurler's syndrome

    h. Osteogenesis imperfecta Type II

    i. Chiari deformation: Abnormality of the brain stem and its location

    j. Dandy Walker syndrome: abnormality of the fourth ventricle

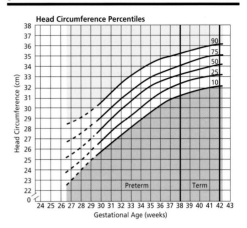

FIGURE 7-2 ■ Head circumference intrauterine growth curve.

Head Circumference Percentiles

Adapted from: Lubchenco LO, Hansman C, and Boyd E. 1966. Intrauterine growth in length and head circumference as estimated from live births at gestational ages from 26 to 42 weeks. *Pediatrics* 37(3): 403. Reprinted by permission.

DIFFERENTIAL DIAGNOSIS

A. Hydrencephaly

B. Holoprosencephaly

C. Ventriculomegaly with loss of brain tissue (hydrocephalus ex-vacuole)

D. Familial macrocephaly

DIAGNOSIS

A. Ultrasound is now the most common means of screening for IVH and PHH.[16,22]

  1. Two to four screening exams are done in high-risk populations of patients <30–32 weeks gestational age and <1,500 gm birth weight. The first exam is done as early as day 3–10 of life.[22]

B. A computed tomography (CT) scan can be used.

C. Magnetic resonance imaging (MRI) may be performed.

D. A lumbar puncture (LP) or ventricular tap may be done for "opening" or initial pressure upon entry into the CSF space, and studies may be made to determine the etiology, such as infection or bleeding.

TREATMENT OPTIONS AND NURSING CARE

A. Treatment depends upon the underlying lesion, outcome, and family wishes.

B. Nontreatment of progressive hydrocephalus regardless of etiology usually results in death of the neonate from increased intracranial pressure.
   1. Some types of hydrocephalus, such as PHH, have been known to resolve spontaneously or after controlling CSF volume.
C. Medical management may include using diuretics and intermittent LPs.
   1. There is no direct evidence that administration of furosemide or acetazolamide to reduce CSF production alters the need for a ventriculoperitoneal shunt.[23,24]
   2. There is no significant randomized control trial evidence that serial LPs for CSF removal reduce the need for a ventriculoperitoneal shunt.[11,25]
D. Medical management of the acute effects of increased intracranial pressure (IICP) may include the following.
   1. Mechanical ventilation if apnea occurs
   2. Diuretics
   3. Nothing by mouth (NPO)
   4. Intravenous (IV) fluids if the infant is unable to eat or has severe emesis
E. Underlying medical conditions such as infection may require treatment.
F. Care for transport includes the following.
   1. Position and support the cranium to prevent injury or airway obstruction.
   2. Protect any associated lesions.
G. Delayed or palliative management is an option.
   1. Compassionate care may be performed if the underlying cause is considered terminal and immediately life threatening (such as hydrencephaly).
   2. A CSF diversion device can be placed as a palliative care intervention to enable home care.
H. Nursing preoperative management includes the following.
   1. Observe for signs and symptoms of IICP and infection.
   2. Some neurosurgeons prefer presurgery body and scalp wash, depending upon the procedure.[26]
   3. Use head positioning, padding, and support to ensure no pressure injury or airway compromise occurs.
      a. The patient may require significant body support if his head is very large.
      b. Patients often do best when nursed flat.
   4. The patient should be NPO in the immediate preoperative period.
   5. Support the family.
      a. Explain the procedure that will be done and the device that is to be used.
      b. Provide family counseling and support, especially if a permanent device is being implanted.

SURGICAL MANAGEMENT

A. The underlying etiology guides which procedure is used.
B. Diversion of CSF
   1. This is an emergency only if there are signs of increased/increasing intracranial pressure.
   2. A temporary device is used if there are contraindications to placement of a long-term shunt.
      a. Size
      b. Characteristics of the CSF (levels of blood, protein, debris, and so on)
   3. There are two main classes of devices.
      a. Ventricular access device (VAD)

b. Ventriculostomy catheter

C. VAD

1. Insertion into a subcutaneous pocket, usually over the posterior parietal bone, of an appliance that consists of a port or reservoir with a short catheter that resides in the lateral ventricle

   a. This can be done at the bedside or in the operating room.

   b. The VAD is accessible immediately after surgery if needed.

   c. Intermittent taps can be done.

      1) With intermittent approaches, one may try to remove 5–10 ml/kg per tap to accomplish the following.

         a) Decrease intracranial pressure to <3 cm H_2O.

         b) Control head growth.

         c) Obviate clinical signs.

      2) More than one access a day may be necessary.

      3) The taps continue until one of the following occurs.

         a) The infant meets surgical criteria in body size and quality of CSF.

         b) Removal of debris, along with time, allows for re-establishment of CSF absorption sufficient to control head growth and ICP. Placement of a permanent shunt can be avoided in 20–40 percent of cases.[11]

         c) The infant can be discharged with a VAD still in place for later access or removal.

D. Ventriculostomy catheter (external ventricular drainage [EVD])

   1. A silastic catheter is inserted through a craniostomy, usually into the frontal portion of one of the lateral ventricles of the brain.

   2. The catheter is then connected to a sterile, closed, continuous EVD to permit controlled drainage of CSF.

      a. EVD system (Figure 7-3)

FIGURE 7-3 ■ EVD system.

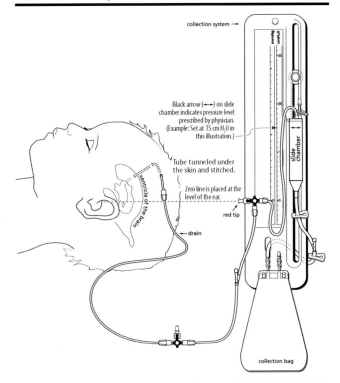

collection system →

Black arrow (←→) on slide chamber indicates pressure level prescribed by physician. (Example: Set at 15 cm H_2O in this illustration.)

Tube tunneled under the skin and stitched.

Zero line is placed at the level of the ear.

red tip

←drain

ventricle of the brain

slide chamber

collection bag

Courtesy of Primary Children's Medical Center Pediatric Education Services, Salt Lake City, Utah. Reprinted by Permission.

      1) This is a self-contained system with a hydrostatic flow control valve (stopcocks and a pressure manometer) and a collection container (Becker drain).

          a) The position of the collection container provides the system pressure (similar to the water seal in thoracostomy drainage setups). The pressure is usually positive: 2–5 cm H_2O.

   3. The EVD can be used for up to two weeks before the incidence of infection increases.[6]

   4. There are two goals for use of an EVD.

     a. Drainage of debris

     b. Control of ICP (usually <10 cm H_2O)[11]

   5. Complications may occur.

     a. Device failure through obstruction or entry site leakage

     b. Infection

     c. Hemorrhage

     d. Overdrainage with the potential for significant circulatory disturbances

     e. Hyponatremia and hypoproteinemia

E. Ventriculoperitoneal CSF shunt[11,26,27]

   1. Main long-term device to move CSF out of the cranial vault to be reabsorbed in another structure or cavity

   2. Timing issues

     a. Infants with uncomplicated diagnoses of the following can be shunted within the first few days of life.

        1) Aqueductal stenosis

        2) Dandy Walker and other posterior fossa cysts

        3) Hydranencephaly

     b. The infant with hydrocephalus secondary to other causes, such as myelomeningocele (spina bifida), may have to wait for completion of the primary repair before a shunt can be done.

     c. Infants with PHH may have to wait for shunt placement until the protein level or level of debris in the CSF has subsided to the point where risk of obstruction is minimized.

        1) What the protein level or level of debris must be to minimize this risk is not known (other than a normal value).

     d. Patient size is a factor.

        1) There must be enough absorptive surface in the peritoneum to handle CSF flow.

        2) Usually this is not a problem in infants who weigh >2 kg; some programs place shunts in patients as low as 1.5 kg.[11]

   3. Procedure (Figure 7-4)

     a. Hair removal is currently the surgeon's preference.[11]

     b. Locations of the shunt can vary.

        1) Usually an occipital or frontal ventricular catheter is tunneled subcutaneously to the peritoneum.

        2) The catheter can also drain from the lumbar space to the peritoneum.

        3) Tubing lengths of 90–120 cm can be placed in the peritoneal cavity.

        4) Alternative drainage sites include the pleural space and the atrium when the peritoneal space is not available.

           a) CSF is absorbed across the pleural space, but at a slower rate then the peritoneum.

b) CSF returns directly to the bloodstream when the shunt is placed in the atrium, but this is a site of more complications.

c. A valve system is used to control the fluid to prevent siphoning.
   1) A low to medium (4–10 cm H_2O) valve set is usually used.
   2) For slow decompression, a high-pressure valve is used.
   3) Valveless sets are used when a high debris level is present.
      a) Flow depends on position.

F. Third ventriculostomy[27,28]
   1. This makes a connection between the third ventricle and the subarachnoid space by placing a hole in the floor of the third ventricle.
   2. It is currently performed via endoscopy.
   3. It may be placed in combination with a ventriculoperitoneal shunt, especially with a trapped ventricle. It is only rarely used in neonates because the success rate is lower in this population than in infants greater than two years of age.

G. Ventriculosubgaleal shunt
   1. Similar to a ventricular access device, but drains into a pocket made in the subgaleal space[29]
   2. Works well for some patients with low CSF output, but usually still a temporary device
   3. Can also be directly tapped

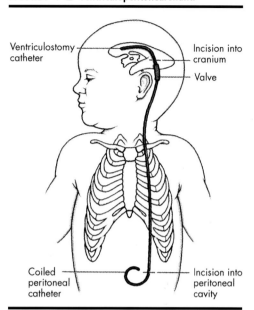

FIGURE 7-4 ■ Ventriculoperitoneal shunt.

Ventriculostomy catheter

Incision into cranium

Valve

Coiled peritoneal catheter

Incision into peritoneal cavity

From: Hill CJ. 1987. *Nursing Management of Children*, Servonsky J, and Opas SR, eds. Sudbury, Massachusetts: Jones & Bartlett, 1297. Reprinted by permission.

COMPLICATIONS[27]

A. Shunt failure is the main source of complications for infants with hydrocephalus.[30]
   1. Most failures occur within six months of placement.
   2. Within one year of placement, 40–50 percent fail.[31]
   3. There are two major causes of failure.
      a. Obstruction
      b. Infection[31]
         1) Infection develops in 5–12 percent of shunts.
         2) The incidence can be as high as 20 percent, depending on surgeon experience (inversely related).
         3) Most infections occur in the first 36 months of life.
   4. The younger the patient is at the time of insertion, the higher the failure risk.

   a. Preterm infants have a failure rate two and a half times greater than infants who are older than one year at the time of shunt placement.

  5. All shunts placed in infants have a limited life because of body growth and the amount of tubing placed in the abdomen.

   a. Usually a shunt will be "outgrown" by three years of age.

B. Overdrainage may occur.

  1. Overdrainage is caused by the siphon effect: effects of gravity and pressure.

  2. Overdrainage can cause the following.

   a. Slitlike ventricles

   b. Subdural hemorrhage

  3. Use of valves has improved, but not prevented, this problem.

POSTOPERATIVE NURSING CARE

A. Provide wound care.

  1. Open site care

  2. Dry, nonadherent dressing

B. Observe for subcutaneous tunnel erythema.

C. Position the infant, depending upon the position of the valve and the underlying pressure, from flat to 15–30 degrees elevation of the head of the bed unless the infant has a high-pressure valve.

D. Provide prophylactic antibiotics as ordered.

E. Provide pain relief.

  1. Major procedures with significant bone and skin manipulation will require pain relief with narcotics, usually for the first two days.

  2. Minor procedures, such as device implantation and removal, may require narcotics for the first day.

   a. Pain can then usually be controlled with nonnarcotic analgesics.

   b. Adjunctive and support therapies are used.

    1) As appropriate for gestational age

    2) As the patient's condition allows

  3. Local anesthesia (such as EMLA [eutectic mixture of local anesthetics]) may be sufficient for intermittent procedures such as ventricular reservoir taps.

  4. Individual assessment is the key.

F. Employ postoperative imaging to ensure ventricles are decreasing in size and assess for overdrainage.

G. Feed as soon as gastrointestinal (GI) function returns.

  1. Nutritional support is based on the following.

   a. Gestation

   b. Underlying medical complicating problems

  2. The infant can breastfeed ad lib as able.

H. Shunt care teaching must be done.

  1. Discharge can occur within two to five days if there are no other issues.

  2. Discharge teaching must occur before surgery or soon after.

I. Follow-up is institution specific, but usually four to six weeks postprocedure.

OUTCOMES

A. See COMPLICATIONS.

B. Infants with hydrocephalus that is left untreated:

  1. Forty-six percent survive infancy, but only 38 percent of the survivors have normal intelligence.

C. Infants with hydrocephalus that is not related to IVH:
    1. Ninety-five percent of treated infants survive.
    2. Seventy percent of survivors have normal intelligence.[14]

D. Infants with PHH:
    1. They are more influenced by the underlying IVH.
    2. The outcome worsens with the need for multiple shunt revisions and/or with infections.[32,33]
    3. There is no direct evidence that treatment of ventriculomegaly improves the infant's outcome.[11,25]
        a. However, if ventriculomegaly is present when the baby is postconceptional term age, there is an increased risk of cerebral palsy and developmental delay.[34]

Myelomeningocele (Spina Bifida)

DEFINITION[35]

A variety of neural tube, bone, and skin defects that can include various neural elements

PATHOPHYSIOLOGY

A. Some lesions may have skin covering the sac.
B. The meningeal sac and contents bulge out.
C. The sac may be intact or ruptured.
D. The lesion may span one to many vertebrae in length, though most involve a single vertebra.

ETIOLOGY

A. Embryologic[36]
    1. The spinal cord closes by 32 days gestation.
        a. Closure occurs in a bidirectional manner, probably in five distinct segments with the caudal (lumbar-sacral) region to close last.[37]
    2. The embryopathy is probably failure of closure.
        a. The role of folate may be related to its impact on various subprocesses, rather than pure deficiency.
        b. Failure of closure can be induced by drugs.
            1) Chemotherapeutics
            2) Calcium channel blockers
            3) Aminopterin
        c. If the neural tube fails to close, generally so do corresponding vertebrae and the overlying muscle and skin. However, there may be a lesion without any significant external evidence (spina bifida occulta).

B. Genetic
    1. There may be genetic factors with the "PAX-3" gene. This gene is located on chromosome 2 and is involved in the control and function of the neural crest cells that help to form the central nervous system.[38]

INCIDENCE

A. Population-dependent epidemiology[17]
    1. Incidence varies.
        a. Overall: 0.7–0.8/1,000 live births
        b. United Kingdom: 0.7–2.5/1,000 live births

    c. U.S.: 0.4–1.43/1,000 live births
      1) Lower in African-Americans
      2) Lower in Native Americans at 0.1/1,000 live births
      3) Overall U.S. rate dropping
B. Recurrence risk
    1. The recurrence risk is 1–2 percent if parents have one child with this defect.
    2. There is a 10 percent risk of further recurrence if two children have been affected.
    3. If a parent had a myelomeningocele, there is a 3 percent chance of the child having the lesion.

Clinical Presentation

A. Spina bifida occulta
    1. Mildest form of the lesion, with a gap in one or more vertebral bodies
    2. May manifest by a dermal sinus or dimple with a hair patch or pigmented nevus above it
    3. Occurs in approximately 1 percent of the normal population without outward symptoms[39]
B. Myelomeningocele
    1. The sac can be completely or partially skin covered.
    2. If the lesion is visible, one of the following is the case.
      a. The sac is covered.
      b. The sac is ruptured, with contents exposed.
    3. The sac (meninges) can contain either of the following.
      a. Fluid only
      b. Fluid and neural elements
    4. This lesion is most often found in the lumbar area of the spine, but it can be found all along the spine.

Associations

A. Congenital heart disease[40,41]
    1. Atrial septal defect
    2. Ventricular septal defect
B. Orthopedic anomalies
    1. Kyphosis (40 percent)
    2. Scoliosis (30 percent)
    3. Congenital hip dysplasia
    4. Clubfoot
C. Occasionally in other syndromes and sequences
    1. Amnion rupture sequence
    2. Caudal dysplasia sequence
    3. Cerebrocostomandibular syndrome
    4. Congenital hemidysplasia with ichthyosiform erythroderma and limb defects (CHILD syndrome)
    5. Fanconi's pancytopenia syndrome
    6. Fetal alcohol syndrome
    7. Fraser's syndrome
    8. Triploidy syndrome
    9. Trisomy 13 (<50 percent of cases)
    10. Trisomy 18 (<10 percent of cases)

11. Warrensburg syndrome[4,21]

12. Imperforate anus

Differential Diagnosis

A. Spina bifida

    1. Dermal sinus or tract

B. Myelomeningocele

    1. Teratoma

    2. Encephalocele, especially if in cervical area of spine

Diagnosis (Postnatal)

A. A CT scan or MRI is used to identify associated lesions (e.g., Chiari, Dandy Walker) and the degree of hydrocephalus and hindbrain herniation prior to surgery.

B. Some institutions may use ultrasound.

C. An echocardiogram may be performed.

    1. In a study of 105 patients with spina bifida referred to a children's hospital, 37 percent had congenital heart disease, with atrial septal defects being the most common. The physical exam was sensitive for identifying those with congenital heart disease.[40,41]

D. Assess neurologic function on physical exam.[42]

    1. Assess the level of motor injury by muscle function and physical deformities.

        a. Hip flexion with extended knees and clubfoot indicate an L1–3 lesion.

        b. Hip flexion, hip adduction, extended knees, and an inverted foot are indicative of a lesion at L2–4.

        c. Hip flexion, hip adduction, knee extension, and flexion with dorsiflexed feet indicate a lesion usually at L5–S2.

        d. If the infant can move his hips, but has plantar flexion, weak foot and pelvic floor muscles, and rocker bottom feet, the lesion is usually at the sacrum and below S2.

    2. Assess the sensory level with pin pricks.

    3. Assessment can include formal muscle evaluation by a physical therapy specialist.

    4. Assess anal function and urinary continence.

        a. These do not predict postsurgery function.

Treatment Options and Nursing Care

A. The mode of delivery may affect the infant's outcome, depending on perinatal factors that include the level of lesion and fetal movement.[43]

    1. Cesarean section without labor may preserve function in certain patients.[44]

B. Protect the lesion.

    1. Cover it with warm, saline-moistened, nonadherent gauze and plastic wrap.

    2. Reduce physical stress on the lesion.

        a. Keep the infant prone.

        b. Elevate the head, body, and trunk so the hips can be flexed to a 90-degree angle.

        c. The infant can be held prone if the sac/lesion is protected.

    3. Place a barrier between the anus and lesion to prevent soiling.

    4. Prevent latex sensitization.[45]

        a. Thirty-six to 80 percent of these infants will develop latex allergy.[42,46,47]

        b. Initiate a latex-free environment, including in the following.

1) Gloves
2) Catheters
3) Nipples
4) Pacifiers
5) Syringes
6) IV tubing
7) Blood pressure cuffs
8) Stethoscope tubing

C. Place an indwelling, latex-free Foley catheter into the infant's bladder.
   1. There is a high incidence of urinary retention in these infants.
      a. Ninety percent have neurogenic bladder with subsequent risk for infection both while the infant is in the hospital and after discharge.

D. Observe for a CSF leak.

E. Coordinate multispecialty consultations.
   1. Renal
   2. Orthopedic
   3. Physical therapy and/or occupational therapy
   4. A spina bifida clinic through which all care is coordinated

F. If the infant is to be transported to a Level III facility, do the following.
   1. Place him prone.
   2. Protect the lesion.
   3. Do not allow latex products to be used for this infant.
   4. Start antibiotics if not already begun.
   5. Place NPO and start IV fluids if not already begun.

G. Delayed management
   1. Repair of the lesion can be delayed 24–72 hours, depending on leakage of CSF.

H. Nursing preoperative management includes the following.[43]
   1. Protect the lesion **(see B above).**
   2. Ensure preoperative imaging is done as ordered.

SURGICAL MANAGEMENT (FIGURE 7-5)

A. The goals of surgery are as follows.
   1. Constructing the neural tube and spinal column
   2. Preserving the nerve roots

FIGURE 7-5 ■ Conceptual steps in surgical repair of the myelomeningocele.

A. Axial cross-section of the myelomeningocele. Note the placode mimics an open book, with the ventral roots lying medially and the dorsal roots lying laterally. **B.** Reconstruction of the neural tube. The placode is dissected from the surrounding tissue by incising the junctional zone. All dermal remnants are resected, and the neural tube is reconstituted by closing the pia with a 7-0 monofilament suture. **C.** Reconstruction of the thecal sac. The dura is dissected free from its junction with the fascia and skin. The goal is a watertight closure without causing constriction of the closed neural placode. **D.** Midline fascial closure. Relaxing incisions may be necessary to mobilize an adequate amount of fascia. **E.** Midline skin closure.

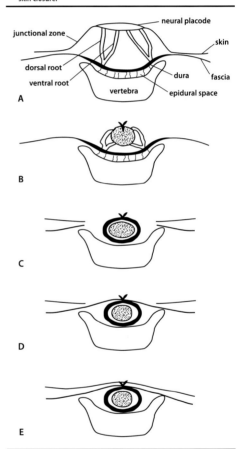

Redrawn from: Cohen AR, and Robinson S. 2001. Early management of myelomeningocele. In *Pediatric Neurosurgery*, 4th ed., McLone DG, ed. Phiadelphia: Saunders, 241. Reprinted by permission.

3. Achieving skin closure
4. Obtaining a watertight seal to prevent CSF leakage
5. Reducing the risk of a tethered cord
6. Placing a CSF shunt as is deemed necessary
   a. Eighty to 85 percent of patients will need a shunt.[48]

B. The infant may require skin flaps if the lesion is too large for primary closure.

COMPLICATIONS[42]

A. Near zero operative mortality
B. Wound complications
   1. Dehiscence
   2. Infection
C. CSF leak
D. Complications from Chiari malformation and hindbrain herniation
   1. Respiratory: Central and obstructive apnea
   2. Swallowing impairment
E. Shunt complications
   1. Infection
   2. Blockage
F. Tethered cord
G. Urinary tract infection (UTI)

POSTOPERATIVE NURSING CARE[43]

A. Infants without other significant disease are usually stable postoperatively, so medical care can follow protocol with appropriate individualization.
   1. Ensure recovery with stable cardiopulmonary status.
   2. Provide short-term IV fluids.
   3. Initiate feedings as soon as GI function allows.
   4. Monitor and treat any UTI.
      a. Urinary tract prophylaxis (amoxicillin 10 mg/kg/day for eight weeks) may be started.
B. There are several nursing interventions.
   1. Maintain the infant in a prone or side-lying position until the incision is adequately healed.
   2. Oral feedings may be initiated when the patient is awake and alert.
      a. Maintain the IV for 24 hours postoperatively to complete the antibiotic administration. However, if the patient is feeding well, the IV can be changed to a heparin lock.
      b. The infant should be fed prone or side-lying.
   3. Maintain the plastic barrier ("mud flap") between the surgical site and the patient's buttocks.
   4. Keep the incision site open to air unless otherwise ordered.
   5. Monitor the infant for signs of hydrocephalus.
      a. Daily OFC
      b. Frequent neurologic exam (checks)
C. Consultations and tests to be done after closure of the sac include the following.
   1. Cranial CT as needed before/after shunt insertion
   2. Other x-rays and scans ordered as needed on an individual basis
   3. Ultrasound of the kidney and a voiding cystourethrogram (VCUG) on the fourth to sixth postoperative day

   a. Remove the Foley catheter after the VCUG.
   b. Check postvoid residual after the VCUG.
      1) Observe the diaper every 15 minutes after the procedure until the diaper is wet.
      2) Use a straight catheter to then immediately catheterize the infant to measure residual volume in the bladder.
      3) Repeat the procedure again in four hours.
      4) Notify the urologist if the residual is >30 ml.
D. Consultations prior to discharge
   1. Orthopedic consultation
   2. Repeat of the manual muscle test before discharge and review of basic therapy with the family by the physical therapist
   3. Audiology consultation for newborn hearing screen
   4. Multidisciplinary follow-up (The first appointment is usually two to four weeks after discharge.)
   5. Maternal counseling on the benefits of folic acid (at least 400 mcg/day preconception) to reduce the risk of recurrence or as primary prevention[35]

OUTCOMES

A. The location of the lesion with or without hydrocephalus may not predict function and outcome.
   1. Cognitive function is not affected by the lesion *per se*, but rather by associated conditions and complications.
B. The ability to ambulate is dependent on the level of the lesion.
C. Function is not gained after surgery; the goal is to prevent its further loss.
D. Bowel and bladder incontinence occur with all major lesions, but to varying degrees.

Tethered Cord[49,50]

DEFINITION

A. Congenitally fixed or "tethered" cord with traction that leads to progressive neurologic and urologic dysfunction
B. Most recently defined as low conus with thickened filum terminale measuring 2 mm or more in diameter, usually occurring below the second lumbar vertebra[51]

PATHOPHYSIOLOGY

A. Initial tethering occurs with a primary lesion or as a result of a repair.
   1. Growth and skeletal motion produce stretch and tension of neuronal structures, which cause vascular, neuronal, and axonal changes leading to sensory and muscular anomalies.[52]
   2. This leads to the following symptoms, which may take years to develop.
      a. Dysfunction in bowel and bladder control
      b. Pain
      c. Deformity of lower extremities
      d. Muscle weakness

ETIOLOGY

A. Embryologic
   1. The usual termination of the cord is at the level of L1–2 by term.
      a. The end is free floating.

2. Failure of normal cord regression from the level of L5 to L1–2 usually occurs around three to four weeks gestation.
   a. The end is not free.

INCIDENCE

A. The true incidence is unknown because many infants are asymptomatic.
B. As part of occult spinal dysraphism, tethered cord may occur at a rate of 0.05–0.25/1,000 live births.[53]

CLINICAL PRESENTATION

A. There is no direct presentation in the neonate.
B. The health care provider should have a high index of suspicion with associated anomalies and syndromes (see ASSOCIATIONS).

ASSOCIATIONS

A. Diastematomyelia
B. Lipomyelomeningocele
C. Myelomeningocele
D. Leptomyelolipoma
E. Spinal tracts and sinuses
F. Cutaneous anomalies
   1. Hypertrichosis (excessive hairiness)
   2. Capillary hemangioma
   3. Dermal sinus
   4. Bumps/lump/tails (lipoma, atretic meningocele)
G. Foot deformities
H. UTI
I. Imperforate anus

DIFFERENTIAL DIAGNOSIS

A. Other types of spinal dysraphism, especially diastematomyelia

DIAGNOSIS

A. Ultrasound[54,55]
   1. Shows location and termination level of the cord and whether it is free floating
   2. Should be done by the third or fourth month of life before significant bone ossification prevents ultrasonic imaging
B. MRI
   1. For better definition of anatomy and vascular structures
   2. Can show
      a. Tethering level
      b. Intradural fat
      c. Distal syrinxes
      d. Thickened filum terminale
C. Plain x-ray films for vertebral or sacral anomalies
D. Clinical exam and a high index of suspicion[49,50]
   1. Seventy percent of infants with some type of occult spinal dysraphism have a tethered cord; only 3 percent of normal infants do.
   2. The lower extremity neurologic exam reveals abnormality.
   3. Bladder and bowel function studies may both identify patients with tethered cord and guide postoperative assessment.

TREATMENT OPTIONS AND NURSING CARE

A. Manage conservatively with close observation.[54,56]
   1. Make a careful baseline neurologic assessment.
      a. Especially note bladder and bowel function and muscle tone and strength.
   2. These observations are necessary so that changes secondary to surgery and recovery of function can be identified.
B. Educate and support the parents.
   1. Parents need to understand that if neurologic changes have occurred, they may not be reversed by surgery.
C. The infant should be managed surgically before significant deficits occur; however, surgery on asymptomatic patients is controversial.[53]

SURGICAL MANAGEMENT

A. Careful dissection to free up conus
B. Closure of dura to allow free conus movement
C. Possibly perioperative steroids to reduce local edema and adhesions

COMPLICATIONS

A. Retethering (15–20 percent of infants)
B. Failure to recover function or prevent further loss of function
C. Scoliosis

POSTOPERATIVE NURSING CARE

A. Positioning the infant flat for a period of days may be required to reduce the hydrostatic pressure of the CSF on the repair.
B. Frequently assess neurologic status to identify changes in function, especially of bowel and bladder.
C. Passive range of motion exercises are necessary to prevent contractures that may be seen secondary to flat positioning.
D. Intervene to prevent pressure injuries, such as prone positioning on an antipressure mattress.
E. Provide pain management and sedation as needed.
   1. Usually only mild to moderate pain control is needed, but it may include opioids.

OUTCOMES

A. Various outcomes are possible, depending on the underlying problems and the timing of surgery.
B. Motor weakness, sensory improvement, and bladder dysfunction either remain the same or improve in up to 40 percent of patients.[53,57]

Spinal Dimples and Sinuses[36,49,58]

DEFINITION

A. A dimple refers to a depression in the tissue over the spine.
B. A sinus refers to a tract of cutaneous ectoderm from the dorsal midline skin into the underlying mesenchymal tissue.
   1. The tract may penetrate the adjacent dura or the neural tube.
   2. Sixty percent end in a dermoid or epidermoid tumor or cyst.

PATHOPHYSIOLOGY

A. Neural folds remain attached to cutaneous ectoderm, dragging a piece of future skin into the tract.
B. They may occur anywhere along the spine.
   1. They predominate in the lumbar region, midline, and caudal to the gluteal cleft.
   2. Neural folds do not usually occur in the intergluteal fold.
C. They also can arise along other midline structures, such as the following.
   1. Nasal dermal sinus tracts
   2. Base of the skull
D. They often cause spinal cord tethering.

FIGURE 7-6 ■ Benign sacral dimple.

Over coccyx, points caudally and is in the intergluteal folds.

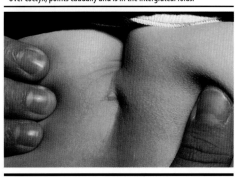

From: Drolet BA. 2001. Developmental abnormalities. In *Textbook of Neonatal Dermatology*, Eichenfield LF, Frieden IJ, and Esterly NB, eds. Philadelphia: Saunders, 125. Reprinted by permission.

ETIOLOGY

A. Embryologic tract in the cutaneus ectoderm into the mesenchymal tissue forming by eight weeks gestation

INCIDENCE

A. The specific incidence is not known.

CLINICAL PRESENTATION

A. Presents as an isolated finding or as a collection of multiple skin and bone abnormalities (**see ASSOCIATIONS**).
B. Location is variable, but they are mostly over the lower back above the gluteal cleft.

ASSOCIATIONS

A. Skin dimples
B. Hemangiomas
C. Tufts of hair
D. Bifid vertebrae
E. Deviated gluteal fold

DIFFERENTIAL DIAGNOSIS

A. The lesion, with its spinal tract connection, must be distinguished from an innocent coccygeal dimple, which is a simple blind pouch with no associated cutaneous anomalies.
B. An isolated sacral dimple or sacrococcygeal pit that lies in the intergluteal fold directly over the coccyx and points caudally does not need imaging (Figure 7-6).[49]

DIAGNOSIS

A. Nurses often make the initial finding on physical examination.

B. Assess for the presence of underlying spinal tract abnormalities.
1. Ultrasound
   a. Should be done by the third to fourth month of life before significant bone ossification obliterates the acoustic window
2. MRI
   a. Will further identify if a tract enters the dura mater and any tumor

TREATMENT OPTIONS AND NURSING CARE

A. Protect the site.

B. Assess for signs that can indicate that the dimple or sinus is an occult spinal cord lesion.
1. Neurologic
   a. Limb weakness
   b. Abnormal deep tendon reflexes
2. Urinary
   a. Retention
3. Physical
   a. Abnormal cutaneous pigmentation
   b. Tufts of hair
   c. Deviation from the midline
   d. Placement above the intergluteal fold

C. Identify infection early.
1. Repair should occur before the tract is infected.

D. Coordinate diagnostic studies.

E. Educate and support the parents.

SURGICAL MANAGEMENT

A. Dissection and removal of the tract and any associated tumor
1. Repair of any found anomalies like tethered cord.

B. Reconstruction of the dura to ensure
1. Adequate space to reduce the risk of tethering
2. A watertight seal

C. Possibly extensive surgery, depending upon the presence and extent of a tumor

COMPLICATIONS

A. Infection
1. If the diagnosis is a dermal sinus, infection can lead to meningitis.
2. If the diagnosis is a dimple or pit, infection will be local only.

B. Tethering of the cord

C. Residual tumor

D. Deterioration of distal neurologic function
1. Bowel
2. Bladder
3. Extremities

POSTOPERATIVE NURSING CARE

A. Recovery is usually simple if surgery is only excision of tissue.
1. May have a small dressing.
   a. Observe for leaking CSF.
   b. Protect the surgical area from stool contamination.

2.   If extensive surgery is required, the infant will have a greater need for pain relief medications.
B. The infant will be NPO.
   1.   Will require IV fluids
   2.   Should be able to eat as soon as GI function returns
C. Assess for infection.
D. Assess bowel and bladder function.
   1.   Assess for impaired bladder emptying.
      a.   Check urinary residuals on patients with extensive repairs.
E. Assist with follow-up MRI or ultrasound.

OUTCOMES

A. Infants usually do very well.
B. If complicated by another lesion, the outcome may depend on that lesion.
C. Tethering of the cord may be an issue if the dura mater had to be repaired.
D. A persistent dimple will need continuous hygiene to prevent infection.

Encephalocele[59,60]

DEFINITION

A. The term *encephalocele* encompasses a group of defects, usually along the midline, that consists of a skull defect with protrusion of various brain contents.
   1.   Cranium bifidum is a skull defect only.
   2.   Cranial meningocele contains CSF and meninges.
   3.   Encephalomeningocele contains neural elements, meninges, and CSF.

PATHOPHYSIOLOGY

A. Brain components herniate through an opening, usually along the midline.
B. The sac contains various structures.
C. The dysphasic brain does not function normally.
D. With subsequent trauma, infection, or bleeding, herniated structures may affect the future development of other structures.[61]

ETIOLOGY

A. Embryologic
   1.   Postneurulation malformation with failure of bone closure
   2.   Possibly malformed underlying brain
B. Genetic
   1.   Frequently seen with
      a.   Meckel-Gruber syndrome
      b.   Walker Warburg syndrome
   2.   Occasionally seen with[4,21]
      a.   Adams Oliver syndrome
      b.   Amnion rupture sequence
      c.   Cervico-oculo-acoustic syndrome (occipital)
      d.   Frontonasal dysplasia sequence (anterior basal)
      e.   Limb–body wall complex
      f.   Oculo-auriculo-vertebral spectrum (occipital)
      g.   Pallister-Hall syndrome
      h.   Roberts-SC phocomelia (frontal)
C. Pathophysiologic

INCIDENCE

A. Encephaloceles occur in about 1/5,000 live births.

B. Most defects occur along the midline structures from the tip of (or inside) the nose to the base of the skull, perhaps into the middle ear.

C. The location of the defect is influenced by geography and sex. In the Western Hemisphere, 85 percent of encephaloceles are occipital; 70 percent occur in males.

CLINICAL PRESENTATION

A. The lesion is found either by physical exam or imaging.

B. The size of the lesion varies.

C. It may be in the usual midline location or hidden, as with nasal encephaloceles.

D. Seventy to 80 percent are usually found in the occipital region.

E. A sac of meningeal tissue, intact or ruptured, will be present.

F. There may be leakage of CSF.

ASSOCIATIONS

A. See ETIOLOGY: B. Genetic above.

B. There may be various developmental brain and structural malformations, depending upon the size and location of the encephalocele.

C. Micrognathia can occur with or without cleft lip.

DIFFERENTIAL DIAGNOSIS

A. Scalp edema

B. Cystic hygroma

C. Hemangioma

D. Myelomeningocele

E. Nasal hamartoma

DIAGNOSIS

A. MRI

    1. It looks at changes in water and fat when exposed to a magnetic field, providing both structural and functional information. MRI is especially useful for vascular and perfusion imaging and new spectroscopic techniques. It can provide finer detail than a CT scan of certain tissues. Limitations include the need for sedation and life-support equipment.

    2. MRI will reveal the following.

        a. Contents of sac

        b. Neural elements

        c. Vascular anatomy

B. CT

    1. This test can provide anatomic details and relationships.

    2. It is currently a second choice because it is not able to provide the detail that an MRI can.

TREATMENT OPTIONS AND NURSING CARE

A. Immediate intervention

    1. Support the airway if compromised.

    2. Protect the lesion.

        a. Warm, moist covering (saline-soaked, *nonadherent* gauze as the first layer) and a vapor barrier

3. Prevent any local pressure or twisting.
4. Avoid infection.
5. Assess for other life-threatening or limiting problems that can influence the repair decision.

B. Delayed or palliative management
   1. The management of the infant will depend on the contents of the encephalocele.
      a. If the content of the brain in the sac exceeds that in the cranium, nonintervention may be a consideration.
   2. If associated anomalies or syndromes are significant when factored with the aspects of the lesion, nonintervention may be considered.

C. Nursing management preoperatively or with nonintervention
   1. Protect the lesion from disruption and desiccation (moist, warm, saline–soaked, nonadherent gauze with covering and vapor barrier).
   2. Position the infant to prevent pressure or torsion on the lesion.
   3. If the lesion is large, observe for other facial anomalies, especially micrognathia and clefts.
   4. Support nutrition and hydration according to the size of the lesion and the impact of other disease states that may exist.
   5. Assess the infant for the need for sedation and airway protection for diagnostic studies.
   6. Support the family.
      a. This lesion is not always identified antenatally.
      b. Nonintervention may be elected.

SURGICAL MANAGEMENT

A. The goals of surgery are to do the following.
   1. Remove the sac.
   2. Limit the amount of tissue removed, and return the contents into the cranium as much as is possible.
   3. Seal the dura; close the cranium and skin.

B. CSF diversion (a shunt) may be needed at the time of initial surgery or later.

COMPLICATIONS

A. CSF leak
B. Bleeding
C. Infection
D. Hydrocephalus
E. Developmental and motor delay in about 60–70 percent of infants
F. Need for gastrostomy feedings and possible anti–gastroesophageal reflux (GER) surgery (Prolonged inability to orally feed and GER are related to profound developmental delay.)

POSTOPERATIVE NURSING CARE

A. Postoperative respiratory support depends on the degree of repair and underlying neurologic function.
B. Assess the cardiovascular system.
   1. Extensive bleeding may have occurred in surgery.
C. A small lesion may require limited standard care.
   1. Pain control
   2. IV fluids until bowel function returns

D. A CSF diversion device may have been placed at initial surgery.
  1. Observe for bleeding and CSF leak.

OUTCOMES

A. Developmental delay as noted above
B. Early death due to complications of the lesion (e.g., infection, aspiration)
C. Small lesions with limited neural elements may be developmentally normal.

Skull Fracture[62,63]

DEFINITION

A. There are three types of skull fractures.
  1. Linear skull fractures are one main type.
    a. A thin break in the bone
    b. Rarely separated edges
  2. Depressed skull fractures are the other main type.
    a. "Ping-Pong" type (looks like an indented Ping-Pong ball)
    b. Only rare bone discontinuity
  3. Basilar fractures at the base of the brain are a rare subset of skull fractures.
    a. This type of fracture may cause significant hemorrhage and brain stem dysfunction.[64]

PATHOPHYSIOLOGY

A. Force applied to the bone exceeds the tensile strength of the bone.
  1. It may be from excessive force over a wide area or concentrated force.
  2. It may occur when the normal force is applied to abnormal or underossified bone.
  3. It may be a combination of both.

ETIOLOGY

A. Skull fractures are seen secondary to the following.
  1. Trauma from internal forces against maternal bony prominences
    a. Pressure exerted on the fetal head during normal delivery ranges between 38 and 390 mmHg.[62]
  2. External trauma from operative delivery techniques (forceps/vacuum)
  3. Direct trauma (falls or nonaccidental trauma)
B. A skull fracture may be a presenting sign (along with other fractures) of congenital abnormalities of bone formation.
  1. Osteogenesis imperfecta
  2. Hypophosphatasia
C. Depressed skull fracture has been estimated to occur in 1/1,000 live births and is the most common head injury in neonates (Figure 7-7).[65]

INCIDENCE

A. Skull fractures are rare in the newborn.
  1. The skull bones are pliable.
  2. The sutures are open.
  3. The bone inner and outer layers (tables) do not densely ossify until approximately age four.

CLINICAL PRESENTATION

A. Symptoms are rarely seen with linear fractures unless there is underlying dural injury.

B. Depressed skull fractures may have the following characteristics.
   1. Be asymptomatic
   2. Present with signs and symptoms of underlying injury
      a. Hemorrhage
      b. CSF leak
      c. Alteration in vital signs

ASSOCIATIONS

A. Cephalohematoma

B. Intracranial hemorrhage

C. Osteogenesis imperfecta

D. Hypophosphatasia

DIFFERENTIAL DIAGNOSIS

A. Extreme molding

B. Caput succedeum

DIAGNOSIS

A. Most infants are asymptomatic.

B. Depression or painful area of the skull may be found on physical examination.

C. Plain skull films can aid diagnosis.

D. CT scan can be helpful.

FIGURE 7-7 ■ Large depressed left parietal skull fracture in a newborn secondary to forceps delivery.

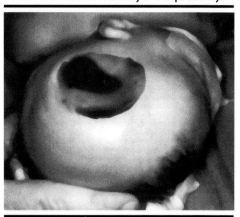

From: Harpold TL, McComb JG, and Levy ML. 1998. Neonatal neurosurgical trauma. *Neurosurgery Clinics of North America* 9(1): 144. Reprinted by permission.

TREATMENT OPTIONS AND NURSING CARE

A. Immediate interventions are unnecessary unless the infant shows signs of acute deterioration.

B. Observe for underlying injury.

C. If the infant must be transported, do the following.
   1. Protect injured bone with padding
   2. Observe for
      a. CNS compromise
      b. Cardiopulmonary decompensation

D. Delayed or palliative management
   1. Linear fractures heal within one to two months without treatment.
   2. Small (<2 cm) "Ping-Pong"-type depressed fractures can be observed for the following.
      a. Extension
      b. CNS deterioration
      c. CSF leak
      d. Blood loss
   3. Nonsurgical treatment can include use of lateral pressure or vacuum to elevate the fracture.

E. Preoperative nursing care includes the following.
   1. Protect the injured site.

FIGURE 7-8 ■ Sites of extracranial hemorrhage: caput, subgaleal hemorrhage, and cephalhematoma.

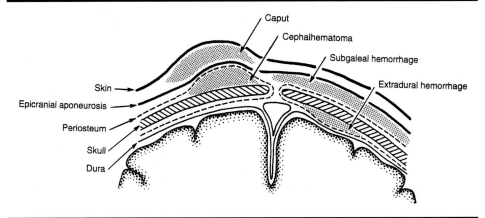

From: Volpe JJ. 2001. *Neurology of the Newborn,* 4th ed. Philadelphia: Saunders, 814. Reprinted by permission.

2. Observe for signs of the following.
   a. Clinical deterioration
   b. Hemorrhage
   c. Seizures
3. Support parents because they may have significant feelings of blame and guilt related to what they believe caused the injury.

SURGICAL MANAGEMENT

A. Indications for surgery include the following.
   1. Bone fragments
   2. Hemorrhage
   3. CSF leak
   4. Neurologic deficits
   5. Seizures
B. Procedure varies based on the underlying involvement of the brain.
   1. The following may be required.
      a. Physical elevation of bone
      b. Piecing bone fragments together
      c. Debridement
   2. Bleeding and hematomas are removed as needed.
   3. The scalp wound is cleaned and repaired as well.

COMPLICATIONS

A. May result from the fracture or the surgery
B. Linear fractures
   1. Can widen into "growing fractures"
   2. Can develop a leptomeningeal cyst
C. Seizures
D. Hidden hemorrhage or new hemorrhage postoperatively
E. Developmental delay, ranging from none to extensive, depending on:
   1. The extent of underlying injury
   2. Related birth depression

Neonatal Surgical Procedures: A Guide for Care and Management

Postoperative Nursing Care

A. General care
  1. Protect the site from further trauma.
  2. Observe the site of the surgery for the following.
     a. CSF leak
     b. Incisional bleeding
     c. Dehiscence (caused by swelling of the brain)
  3. Observe for general clinical deterioration and changes in neurologic status.
     a. Further bleeding
     b. Seizures
     c. Change in level of consciousness
  4. Provide medications for pain control if the incision is extensive.
     a. Usually mild analgesics such as acetaminophen will provide effective relief.
     b. Occasionally narcotics are needed.
  5. Avoid IV placement in the head.
B. Specific nursing care, depending on the extent of the surgery
  1. It is critical to prevent or treat any hemorrhage that may occur.
  2. Treat seizures.
  3. Observe and appropriately restrict fluids if syndrome of inappropriate antidiuretic hormone secretion (SIADH) occurs.

Outcomes

A. Uncomplicated linear and depressed fractures resolve within three to four weeks.
B. Complicated fractures with underlying brain injury have a worse prognosis that depends on the underlying injury.

Extra- and Intracranial Hemorrhage[62–64]

Definition

A. This is bleeding that occurs in the following spaces.
  1. Extracranial (Figure 7-8)
     a. Caput succedaneum
     b. Subgaleal
     c. Between the periosteum of the skull and the bone (cephalhematoma)
  2. Intracranial
     a. Epidural
     b. Subdural
        1) Blood mainly above the tentorium cerebelli is known as a supratentorial hemorrhage
        2) Blood mainly below the tentorium cerebelli is known as a subtentorial hemorrhage or posterior fossa hemorrhage
     c. Subarachnoid
     d. Intraventricular **(See Hydrocephalus: Etiology.)**
     e. Intracerebral
     f. Intracerebellar
B. Blood can collect in all spaces as well as in the brain parenchyma.

PATHOPHYSIOLOGY

A. Hemorrhage can occur during the birth process secondary to an imbalance between forces applied to the skull and the strength of the underlying blood vessels and dura mater.

   1. These forces are especially focused on the posterior fossa at the falcotentorial junction.[66]

   2. The forces may be the following.

      a. Natural (labor)

         1) Molding

         2) Stretching

         3) Pulling

      b. Secondary to operative delivery

         1) Forceps

         2) Vacuum extractors

B. The amount of bleeding can be small or large, depending on two factors.

   1. Location

      a. Some **subdural** hemorrhages can be very large, especially if large vessels or sinuses are injured.

      b. Bleeding in the **subgaleal** space may mimic a caput succedaneum, but can progress to contain a massive amount of blood (i.e., potentially the entire baby's blood volume); the bleeding can extend from the nape of the neck to the bridge of the nose.[67]

   2. Type of injury

ETIOLOGY

A. Hemorrhage may occur in an infant with the following.

   1. An unknown bleeding defect such as

      a. Thrombocytopenia

      b. Hemophilia

   2. An unknown vascular abnormality

B. Bleeding may occur secondary to other factors.

   1. Reperfusion after a stroke

   2. Administration of vasoconstrictors

   3. Thrombus formation from a hypercoagulable state, leading to venous hypertension with resultant bleeding or frank infarct with bleeding on reperfusion

INCIDENCE

A. Intracranial hemorrhage is a fairly frequent occurrence.

B. The exact incidence is not known because many hemorrhages are asymptomatic.

C. Hemorrhage can occur in both term and preterm infants.

D. They occur with the following frequency.

   1. They are effected by the mode of delivery from 1/900–1,900 live births.[68]

   2. The most common type of hemorrhage is **subarachnoid**, but the exact incidence is not known.

   3. **Subgaleal** hemorrhage is very rare (0.02/1,000 live births).[67]

CLINICAL PRESENTATION

A. Frank bleeding is rarely visible.

B. Frank swelling and changes in consistency may occur.

C. As bleeding persists, the infant develops shock or seizures.

D. Various degrees of anemia may be present.

ASSOCIATIONS

A. Skull fracture

B. Occipital osteodiastasis

C. Macrosomia (in large-for-gestational-age infants)

D. Macrocephalus

E. Breech delivery

F. Arteriovenous malformation

DIFFERENTIAL DIAGNOSIS

A. Hypoxic-ischemic encephalopathy

B. Stroke

C. Anemia from other bleeding

D. Seizures from other causes

E. Meningitis

F. Cardiovascular collapse from left heart obstruction

DIAGNOSIS

A. Maintain a high index of suspicion in infants with risk factors, though this can occur in infants with no risk factors.
   1. Operative deliveries, especially vacuum assisted (for **subgaleal** hemorrhage)[67,68]
   2. Macrosomia
   3. Macrocephaly
   4. Precipitous delivery
   5. Breech
   6. Prematurity

B. Do frequent physical examinations that include the nape of the neck.

C. Assess for the following.
   1. Anemia
   2. Coagulopathy
      a. If bleeding is thought to be secondary to hemorrhage after a stroke, obtain blood for evaluation of a possible hypercoagulable state.

D. CT is the preferred method of diagnosis.

E. Ultrasound can be used for diagnosis if the infant is unstable or CT is not available.
   1. Ultrasound will not pick up all hemorrhages because the peripheral cranial vault and the posterior fossa space are not easily seen.

F. CSF examination may be performed.
   1. *Caution:* An LP is avoided if the infant is at risk for a **posterior fossa subdural** hemorrhage. Doing an LP may result in herniation of the brain stem with acute cardiopulmonary decompensation.[18]

G. If stroke is present, obtain blood to be tested for substances of abuse because the etiology may be illicit vasoconstrictors.

TREATMENT OPTIONS AND NURSING CARE

A. Immediate intervention
   1. For **subgaleal** and **posterior fossa subdural** hemorrhages, early identification is vital to prevent shock and death.
      a. Initially, there may be no abnormal signs.
      b. These types of hemorrhages progress, usually within 24 hours, as the clot gets bigger and more brain stem compression occurs.
      c. **Subgaleal** hemorrhages need aggressive medical management for shock and coagulopathy because there is no effective neurosurgical procedure to stop the bleeding.
      d. Acute **subdural** hemorrhage may be initially treated with needle aspiration.
   2. A **subarachnoid** hemorrhage rarely causes clinical signs (seizures, anemia, hypotension), unless it is large.
      a. When large, this type of hemorrhage can be fatal.
      b. Emergency CSF diversion and/or surgical evacuation may be undertaken if there are significant and progressive neurologic signs.
         1) IICP
         2) Apnea
         3) Bradycardia
         4) Fixed pupils
      c. If there are no significant and progressive neurologic signs, then frequent clinical and laboratory assessments for shock and coagulopathy are needed.
   3. Seizures may be a presenting sign.
      a. Treat with anticonvulsant medications.
      b. Evaluate for cranial hemorrhage (especially **subarachnoid**).
B. Interventions prior to transport
   1. Identify patients at risk for large **subdural** or **subgaleal** hemorrhages, and make arrangements for rapid transfer.
   2. Manage symptoms as they arise.
   3. Anticipate and prepare for acute and severe deterioration.
      a. Shock
      b. Anemia
C. Medical management
   1. A conservative approach is warranted unless the hemorrhage is extensive.
      a. Observe for changes in the following.
         1) Neurologic status and exam
         2) Cardiovascular status and exam
      b. Frequently monitor the infant for anemia and coagulopathy.
D. Nursing management
   1. Frequently assess the infant for the following.
      a. Changes in vital signs
         1) Early identification of acute brain stem dysfunction (bradycardia and hypertension)
         2) Early identification of shock
      b. Changes in neurologic status
         1) Seizures
         2) Level of consciousness
         3) Size and reaction of pupils
         4) Fontanel tension

    c. Anemia
      1) Close follow-up on blood test results
    d. Changes in OFC measurement
  2. Infants at risk for **subgaleal** hemorrhage require the following.
    a. Frequently examine the occiput and nape of the neck because this is where blood tends to pool.
  3. Administer blood products (possibly rapidly) to combat coagulopathy and shock.
  4. Ensure that the infant has received a vitamin K injection at birth.
  5. Rapidly complete presurgical procedures and paperwork should emergency surgery be needed.

SURGICAL MANAGEMENT[69]

A. Surgery is usually necessary for these conditions.
  1. Clinical deterioration
  2. Midline shift
  3. Persistent bleeding
  4. Effusion
B. The following types of procedures may be done.
  1. CSF diversion
  2. Direct subdural taps for symptomatic **subdural** hematoma
  3. Frontal-parietal flap procedure for **supratentorial** hematoma
  4. Small suboccipital craniectomies for **posterior fossa** hemorrhages

COMPLICATIONS[18,66,69]

A. **Posterior fossa** hemorrhage
  1. Five to 10 percent die.
  2. Fifteen percent develop hydrocephalus.
  3. Eighty to 90 percent have a good outcome.
B. **Supratentorial** hemorrhage
  1. Fifty to 90 percent do well, but can develop hydrocephalus and/or chronic effusions.
C. **Subarachnoid** hemorrhage
  1. These are complicated by hydrocephalus.
  2. Infants who have suffered these do well unless the hemorrhage is catastrophic (very large).

POSTOPERATIVE NURSING CARE

A. Take frequent vital signs for early identification of the following.
  1. Acute brain stem dysfunction
  2. Shock
B. Identify changes in the neurologic exam (as above), indicating the need for further surgery.
C. Observe for these conditions.
  1. Coma
  2. Progressive apnea
  3. Bradycardia
  4. Hypertension
D. Observe for seizures.
E. Observe for further bleeding.
  1. Administer blood products as ordered.

F. Care for the ventricular drain as needed.

G. Observe for signs of hydrocephalus.

H. Administer medication for pain as ordered.

I. Manage control of ICP as ordered by the following.
   1. Fluid restriction
   2. Sedation
   3. Paralysis

J. Control the infant's movements as needed.

K. Monitor mechanical ventilation as needed.

L. Care for the parents in this situation where delivery issues may cause added guilt, anger, and stress.

OUTCOMES

See COMPLICATIONS.

Traumatic Spinal Cord Injury

DEFINITION

A. Direct injury to the spinal cord
   1. The spectrum of presentation can range from no signs to varying degrees of weakness and paralysis.
   2. Which systems are affected is based on the level and extent of the injury.

PATHOPHYSIOLOGY

A. Excessive shear and twisting forces can lead to the following.
   1. Stretching of the spinal cord
   2. Avulsion (tearing)
   3. Transection of individual fibers
   4. Focal necrosis (ischemia)
   5. Compression from bone or clot

B. The injury is compounded by the following as either the primary event or the secondary effect.
   1. Local
      a. Hemorrhage
      b. Ischemia
      c. Edema
   2. Release of various substances (such as excitotoxic neurotransmitters and cytokines) that lead to cell death

ETIOLOGY

A. Many injuries have no identifiable etiology.

B. The main pathogenesis of most injuries is trauma from forces applied during birth.
   1. This includes forces due to the following.
      a. Forceps
      b. Vacuum extractors
      c. Dysfunctional labor
   2. These forces result in excessive longitudinal or lateral pulling on the spine or excessive rotation of the spine or head.[18]
      a. Hyperextension of the fetal head

C. Other causes of injury include the following.
   1. Embolism
      a. Air or clot from various types of catheters
         1) Umbilical arterial catheter
         2) Peripherally inserted central catheter placed into a vertebral artery or vein
   2. Vascular anomalies or thrombus
   3. Tumor[70]

INCIDENCE

A. Incidence is not clearly known.
   1. Significant injury is rare, but in some settings can occur more frequently.
      a. Twenty-two injuries in 20 years in one referral hospital[71]
   2. There is a higher incidence of injury in infants born breech.
      a. Spinal hemorrhages were seen in 46 percent of those on autopsy.[18]
B. Most traumatic lesions are cervical; lesions from other causes may be thoracolumbar.

CLINICAL PRESENTATION

A. Most injuries present at birth through the first 24 hours.
   1. Some infants with mild injury can present months later.
B. Neonates present with varying degrees of spinal shock.
   1. Flaccidity or weakness
   2. Decrease or absent spontaneous movements
   3. Apnea
   4. Weak respirations or respiratory distress
   5. Various levels of sensory response
C. Signs of injury progress as swelling and necrosis progress; they subside as recovery occurs.

ASSOCIATIONS

A. Macrosomia
B. Shoulder dystocia
C. Breech presentation
D. Hypoxic-ischemic encephalopathy
   1. Especially with high lesions
E. Inadvertent anticoagulation

DIFFERENTIAL DIAGNOSIS

A. Hypoxic-ischemic encephalopathy
B. Discrete brain stem lesions
C. Spinal tumors
D. Myopathies

DIAGNOSIS[70,71]

A. X-ray
   1. The neck is often included in the chest radiograph.
   2. Vertebral spaces should be examined to discover any unusual gaps.
B. CT with or without contrast

C. Ultrasound
1. Ultrasound study has a high positive predictive value and can be done at the bedside.[71]
D. MRI (Figure 7-9)
1. This provides specific anatomic data, including the ability to do angiography. It is important in evaluation for other causes of weakness.

TREATMENT OPTIONS AND NURSING CARE

A. Immediate intervention
1. Treatment of respiratory insufficiency
2. Neck and back stabilization
3. Possible role for steroids for spinal shock[18]
4. Identification and treatment of any coagulopathy
B. Preoperative nursing management
1. Maintain a neutral spine and neck position throughout admission and care procedures.
   a. May require sandbags or fashioning a type of neck collar
   b. Controlled, log-type rolling for position changes
   c. Control of spontaneous movement with
      1) Sedation
      2) Pain medication at a level to control pain, but still allow complete neurologic assessment
2. Monitor for neurologic changes, especially in respiratory drive and muscle function.
   a. Weakness may be progressive as cord edema progresses.
3. Protect from tissue injury as sensory responses are impaired.
4. Protect the infant from developing pressure sores by using appropriate padding.
5. Do range of motion exercises to prevent contractures.

FIGURE 7-9 ■ Neonatal spinal cord injury: MRI scan obtained at five days of age.

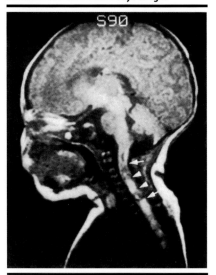

From: Minami T, et al. 1994. A case of neonatal spinal cord injury: Magnetic resonance imaging and somatosensory evoked potentials. *Brain & Development* 16(1): 57. Reprinted by permission.

SURGICAL MANAGEMENT

A. Surgical procedures for spinal cord injury are rarely done.
B. There are two possible procedures.
1. Vertebral fusion and stabilization
2. Clot removal and laminectomy for focal pressure phenomena

COMPLICATIONS

A. Complications of spinal cord injury are dependent upon the level of the injury and may include the following.
1. Additional nerve root injury
2. Autonomic dysreflexia
3. Immobility contractures

   4. Stasis pneumonia
   5. Respiratory insufficiency
   6. Skin breakdown

Postoperative Nursing Care

A. Treatment of spinal shock if extensive surgical manipulations occurred
B. Mechanical ventilation as needed
   1. Support respiratory function with good pulmonary toilet.
   2. Assist the physician in evaluating for phrenic nerve pacing if there is diaphragmatic paralysis.
      a. Most infants are not candidates.
C. Observation for and treatment of autonomic dysreflexia, a local imbalance of sympathic and parasympathic tone causing hypertensive crisis
   1. Observe for hypertension as an early sign of autonomic dysreflexia.
   2. Observe for the following.
      a. Muscle spasms
      b. Tachycardia
      c. Bradycardia
      d. Sweating
D. Stabilization of neck and spine
   1. Gel mattress
   2. Log roll turning
E. Skin care
   1. Protect the infant from pressure injury.
      a. Mobility
         1) Limited mobility both pre- and postprocedure may increase the risk of skin breakdown.
            a) The limitations may be secondary to the spinal lesion itself or as a consequence of the procedure.
         2) Frequent turning or position alteration (every two to four hours) is necessary.
            a) It is especially needed in situations where there is specific limb or total body immobility.
            b) Turning can be limited by specific procedures or lesion.
            c) Special appliances may be necessary.
               • Various gel pillows and protective mattresses can be employed to change the pressure amounts and contact points.
               • Local padding or skin protection can be provided through the use of gauze pads, pectin-based barriers, and semipermeable adhesive membranes.
   2. Skin covering the lesion (if present) may be abnormal and more easily damaged.
F. Range of motion exercises to prevent contractures
G. Assessment of bowel and bladder function
   1. Catheterize and give enemas as necessary.
H. Function assessment for prognosis
   1. Especially important at 24 hours and three months of age

OUTCOMES[70,71]

A. Motor disability includes the following.
1. Paraplegia
2. Quadriplegia
   a. Many infants will be fully or partially ventilator dependent.
B. Two-thirds of infants with injuries have prolonged sphincter dysfunction.
C. One-third of infants with injuries have scoliosis.
D. There may be partial to complete transection of the spinal cord.
1. The outcome was best predicted by breathing movements on day 1 and the rate of recovery of limb movements.
   a. Apnea on day 1 and no recovery of limb movements by three months was associated with ventilator dependency and quadriplegia.[71]
E. Ambulation of some type can occur in 40 percent of survivors.
F. Full recovery occurs in less than 5 percent of survivors.
G. Death occurs in as high as 20–35 percent of infants.
1. Death is usually the result of respiratory failure.
H. Autonomic dysreflexia persists if the lesion is above T-7.

Latex Allergy

Latex allergy is a problem for both patients and caregivers. It is secondary to sensitization by antigens from natural rubber or latex (the sap from which rubber is made). Repeated exposure leads to hypersensitivity and, in severe cases, anaphylaxis. Patients at risk are those requiring frequent surgeries or frequent contact with latex devices (gloves, catheters), making neonates with neurosurgical conditions a very high-risk population. Infants with spina bifida are at the highest risk. As many as 60–80 percent have a positive skin test indicating allergy to latex proteins.[47,52] Unfortunately, sensitization can occur with very limited exposure soon after birth.[47] Other high-risk infants are those requiring frequent shunt surgery. Although the shunt itself does not contain latex, the operating room environment does.

Ethical Considerations and Summary[11,72,73]

Prior to World War II, patients who presented with neurosurgical lesions that did not need significant intervention had the best outcomes. Nonintervention at that time, generally, was related to technical issues. After 1960, when ventriculoperitoneal shunts became available, there was more controversy concerning treatment.

In 1973, Roe v Wade established legal definitions of viability and when legal termination of pregnancy could occur for various neurosurgical lesions. And in 1983, Baby Jane Doe was born with spina bifida and her parents declined surgical treatment. Civil involvement led to Baby Doe regulations, which required treatment without consideration of handicap.

These regulations were struck down in 1986. The Child Abuse and Treatment Act of 1984 now defines withholding of treatment. Table 7-1 provides a general ethical framework.

The care of the neonate with a neurosurgical condition builds on the care of all neonatal patients with and without surgical conditions. The same nursing process is used, with attention to the unique features of the neonate with a neurosurgical diagnosis as compared to other populations.[74]

All neurosurgical disorders create psychological support and education needs for the parents and family. Adult learner concepts should be employed. Support the

TABLE 7-1 ■ Salient Points in Building an Ethical Framework[73]

1. The framework builds on basic principles and adjusts to the unique situation of the fetus or newly born baby.

2. The parental role as key baby decision maker is supported (autonomy).

3. Treatments that will prolong dying or that are virtually futile or inhumane (nonmaleficence) do not have to be provided.

4. Decisions for or against treatment should not consider future handicap or retardation, but rather how the treatment could help the patient. If there is a reasonable degree of uncertainty, then the patient should have the benefit of the doubt (beneficence).

5. Clinical interventions can be discontinued after a period of time that allows for observation and reflection on the decision (nonmaleficence).

family in crisis by explaining, listening, and offering referrals to support groups, clergy, and social services.

Education and counseling regarding the lesion, proposed treatment, operative course, outcome, home care, and follow-up must be provided, often repetitively. Education and counseling may build on that already accomplished after a prenatal diagnosis. Education should be multidisciplinary and continuous. It is vital that the nurse be involved in these discussions to ensure consistency of the communication and information shared.

REFERENCES

1. Shaw N. 2002. *Neonatal Embryology: A Course for Neonatal Nurses and Nurse Practitioners.* Salt Lake City, Utah: Nancy Shaw.

2. Moore KL, and Persaud TVN. 2003. *The Developing Human: Clinically Oriented Embryology,* 7th ed. Philadelphia: Saunders, 427.

3. Moore KL, Persaud TVN, and Shiota K. 2000. *Color Atlas of Clinical Embryology,* 2nd ed. Philadelphia: Saunders, 232.

4. Jorde LB, Carey JC, and Bamshad MJ. 2005. *Medical Genetics,* 3rd ed. St. Louis: Mosby.

5. Sarnat H. 2002. The central nervous system: Embryology and malformations of the CNS. In *Neonatal-Perinatal Medicine: Diseases of the Fetus and Infant,* 7th ed., Fanaroff AA, and Martin RJ, eds. St. Louis: Mosby, 816–846.

6. Walker MJ. 1988. Personal communication. CSF production in neonates.

7. McComb JG, and Zlokovic BV. 2001. Cerebrospinal fluid and the blood-brain interface. In *Pediatric Neurosurgery,* McLone DG, and Marlin AE, eds. Philadelphia: Saunders, 180–198.

8. Lancon JA, et al. 2001. Cerebral blood flow and metabolism. In *Pediatric Neurosurgery,* McLone DG, and Marlin AE, eds. Philadelphia: Saunders, 163–175.

9. Tyszczuk L, et al. 1998. Cerebral blood flow is independent of mean arterial blood pressure in preterm infants undergoing intensive care. *Pediatrics* 102(2 part 1): 337–341.

10. Vannucci RC. 2002. The central nervous system: Disorders in head size and shape. In *Neonatal-Perinatal Medicine: Diseases of the Fetus and Infant,* 7th ed., Fanaroff AA, and Martin RJ, eds. St. Louis: Mosby, 911–915.

11. Frim DM, Scott RM, and Madsen JR. 1998. Surgical management of neonatal hydrocephalus. *Neurosurgery Clinics of North America* 9(1): 105–110.

12. McAllister JP II, and Chovan P. 1998. Neonatal hydrocephalus: Mechanisms and consequences. *Neurosurgery Clinics of North America* 9(1): 73–95.

13. Papile L, et al. 1978. Incidence and evolution of subependymal and intraventricular hemorrhage: A study of infants with birth weights less than 1,500 gm. *Journal of Pediatrics* 92(4): 529–534.

14. Punt J. 2001. Neurosurgical management of hydrocephalus. In *Fetal and Neonatal Neurology and Neurosurgery,* 3rd ed., Levene MI, Chervenak FA, and Whittle MJ, eds. London: Churchill Livingstone, 753–763.

15. Kirby CL. 2002. Posthemorrhagic hydrocephalus: A complication of intraventricular hemorrhage. *Neonatal Network* 21(1): 59–68.

16. Paneth N, et al. 1993. Incidence and timing of germinal matrix/intraventricular hemorrhage in low birth weight infants. *American Journal of Epidemiology* 137(11): 1167–1176.

17. Marks JD, and Khoshnood B. 1998. Epidemiology of common neurosurgical diseases in the neonate. *Neurosurgery Clinics of North America* 9(1): 63–72.

18. Volpe JJ. 2001. *Neurology of the Newborn,* 4th ed. Philadelphia: Saunders, 397–427, 440–455, 820–825.

19. Rodriguez Criado G, et al. 2003. X-linked hydrocephalus: Another two families with an L1 mutation. *Genetic Counseling* 14(1): 57–65.

20. Haverkamp F, et al. 1999. Congenital hydrocephalus internus and aqueduct stenosis: Aetiology and implications for genetic counseling. *European Journal of Pediatrics* 158(6): 474–478.

21. Jones KL. 1996. *Smith's Recognizable Patterns of Human Malformation,* 5th ed. Philadelphia: Saunders, 875.

22. Perlman J, and Rollins N. 2000. Surveillance protocol for the detection of intracranial abnormalities in premature neonates. *Archives of Pediatrics & Adolescent Medicine* 154(8): 822–826.

23. Volpe JJ. 1998. Neonatal neurologic evaluation by the neurosurgeon. *Neurosurgery Clinics of North America* 9(1): 1–16.

24. Whitelaw A, Kennedy CR, and Brion LP. 2001. Diuretic therapy for newborn infants with posthemorrhagic ventricular dilatation (Cochrane Review). *The Cochrane Database of Systematic Reviews* (2): CD002270.

25. Whitelaw A. 2001. Repeated lumbar or ventricular punctures in newborns with intraventricular hemorrhage (Cochrane Review). *The Cochrane Database of Systematic Reviews* (2): CD000216.

26. Drake JM, and Iantosca MR. 2001. Management of pediatric hydrocephalus with shunts. In *Pediatric Neurosurgery,* 4th ed., McLone DG, ed. Philadelphia: Saunders, 505–522.

27. Chumas P, Tyagi A, and Livingston J. 2001. Hydrocephalus—what's new? *Archives of Diseases in Childhood. Fetal and Neonatal Edition* 85(3): F149–F154.

28. Brockmeyer D, et al. 1998. Endoscopic third ventriculostomy: An outcome analysis. *Pediatric Neurosurgery* 28(5): 236–240.

29. Fulmer BB, et al. 2000. Neonatal ventriculosubgaleal shunts. *Neurosurgery* 47(1): 80–84.

30. Tuli S, et al. 2000. Risk factors for repeated cerebrospinal shunt failures in pediatric patients with hydrocephalus. *Journal of Neurosurgery* 92(1): 31–38.

31. Cochrane DD, and Kestle J. 2002. Ventricular shunting for hydrocephalus in children: Patients, procedures, surgeons and institutions in English Canada, 1989–2001. *European Journal of Pediatric Surgery* 12(supplement 1): S6–S11.

32. Resch B, et al. 1996. Neurodevelopmental outcome of hydrocephalus following intra-/periventricular hemorrhage in preterm infants: Short- and long-term results. *Child's Nervous System* 12(1): 27–33.

33. Reinprecht A, et al. 2001. Posthemorrhagic hydrocephalus in preterm infants: Long-term follow-up and shunt-related complications. *Child's Nervous System* 17(11): 663–669.

34. Ment L, et al. 1999. The etiology and outcome of cerebral ventriculomegaly at term in very low birth weight preterm infants. *Pediatrics* 104(2 part 1): 243–248.

35. Botto LD, et al. 1999. Neural-tube defects. *New England Journal of Medicine* 341(20): 1509–1519.

36. Dias M. 1999. Myelomeningocele. In *Pediatric Neurosurgery*, Choux M, Hockley AD, and Di Rocco C, eds. London: Churchill Livingstone, 33–60.

37. Van Allen MI, et al. 1993. Evidence for multi-site closure of neural tube in humans. *American Journal of Medical Genetics* 47(5): 723–743.

38. Genetics Home Reference. 2005. PAX3. U.S. National Library of Medicine, September 30.

39. Northrup H, and Volcik KA. 2000. Spina bifida and other neural tube defects. *Common Problems in Pediatrics* 30(10): 313–332.

40. Nickel RE, et al. 1994. Velo-cardio-facial syndrome and DiGeorge sequence with meningomyelocele and deletions of the 22q11 region. *American Journal of Medical Genetics* 52(4): 445–449.

41. Ritter S, et al. 1999. Are screening echocardiograms warranted for neonates with meningomyelocele? *Archives of Pediatrics & Adolescent Medicine* 153(12): 1264–1266.

42. Cohen AR, and Robinson S. 2001. Early management of myelomeningocele. In *Pediatric Neurosurgery*, 4th ed., McLone DG, ed. Philadelphia: Saunders, 241–259.

43. Peterson P, and Hardy R. 2002. *Protocol for Management of a Newborn with Myelomeningocele*. Salt Lake City, Utah: Primary Children's Medical Center, 2.

44. Luthy DA, et al. 1991. Cesarean section before the onset of labor and subsequent motor function in infants with meningomyelocele diagnosed antenatally. *New England Journal of Medicine* 324(10): 662–666.

45. Peterson P. 2002. *Latex Allergy or Latex Precautions: Care of the Patient*. Salt Lake City, Utah: Primary Children's Medical Center, 2.

46. Kinnaird SW, McClure N, and Wilham S. 1995. Latex allergy: An emerging problem in health care. *Neonatal Network* 14(7): 33–38.

47. Szepfalusi Z, et al. 1999. Latex sensitization in spina bifida appears disease-associated. *Journal of Pediatrics* 134(3): 344–348.

48. Rintoul NE, et al. 2002. A new look at myelomeningoceles: Functional level, vertebral level, shunting, and the implications for fetal intervention. *Pediatrics* 109(3): 409–413.

49. Iskandar BJ, and Oakes WJ. 2001. Anomalies of the spine and spinal cord. In *Pediatric Neurosurgery*, 4th ed., McLone DG, ed. Philadelphia: Saunders, 307–323.

50. Warf BC. 2001. Pathophysiology of tethered cord syndrome. In *Pediatric Neurosurgery*, 4th ed., McLone DG, ed. Philadelphia: Saunders, 282–287.

51. Hoffman HJ, Hendrick EB, and Humphreys RP. 1976. The tethered spinal cord: Its protean manifestations, diagnosis and surgical correction. *Child's Brain* 2(3): 145–155.

52. Reigel DH, Ammerman RT, and Rothenstein D. 2001. Health care of the adult with spina bifida. In *Pediatric Neurosurgery*, 4th ed., McLone DG, ed. Philadelphia: Saunders, 266–278.

53. Warder DE. 2001. Tethered cord syndrome and occult spinal dysraphism. *Neurosurgical Focus* 10(1): 1–9.

54. Raghavendra BN, et al. 1983. The tethered spinal cord: Diagnosis by high-resolution real-time ultrasound. *Radiology* 149(1): 123–128.

55. Korsvik HE. 1994. Ultrasound assessment of congenital spinal anomalies presenting in infancy. *Seminars in Ultrasound, CT, and MR* 15(4): 264–274.

56. Jamil M, and Bannister CM. 1992. A report of children with spinal dysraphism managed conservatively. *European Journal of Pediatric Surgery* 2(supplement 1): S26–S28.

57. Hudgins RJ, and Gilreath CL. 2004. Tethered spinal cord following repair of myelomeningocele. *Neurosurgical Focus* 16(2): E7.

58. Cheek WR. 2001. Dermal sinus tract repair. In *Pediatric Neurosurgery*, 4th ed., McLone DG, ed. Philadelphia: Saunders, 328–331.

59. Partington MD, and Petronio JA. 2001. Malformations of the cerebral hemispheres. In *Pediatric Neurosurgery*, 4th ed., McLone DG, ed. Philadelphia: Saunders, 201–208.

60. Drake JM, and MacFarlane R. 2001. Encephalocele Repair. In *Pediatric Neurosurgery*, 4th ed., McLone DG, ed. Philadelphia: Saunders, 209–213.

61. Tubbs RS, et al. 2003. Neurological presentation and long-term outcome following operative intervention in patients with meningocele manque. *British Journal of Neurosurgery* 17(3): 230–233.

62. Medlock MD, and Harrigan WC. 1997. Neurologic birth trauma. Intracranial, spinal cord, and brachial plexus injury. *Clinics in Perinatology* 24(4): 845–857.

63. Dutcher S, et al. 2001. Skull fractures and penetrating brain injury. In *Pediatric Neurosurgery*, 4th ed., McLone DG, ed. Philadelphia: Saunders, 573–583.

64. McGee S, and Burkett KW. 2000. Identifying common pediatric neurosurgical conditions in the primary care setting. *Nursing Clinics of North America* 35(1): 61–85.

65. Harpold TL, McComb JG, and Levy ML. 1998. Neonatal neurosurgical trauma. *Neurosurgery Clinics of North America* 9(1): 141–154.

66. Piatt JH, and Kernan JC. 2001. Intracranial hematomas. In *Pediatric Neurosurgery*, 4th ed., McLone DG, ed. Philadelphia: Saunders, 634–645.

67. Center for Devices and Radiologic Health. 1998. Need for CAUTION when using vacuum assisted delivery devices. Rockville, Maryland: U.S. Food and Drug Administration. Available at www.fda.gov/cdrh/fetal598.html.

68. Towner D, et al. 1999. Effect of mode of delivery in nulliparous women on neonatal intracranial injury. *New England Journal of Medicine* 341(23): 1709–1714.

69. Aronyk KE. 2001. Subdural and epidural hematomas. In *Pediatric Neurosurgery*, 4th ed., McLone DG, ed. Philadelphia: Saunders, 646–654.

70. Ruggieri M, Smarason AK, and Pike M. 1999. Spinal cord insults in the prenatal, perinatal, and neonatal periods. *Developmental Medicine and Child Neurology* 41(5): 311–317.

71. MacKinnon JA, et al. 1993. Spinal cord injury at birth: Diagnostic and prognostic data in twenty-two patients. *Journal of Pediatrics* 122(3): 431–437.

72. Chervenak FA, and McCullough LB. 2001. Issues for the obstetrician. In *Fetal and Neonatal Neurology and Neurosurgery*, 3rd ed., Levene MI, et al, eds. London: Churchill Livingstone, 822–827.

73. Stephenson T. 2001. Ethical dilemmas: Issues for the neonatologist. In *Fetal and Neonatal Neurology and Neurosurgery*, 3rd ed., Levene MI, et al., eds. London: Churchill Livingstone, 828–832.

74. Keener KE, et al. 2000. The surgical neonate. In *Nursing Care of the General Pediatric Surgical Patient*, Wise BV, et al., eds. Gaithersburg, Maryland: Aspen, 443–445.

8

Surgical Repair of Defects and Injuries of the Extremities in the Neonatal Period

Diane B. Longobucco, RNC, MSN, APRN, NNP
Erica Siddell, PhD, RN

Congenital defects and injuries of the upper and lower extremities are relatively uncommon. Their expression runs the gamut from mild and inconsequential to extremely severe and disabling. Many times, correction, if it is possible, requires several surgeries over a period of months or years. In very few circumstances do these defects require surgical intervention in the immediate neonatal period. Often, the best surgical results require additional growth of the infant before surgery is attempted.

The purpose of this chapter is to help the neonatal nurse understand the origin of these defects so she may assist the physician in case finding or in preserving the integrity of the affected limb prior to treatment. In many cases, the primary role for the neonatal nurse is parent support and education. The birth of an infant with a congenital defect or brachial plexus injury can be overwhelming for many families. Helping parents accept the infant and make informed treatment decisions is a significant component of the care the family will require.

Embryology

BEGINNINGS OF THE SKELETAL SYSTEM[1-5]

A. Weeks 1–2
  1. The embryonic disc, which develops in the second week of gestation, consists of three layers of cells: The outer ectoderm, the mesoderm, and the inner layer, the endoderm.
    a. These layers of cells give rise to the tissues and structures that will form the fetus.

FIGURE 8-1 ■ **Drawing illustrating formation of the limb buds.**

A. An embryo at about 28 days, showing the early appearance of the limb buds. B. Longitudinal section through an upper limb bud. The apical ectodermal ridge has an inductive influence on the mesenchyme in the limb bud; it promotes growth of the mesenchyme and appears to give it the ability to form specific cartilaginous elements. C. Similar sketch of an upper limb bud at about 33 days, showing the mesenchymal primordia of the forearm bones. The digital rays are mesenchymal condensations that undergo chondrification and ossification to form the bones of the hand. D. Upper limb at six weeks, showing the cartilage models of the bones. E. Later in the sixth week, showing the completed cartilaginous models of the bones of the upper limb.

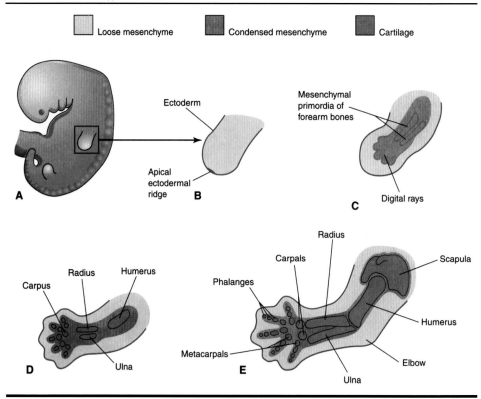

From: Moore KL, and Persaud TVN. 2003. *The Developing Human: Clinically Oriented Embryology,* 7th ed. Philadelphia: Saunders, 396. Reprinted by permission.

    b. The skeletal system develops from the mesoderm and neural crest cells.

B. Week 3

1. Early in the third week, development of the future central nervous system and axial skeleton begins.

2. The nervous system arises from a thickening of the ectoderm known as the neural plate.

3. Elevations of ectodermal tissue, the neural folds develop along a central groove in the neural plate.

4. The folds fuse at the junction of the future brain and spinal cord, creating the neural tube and the major divisions of the brain.

    a. Forebrain

    b. Midbrain

    c. Hindbrain

5. Ectodermal cells next to the neural fold form the neural crest cells, which migrate throughout the embryo.

    a. Most connective and skeletal tissue is derived from neural crest cells.

6. At the same time, mesenchymal cells form the notochordal process, which forms a plate and eventually folds inward to form the notochord around which the skeleton forms.

7. Lateral to the neural tube and notochord, tissue from the mesoderm thickens to form two columns known as the paraxial mesoderm, which then divide into blocks known as somites.

8. Somites differentiate into cells that will form:
   a. The vertebrae and ribs
   b. Muscle and skin

9. The mesenchyme (connective tissue) comes from mesodermal cells.
   a. This tissue differentiates to form:
     1) Fibroblasts
     2) Chondroblasts
     3) Osteoblasts

C. Week 4

1. Upper limb buds become visible as swellings on the ventrolateral body wall.[1]
   a. Buds consist of a mass of mesenchyme covered by a thick band of ectoderm.
   b. These buds appear low due to cranial development.

2. By the end of the fourth week, lower limb swellings are noted in three regions:
   a. Thigh
   b. Leg
   c. Foot

3. Homeobox-containing (Hox) genes regulate positioning of limbs and the types and shapes of bones of the limbs.[1,2]

D. Week 5

1. The upper limbs continue to develop as condensations of mesenchyme appear in limb buds (Figure 8-1).[3]

2. Upper limbs become paddlelike while the lower limbs appear more like flippers.

3. A flat, rounded, foot disc appears and then rotates inward.

4. Chondrification centers, which will eventually result in cartilaginous models of the bones in the extremities, develop.

E. Week 6

1. Hand plates appear, and elbows can also be identified (Figure 8-2).

2. Structures known as digital rays develop on the hands.

3. The five foot rays (precursors to the toes) develop.

4. Joint development begins.

F. Week 7

1. Limbs extend ventrally.

2. Upper limbs rotate laterally through 90 degrees on longitudinal axes so that the elbows project posteriorly.
   a. Lateral and posterior aspects of the arms develop extensor muscles.
   b. Thumbs lie laterally.

3. Lower limbs rotate 90 degrees medially—one to two days behind upper limbs in development.
   a. Knees face medially.
   b. Anterior aspects of the legs develop extensor muscles.

FIGURE 8-2 ■ Drawing illustrating embryologic development of the limbs (32–56 days).

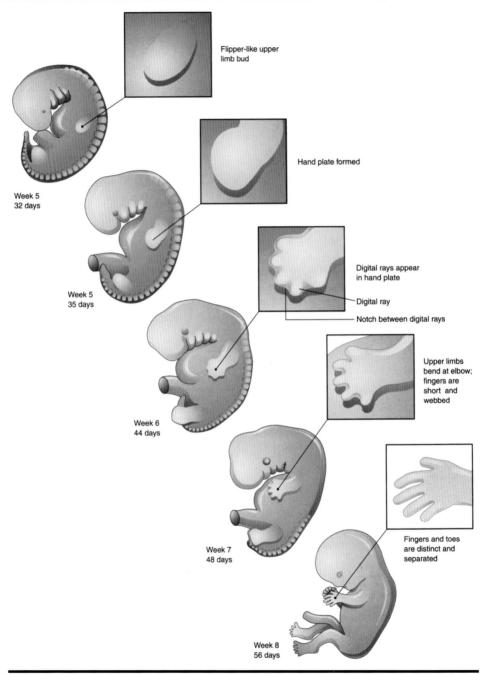

From: Moore KL, and Persaud TVN. 2003. *The Developing Human: Clinically Oriented Embryology,* 7th ed. Philadelphia: Saunders, 413. Reprinted by permission.

    4. Notches appear on the digital rays where fingers will eventually develop.
      a. By the end of week 7, webbed fingers can be seen.
    5. Ossification of the upper limbs begins within the diaphysis of each cartilaginous model.
    6. Fan-shaped feet are visible with toe buds developing into toes.
G. Week 8
    1. All aspects of the limbs have developed, and the first purposeful movements are noted.
    2. Webbing between the fingers disappears, and the fingers lengthen.
    3. Joints begin to resemble those of an adult.[1,3]
    4. Chondrification proceeds, now reaching the distal phalanxes.
    5. Ossification of the lower limbs begins.[1,3]
      a. Bone formation begins at the center of the diaphysis (shaft), the femur.
H. Weeks 9–12
    1. Primary ossification centers can be seen in the skull and long bones.
    2. The upper limbs reach their full length, but the lower limbs have not yet reached their full length.
I. Weeks 13–16
    1. Lower limb length has increased, approaching full relative length.
    2. The foot pronates with a slight degree of metatarsus varus remaining.
    3. Limb movements become more coordinated around 14 weeks, but are still imperceptible to the mother.
    4. Skeletal ossification is ongoing during this period.
J. Weeks 17–20
    1. Fetal movements become evident to the mother.
    2. The limbs achieve their full length.

FORMATION OF BONES AND CARTILAGE[1-5]

A. Bones begin as condensations of mesenchymal cells. Two types of bone development occur.
    1. Intramembranous bone formation. Flat bones form from mesenchyme with preexisting membranous sheaths.
    2. Endochondral bone formation. Limb bones form from cartilage bone models (hyaline cartilage models).
B. Ossification occurs.[1,3]
    1. This begins at the end of the embryonic period (about week 8).[1-3]
    2. There is a high demand for calcium and phosphorus.[1,3]
    3. In the primary ossification centers, bone formation at the center of the diaphysis (shaft) of a long bone appears between 7 and 12 weeks gestation.[1,3]
    4. Secondary ossification centers, located in epiphyses of long bones, are cartilaginous at birth.[1-3]
    5. Bones continue to ossify and grow until completion of growth, when the epiphyses and diaphysis have fused (about 20 years of age) and the epiphyseal plate is replaced by bone development.[1-3]
C. Cartilage develops.[1,3]
    1. Cartilage develops from mesenchyme and appears during the fifth week of life.
    2. Three types of cartilage are formed.
      a. Hyaline cartilage
        1) This is widely distributed in the body.

   2) It is found in the joints.
  b. Fibrocartilage
   1) This makes up the intravertebral discs.
  c. Elastic cartilage
   1) This is found in the auricle of the ear.

Abnormalities of Limb Development

INTRINSIC AND EXTRINSIC LIMB REDUCTION DEFECTS

Definition

"A congenital deficiency of a part of a limb, with at least (part of) a bone structure absent" (p. 243)[6]

Pathophysiology

A. Intrinsic or extrinsic limb reduction defects occur as:[7–9]
   1. Isolated defects, including sporadic, nonhereditary defects
   2. Autosomal dominant inheritance defects
   3. Malformation syndromes
   4. Part of generalized skeletal dysplasia
   5. Constriction band defects
B. Developmental factors include the following:[1,10]
   1. Defects early in gestation are more likely to occur with complex syndromes, involve multiple limbs, and be associated with maternal medical problems.[10]
   2. Middle- or late-stage limb reduction defects are more likely to occur with syndactyly and occur more often in nonwhite infants.[10]
   3. Perinatal complications such as prematurity and low birth weight are associated with any category of defect.[10]
   4. Upper limb defects occur earlier in gestation than lower limb defects.[10]
   5. The most critical time in limb development is 24–36 days after fertilization.[1]
   6. The timing of disturbance in limb development is crucial to determining the characteristics of the defect.[10]
      a. Insults occur most commonly from 3.5 to 8.5 weeks after maternal ovulation.[10]
      b. The majority (81.1 percent) occur between 6 and 7.5 weeks gestation.[1,10]
C. Causes include the following:[9]
   1. Positional limb anomalies resulting from fetal constraint
   2. Vascular disruption—loss of previously normally formed tissue
      a. Extrinsic vascular compression
      b. Intrinsic vascular occlusion
         1) Early amnion rupture

Etiology

A. Risk factors/complications associated with development of limb reduction defects include:[10,11]
   1. Threatened abortion
   2. Family history
   3. Previous malformations
   4. Prematurity or low birth weight
   5. Low placental weight
   6. Maternal influenza early in the pregnancy

7. Alcohol consumption
8. Smoking during pregnancy
9. Chorionic villus sampling prior to ten weeks gestation
10. Thalidomide use
11. Chemotherapy agents
12. Poorly controlled diabetes

Incidence

A. Incidence is difficult to ascertain because a variety of classification systems has been applied to the description of these anomalies.[12]
B. Estimates of the occurrence of limb reduction defects range from 3.9–7/10,000 live births.[6,9,10]

Clinical Presentation[1,9] (See the specific defect presentation in this chapter.)

A. Amelia—absence of limb or limbs[1]
B. Meromelia—partial absence of limb or limbs[1]
C. Variable degree of absence of arterial and nervous structures[7]
D. Shortened or malformed extremity noted with physical examination
E. Varying degrees of elbow, wrist, hand, and thumb function and positioning depending upon defect

Associations

A. Prenatal interventions:
   1. Prenatal use of multivitamins and folic acid is associated with reduced incidence of limb reduction defects.[13,14]
B. Associated syndromes:[6,15]
   1. Fanconi's anemia
   2. Cornelia de Lange
   3. Holt-Oram
   4. Trisomy 18
   5. Thrombocytopenia with absent radius (TAR)
   6. Larsen
   7. Ulnar/radial deficiency
   8. Poland
   9. VACTERL association (an acronym for vertebral defects, imperforate anus, cardiac anomalies, tracheoesophageal fistula, renal dysplasia, limb anomalies)
   10. Trisomy 17
   11. Apert

Differential Diagnosis[6,8]

A. Upper extremity deficiencies
B. Radioulnar synostosis
C. Radial ray defects
D. Ulnar ray defects
E. Constriction rings
F. Radial club hand
G. Apert syndrome[15]
H. Poland syndrome
I. Nager syndrome
J. Holt-Oram syndrome
K. VACTERL association
L. Adams-Oliver syndrome

Diagnosis

A. History
   1. Teratogenic exposure
      a. Thalidomide
      b. Methotrexate
      c. Chemotherapy agents
      d. Alcohol
   2. Evaluation of parents, siblings, and close relatives for similar limb defects
B. Prenatal[16–18]
   1. High-resolution, real-time ultrasonography
   2. May be difficult to diagnose in the first trimester
   3. Easier to diagnose in second and third trimesters, when restriction in motion of the fetal parts is more easily observed
   4. Rate of detection: 18.2 percent[19] (This means that a negative prenatal ultrasound does not guarantee that a fetus is defect free.[20])
C. Physical assessment
   1. Shortened or malformed extremity on examination
   2. Varying degrees of functioning/movement, depending upon the defect
D. Radiodiagnostic studies

Treatment Options and Nursing Care[8]

A. Treatment options are influenced by:
   1. The type and severity of the defect
   2. Associated complications
   3. The functional deficit
B. Treatment is geared toward functional and cosmetic improvement.

Surgical Management—General[8] (See the specific lesion presentation for specific interventions.)

A. Surgical intervention is geared toward functional improvement.
B. It depends upon the severity of the defect.
C. Surgery is seldom an urgent consideration.
D. Soft tissue procedures are done at an earlier age than bone-joint procedures.
E. Bone-joint procedures are best delayed until the child can participate in recovery.
F. Each case is assessed for timing of the surgery.
G. Success includes long-term postoperative supervision and physical therapy.
H. Goals for surgical treatment include:
   1. Promote control for pinch and grasp with an upper limb anomaly.
   2. Improve function.
   3. Promote adequate sensation.
   4. Promote proprioception.
   5. Promote stereognosis.
   6. Address cosmetic issues, including minimizing scarring.

Complications[8]

A. In the immediate postoperative period:
   1. Infection
   2. Swelling
   3. Vascular and neurologic compromise
   4. Loss of joint motion or correction
   5. Neuropraxia

6. Wound necrosis
7. Fixation complications
8. Loss of skin graft

B. Long-term complications as the child grows:
1. Recurrence of wrist flexion
2. Radial deviation deformity
3. Angular deformities
4. Ineffective hand prehension patterns

Postoperative Nursing Care

A. Vital signs
1. Assess every 2–4 hours
   a. Temperature
   b. Heart rate
   c. Respiratory rate
   d. Blood pressure
   e. O_2 saturation

B. Airway management
1. Assess for complications associated with prolonged intubation (due to length of surgery).
   a. Patency of airway
   b. Difficulty extubating
   c. Need for supplemental O_2 via mask or cannula

C. Fluid and electrolyte management
1. Assess for fluid overload in the early postoperative period.

D. Thermoregulation
1. Prevent hypo/hyperthermia.

E. Pain management **(See Chapter 10: Assessment and Management of Postoperative Pain.)**
1. Rate pain with a nonverbal pain scale, dependent upon the age and verbal skill of the child. **(See Appendix E: Infant Pain Scales.)**
2. Assess for signs of pain.
   a. Crying
   b. Grimacing
   c. Irritability
   d. Withdrawal from touch
   e. Altered vital signs
3. Pain management may include the following.
   a. Intravenous (IV) morphine
   b. IV fentanyl
   c. Use of epidural analgesia
4. Pain management goals must be set for postdischarge.
   a. Nonpharmacologic and pharmacologic interventions for home use

F. Assessment of circulation, movement, and sensation in the affected extremity
1. Check circulation every 5–10 minutes initially.
2. Assess every 1–2 hours for 12 hours, then every 4 hours for the following:
   a. Color
   b. Temperature
   c. Capillary refill
   d. Sensation

e. Movement
f. Presence and quality of pulse
3. Complications
a. Impaired circulation
b. Swelling
c. Slippage if in cast
G. Wound care and dressing changes
H. Assessment for signs and symptoms of infection
I. Observation for edema (Position the extremity to promote drainage.)
J. Monitoring for bleeding and/or excessive drainage
K. Parent education
1. Preoperative assessment and teaching
2. Pain management—nonpharmacologic and pharmacologic interventions
3. Skin care—teach parents to assess for:
a. Redness
b. Skin breakdown
1) Edges of the cast
c. Pressure sores
d. Swelling
e. Severe pain
f. Foul odor, drainage, or fever
4. Bathing
5. Dressing
6. Safety
7. Restrictions and adapting routines
8. Promoting normal growth and development
a. Sensory and motor stimulation
b. Sitting and crawling
9. Review of complications
10. Signs and symptoms of infection
a. Possible elevated temperature for the first 48 hours postoperatively
b. Irritability
c. Listlessness
d. Difficulty sleeping
e. Poor feeding
f. Foul odor from incision
11. Follow-up

Outcomes

A. Outcomes are dependent on the defect.
B. Most interventions are geared toward functional and cosmetic improvement, not correction.
C. Depending on the etiology, there is risk of recurrence of the anomaly in a subsequent pregnancy.

FIGURE 8-3 ■ Intrauterine pregnancy prior to tear in amnion.

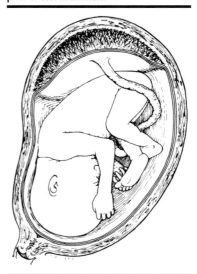

From: Turner BS. 1985. Amniotic band syndrome. *Journal of Obstetric, Gynecologic, and Neonatal Nursing* 14(4): 299. Reprinted by permission.

FIGURE 8-4 ■ Fetal fingers protruding through tear in amnion.

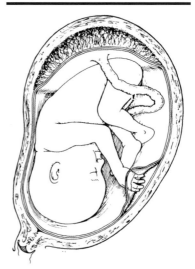

From: Turner BS. 1985. Amniotic band syndrome. *Journal of Obstetric, Gynecologic, and Neonatal Nursing* 14(4): 299. Reprinted by permission.

Amniotic Band Syndrome

Definition

This uncommon complex of physical defects is caused by physical constraint on limb development, usually after normal formation.[16] It is associated with the following synonyms and acronyms:[16] constriction band syndrome, Streeter dysplasia, Simonart bands, congenital ring constriction, ADAM (an acronym for **a**mniotic **d**eformity, **a**dhesions, **m**utilations), and TEARS (an acronym for **t**he **e**arly **a**mnion **r**upture **s**pectrum).

Pathophysiology[17,21]

A. The amnion ruptures and separates from the chorion during pregnancy (Figures 8-3–8-5).
B. Rupture of the amnion causes fluid to escape and increases pressure on the chorion.
 1. This increased pressure may result in further separation of the amnion and chorion and compression of the fetus and fetal parts.
C. Fetal parts or the complete fetus may exit the amnion and enter the chorionic cavity and become entangled.
D. Bands are short and fine with early rupture.
 1. Defects may be severe.
 2. Defects may be due to compression or adherence to the amnion rather than bands.
E. Bands are stronger and longer with a rupture later in pregnancy.
 1. Cause greater damage
 2. Exert greater pressure around extremity
 3. Usually restricted to extremity

Etiology

A. Whether the pathogenesis of amniotic band syndrome results from intrinsic causes (pathogenic mechanism)[22,23] or from extrinsic events (family susceptibility, insult compromises vascular integrity) is controversial.[9,16,24,25] The syndrome likely results from a multifactorial process. Theories proposed to explain the defects associated with amniotic band syndrome include:[15,16,21–25]
 1. Intrinsic disruptions in embryonic morphogenesis
 2. Mechanical deformations caused by early rupture of the amnion
 3. Deformations caused by vascular compromise and secondary disruption of normally developing structures
B. The theory of early amniotic rupture, first proposed during the nineteenth century, still receives the most support in the scientific literature.[16,22,25]
 1. As restated by Torpin in 1968, a tear occurs in the amnion at some point during gestation, allowing passage of fluid between the amnion and chorion.[25]
 2. Separation of the amnion and chorion, with loss of amniotic fluid, results in secondary oligohydramnios and compression of the fetus.

FIGURE 8-5 ■ Fingers entrapped in amnion bands.

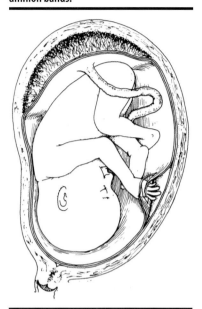

From: Turner BS. 1985. Amniotic band syndrome. *Journal of Obstetric, Gynecologic, and Neonatal Nursing* 14(4): 299. Reprinted by permission.

3. Tearing of membranes creates fibrous strands that entangle fetal parts.
4. The fetus (or fetal parts) may escape through the tears in the amnion and become caught where the rupture occurred.
5. Early rupture of the amnion results in bands that are short and fine, so small fetal parts are trapped.[17,21,25] These types of bands can cause compression injuries to fingers or toes, pseudosyndactyly, or actual amputation.
6. Rupture later in the pregnancy may result in longer, stronger bands capable of exerting greater force on fetal extremities, causing greater damage.[17,21]

FIGURE 8-6 ■ **Comparison of constriction band images.**

A. Two-dimensional ultrasound image. B. Three-dimensional surface-rendered image. C. Photograph at birth of the constriction band. Arrows indicate the site of the constriction in A and B. Note the minus posture of the hand in B.

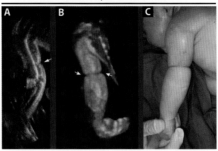

From: Paladini D, et al. 2004. Congenital constriction band of the upper arm: The role of three-dimensional ultrasound in diagnosis, counseling, and multidisciplinary consultation. *Ultrasound in Obstetrics and Gynecology* 23(5): 521. Copyright John Riley and Sons, Ltd. Reprinted by permission.

Incidence

A. The incidence of amniotic band syndrome is unclear because of misdiagnosis.
B. Limb reduction defects with amniotic or constriction bands are more likely to occur between 6.6 and 7.5 postovulatory weeks.[1,10]
C. It occurs anywhere from 1/1,200–15,000 live births. The incidence appears to be increasing.
D. Occurrence is sporadic; it is not usually associated with genetic or chromosomal disorders.[16]
E. It more commonly occurs in infants of young, African-American multigravidas.
F. Malformations of the hand are twice as common as those involving the foot.
G. Recurrence in siblings is very low.
H. It is more frequent in monozygotic twins.[17]

Clinical Presentation[16]

A. This is a result of external compression and/or disruption.
B. No two anomalies are alike.
C. Internal anomalies are not known to occur simultaneously.
D. Features on external examination are usually the only abnormalities.
E. The most common manifestations include:
1. Distal ring constriction
2. Intrauterine amputation
3. Acrosyndactyly—most common finding in distal aspects of extremities
4. Syndactyly
5. Progressive lymphedema
6. Limb length discrepancies
7. Phalangeal hypoplasia
8. Umbilical cord constriction

Associations

A. Familial associations are rare[16]

B. Deformational defects secondary to decreased movement, tethering, or constraint[26]

1. Scoliosis
2. Foot abnormalities
3. Necrosis
4. Edema
5. Resorptive necrosis

C. Robin sequence[17]

D. Connective tissue disorders[17]

E. Increased incidence in mothers who have discontinued use of oral contraceptives within one month of conception[27]

F. Significant abdominal trauma

Differential Diagnosis

A. Limb-body wall complex[26,28]

1. Defects involving facial clefts and thoraco- and/or abdominoschisis, exencephaly/encephalocele, also associated with amelia, sirenomelia, limb disruptions, or amputations
2. Incorrectly attributed to amniotic band syndrome
3. Thought to occur as a result of flawed lateral and caudal folding of the embryonic disc resulting in retention of the extraembryonic coelom (Amnion is continuous with the edge of the defect, resulting in limb malformations similar to amniotic band syndrome.)
4. High incidence of associated anomalies of internal organs

Diagnosis

A. Prenatal[16–18,29]

1. High-resolution, real-time ultrasonography (Figure 8-6) is useful.
   a. Two-dimensional
   b. Three-dimensional[29]
2. Bands are difficult to diagnose in the first trimester, especially if they are limited to the extremities.
3. Bands are easier to diagnose in the second and third trimesters, when restriction in motion of the fetal parts is more easily observed.
4. Visualization of bands is not in and of itself diagnostic of amniotic band syndrome.
5. The rate of detection for limb reduction defects is 18.2 percent.[19] This means a negative prenatal ultrasound does not guarantee that a fetus is defect free.[20]
6. So-called amniotic sheets or innocent bands have been described. These strands or sheets of tissue originating in the amnion and chorion have a free end and do not restrict the growth or movement of the fetus.[16,17]
7. The advantage of a prenatal diagnosis, when it can be made, is that parents have more time to make informed decisions regarding their child.

Treatment Options and Nursing Care

A. Treatment depends on the severity of the defect(s).

1. Two classification systems describe manifestations of amniotic band syndrome.
   a. Hall classification system[30]

1) Mild constriction (no lymphedema present)
2) Moderate constriction (lymphedema present)
3) Severe constriction (amputation)
   b. Weinzweig classification system[31]
1) Stage 1—mild constriction (no lymphedema present)
2) Stage 2a—moderate constriction with:
   a) Distal deformity syndactyly *or*
   b) Discontinuous neurovascular or musculotendinous components
   c) No vascular compromise or lymphedema present
3) Stage 2b—same as Stage 2a, with lymphedema present
4) Stage 3a—severe constriction with progressive lymphaticovenous or interference in arterial blood flow, but without soft tissue damage
5) Stage 3b—same as Stage 3a, with soft tissue damage present
6) Stage 4—constriction deep enough to cause intrauterine amputation
B. Prenatal intervention may be possible.
   1. There are reports of successful lysis of constriction bands *in utero*.[32]
   2. Fetoscopic laser release *in utero* may prevent limb amputation.[33]

Surgical Management

A. Surgical corrections require the release of both deep and superficial structures.[16,31,34–36]
   1. Fibrous bands around fingers or toes may be unwound and removed.
   2. Indentations or deep grooves in the soft tissues are treated by excising the bands and recontouring the tissue (Figure 8-7–8-9).
      a. Z- or W-plasty techniques refer to the shape of the incision or skin flap, combined with tissue debulking when necessary.
      b. These allow lengthwise expansion of the surgical scar.

FIGURE 8-7 ■ Deep constriction band.

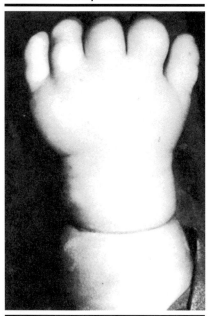

From: Di Meo L, and Mercer DH. 1987. Single-stage correction of constriction ring syndrome. *Annals of Plastic Surgery* 19(5): 470. Reprinted by permission.

FIGURE 8-8 ■ Circumferential excision and multiple Z-plasty repair in a single stage.

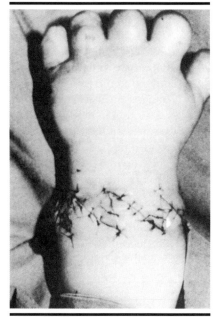

From: Di Meo L, and Mercer DH. 1987. Single-stage correction of constriction ring syndrome. *Annals of Plastic Surgery* 19(5): 470. Reprinted by permission.

3. Amputation of the limb is recommended when band constriction results in:
   a. Gross motor and sensory deficits
   b. Vascular compromise
   c. Infection (osteomyelitis)[16]
4. Syndactyly may occur in amniotic band syndrome.[34]
   a. It is usually the result of distal binding of adjacent digits (acrosyndactyly).
   b. It is characterized by the presence of an interdigital sinus.
   c. The sinus is excised when the adjacent digits are released. Grafting may be required.
   d. Release will increase the functional length of the digits and improve their independent function.
B. Surgeries are staged to avoid vascular embarrassment to the distal segment of the limb.
   1. A single-stage correction of constriction bands is used to avoid the need for multiple surgeries in infants.
   2. Whether the correction is done in a single-stage procedure or in multiple stages depends on the nature of the constriction and the presence of sepsis, lymphedema, or neuropathy.
C. Several factors affect the decision regarding the timing and number of operations.
   1. Soft tissue procedures tend to be performed early.
   2. Procedures involving bone are done later.
   3. Defects involving the hand are usually corrected before the child's first birthday because hand prehension patterns develop by the end of the first year.[8]

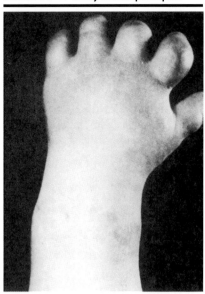

FIGURE 8-9 ■ Thirty months postrepair.

From: Di Meo L, and Mercer DH. 1987. Single-stage correction of constriction ring syndrome. *Annals of Plastic Surgery* 19(5): 470. Reprinted by permission.

Complications

A. Scar deformity
B. Loss of the skin graft
C. Failure to achieve satisfactory correction
D. Neurologic and/or vascular compromise
E. Infection
F. Loss of joint motion or correction
G. Severe swelling
H. Tissue necrosis

Postoperative Nursing Care

See Postoperative Nursing Care in INTRINSIC AND EXTRINSIC LIMB REDUCTION DEFECTS at the beginning of this chapter.

Outcomes

A. There is a small risk of recurrence of amniotic band syndrome in a subsequent pregnancy.[6,16]

   1. The risk is very low in siblings of the affected infant. Karyotypes of affected children are almost always normal.

   2. Any rare familial associations are probably due to chance and not likely to recur in subsequent children.

ABSENT RADIUS

Definition

A very rare condition where there is nondevelopment of the radius

Pathophysiology

A. The radial ray consists of the following.

   1. Radius

   2. Scaphoid bone

   3. Trapezium

   4. First metacarpal bone

   5. Two phalanges of the thumb

B. The radius provides the main support for the hand.

   1. When it is absent or deficient, the wrist deviates radially toward the forearm, resulting in a deformity called clubhand.[7,8]

   2. The severity of the deformity depends on the amount of radial deficiency present.[8]

C. Radial dysplasia can be categorized into four types.[8]

   1. Type I—short distal radius

     a. There is good support for the thumb and little deformity.

     b. Elbow function is generally normal.

   2. Type II—hypoplastic distal radius

     a. Growth was abnormal at both the proximal and distal epiphyses.

     b. The ulna is thick and bowed toward the radial side.

   3. Type III—partial absence of the radius

     a. The radius may be absent in the proximal, middle, or distal ends.

     b. The hand is unsupported and deviated toward the radius.

   4. Type IV—absent radius

     a. This is the most common manifestation of the defect.

     b. The hand is completely unsupported; the ulna is bowed and thickened.

     c. The elbow may be rigid.

     d. The infant may present severe deficiencies of the thumb.

Etiology

A. Results from failure of the mesenchymal primordium of the radius to form

B. Occurs during the fifth week of gestation

C. Usually caused by genetic factors

FIGURE 8-10 ■ Congenital absence of the radius.

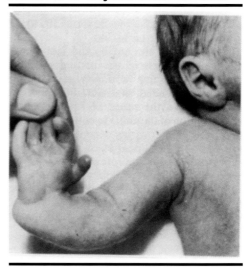

From: Griffin PP, and Robertson WW Jr. 1999. Orthopedics. In *Neonatology: Pathophysiology and Management of the Newborn*, 5th ed., Avery GB, Fletcher MA, and MacDonald MG, eds. Philadelphia: Lippincott Williams & Wilkins, 1273. Reprinted by permission.

Incidence[8]

A. Radial clubhand occurs in approximately 1/100,000 live births.

B. It occurs spontaneously and in association with different syndromes, some genetic.

C. The defect is bilateral in 50 percent of cases.

D. When it occurs unilaterally, it affects the right side more often than the left.

E. Both males and females are equally affected.

Clinical Presentation

A. The radius is partially or completely absent (Figure 8-10).[1]

B. The hand deviates laterally.[1]

C. The ulna bows on the lateral side of the arm because of the concavity.[1]

D. Arterial and nervous system structures are absent to a variable degree.[8]

E. Ulnar muscles are deficient or absent.

F. Radial forearm flexor and extensor muscles are severely affected.[7]

G. The thumb is unstable or absent.

Associations[26,37]

A. Associations with autosomal recessive syndromes include:
1. TAR[26,38,39]
2. Fanconi pancytopenia (also referred to as Fanconi's anemia)[26]
3. Roberts/SC phocomelia
4. Baller-Gerold
5. Aase
6. Seckel

B. Associations with autosomal dominant syndromes include:[37]
1. Holt-Oram
2. Levy Hollister
3. Nager

C. Radial dysplasia also occurs sporadically with:[28,37]
1. VACTERL association
2. Fetal valproate
3. Cat's eye
4. Trisomy 13 and trisomy 18

D. Unlike limb reduction defects caused by amniotic band syndrome, anomalies seen with syndromes associated with radial ray defects complicate the prognosis for affected children.[26,37]

Differential Diagnosis

A. Radial ray defects

B. Ulnar ray defects

C. Radioulnar synostosis

D. Short distal radius

E. Hypoplastic distal radius

F. Partial absence of the radius

Diagnosis[37,38]

A. Radial dysplasia can be diagnosed prenatally through ultrasonography.

B. A careful family history is taken, noting any family members with similar limb anomalies.

C. Physical assessment may reveal the following.
1. The hand inclines toward the forearm if left unsupported—clubhand.

2. The ulna is thick and bowed toward the radial side.
3. There is abnormal growth of the affected arm.
4. The elbow may be rigid.
5. There may be deficiencies of the thumb.
   a. Absent
   b. Unsupported
D. Genetic testing may reveal the following.[37,38]
   1. Autosomal dominant disorders like Holt-Oram syndrome carry a high risk of transmission to subsequent offspring.
   2. Autosomal recessive disorders like TAR syndrome and Fanconi's anemia may be mistaken for other conditions with radial defects, including the VACTERL association.
   3. The presence of hematologic changes and increased chromosomal breakage can differentiate Fanconi anemia from other syndromes.

Treatment Options and Nursing Care

A. Treatment is influenced by several factors.[8,15]
   1. The presence of complicating factors
   2. The age of the child
   3. Severity of the defect
   4. Any functional deficit
B. The first option is no treatment. This would be considered in the following cases.
   1. The child is older, has accepted the defect, and has compensated accordingly.
   2. There is adequate length of the radius and support of the hand for functional use of the limb.
   3. The radial defect is complicated by a fixed elbow and not amenable to treatment.
   4. Associated anomalies are incompatible with long-term survival.
C. Casts and splints may be useful for children with mild defects and soft tissue contractures.
D. The use of prosthetics in children is a possibility.[15,40]
   1. Because both amniotic band syndrome and radial ray defects can result in congenital absence or surgical loss of part or all of a limb, some children benefit from a prosthetic device.
   2. Consideration of prosthetics is unlikely to occur during the immediate neonatal period; however, for the following reasons, NICU nurses should be aware that these options exist.
      a. To help parents with anticipatory guidance
      b. To assist with referrals to other health care professionals
      c. To help plan and promote optimal achievement of developmental milestones
         1) Infants who lack functional upper limbs cannot develop motor skills normally.
         2) The infant will not be able to crawl, and the development of elevation activities such as pushing to sit or pulling to stand will be affected without prosthetic assistance.
   3. Children with lower limb defects tend to benefit from prostheses more than children with upper limb defects.[39-41]

4. Controversy exists regarding the use of cosmetic versus functional prosthetics.
    a. Many children with partial absence/loss of a limb do better with adaptive devices because the defect involves weakness of upper body musculature.
    b. When the device is appropriate, the child should be fitted with a prosthesis at the earliest possible developmental stage in order to match motor readiness.
5. Myoelectric and externally powered prosthetic devices may be appropriate.[42–44]
    a. These are used with greater frequency and with greater success in younger and younger children.
    b. Children less than two years of age have been successfully fitted with electric prosthetic devices.

Surgical Management

A. Surgery should be considered for:
1. Children who lack sufficient support for the hand
2. Children with thumb and/or finger deformities
3. Children with soft tissue contractures that cannot be treated with casting or splinting
B. Treatment of the radial defect should be initiated early in the neonatal period for best results.[8]
1. Serial stretching and casting of the limb improve alignment of the bones.
2. External fixation devices are used to facilitate soft tissue stretching and lengthening.
3. Surgery to centralize the hand over the ulna is delayed until the infant is about six months old.
4. Multiple procedures may be required to correct defects to the thumb or improve function of the hand.

Complications

A. Failure to achieve a satisfactory correction
B. Loss of joint motion or correction
C. Vascular or neurologic compromise caused by swelling or infection
D. Fixation complications
E. Residual ulnar distortion
F. Severe swelling
G. Infection as a result of skin necrosis or wire fixation
H. Wires that break or slide out

Postoperative Nursing Care

See Postoperative Nursing Care in INTRINSIC AND EXTRINSIC LIMB REDUCTION DEFECTS at the beginning of this chapter.

Outcomes

A. Prognosis varies according to the disorder involved.
B. Radial clubhand may recur after surgery related to technical difficulties of the surgery.

TALIPES EQUINOVARUS (CLUBFOOT)

Definition

A. A congenital condition of the foot and ankle characterized by (Figure 8-11):[45–47]

   1. Adducted forefoot—forefoot curls toward heel
   2. Hindfoot varus—heel turns inward
   3. Ankle equinus—foot points downward and entire foot is rotated upward (supinated)

B. Includes deformities of soft tissue structures and multiple bone abnormalities described according to the position of the foot[45]

FIGURE 8-11 ■ Deformities of talipes equinovarus.

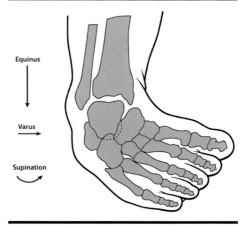

Illustration by Briar Lee Mitchell.

Pathophysiology

A. History

   1. Documented cases of clubfoot date back to ancient civilization, including drawings and writing of the nineteenth dynasty pharaoh, Siphtah, circa 1300 BC, and Ajur-Veda, circa 1000 BC.[48]
   2. The Chinese tradition of foot binding caused development of clubfoot.[49]
   3. Hippocrates (460–377 BC) discussed clubfoot and other congenital orthopedic conditions in his writing.[48,50]
      a. He first described the difference between congenital and acquired clubfoot and proposed that the deformity was caused by intrauterine pressure and rapid skeletal growth.
      b. He recommended early treatment using repeated manipulation and bandaging.
   4. In the late 1800s in the U.S., manipulation and bandaging were routine practice.[48]
   5. In 1939, Kite published nonoperative methods to correct clubfoot, including the following.[51]
      a. Shaping
      b. Taping
      c. Wedging
      d. Casting
   6. In 1971, Turco reported on an operative procedure known as "one-stage posteromedial soft tissue release with internal fixation" (p. 477). This continues to be the basic surgical treatment of choice.[52]

B. Structure

   1. There is an abnormal relationship of tarsal bones, with a medial displacement of the navicular and calcaneus around the talus (Figure 8-12).
   2. The expression of the deformity is dependent on the severity of articular malalignment.

3. Soft tissues (muscles, tendons, tendon sheaths, ligaments, and joint capsules) on the medial plantar, subtalar, posterior, and plantar aspects of the foot, ankle, and distal leg may be hypertrophied, contracted, fibrosed, or shortened.
   a. These affect the position and rigidity of the foot and may impact resistance to anatomic reduction and correction.[48,53–55]
   b. Soft tissues are often stretched tight on the lateral side of the ankle and foot and contracted on the medial side.[45]

FIGURE 8-12 ■ Normal and talipes equinovarus (clubfoot) structure.

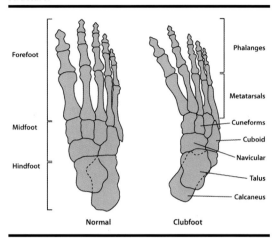

Illustration by Briar Lee Mitchell.

4. Vimentin and microfibroblast-like cells in the thick, tight, and shortened medial and posterior tarsal ligaments play a role in both the pathogenesis and relapse of the deformity.[56]
   a. Shortening and fibrosis are also seen in the posterior tibial muscle and the gastrocsoleus and their respective tendons.[57]
5. Osseous structures, such as the talus, are reduced in size with malalignment and angulation in a plantar-medial direction.[48]
   a. The talus is anteriorly positioned out of the ankle mortise, and plantar fixed.[48]
6. Malrotation of talocrural, talocalcaneal, talonavicular, and calcaneocuboid joints also occurs.[48]
7. The Achilles tendon is contracted.[48]
8. The calcaneus bone is shortened and flattened.[45,51]
9. The calf muscles are shortened and underdeveloped, with generalized muscle atrophy.[47]
10. Soft tissues, including blood vessels, nerves, and skin, are shortened on medial and posterior aspects of the foot.[45]
C. Smaller affected leg and foot in a unilateral presentation[45,47]
D. Categories[46,58,59]
   1. Mild—the positional disorder resulting from intrauterine positioning
      a. The foot is flexible and easily manipulated into a straight position.[47]
      b. The heel of the foot is normal in size and appearance.
      c. Calf and leg atrophy are minimal or nonexistent.[60]
      d. This resolves spontaneously or with the application of serial casts or passive exercises beginning after birth and continuing until overcorrection is achieved.
   2. Tetralogic—associated with other conditions
      a. The deformity is often severe and resistant to treatment.
      b. It recurs after initial correction.

3. Idiopathic—true clubfoot or talipes equinovarus (Figure 8-13)
   a. The foot is rigid and cannot be easily manually realigned to a normal position.[47]
   b. This may require nonoperative and operative intervention to correct.

Etiology

A. Exact cause unknown
B. Influence of multifactorial genetics, environmental factors, and polygenic mode of inheritance[45,46,61-63]
   1. Nongenetic causes may include the following.
      a. Amniotic bands
      b. Drug exposure
      c. Small uterine cavity causing compression
      d. Paralysis of mother[61]
      e. Oligohydramnios[64]
   2. There are at least six well-established proposed theories of etiology.[48]
      a. Chromosomal
         1) The defect is in the unfertilized germ cell and exists before fertilization.
         2) The head and neck of the talus are affected.[65-67]
      b. Embryonic (primary germ plasm defect)[47,67-69]
         1) The defect occurs after fertilization, within the first 12 weeks of fetal development.
         2) The malformation is in the cartilaginous anlage of the tarsal bones.
      c. Otogenic (arrested skeletal and soft tissue development)
         1) The result of a temporary arrest of normal fetal development in the fibular phase by an intrauterine environmental factor
            a) Arrest during seven to eight weeks gestation results in a markedly rigid clubfoot.
            b) Arrest during 9 to 12 weeks gestation results in a mild to moderately flexible clubfoot.[70-72]
      d. Neurogenic (neuromuscular dysfunction)[47,73-77]
         1) A defect in neurogenic tissue creates the predominance of Type I muscle fibers (slow twitch, high tension, tonic fiber) and an increase in the total number of muscle fibers.
         2) This leads to contractile imbalances, which cause a collapsing deformity of the foot in which bony changes are secondary.
      e. Myogenic (muscle abnormalities)[53-55,77]
         1) This defect in muscle and connective tissue (myofibroblast-like cells) causes an imbalance between the muscle on the posterior medial aspect of the foot and the muscles on the lateral side of the foot.
         2) This pulls the forefoot and midfoot into an equinovarus position.
      f. Vascular[47,78-80]
         1) Absence or underdevelopment of the dorsalis pedis and anterior tibial arteries results in medial foot and ankle tethering.

FIGURE 8-13 ■ Congenital idiopathic talipes equinovarus (clubfoot).

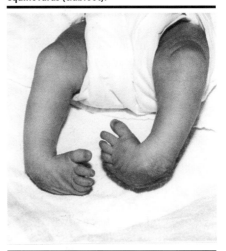

Courtesy of Carol Trotter, St. John's Mercy Medical Center, St. Louis, Missouri.

2) Blockage of one or more arterial branches at the level of the sinus tarsi diminishes blood flow and increases tissue damage in early fetal development.

Incidence

A. 1–3/1,000 live births[45,46,48,61,81,82]

B. Ethnicity[48,60,83]

1. Asian
   a. Lowest incidence at 0.57/1,000 live births
2. Hawaiian/Polynesian descent
   a. Highest incidence at 6.8/1,000 live births
3. South African black
   a. 3.5/1,000 live births
4. Caucasian
   a. 1–5/1,000 live births

C. Male to female predominance: 2–2.5 to 1[48]

D. Bilateral involvement in 50 percent of cases

E. Previous child with this defect: Increases the probability (3–4 percent) of having a second child with the defect

F. A parent with a clubfoot: One in ten chance of having a child with this disorder[46]

Clinical Presentation

A. There are several characteristic deformities of idiopathic clubfoot.[45–48]

1. Metatarsus adductus—adducted forefoot (turns toward heel)
2. Inverted hindfoot ([varus] occurs in talocalcaneonavicular joint)—heel turns inward
3. Ankle equinus (midfoot points downward)—entire foot rotated upward
4. Talocalcaneonavicular subluxation
5. Lateral rotation of the talus in the ankle mortise (often smaller with the head deviated medially)

Associations

A. Disorders classified as tetralogic are associated with other conditions such as:[76]

1. Myelodysplasia (defective spinal cord development)
2. Arthrogryposis multiplex congenita (joint remains in fixed position due to muscular contraction or adhesions)
3. Cerebral palsy
4. Neuropathies
5. Chromosomal anomalies
6. Freeman-Sheldon syndrome
7. Diastrophic dwarfism
8. Larson syndrome

Differential Diagnosis

A. Postural clubfoot deformity
1. This resolves spontaneously or with application of a series of casts.

B. Teratologic foot deformity
1. Associated syndromes and diagnoses must be ruled out before a diagnosis of idiopathic clubfoot can be made.
2. Teratologic foot deformity is difficult to treat.
3. There is a high incidence of recurrence with teratologic deformity.

Diagnosis

A. History
1. Prenatal history, family history
2. Pregnancy, labor, and delivery history
3. Medical history
4. Deformity, presentation, and any prior treatment
B. Physical assessment[48]
1. Evaluate within 24–48 hours of birth.
2. Perform a musculoskeletal examination.
   a. Examine the following.
      1) Foot
      2) Skin
      3) Muscles
      4) Degree of flexibility
      5) Back
      6) Hips
   b. A thorough hip evaluation should be done.
      1) Ultrasound is the method of choice for infants <3 months of age.[83,84]
3. Assess for the following.
   a. Sacral abnormalities
   b. Muscle tone
   c. Motor function
   d. Sensation
   e. Reflex activity
   f. Motion
   g. Gait (if appropriate)
4. Check angular measurements.
5. Classify the deformity based on its cause and nature.
6. Determine and initiate treatment.
C. Radiographic evaluation
1. This can show the type and degree of articular alignments (Figures 8-14 and 8-15).[46,56]
2. Not every deformity is visible because of the degree of ossification in infancy.
D. Limited application in diagnosis[48]
1. Tomography
2. Arthrography
3. Three-dimensional CAT modeling
4. Magnetic resonance imaging (MRI)[48]

Treatment Options and Nursing Care

A. Early evaluation and initiation of treatment (24–48 hours after birth)[48,61,76]
1. The goal of treatment is to reduce or eliminate deformity so that the infant will have a functional, pain-free, plantigrade foot with good mobility.

FIGURE 8-14 ■ X-ray showing normal angle (approximately 30–35 degrees) and orientation of the talus and calcaneus.

The foot was inadvertently positioned into a slight hyperflexion posture.

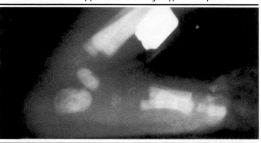

From: Swischuk LE. 2004. *Imaging of the Newborn, Infant, and Young Child,* 5th ed. Philadelphia: Lippincott Williams & Wilkins, 757. Reprinted by permission..

B. Serial manipulation and casting to midthigh[48,51,62]

1. Ligaments and soft tissues are pliable and easy to stretch in the first few weeks.

2. Manipulation is stretching performed with intermittent application of gentle but firm force over 10–15 minutes prior to casting. Casting is done after the correct position is achieved.[48]

3. Maintain serial manipulation and casting to gently elongate ligaments, tendon sheaths, capsules, and other soft tissues around the joint to reduce subluxation in talocalcaneal and midtarsal joints.

4. Maintain the foot in proper position in the cast until the foot has grown enough for surgical intervention.

5. Manipulation and serial casting is done weekly for the first one to two months, then every 10–14 days until two to three months of age.

6. Clinical and radiographic evaluation is done at three months of age.

   a. If the reduction is satisfactory, the foot is held in an overcorrected position (so it will stay in the corrected position without a cast) with a series of casts that are changed periodically for six to eight months to allow for maximum correction.[55]

C. Ponseti casting technique[82,85–93]

1. This nonsurgical technique has a high reported success rate (90 percent) without posteromedial release (PMR) surgery necessary.[85]

2. It uses gentle manipulation followed by several basic long-leg cast types. Each cast has a specific purpose, with the number of casts varying by response.[57,83,85–87]

3. It is believed that this method of correction reverses the order of the formation of the deformity *in utero,* with the correction of the equinus last.[57]

4. This casting technique proceeds as follows.[57]

   a. The first cast attempts to correct pronation of the first metatarsal and cavus together with the adduction, by supinating and abducting the forefoot to bring it into proper alignment with the hindfoot.

   b. Weekly manipulations of the foot are done to promote proper alignment of the foot and bones (specific to the Ponseti method).[57]

   c. Well-molded, plaster, toe-to-groin casts are applied weekly after manipulations.

      1) These increase the amounts of abduction to achieve maximal correction of 70 degrees.

      2) Four to seven long-leg casts are usually sufficient to maintain correction.

   d. Heel varus is corrected after the entire foot is fully abducted under the talus.

      1) There is no direct manipulation of the calcaneus.

      2) The heel is not touched.

FIGURE 8-15 ■ X-ray lateral view shows that the angle between the talus and calcaneus is retained or slightly increased in the metatarsus varus deformity.

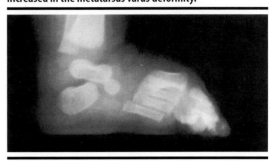

From: Swischuk LE. 2004. *Imaging of the Newborn, Infant, and Young Child,* 5th ed. Philadelphia: Lippincott Williams & Wilkins, 758. Reprinted by permission.

      e. The last cast involves correcting the equinus (inability to dorsiflex at the ankle) by dorsiflexing the foot.

         1) A percutaneous tenotomy of the Achilles tendon may be necessary to facilitate this position. (This may be done as an outpatient procedure in the physician's office.)

         2) The foot is kept in this position (70 degrees of abduction and 20 degrees of ankle dorsiflexion) for three weeks to allow healing.

         3) During this time, the tendon regenerates to the proper length without scarring.

         4) When treatment occurs shortly after birth, the infant is out of casts in approximately two months.[90]

      f. The final phase involves foot abduction orthosis with straight-laced shoes and foot abduction bar (Denis Browne style bar without Denis Browne plates) set at 30 degrees of outward rotation and neutral dorsiflexion for the normal foot and 70 degrees of outward rotation and 15 degrees of dorsiflexion for the clubfoot.

         1) These shoes are worn full-time for three months.

         2) The bar is kept in place at night and during naps until the child is two to four years of age.

         3) The last two interventions are crucial to avoid relapse of the treated foot. Failure is attributed to noncompliance with the use of the orthosis after correction has been obtained.[88,89]

         4) Infants with very loose ligaments should have the abduction bar removed shortly after walking commences to prevent overcorrection.

      g. MRI evaluations show marked improvement or complete correction of the following, thought to be due to changes in the mechanical loading of fast-growing tissues.[57]

         1) Abnormal relationships

         2) Abnormal shapes of tarsal bones

D. Physical therapy

  1. Various methods of manipulation of the foot (Bensahel, Dimeglio) are performed by a physical therapist with splinting between treatments.

  2. Therapy is continued for months with limited success.

    a. The need for surgery is not necessarily eliminated.[94–96]

E. Bivalved casts

  1. Denis Browne (D-Bar) splint with attached open toe tarso pronator shoes to maintain correction (Figure 8-16).

    a. This is worn 24 hours a day, removed for exercises.

    b. It is used until replaced by prewalker-type, straight-laced shoes once walking. The D-Bar is then used at nap time and nighttime.

    c. The child is evaluated at frequent intervals for several years (up to age seven) to make certain the correction is maintained.[55]

F. Botulinum toxin type A (BTXA [Botox])[97–99]

  1. Derived from bacterium *Clostridium botulinum*

  2. Injected into the gastrocnemius soleus and/or posterior tibial muscles[97]

  3. Injected into the triceps surae muscle complex at hindfoot stall to relax the function[98]

  4. Causes reversible muscle denervation by blocking release of acetylcholine at the neuromuscular junction[100]

5. Leads to muscle relaxation and reduction in tone, which may facilitate the lengthening achieved by manipulative stretching

6. Concurrent physical therapy with daily manipulation:
   a. Positive changes in growing muscle
   b. May reduce the need for ongoing management or surgical correction

7. May require reinjection after three to four months

8. Standardized pediatric dose of BTXA not yet established
   a. Doses ranging from 5 to 15 units/kg in the pediatric population have been reported in the literature.[97–99,101–103]
   b. The Spasticity Study Group recommends 10 IU/kg.[99]
   c. The total dose is divided equally between legs in patients with bilateral clubfeet.

9. Considerations when determining the appropriate dose to be given:[97]
   a. Weight
   b. Age
   c. Muscle size
   d. Response to dose

FIGURE 8-16 ■ Denis Browne splint.

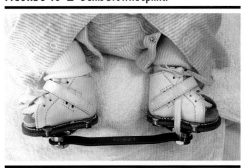

From: Hart ES. 2003. Pediatric orthopaedic ailments: Clubfoot (talipes equinovarus). Boston: Massachusetts General Hospital. Retrieved September 16, 2005, from http://www.mgh.harvard.edu/ortho/clubfoot.htm. Reprinted by permission.

Surgical Management

A. Soft tissue release may be done.
   1. This procedure is performed if there is no improvement either clinically or on radiographic evaluation after one month of manipulation and casting.
   2. Serial casting is done prior to surgery to maintain the foot in optimal position.
   3. Procedures may involve releasing or lengthening tight, deformed, soft tissue structures as well as tendon transfers to remove deforming forces or correct muscle imbalances.[59]

B. The preferred timing of the release varies.
   1. Early soft tissue release[57,59,104,105]
      a. Early surgery necessitates a thorough comprehension of pathoanatomy and meticulous surgical technique to prevent excessive scarring and damage to cartilage.
      b. Some practitioners recommend release between 3 and 6 months or "late" between 9 and 12 months.[57] Others use a foot size of 8 cm or larger as one of the criteria.[105–107]
      c. Proponents of early surgery argue that there is a great deal of growth and remodeling potential in the first year of life.[57]
   2. Complete soft tissue release between one and two years of age
      a. Turco recommends one-stage soft tissue posteromedial release later, with use of a D-Bar splint as the holding device prior to surgery to prevent increasing deformity.[55,108]

    b. Turco reports a higher incidence of operative failure when operative treatment is performed at an earlier age.

      1) The small size of the foot means loss of correction in plaster is more likely to occur following removal of internal fixation.

      2) Overcorrection is more likely to occur due to growth.

      3) Tarsal remodeling is stimulated by weight bearing in older children.

      4) There is a greater likelihood of treating an unrecognized nonidiopathic clubfoot that could have been treated nonsurgically.[108]

Complications[47,109,110]

A. Vascular compromise

B. Neuromuscular impairment

C. Excessive bleeding

D. Infection

E. Wound dehiscence

F. Overcorrection of clubfoot

G. Injury to vascular bundle

H. Recurrence of deformity

I. Long-term complications[51,111]

    1. Stiffness and weakness leading to premature arthritis of the foot

    2. Reduced ankle plantar flexion motion

    3. Diminished push-off strength

Postoperative Nursing Care

A. See Postoperative Nursing Care under Intrinsic and Extrinsic Limb Reduction Defects at the beginning of this chapter.

B. Position

    1. Elevate the extremity for 24–48 hours.

    2. Position the infant so pressure points do not cause indentations in the wet cast.

    3. Reposition the infant every two to four hours to help prevent pressure on the cast and complications caused by immobility.

C. Casts[112]

    1. Surgical pin fixation is done, and a padded long-leg cast is applied and bivalved anteriorly to the knee to accommodate postoperative swelling.

    2. Casts are usually left in place for three to six weeks.

    3. Percutaneous pins are removed at six weeks.

    4. A short-leg cast is worn continuously for three months postoperatively.

    5. The cast is bivalved before removal and used at night as splints.

    6. Prewalker-type, straight-laced shoes are used during the day.

    7. Yearly radiologic and clinical evaluations are done until skeletal maturity.

D. Parent education

    1. Use and care of appliance or cast

    2. Review of possible cast complications

      a. Impaired circulation

      b. Lack of feeling or sensation

      c. Inability to move toes or fingers

      d. Cast slippage or malposition

      e. Objects getting into cast

E. Cast removal
   1. Soak cast in solution (1 teaspoon vinegar/1 gallon water). Use marker tabs to unwind in opposite direction of application.
   2. Casting for 4–6 weeks. Ankle orthosis is usually worn for six months after casting removal. Follow up and adhere to treatment regimen to prevent recurrence.[64]

Outcomes

A. Serial manipulation and casting have the following response rates.
   1. 90 percent with Ponseti method
   2. 50 percent with other methods
B. Those who do not respond to serial manipulation and casting require some degree of surgical intervention.
   1. The best long-term outcome is achieved when all components of the deformity are released simultaneously (variations of Turco one-stage posteromedial release with internal fixation).
   2. Positive results and level of range of motion are inversely proportional to the number of surgeries.
C. Long-term follow-up indicates that children who have had Ponseti's manipulation followed by open heel cord lengthening and limited posterior ankle release have better results than those who had other manipulation techniques followed by extensive PMR of the foot.[91]
D. Functional and anatomic normalcy may not be possible because of the abnormal anatomy of the clubfoot and surrounding bony structures.
   1. In most cases, a functional foot that will not require activity restriction and will result in little or no pain can be achieved.
   2. Cosmetically, the foot may not appear perfect because slight under- or overcorrection is frequent.
   3. The corrected clubfoot is usually one-half shoe size smaller than the unaffected foot.
      a. The affected calf is 10 percent smaller that the normal extremity.[69]
E. The parents should be made aware prior to surgery of the possibility of recurrence of the deformity and the need for future surgeries, which may include the following.[48,55]
   1. Soft tissue release
   2. Multiple tendon lengthening
   3. Cutting of ligaments and joint capsules
   4. Pinning and realignment of bones

DEVELOPMENTAL DYSPLASIA OF THE HIP (DDH)

Definition

Abnormal formation of hip joint between organogenesis and maturity as a result of joint instability[113]

Pathophysiology

A. Dysplasia
   1. This is an abnormality in development.
   2. There is a continuum of presentation.
   3. The term refers to abnormal formation of tissue, including acetabulum, femur, and soft tissue.[113]

B. Terms
1. Dislocated hip
   a. The cartilage of the acetabulum and the femoral head are not in contact.
   b. The femoral head lies completely out of the acetabulum.
2. Dislocatable hip
   a. The femoral head can be manually displaced with stress but returns to the acetabulum once the stress ceases.
3. Subluxation of the hip
   a. The femoral head is partially out of the acetabulum and positioned away from the floor of the acetabulum.[113,114]
4. Subluxable hip
   a. The tight fit between the femoral head and the acetabulum is lost, and the femoral head is within or at the outside edge of the acetabulum, but is not dislocated.[115,116]
5. Teratologic dislocation[117]
   a. This irreversible malformation occurs *in utero* and is often associated with chromosomal or neuromuscular abnormalities.

Etiology
A. No recognized cause, except teratologic dislocation **(see above)**.
B. Multifactorial influences
1. Mechanical factors
   a. "Packaging" issues causing intrauterine compression and abnormal intrauterine positioning
   b. Oligohydramnios[116]
   c. Primiparous (Unstretched uterus and tight abdominal muscles may limit fetal movement.)
   d. Frank breech presentation
   e. Large for gestational age (>4,500 gm)[112]
2. Primary acetabular dysplasia
   a. This predisposes the hip to dislocation.
   b. There is an increased rate of acetabular dysplasia in biologic parents of patients with late DDH.
   c. A shallow, cartilaginous acetabulum provides poor structural support to the femoral head, allowing the head to move and stretch the supporting ligamentous structures.[118]
3. Ligamentous laxity
   a. Hormonal effects of relaxin on the collagenous structures of the infant cause a laxity that results in pathologic change.
   b. This tendency, combined with mechanical factors such as malpositioning, can cause the femoral head to move out of the acetabulum.
      1) This results in deterioration of the acetabulum, cartilage, and osseous structures.
      2) This abnormal motion prevents normal ossification of the hip.
   c. Females may be more sensitive to the effects of relaxin than males.
4. Embryologic factors
   a. The hip joint develops from cartilaginous anlage; the femoral head is completely encircled by the acetabulum cartilage.
      1) By 11 weeks gestation, development of the hip joint is complete.[116]

2) During gestation, the femoral head grows at a more rapid rate than surrounding cartilage, resulting in less than 50 percent of it being covered at birth.
   b. Cartilage develops rapidly in first few weeks after birth.
   c. Because maturation occurs later in gestation and during the first few postnatal months, there is less structural support for the femoral head from the acetabulum, resulting in a high risk for subluxation or dislocation.
   d. The addition of environmental influences, such as oligohydramnios and breech presentation, can result in adduction of the femoral head away from the central position of the acetabulum.[118]

Incidence

A. 1–2/1,000 live births[119]
B. Increased incidence in Lapps and Native Americans
C. Decreased incidence in African-Americans, Koreans, and Chinese
D. Common in cultures that practice swaddling or use of cradle boards[120,121]
E. Females four times more likely to be affected than males
F. Manifestation of 60 percent of cases on the left side, 20 percent on the right, and 20 percent bilateral[113,120,122]
G. Familial history
   1. Sibling (2–10 percent)
   2. Biologic parent (1–2 percent)

Clinical Presentation

A. Emphasis has changed focus from "congenital" to "developmental."
B. Not all cases present and/or are diagnosed at birth. Many cases may not appear abnormal until later or may be undetected for a few months.[113,118,123,124]

Associations

A. Birth-related factors
   1. Torticollis
   2. Breech presentation (16–25 percent)
   3. Talipes equinovarus
   4. Metatarsus adductus
   5. Female[125]
   6. Family history[125]
   7. Ligamentous laxity[125]
   8. Caucasian female[126]
   9. Myelomeningocele
   10. Neuromuscular disorders
B. Intrauterine environment (compression)
   1. Oligohydramnios
   2. Bicornuate uterus
   3. Uterine anomaly
   4. Multiple gestation
   5. Primiparous

Differential Diagnosis[127]

A. Arthrogryposis
B. Teratologic hip dysplasia
C. Septic arthritis
D. Traumatic hemarthrosis

E. Connective tissue disorder
   1. Ehlers Danlos syndrome
F. Congenital coxa vara

Diagnosis

A. History
   1. Risk factors
      a. Race
      b. Sex
      c. Family history
      d. Firstborn
      e. Breech presentation
B. Newborn to three to four months of age—physical assessment
   1. Observe gluteal folds for symmetry.
   2. Place infant supine on a firm surface. Flex both of the infant's knees and cradle them between the thumb and first finger for Ortolani and Barlow maneuvers.
      a. Ortolani maneuver (Figure 8-17)
         1) This detects dislocation.
         2) Emphasis is on the "pull" to reposition (reduce) the femoral head anteriorly back into place.[113]
         3) Hips are gently flexed to approximately 90 degrees as the examiner's third, ring, and little fingers are placed over the greater trochanter of the infant. The thumb rests on the inner thigh. The hip is then brought slowly from a neutral abduction to full abduction. A gentle upward and medially directed pressure is placed on the greater trochanter in an attempt to lift the dislocated hip into the acetabulum. A positive Ortolani maneuver is appreciated when the examiner feels a "clunk" as the femoral ball pops back into the acetabulum.
      b. Barlow maneuver (Figure 8-18)
         1) This detects the subluxable or dislocatable hip.
         2) Emphasis is on the "push" to try to move the femoral head posteriorly.[113]
         3) If the Ortolani maneuver is negative, the Barlow maneuver is employed during the return of the hip to the neutral position.
         4) A downward force is applied by the examiner's thumb to the medial side of the femur.
   3. Each maneuver may be repeated several times until the tests are determined to be positive or negative. If done gently, neither maneuver should be painful or harmful to the infant.[122]

FIGURE 8-17 ■ Ortolani maneuver.

A. The dislocated left femoral head reduces into the hip socket with gentle hip abduction. B. This produces a palpable clunk.

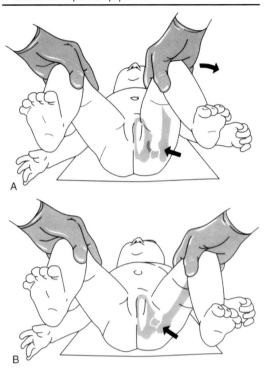

From: Wall EJ. 2000. Practical primary pediatric orthopedics. *Nursing Clinics of North America* 35(1): 96. Reprinted by permission.

C. After four months of age—
physical assessment
   1. Secondary soft tissue
      contractions develop
      and prevent reduction
      of the femoral head into
      the acetabulum. The
      performance and reliability
      of Ortolani and Barlow
      maneuvers decrease.
   2. During assessments at each
      well-child visit until the child
      is walking normally, observe
      for the following.
      a. Asymmetrical inguinal,
         gluteal, or thigh folds
         (better observed prone)
      b. Flexed hips
      c. Widening of the perineum
         (bilaterally)
      d. Limited abduction of less
         than 45 degrees (spreading
         of hips during diaper
         changes)
      e. Abnormally wide-based,
         waddling gait
      f. Unilateral shortening of the
         extremity
      g. Galeazzi sign—the
         appearance of abnormally
         short thigh segments for
         the child's overall size
         (Figure 8-19)[113,116,118]
D. Radiographic findings
   1. Birth to four months
      a. The secondary center of ossification of the femoral head has not yet
         developed, making visualization difficult.
      b. The relationship between the upper end of the femur and acetabulum may
         not be apparent unless the femoral head lies in an abnormal position at rest.
   2. Four to six months
      a. Femoral head ossification is complete.
      b. Abnormalities and asymmetries are apparent on a radiograph.
   3. Acetabular index on x-ray
      a. Angle that the slope of the acetabular roof makes with a horizontal line
         drawn through comparable points on the triradiate cartilage
      b. Index greater than 40 degrees[123]
   4. Ultrasonography
      a. Two views used in the American College of Radiology standard for
         examination of the hip using ultrasound[128]
         1) Coronal view:

FIGURE 8-18 ■ Barlow maneuver.

A. The femoral head, which is initially reduced in the hip socket, is tested for instability with a gentle posterior force applied to the femur in the adducted position. B. The examiner feels a clunk as the femoral head dislocates out of the socket.

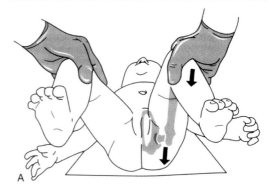

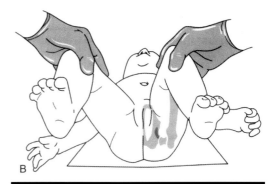

From: Wall EJ. 2000. Practical primary pediatric orthopedics. *Nursing Clinics of North America* 35(1): 97. Reprinted by permission.

a) Standard plane at rest with hip in flexed position

b) Performance of stress (application of gentle posteriorly directed force to assess stability) in view, optional

2) Transverse flexion view with hip flexed:

a) Femur at rest with passive abduction and adduction

b) Femur in flexion

c) Femur with gentle posteriorly directed force (to assess stability)

b. Static technique—using Graf classification (Figure 8-20 and Table 8-1)[118,129–131]

c. Dynamic test—performed in real-time during Ortolani and Barlow maneuvers[113,132]

1) Has replaced the static technique in North America[133]

5. MRI[134]

FIGURE 8-19 ■ **Galeazzi sign.**

With both hips flexed to 90 degrees, there is a noticeable difference in the patient's thigh length, which signifies a dislocated right hip.

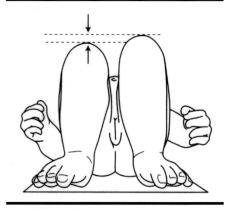

From: Wall EJ. 2000. Practical primary pediatric orthopedics. *Nursing Clinics of North America* 35(1): 98. Reprinted by permission.

FIGURE 8-20 ■ **Graf classification.**

Illustrations of coronal ultrasound images obtained using the Graf method. **A.** The Type I hip is a normal or fully mature hip and has as its hallmarks a deep acetabular cup with the femoral head completely contained beneath the acetabular roof. **B.** The Type II hip is immature (less than three months of age) or mildly dysplastic (more than three months of age) and has a more shallow acetabulum with a round rim. **C.** The Type III hip is dislocated. The acetabulum is very shallow, and the cartilaginous roof is displaced with eversion of labrum. **D.** The Type IV hip is a high dislocation. The acetabular cup is flat, the femoral head is laterally and superiorly displaced, and the labrum is interposed between the femoral head and the lateral wall of the ilium.

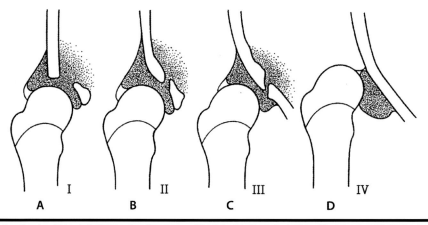

From: Donaldson J, and Feinstein K. 1997. Imaging of developmental dysplasia of the hip. *Pediatric Clinics of North America* 44(3): 595. Reprinted by permission.

Treatment Options and Nursing Care

A. Goals of treatment
  1. Hip reduction
     a. Cartilage of the surface of the femoral head must lie directly on the cartilage floor of the acetabulum with no soft tissue or space between them.
  2. Stability
     a. Achieve and maintain proper positioning.
     b. Prevent movement that may cause dislocation or subluxation.
     c. Promote development of normally shaped socket and femoral head, and promote development of bony and cartilaginous components over time to ensure long-term stability.
  3. Resolution of dysplastic bone and cartilage
     a. Resolution occurs when the femur head is stable in the acetabulum.
     b. Changes that result in resolution occur slowly, but are long lasting.
     c. Characteristics to be resolved include:
        1) Flattening of the femoral head
        2) Misshapen acetabulum
        3) Abnormal shape of the proximal femur
B. Newborn to six months
  1. Splints to position and stabilize hips
     a. Barlow splint
     b. Von Rosen splint
     c. Frejka pillow (abduction) (preferred method in Europe)[135–137]
     d. Pavlik harness (preferred device in U.S.) (Figure 8-21)[138]
        1) Advantages
           a) Less restrictive than a cast
           b) Less costly than a cast
           c) More comfort and freedom of movement for the child
           d) Does not interfere with perineal care
           e) Less likely to cause skin breakdown
           f) Easy to use
           g) Does not rigidly immobilize hips, but maintains flexion greater than 90 degrees and abduction of 40–60 degrees while not allowing extension, adduction, or hyperabduction
           h) Encourages unstable hips to "tighten up" and dislocated hips to reduce[114]

TABLE 8-1 ■ Graf Classification

Type	Description
I	Normal hip
II (<3 months)	Physiologic immaturity
II (>3 months)	Mild dysplasia
III	Dislocation
IV	High dislocation

From: Donaldson J, and Feinstein K. 1997. Imaging of developmental dysplasia of the hip. *Pediatric Clinics of North America* 44(3): 596. Reprinted by permission.

FIGURE 8-21 ■ Pavlik harness.

A Pavlik harness holds the child's legs in the flexed and abducted position. This reduces the femoral head into the socket.

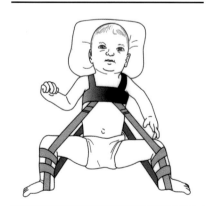

From: Wall EJ. 2000. Practical primary pediatric orthopedics. *Nursing Clinics of North America* 35(1): 100. Reprinted by permission.

    2) Length of treatment
       a) Recommend starting before the infant is two months of age
       b) Minimum of six weeks (usually two to three months)[133]
       c) Frequent adjustments (approximately every two weeks) to accommodate growth and maintain position[122]
    3) Closed reduction and spica cast necessary in 10–15 percent of infants treated with the Pavlik harness[122]

C. Closed reduction[113,119]
   1. This is often done in infants over 6 months of age because the Pavlik harness is no longer effective.
   2. Preliminary traction is used by many to aid in stretching out the soft tissue around the hip.[139,140]
   3. Reduction is done under general anesthesia with correction confirmed by arthrogram or ultrasound.
   4. Percutaneous adductor tenotomy may be performed to release contraction of the adductor to avoid any forces that could lead to redislocation or avascular necrosis (decreased blood supply to the femoral head).
   5. A hip spica cast is applied to maintain hip abduction and flexion of 90 to 100 degrees.
      a. Casts are changed every four to six weeks until the hip is stable and reduced, usually after two to three casts.
      b. Casts are changed under general anesthesia.
      c. A flexion-abduction brace is applied after the final cast removal to remold dysplastic structures.

Surgical Management

A. Open surgical reduction
   1. If closed reduction unsuccessful or if the child is diagnosed and treated after 18 months of age, surgery is required.
   2. An attempt may be made to stretch contracted soft tissue with skin traction for several weeks prior to surgery to facilitate reduction without disruption of blood supply to the femoral head.[113,141]
   3. A medial approach is recommended in children under one year of age, although techniques vary.[142]
      a. Anteriomedial[143–145]
      b. Posteriomedial[146]
      c. Variation of medial approach[144–147]
   4. Immobilization following surgery is achieved with a spica cast for six to eight weeks, followed by abduction casts for an additional four weeks.[133]

Complications[124,148–151]

A. Loss or lack of complete, concentric reduction
B. Residual subluxation
C. Acetabular dysplasia
D. Failure of dysplastic components to easily remold, requiring a prolonged time in splints or surgery
E. Failed reduction, requiring repeated operative procedures
F. Avascular necrosis
   1. The femoral head vessels may occlude between the femoral head and the acetabulum.

2. This is associated with aggressive reduction and abduction or improper application of the harness.[138,141]

3. It results from pressure on the femoral head following reduction.[150,151]

4. This continues to be the most serious complication following treatment for hip dysplasia.[126]

5. Avascular necrosis may occur months to years after treatment.[149]

6. It is graded in terms of severity.

G. Nerve paralysis

H. Infection

I. Early arthrosis[126]

J. Decreased range of motion, limping[126]

K. Leg length discrepancy—growth disturbances of the proximal femur[126]

L. Pain

Postoperative Nursing Care

A. See Postoperative Nursing Care under Intrinsic and Extrinsic Limb Reduction Defects at the beginning of this chapter.

B. Harness
1. Proper positioning
2. Application and removal
3. Diapering
4. Care and maintenance of device
5. Skin care
6. Bathing

C. Care of spica cast
1. Compliance with casting/harnessing
2. Observe for
   a. Impaired circulation
   b. Lack of feeling or sensation
   c. Inability to move toes or fingers
   d. Cast slippage or malposition
   e. Objects getting into cast
3. Cast removal

Outcomes

A. With early detection and treatment, 96 percent of infants develop normal hips, both functionally and radiographically.[141]

B. With late detection, bone and tissue damage is seen. The infant may experience:
1. Leg length discrepancies
2. Abnormal gait
3. Limited hip motion
4. Continuing pain issues

C. Untreated DDH can result in:[119,122]
1. Progressive deformity with growth
2. Early onset of osteoarthritis
3. Degenerative joint disease in the fourth and fifth decades of life

Injury

BRACHIAL PLEXUS INJURIES

Definition

Paralysis of the arm muscles most commonly caused by injury to the fifth and sixth cervical nerves (C5 and C6), up to and including C8 and T1.[152]

Pathophysiology

A. First described in 1764, later elaborated by Erb, Eng, and Klumpke[153–155]

   1. Upper plexus palsy—Erb's palsy, involves the nerve roots at C5 and C6 (Figure 8-22) and affects elbow and shoulder function (nearly 80 percent of all injuries[155]). C7 may be involved, affecting wrist and finger extension.[156]

   2. Total plexus palsy—Erb-Duchenne-Klumpke palsy, involves the nerve roots at C5–T1 and involves shoulder and elbow dysfunction, including paralysis of wrist and hand.[157]

   3. Lower plexus injury—Klumpke's palsy, affects roots C8–T1 and is frequently associated with Horner's syndrome (sympathetic loss, paralysis of diaphragm).

Etiology

A. There is excessive lateral traction on the neck and head when the shoulder is trapped behind the pubic ramus during delivery.[158] This force tears or avulses cervical nerve roots from the spinal cord.

B. There is intrauterine maladaptation.

   1. Associated with young maternal age:
      a. <20 years
      b. Nulliparity

   2. Factors associated with a higher incidence of intrauterine compression:
      a. Fibroids
      b. Bicornuate uterus

   3. Also cited as a causative factor in nerve impairment, where there is no evidence of shoulder dystocia or extreme lateral traction on the head or other risk factors[159–163]

C. Nearly half of all brachial injuries may not be associated with management of shoulder dystocia, but rather attributed to an unavoidable antepartum/intrapartum event.[159]

   1. This injury often involves the posterior shoulder as it passes out of the sacral promontory in utero.

   2. There is a higher rate of persistence of this injury at one year of age than in those with identified shoulder dystocia.[159]

D. Unusually forceful expulsive efforts and rapid deliveries in the absence of shoulder dystocia are also cited as factors in the development of brachial plexus injuries.[160,161]

E. Perinatal risk factors are those associated with a difficult delivery.

   1. Macrosomia
   2. Infant of a diabetic mother
   3. Prolonged second stage of labor
   4. Postmaturity
   5. Shoulder dystocia
   6. Multiparity

FIGURE 8-22 ■ The nerves of the brachial plexus.

The ventral rami of the spinal nerves from C5 to C8, together with the T1 thoracic spinal nerve, join together to form the brachial plexus. The nerve elements combine, divide, and combine again to mix together the various components that lead into the major nerves of the shoulder, arm, and hand (musculocutaneous, axillary, radial, median, and ulnar nerves).

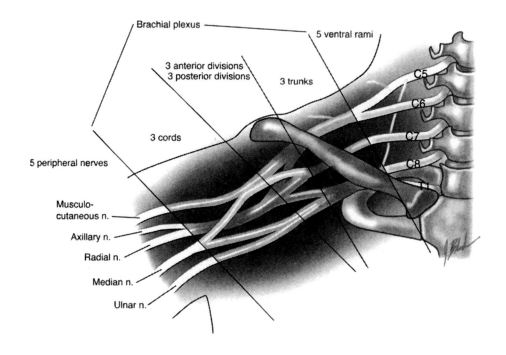

From: Filler AG. 2004. *Do You Really Need Back Surgery? A Surgeon's Guide to Neck and Back Pain and How to Choose Your Treatment.* Oxford: Oxford University Press, 75. Reprinted by permission.

   7. Breech presentation
       a. Five times greater risk, including a high risk in premature infants[164]
   8. Prolonged occiput posterior position[165]
   9. Assisted delivery[166–170]
       a. Forceps
       b. Vacuum extraction

Incidence

A. 0.6–2.5/1,000 live births[157,168,171–174]
B. Most common peripheral nerve injury associated with vaginal delivery[158]

Clinical Presentation[175]

A. Position
   1. Affected extremity held flaccidly extended along the infant's side (Figure 8-23).
   2. Tight adduction of the arms
   3. Internal rotation at the shoulder instead of a normal flexed position
   4. Extended elbow
   5. Pronated forearm
   6. Often flexed wrist

 7. Occasionally flexed fingers

B. Impaired sensory function of the infant's extremity

Associations

A. Horner syndrome
   1. This is associated with brachial plexus trauma.
   2. Elevated diaphragm, winged scapula, or both may mean nerve avulsion close to the spinal cord.
B. Concomitant injuries
   1. Known to occur presumably as a result of the same trauma and may include:[154]
      a. Fractured clavicle
      b. Facial paralysis
      c. Fractured humerus
      d. Separation of the humeral epiphysis
      e. Spinal cord damage without bone injury
      f. Cervical spine injury
      g. Paralysis of the diaphragm, and torticollis

Differential Diagnosis

A. Fractures of clavicle or humerus
   1. Plexus injuries are painless
   2. Crepitus
   3. Pain on movement
   4. X-ray:
      a. Can confirm fractured clavicle
      b. May be missed until callus is felt two to four weeks after the injury[157]
B. Fracture, dislocation, or subluxation of shoulder joint[176]
   1. X-rays of the cervical spine, affected shoulder, and clavicle
C. Pseudoparalysis
   1. Results from swelling in the neck and shoulder
   2. Mimics brachial plexus palsy
D. Phrenic nerve damage and paralysis of the hemidiaphragm[175]
   1. Abdominal asymmetry
E. Cerebral palsy
F. Cervical spine injury
G. Septic shoulder

Diagnosis

A. History
   1. Review of perinatal and intrapartum information for risk factors
   2. Mode of delivery
   3. General health of the infant
B. Physical assessment
   1. Affected arm
      a. Position
         1) Extended along the infant's side
         2) Tight adduction of the arms and internal rotation at the shoulder
         3) Extension of the elbow and pronation of the forearm
         4) Injury to C5–T1: More severe positioning with a clawed hand and little ability to feel sensation[175]

FIGURE 8-23 ■ Characteristic postures of a child with perinatal brachial plexus palsy.

A. "Waiter's tip" posture. B. "Trumpet sign" posture.

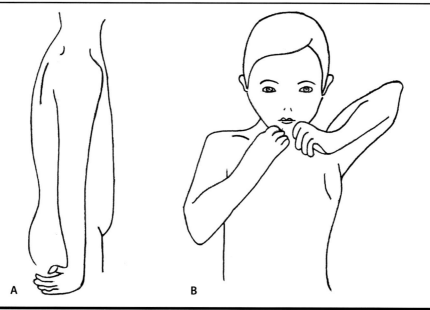

From: Dodds SD, and Wolfe SW. 2000. Perinatal brachial plexus palsy. *Current Opinion in Pediatrics* 12(1): 41. Reprinted by permission.

  b. Tone
    1) Hypotonic, flaccid
  c. Active and passive range of motion
    1) Assess differences and establish a baseline for future examinations.
    2) Hand movement may be affected if there is a lower plexus injury with the pull of the flexors against the wrist and finger extensions, giving the "waiter's tip" posture (injury to C7) (see Figure 8-23).[154,177]
  d. Motor and sensory function
    1) Reaction to touch
      a) The patient may demonstrate a sensate arm by ignoring one side of his body and turning his head away from the affected side.[178]
 2. Moro response
  a. Diminished on affected side
  b. No active motion, but full passive range of motion
 3. Underlying bony injury
  a. A fractured clavicle or humerus may be present.
 4. Motor function
  a. Several scales are described in the literature.[166,178–184]
  b. Consistency in the use of an assessment protocol is necessary to accurately gauge improvement.
  c. Michelow and associates assessed the following.[179]
    1) Clinical parameters, with indications for nerve reconstruction
      a) Shoulder abduction
      b) Elbow flexion
      c) Wrist extension

            d) Finger extension

            e) Thumb extension

        2) Score of 0–2 for each motor function, with 2 being normal function

        3) Active motion against gravity required

        4) Microsurgical repair recommended for a total score of less than 3.5 after three months of age[179]

    d. The Hospital for Sick Children revised its muscle grading system (Active Movement Scale).[178,180,181]

        1) It revised the Michelow grading system to an eight-grade scale.

        2) This scoring system requires full motion with gravity eliminated before muscle strength against gravity is graded.

        3) The following are assessed:

            a) Shoulder movement

            b) Pronation and supination of the forearm

            c) Flexion and extension of the elbow, wrist, fingers, and thumb

    e. The Mallet classification system has been modified.[182,184]

        1) Used to assess the recovery of upper trunk function in infants

        2) Cannot be used to assess hand, wrist, or forearm function

        3) Difficult to use in infants

        4) Five categories of assessment:

            a) Global abduction

            b) Global external rotation

            c) Hand to neck

            d) Hand to spine

            e) Hand to mouth

        5) Scale of 0–5 for each category, with 5 being normal function

    f. The British Medical Research Council developed an evaluation system.[183]

        1) Evaluation of muscle strength

        2) Uses limb segment positioning with and without gravity and manual resistance

        3) Modification of this system by Narakas[166]

C. Electromyography and nerve conduction studies

    1. Examine electrical activity in muscle fibers and speed of impulse conduction

D. Fast-spin MRI

    1. Noninvasive, fast, and decreases the need for general anesthesia for testing[164]

    2. Can be used to help distinguish between intact nerve roots and pseudomeningoceles (indicative of complete avulsion)[185,186]

Treatment Options and Nursing Care

A. Physical therapy

    1. During the first two weeks after injury, the affected arm should be rested at the infant's side to avoid further injury and stretching to already damaged nerves.[177]

    2. Thereafter, passive range of motion (gentle external rotation and abduction) exercises to the shoulder along with flexion of the elbow are begun several times a day until age two to prevent atrophy of muscles and contractures.[154,177]

    3. Hand/wrist splinting may also be done with strengthening exercises introduced later.[187]

B. Botulinum toxin A

    1. Injection therapy used for severe biceps-triceps contractions may show improvement in the arm's range of motion.[188]

Surgical Management

A. Surgical exploration, microsurgical neurolysis of the upper brachial plexus with nerve grafting, may be done in the first year of life, usually between three and six months of age, in infants who do not achieve significant neurologic recovery before three to four months of age.[189,190]

B. Laurent and associates reported that early surgical exploration resulted in an improvement in over 90 percent of patients who had no neurologic improvement by four months of age.[189]

C. Late orthopedic procedures after eight months of age may include joint releases and muscle transfers,[191] along with microsurgical neurolysis bypass nerve grafting and release of associated contractures of the shoulder.[192]

D. Secondary reconstruction (muscle or tendon transfers, nerve transfers, joint fusions, rotational wedge or sliding osteotomies) may be necessary in infants who do not respond to further physical therapy after reconstruction.[175] The goal is to improve function.

Complications[177,193]

A. Infection

B. Contractures of elbows and shoulders

C. Posteromedial subluxation

D. Posterior dislocation of the elbow

E. Burns caused by the operating microscope

Postoperative Nursing Care

A. See Postoperative Nursing Care under Intrinsic and Extrinsic Limb Reduction Defects at the beginning of this chapter.

B. A sling is used for six to eight weeks with the arm loosely secured to the chest.

C. Some surgeons recommend immobilization in a shoulder spica cast[191] or custom fitted body brace for six to eight weeks following secondary reconstruction. The arm is immobilized in external rotation (90 degrees) and abduction (90 degrees) for protection of the transferred tendon or muscle units.[191]

D. Passive range of motion and slow-pulse electrical stimulation may be employed.

E. Occupational therapy and physiotherapy for six months is begun once the splint is removed. Re-evaluation is done by the surgeon over the next few years.

Outcomes

A. Prognosis for spontaneous recovery of motor and sensory function drastically diminished with Horner syndrome[157]

B. Spontaneous recovery

    1. Much of the literature supports a spontaneous recovery figure for infants of more than 70–90 percent.[157,158,172–174,176,179]

        a. Upper plexus injuries are generally less severe.

        b. Lower plexus injuries are more severe, often with incomplete recovery.

    2. The average time to resolution or plateau is three to four months.

C. Stretching- or edema-caused nerve damage

    1. Partial versus total injury

    2. Severity of deficit

    3. Six-month evaluation of status

      a. This will predict complete recovery or severe disability.

D. Impaired function

   1. Five to ten percent experience significant disability.

   2. Forty percent of injuries involving Klumpke's palsy resolve at one year of age.[159]

   3. Failure to receive sensory input in the first three months of life can result in functional impairment even after regeneration of nerve pathways because of the body's inability to establish normal motor patterns of movement and organization of body images.[194]

   4. This impaired motor unit activation results in a developmental apraxia.[195]

   5. The brain and spinal cord do not develop activity-dependent changes that lead from normal motor/neuron recruitment into skilled movements because of the absence of normal movements early in life and their patterns of cutaneous and proprioceptive sensory input.[195]

   6. Functional limitation may exist in the shoulder:

      a. Inability to raise arm above shoulder[179,187,195,196]

E. Bone deformities[171,179,187,197]

F. Winging of scapula (upward and lateral fixation of scapula)[198]

G. Joint contractures

H. Weakness of the deltoid and supraspinatus muscles, involvement of muscles in shoulder, upper arm, forearm, and hand[195]

I. Impaired elbow function, hand grip strength[156]

J. Impaired sensory perception[156]

REFERENCES

1. Moore K, and Persaud TVN. 2003. *The Developing Human: Clinically Oriented Embryology,* 7th ed. Philadelphia: Saunders, 382–399, 410–425.

2. Sadler TW. 2004. *Langman's Medical Embryology,* 9th ed. Philadelphia: Lippincott Williams & Wilkins, 171–197.

3. Moore KL, and Persaud TVN. 2003. *Before We Are Born: Essentials of Embryology and Birth Defects,* 6th ed. Philadelphia: Saunders, 305–320, 330–341.

4. Mooney EK. 2004. Lower limb embryology. *eMedicine.* Retrieved October 14, 2005, from www.emedicine.com/plastic/topic215.htm.

5. Mooney EK, and Maier JP. 2003. Hand, upper extremity embryology. *eMedicine.* Retrieved October 14, 2005, from www.emedicine.com/plastic/topic516.htm.

6. Cobben JM, Hiemstra S, and Robinson PH. 1994. Genetic counseling in limb reduction defects. *Genetic Counseling* 5(3): 243–248.

7. Burge P. 2002. Developmental anomalies of the hand. In *Children's Orthopaedics and Fractures,* 2nd ed., Benson MK, et al., eds. Edinburgh: Churchill Livingstone, 301–315.

8. McCluskey WP, and Costas BL. 1994. Surgery of upper extremity malformations: Complications and management. In *Complications in Pediatric Orthopaedic Surgery,* Epps CH, and Bowen JR, eds. Philadelphia: Lippincott Williams & Wilkins, 309–334.

9. Graham JM Jr. 1986. Causes of limb reduction defects: The contribution of fetal constraint and/or vascular disruption. *Clinics in Perinatology* 13(3): 575–591.

10. Lin S, and Marshall EG. 1996. Comparison of demographic and defect characteristics among different developmental stages of congenital limb reduction defects. *Paediatric and Perinatal Epidemiology* 10(3): 294–308.

11. Aro T, Haapakoski J, and Heinonen OP. 1984. A multivariate analysis of the risk indicators of reduction limb defects. *International Journal of Epidemiology* 13(4): 459–464.

12. Froster UG, and Baird PA. 1992. Upper limb deficiencies and associated malformations: A population-based study. *American Journal of Medical Genetics* 44(6): 767–781.

13. Werler MM, et al. 1999. Multivitamin supplementation and risk of birth defects. *American Journal of Epidemiology* 150(7): 675–682.

14. Czeizel AE. 2000. Primary prevention of neural-tube defects and some other major congenital abnormalities: Recommendations for the appropriate use of folic acid during pregnancy. *Paediatric Drugs* 2(6): 437–449.

15. Watson S. 2000. The principles of management of congenital anomalies of the upper limb. *Archives of Disease in Childhood* 83(1): 10–17.

16. Walter JH, Goss LR, and Lazzara AT. 1998. Amniotic band syndrome. *Journal of Foot and Ankle Surgery* 37(4): 325–333.

17. Diaz MR. 1993. Amniotic band syndrome: A nursing perspective. *Neonatal Network* 12(2): 7–19.

18. Chervenak FA, and Isaacson G. 1986. Diagnosing congenital malformation *in utero:* Ultrasound. *Clinics in Perinatology* 13(3): 593–607.

19. Stoll C, et al. 1995. Evaluation of routine prenatal diagnosis by a registry of congenital anomalies. *Prenatal Diagnosis* 15(9): 791–800.

20. Goncalves LF, Jeanty P, and Piper JM. 1994. The accuracy of prenatal ultrasonography in detecting congenital anomalies. *American Journal of Obstetrics and Gynecology* 171(6): 1606–1612.

21. Turner BS. 1985. Amniotic band syndrome. *Journal of Obstetric, Gynecologic, and Neonatal Nursing* 14(4): 298–301.

22. Lockwood C, et al. 1989. Amniotic band syndrome: Reevaluation of its pathogenesis. *American Journal of Obstetrics and Gynecology* 160(5 part 1): 1030–1033.

23. Streeter GL. 1930. Focal deficiencies in fetal tissues and their relation to intra-uterine amputation. *Contributions to Embryology* 22(126): 1–44.

24. Yang SS. 1990. ADAM sequence and innocent amniotic band: Manifestations of early amnion rupture. *American Journal of Medical Genetics* 37(4): 562–568.

25. Torpin R. 1968. *Fetal Malformations Caused by Amnion Rupture During Gestation.* Springfield, Illinois: Charles C. Thomas.

26. Jones KL. 2006. *Smith's Recognizable Patterns of Human Malformation,* 6th ed. Philadelphia: Saunders, 732–737.

27. Ossipoff V, and Hall BD. 1977. Etiologic factors in the amniotic band syndrome: A study of 24 patients. *Birth Defects Original Article Series* 13(3D): 117–132.

28. Mastroiacovo P, et al. 1992. Absence of limbs and gross body wall defects: An epidemiological study of related rare malformation conditions. *Teratology* 46(5): 455–464.

29. Paladini D, et al. 2004. Congenital constriction band of the upper arm: The role of three-dimensional ultrasound in diagnosis, counseling and multidisciplinary consultation. *Ultrasound in Obstetrics and Gynecology* 23(5): 520–522.

30. Hall EJ, Johnson-Giebink R, and Vasconez LO. 1982. Management of the ring constriction syndrome: A reappraisal. *Plastic and Reconstructive Surgery* 69(3): 532–536.

31. Weinzweig N. 1995. Constriction band–induced vascular compromise of the foot: Classification and management of the "intermediate" stage of constriction-ring syndrome. *Plastic and Reconstructive Surgery* 96(4): 972–977.

32. Quintero RA, et al. 1997. *In utero* lysis of amniotic bands. *Ultrasound in Obstetrics and Gynecology* 10(5): 316–320.

33. Keswani S, et al. 2003. *In utero* limb salvage: Fetoscopic release of amniotic bands for threatened limb amputation. *Journal of Pediatric Surgery* 38(6): 848–851.

34. Light TR, and Ogden JA. 1993. Congenital constriction band syndrome: Pathophysiology and treatment. *Yale Journal of Biology and Medicine* 66(3): 143–155.

35. Muguti GI. 1990. The amniotic band syndrome: Single-stage correction. *British Journal of Plastic Surgery* 43(6): 706–708.

36. DiMeo L, and Mercer DH. 1987. Single-stage correction of constriction ring syndrome. *Annals of Plastic Surgery* 19(5): 469–474.

37. Cox H, et al. 1989. Radial ray defects and associated anomalies. *Clinical Genetics* 35(5): 322–330.

38. Shelton SD, Paulyson K, and Kay HH. 1999. Prenatal diagnosis of thrombocytopenia absent radius (TAR) and vaginal delivery. *Prenatal Diagnosis* 19(1): 54–57.

39. McLaurin TM, et al. 1999. Management of thrombocytopenia-absent radius (TAR) syndrome. *Journal of Pediatric Orthopaedics* 19(3): 289–296.

40. Rosenfelder R. 1980. Infant amputees: Early growth and care. *Clinical Orthopaedics and Related Research* (148): 41–46.

41. Hockenberry MJ, et al. 2003. *Wong's Nursing Care of Infants and Children,* 7th ed. St. Louis: Mosby.

42. Shaperman J, and Sumida CT. 1980. Recent advances in research in prosthetics for children. *Clinical Orthopaedics and Related Research* (148): 26–33.

43. Datta D, and Ibbotson V. 1998. Powered prosthetic hands in very young children. *Prosthetics and Orthotics International* 22(2): 150–154.

44. Sorbye R. 1980. Myoelectric prosthetic fitting in young children. *Clinical Orthopaedics and Related Research* (148): 34–40.

45. Kyzer SP. 1991. Congenital idiopathic clubfoot. *Orthopaedic Nursing* 10(4): 11–18. (Published erratum in *Orthopaedic Nursing,* 1992, 11[1]: 9.)

46. Kyzer SP, and Stark SL. 1995. Congenital idiopathic clubfoot deformities. Part 1. *AORN Journal* 61(3): 492–505.

47. Alexander M, Ackman JD, and Kuo KN. 1999. Congenital idiopathic clubfoot. *Orthopaedic Nursing* 18(4): 47–55.

48. Blakeslee T. 1997. Congenital idiopathic talipes equinovarus (clubfoot). Current concepts. *Clinics in Podiatric Medicine and Surgery* 14(1): 9–56.

49. Lyons AS, and Petrucelli RJ. 1978. *Medicine: An Illustrated History.* New York: Harry N. Abrams, 135.

50. Adams CF. 1939. *The Genuine Works of Hippocrates.* Baltimore: Lippincott Williams & Wilkins.

51. Kite JH. 1939. Principles involved in the treatment of congenital clubfoot. *Journal of Bone and Joint Surgery (Am)* 21(3): 595–606.

52. Turco V. 1971. Surgical correction of the resistant clubfoot. *Journal of Bone and Joint Surgery (Am)* 53(3): 477–478.

53. Fukuhara K, Schollmeier G, and Uhthoff HK. 1994. The pathogenesis of clubfoot: A histomophometric and immunohistochemical study of fetuses. *Journal of Bone and Joint Surgery (Br)* 76(3): 450–457.

54. Isaacs H, et al. 1977. The muscles in clubfoot: A histological, histochemical and electron-microscopic study. *Journal of Bone and Joint Surgery (Br)* 59(4): 465–472.

55. Zimny ML, et al. 1985. An electron microscopic study of the fascia from the medial and lateral sides of clubfoot. *Journal of Pediatric Orthopaedics* 5(5): 577–581.

56. Sano H, et al. 1998. Pathogenesis of soft-tissue contracture in clubfoot. *Journal of Bone and Joint Surgery (Br)* 80(4): 641–644.

57. Ponseti IV. 1996. *Congenital Clubfoot: Fundamentals of Treatment.* New York: Oxford University Press.

58. Coleman SS. 1983. *Complex Foot Deformities in Children.* Philadelphia: Lea & Febiger, 255–265.

59. Cummings RJ, and Lovell WW. 1988. Current concepts review: Operative treatment of congenital idiopathic clubfoot. *Journal of Bone and Joint Surgery (Am)* 70(7): 1108–1112.

60. Tachdijian MO. 1985. *The Child's Foot.* Philadelphia: Saunders.

61. Fernbach S. 1998. Common orthopedic problems of the newborn. *Nursing Clinics of North America* 33(4): 583–594.

62. Turco V. 1981. *Club Foot: Current Problems in Orthopaedics.* New York: Churchill Livingstone.

63. March of Dimes Foundation. 1986. *Public Health Education Information Sheet: Clubfoot.* New York: March of Dimes Foundation.

64. Cummings J, et al. 2002. Congenital clubfoot. *Journal of Bone and Joint Surgery (Am)* 84(2): 290–308.

65. Rebbeck TR, et al. 1993. A single-gene explanation for the probability of having idiopathic talipes equinovarus. *American Journal of Human Genetics* 53(5): 1052–1063.

66. Yang H, Chung CS, and Nemechek RW. 1987. A genetic analysis of clubfoot in Hawaii. *Genetic Epidemiology* 4(4): 299–306.

67. Irani RN, and Sherman MS. 1963. The pathological anatomy of clubfoot. *Journal of Bone and Joint Surgery (Am)* 45(1): 45–52.

68. Kawashima T, and Uhthoff HK. 1990. Development of the foot in prenatal life in relation to idiopathic clubfoot. *Journal of Pediatric Orthopaedics* 10(2): 232–237.

69. Settle GW. 1963. The anatomy of congenital talipes equinovarus: Sixteen dissected specimens. *Journal of Bone and Joint Surgery (Am)* 45(7): 1341–1354.

70. Alderman BW, Takahashi ER, and Lefflier MK. 1991. Risk indicators for talipes equinovarus in Washington state, 1987–1989. *Epidemiology* 2(4): 289–292.

71. Bohm M. 1929. The embryologic origin of clubfoot. *Journal of Bone and Joint Surgery (Am)* 11(2): 229–259.

72. Peretti G, and Surace A. 1986. Clubfoot, classification, etiology, and pathogenesis. *Italian Journal of Orthopaedics and Traumatology. Supplementum* 87(supplement II): S11–S37.

73. Handlesman JE, and Badalamente MA. 1982. Club foot: A neuromuscular disease. *Developmental Medicine & Child Neurology* 24(1): 3–12.

74. Maffulti N, et al. 1992. Histochemistry of the triceps surae muscle in idiopathic congenital clubfoot. *Foot & Ankle* 13(20): 80–84.

75. Sirca A, Erzen I, and Pecak F. 1990. Histochemistry of abductor hallucis muscle in children with idiopathic clubfoot and in controls. *Journal of Pediatric Orthopedics* 10(4): 477–482.

76. White R, and Blasier D. 1994. Clubfoot: Nature and treatment. *Today's OR Nurse* 16(2): 29–35.

77. Gray DH, and Katz JM. 1981. A histochemical study of muscle in clubfoot. *Journal of Bone and Joint Surgery (Br)* 63(3): 417–423.

78. Hootnick DR, et al. 1980. Vascular dysgenesis associated with skeletal dysplasia of the lower limb. *Journal of Bone and Joint Surgery (Am)* 62(7): 1123–1129.

79. Hootnick DR, et al. 1982. Congenital arterial malformations associated with clubfoot. A report of two cases. *Clinical Orthopaedics and Related Research* (167): 160–163.

80. Atlas S, Menacho LC, and Ures S. 1980. Some new aspects in the pathology of clubfoot. *Clinical Orthopaedics and Related Research* (149): 224–228.

81. Cunningham S, and Albert MC. 1993. Congenital clubfoot. *Today's OR Nurse* 15(16): 31–34.

82. Ponseti IV. 2002. The Ponseti technique for correction of congenital clubfoot (letter). *Journal of Bone and Joint Surgery (Am)* 84(10): 1889-1890.

83. Dietz F. 2002. The genetics of idiopathic clubfoot. *Clinical Orthopaedics and Related Research* (401): 39–48.

84. Scherl S. 2004. Common lower extremity problems in children. *Pediatrics in Review* 25(2): 52–62.

85. Cooper DM, and Dietz FR. 1995. Treatment of idiopathic clubfoot. A thirty-year follow-up note. *Journal of Bone and Joint Surgery (Am)* 77(10): 1477–1489.

86. Herzenberg JE, Radler C, and Bor N. 2002. Ponseti versus traditional methods of casting for idiopathic clubfoot. *Journal of Pediatric Orthopedics* 22(4): 517–521.

87. Pirani S, Zeznik L, and Hodges D. 2001. Magnetic resonance imaging study of the congenital clubfoot treated with the Ponseti method. *Journal of Pediatric Orthopaedics* 21(6): 719–726.

88. Roye DP, and Roye BD. 2002. Idiopathic congenital talipes equinovarus. *Journal of the American Academy of Orthopaedic Surgeons* 10(4): 239–248.

89. Dobbs MB, et al. 2004. Factors predictive of outcome after use of the Ponseti method for the treatment of idiopathic clubfeet. *Journal of Bone and Joint Surgery (Am)* 86(1): 22–27.

90. Ponseti IV. 2000. Clubfoot management. *Journal of Pediatric Orthopaedics* 20(6): 699–700.

91. Ippolito E, et al. 2003. Long-term comparative results in patients with congenital clubfoot treated with two different protocols. *Journal of Bone and Joint Surgery (Am)* 85(7): 1286–1294.

92. Ponseti IV. 1992. Treatment of congenital club foot. *Journal of Bone and Joint Surgery (Am)* 74(3): 448–454.

93. Lehman WB, et al. 2003. A method for the early evaluation of the Ponseti (Iowa) technique for the treatment of idiopathic clubfoot. *Journal of Pediatric Orthopaedics. Part B* 12(2): 133–140.

94. Bensahel H, et al. 1990. Results of physical therapy for idiopathic clubfoot: A long-term follow-up study. *Journal of Pediatric Orthopaedics* 10(2): 189–192.

95. Bensahel H, et al. 1994. The intimacy of clubfoot. The ways of functional treatment. *Journal of Pediatric Orthopaedics Part B* 3: 155–160.

96. Dimeglio A, et al. 1996. Orthopaedic treatment and passive motion machine: Consequences for the surgical treatment of clubfoot. *Journal of Pediatric Orthopaedics Part B* 5(3): 173–180.

97. Delgado M, et al. 2000. A preliminary report of the use of botulinum toxin type A in infants with clubfoot: Four case studies. *Journal of Pediatric Orthopedics* 20(4): 533–538.

98. Alvarez C, et al. 2005. Treatment of idiopathic clubfoot utilizing botulinum A toxin: A new method and its short-term outcomes. *Journal of Pediatric Orthopedics* 25(2): 229–235.

99. Brin MR. 1997. Spasticity: Etiology, evaluation, management and the role of botulinum toxin A. *Muscle and Nerve* 20(supplement 6): S61–S91.

100. Borodic G, et al. 1994. Pharmacology and histology of the therapeutic application of botulinum toxin. In *Therapy with Botulinum Toxin*, Jankovic J, and Hallet M, eds. New York: Marcel Dekker, 120–121.

101. Gooch JL, and Sandell TV. 1996. Botulinum toxin for spasticity and athetosis in children with cerebral palsy. *Archives of Physical Medicine Rehabilitation* 77(5): 508–511.

102. Gormley ME, Herring GM, and Gaebler-Spira DJ. 1997. The use of botulinum toxin in children: A retrospective study of adverse reactions and treatment of idiopathic toe-walking. *European Journal of Neurology* 4(supplement 2): S27–S30.

103. Delgado M. 1999. The use of botulinum toxin type A in children with cerebral palsy: A retrospective study. *European Journal of Neurology* 6(supplement 4): S11–S18.

104. DePuy J, and Drennan JC. 1989. Correction of idiopathic clubfoot: A comparison of results of early versus delayed posteromedial release. *Journal of Pediatric Orthopedics* 9(1): 44–48.

105. Carroll NC. 1996. Controversies in the surgical management of clubfoot. *Instructional Course Lectures* 45: 331–337.

106. Simons, GW. 1985. Complete subtalar release in club feet: Part I: A preliminary report. *Journal of Bone and Joint Surgery (Am)* 67(7): 1044–1055.

107. Simons GW. 1985. Complete subtalar release in club feet. Part II: Comparison with less extensive procedures. *Journal of Bone and Joint Surgery (Am)* 67(7): 1056–1065.

108. Turco VJ, and Spinella AJ. 1982. Current management of clubfoot. *Instructional Course Lectures* 31: 218–234.

109. Atar D, et al. 1992. Revision surgery in clubfeet. *Clinical Orthopaedics and Related Research* (283): 223–230.

110. Vizkelety T, and Szepesi K. 1989. Reoperation in treatment of clubfoot. *Journal of Pediatric Orthopedics* 9(2): 144–147.

111. Aronson J, and Puskarich CL. 1990. Deformity and disability from treated clubfoot. *Journal of Pediatric Orthopedics* 10(1): 109–119.

112. Lapunzina P, et al. 2002. Risks of congenital anomalies in large for gestational age infants. *Journal of Pediatrics* 140(2): 200–204.

113. Novacheck T. 1996. Developmental dysplasia of the hip. *Pediatric Clinics of North America* 43(4): 829–848.

114. Fembach S. 1998. Common orthopedic problems of the newborn. *Nursing Clinics of North America* 33(4): 583–594.

115. Coleman SS. 1989. Diagnosis of congenital dysplasia of the hip in the newborn infant. *Clinical Orthopaedics and Related Research* (247): 3–12.

116. American Academy of Pediatrics. 2000. Clinical practice guidelines: Early detection of developmental dysplasia of the hip. *Pediatrics* 105(4): 896–905.

117. Haynes RJ. 2001. Developmental dysplasia of the hip: Etiology, pathogenesis, and examination and physical findings in the newborn. *Instructional Course Lectures* 50: 535–540.

118. Donaldson JS, and Feinstein K. 1997. Imaging of developmental dysplasia of the hip. *Pediatric Clinics of North America* 44(3): 591–614.

119. Shoppee K. 1992. Developmental dysplasia of the hip. *Orthopaedic Nursing* 11(5): 30–36.

120. Kutlu A, et al. 1992. Congenital dislocation of the hip and its relation to swaddling used in Turkey. *Journal of Pediatric Orthopedics* 12(5): 598–602.

121. Churgay CA, and Caruthers BS. 1992. Diagnosis and treatment of congenital dislocation of the hip. *American Family Physician* 45(3): 1217–1228.

122. Mooney JF III, and Emans JB. 1995. Developmental dislocation of the hip: A clinical overview. *Pediatrics in Review* 16(8): 299–304.

123. Ilfeld FW, Westin GW, and Makin M. 1986. Missed or developmental dislocation of the hip. *Clinical Orthopaedics and Related Research* (203): 276–281.

124. Harcke HT. 1994. Screening newborns for developmental dysplasia of the hip: The role of sonography. *American Journal of Roentgenology* 162(2): 395–397.

125. Scherl SA. 2004. Common lower extremity problems in children. *Pediatrics in Review* 25(2): 52–62.

126. Barkin SZ, Kondo KL, and Barkin RM. 2000. Avascular necrosis of the hip: A complication following treatment of congenital dysplasia of the hip. *Clinical Pediatrics* 39(5): 307–310.

127. Witt C. 2003. Detecting developmental dysplasia of the hip. *Advances in Neonatal Care* 3(2): 65–75.

128. American College of Radiology. 2003 (revised). *ACR Practice Guideline for the Performance of the Ultrasound Examination for Detection of Developmental Dysplasia of the Hip.* Reston, Virginia: American College of Radiology. Retrieved October 17, 2005, from www.acr.org/s_acr/bin.asp?CID=539&DID=12230&DOC=FILE.PDF.

129. Holen KJ, et al. 1999. The use of ultrasound in determining the initiation of treatment in instability of the hip in neonates. *Journal of Bone and Joint Surgery (Br)* 81(5): 846–851.

130. Graf R. 1980. The diagnosis of congenital hip-joint dislocation by the ultrasonic Combound treatment. *Archives of Orthopaedic and Trauma Surgery* 97(2): 117–133.

131. Graf R. 1987. *Guide to Sonography of the Infant Hip.* New York: Thieme Medical.

132. Abramson SF. 1992. Real time ultrasonographic evaluation of the hip. *Orthpaedic Nursing* 11(1): 72–73.

133. Willis RB. 2001. Developmental dysplasia of the hip: Assessment and treatment before walking age. *Instructional Course Lectures* 50: 541–545.

134. Kashiwagi N, et al. 1996. Prediction of reduction in developmental dysplasia of the hip by magnetic resonance imaging. *Journal of Paediatric Orthopaedics* 16(2): 254–258.

135. Darmonov AV, and Zagora S. 1996. Clinical screening for congenital dislocation of the hip. *Journal of Bone and Joint Surgery (Am)* 78(3): 383–388.

136. Poul J, et al. 1992. Early diagnosis of congenital dislocation of the hip. *Journal of Bone and Joint Surgery (Br)* 74(5): 695–700.

137. Krikler SJ, and Dwyer NS. 1992. Comparison of results of two approaches to hip screening in infants. *Journal of Bone and Joint Surgery (Br)* 74(5): 701–703.

138. French L, and Dietz F. 1999. Screening for developmental dysplasia of the hip. *American Family Physician* 60(1): 173–184.

139. Joseph K, MacEwen GD, and Boos ML. 1982. Home traction in the management of congenital dislocation of the hip. *Clinical Orthopaedics and Related Research* (165): 83–90.

140. Yamada N, et al. 2003. Closed reduction of developmental dislocation of the hip by prolonged traction. *Journal of Bone and Joint Surgery (Br)* 85(8): 1173–1177.

141. Aiello D. 1989. Congenital dysplasia of the hip: Diagnosis, treatment, nursing care. *AORN Journal* 49(6): 1566–1605.

142. Konigsberg DE, et al. 2003. Results of medial open reduction of the hip in infants with developmental dislocation of the hip. *Journal of Pediatric Orthopaedics* 23(1): 1–9.

143. Ludloff K. 1908. Zurblutigen Einrenkung der angeborenen Huftluxation. *Zeitschrift Orthopaedicae Chirurgica* 22: 272–276.

144. Bicimoglu A, et al. 2003. Six years of experience with a new surgical algorithm in developmental dysplasia of the hip in children under 18 months of age. *Journal of Pediatric Orthopaedics* 23(6): 693–698.

145. Ludloff K. 1913. The open reduction of the congenital hip dislocation by an anterior incision. *American Journal of Orthopedic Surgery* 10: 438–454.

146. Ferguson AB Jr. 1973. Primary open reduction of congenital dislocation of the hip using a median adductor approach. *Journal of Bone and Joint Surgery (Am)* 55(4): 671–689.

147. Weinstein SL. 1987. Anteromedial approach to reduction for congenital hip dysplasia. *Strategies in Orthopaedic Surgery* 6: 2.

148. Weinstein SL. 2001. Developmental hip dysplasia and dislocation. In *Lovell and Winter's Pediatric Orthopaedics,* 5th ed., Morrissey RT, and Weinstein SL, eds. Philadelphia: Lippincott Williams & Wilkins, 905–956.

149. Weinstein SL. 1992. Congenital hip dislocation. Long-range problems, residual signs, and symptoms after successful treatment. *Clinical Orthopaedics and Related Research* (281): 69–74.

150. Binnet MS, et al. 1992. The relationship between the treatment of congenital dislocation of the hip and avascular necrosis. *Orthopedics* 15(1): 73–81.

151. Kruczynski J. 1996. Avascular necrosis of the proximal femur in developmental dislocation of the hip. Incidence, risk factors, sequelae and MR imaging for diagnosis and prognosis. *Acta Orthopaedica Scandinavica. Supplementum* 268: 1–48.

152. Filler AG. 2004. *Do You Really Need Back Surgery?: A Surgeon's Guide to Neck and Back Pain and How to Choose Your Treatment.* Oxford: Oxford University Press, 63–80.

153. Erb W. 1969. On a characteristic site of injury in the brachial plexus (reprinted). *Archives of Neurology* 21: 433–434.

154. Eng GD. 1971. Brachial plexus palsy in newborn infants. *Pediatrics* 48(1): 18–28.

155. Klumpke A. 1885. Contribution à l'étude des paralysies radiculaires du plexus brachial. Paralysies radiculaires totales. Paralysies radiculaires inférieures. De la participation des filets sympathiques oculo-pupillaires dans ces paralysies. *Revue de Médecine* 5: 591–616.

156. Sundholm LK, Eliasson AC, and Forssberg H. 1998. Obstetric brachial plexus injuries: Assessment protocol and functional outcome at age 5 years. *Developmental Medicine and Child Neurology* 40(1): 4–11.

157. Fernbach SA. 1998. Common orthopedic problems of the newborn. *Nursing Clinics of North America* 33(4): 583–594.

158. Gordon M, et al. 1973. The immediate and long-term outcome of obstetric birth trauma. Part 1: Brachial plexus paralysis. *American Journal of Obstetrics and Gynecology* 117(1): 51–56.

159. Gherman R, Ouzounian J, and Goodwin M. 1999. Brachial plexus palsy: An *in utero* injury. *American Journal of Obstetrics and Gynecology* 180(5): 1303–1307.

160. Jennett RJ, and Tarby TJ. 1997. Brachial plexus palsy: An old problem revisited again. Part 2: Cases in point. *American Journal of Obstetrics and Gynecology* 176(6): 1354–1357.

161. Jennett RJ, Tarby TJ, and Kreinick CJ. 1992. Brachial plexus palsy: An old problem revisited. *American Journal of Obstetrics and Gynecology* 166(6 part 1): 1673–1677.

162. Koenigsberger MR. 1980. Brachial plexus palsy at birth: Intrauterine or due to birth trauma? *Annals of Neurology* 8: 228.

163. Dunn DW, and Engle WA. 1985. Brachial plexus palsy: Intrauterine onset. *Pediatric Neurology* 1(6): 367–369.

164. Francel PC, et al. 1995. Fast spin-echo magnetic resonance imaging for radiological assessment of neonatal brachial plexus injury. *Journal of Neurosurgery* 83(3): 461–466.

165. McFarland LV, et al. 1986. Erb/Duchenne's palsy: A consequence of fetal macrosomia and method of delivery. *Obstetrics and Gynecology* 68(6): 784–788.

166. Narakas AO. 1987. Obstetrical brachial plexus injuries. In *The Paralyzed Hand: The Hand and Upper Limb,* vol. 2, Lamb DW, ed. Edinburgh: Churchill Livingstone, 116–135.

167. Medlock MD, and Hanigan WC. 1997. Neurologic birth trauma. Intracranial, spinal cord, and brachial plexus injury. *Clinics in Perinatology* 24(4): 845–857.

168. Jackson ST, Hoffer MM, and Parrish N. 1988. Brachial-plexus palsy in the newborn. *Journal of Bone and Joint Surgery (Am)* 70(8): 1217–1220.

169. Geutjens G, Gilbert A, and Helsen K. 1996. Obstetric brachial plexus palsy associated with the breech delivery. A different pattern of injury. *Journal of Bone and Joint Surgery (Br)* 78(2): 303–306.

170. Hopwood HG. 1982. Shoulder dystocia: Fifteen years experience in a community hospital. *American Journal of Obstetrics and Gynecology* 144(2): 162–166.

171. Bager B. 1997. Perinatally acquired brachial plexus palsy— A persisting challenge. *Acta Paediatrica* 86(11): 1214–1219.

172. Tan KL. 1973. Brachial palsy. *Journal of Obstetrics and Gynaecology of the British Commonwealth* 80(1): 60–62.

173. Greenwald AG, Schute PC, and Shiveley JL. 1984. Brachial plexus birth palsy: A 10-year report on the incidence and prognosis. *Journal of Pediatric Orthopedics* 4(6): 689–692.

174. Sjoberg I, Erichs K, and Bjerre I. 1988. Cause and effect of obstetric (neonatal) brachial plexus palsy. *Acta Paediatrica Scandinavica* 77(3): 357–364.

175. Dunham EA. 2003. Obstetrical brachial plexus palsy. *Orthopaedic Nursing* 22(2): 106–116.

176. Dodds SD, and Wolfe SW. 2000. Perinatal brachial plexus palsy. *Current Opinion in Pediatrics* 12(1): 40–47.

177. Aston JW. 1979. Brachial plexus birth palsy. *Orthopedics* 2(6): 594–601.

178. Clarke HM, and Curtis CG. 1995. An approach to obstetrical brachial plexus injuries. *Hand Clinics* 11(4): 563–581.

179. Michelow BJ, et al. 1994. The natural history of obstetrical brachial plexus palsy. *Plastic and Reconstructive Surgery* 93(4): 675–680.

180. Clark HM, et al. 1996. Obstetrical brachial plexus palsy: Results following neurolysis of conducting neuromas-in-continuity. *Plastic and Reconstructive Surgery* 97(5): 974–982.

181. Curtis C, et al. 2002. The Active Movement Scale: An evaluative tool for infants with obstetrical brachial plexus palsy. *Journal of Hand Surgery (Am)* 27(3): 470–478.

182. Gilbert A, and Tassin JL. 1984. Surgical repair of the brachial plexus in obstetric paralysis [French] *Chirurgie* 110(1): 70–75.

183. Medical Research Council. 1942. *Aids to the Investigation of the Peripheral Nerve Injuries*. London: His Majesty's Stationary Office.

184. Waters P. 1997. Obstetric brachial plexus injuries: Evaluation and management. *American Academy of Orthopedic Surgeons* 5(4): 205–214.

185. Miller SF, et al. 1993. Brachial plexopathy in infants after traumatic delivery. Evaluation with MR imaging. *Radiology* 189(2): 481–484.

186. Urabe F, et al. 1991. MR imaging of birth brachial palsy in a two-month-old infant. *Brain and Development* 13(2): 130–131.

187. Eng GD, et al. 1996. Obstetrical brachial plexus palsy (OBPP) outcome with conservative management. *Muscle and Nerve* 19(7): 884–891.

188. Rollnik JD, et al. 2000. Botulinum toxin treatment of cocontractions after birth-related brachial plexus lesions. *Neurology* 55(1): 112–114.

189. Laurent JP, et al. 1993. Neurosurgical correction of upper brachial plexus birth injuries. *Journal of Neurosurgery* 79(2): 197–203.

190. Slooff AC. 1993. Obstetric brachial plexus lesions and their neurosurgical treatment. *Clinics in Neurological Neurosurgery* 95(supplement): S73–S77.

191. Grossman JA, et al. 2003. Outcome after later combined brachial plexus and shoulder surgery after birth Trauma. *Journal of Bone and Joint Surgery (Br)* 85(8): 1166–1168.

192. Waters PM. 1999. Comparison of the natural history, the outcome of microsurgical repair, and the outcome of operative reconstruction in brachial plexus birth palsy. *Journal of Bone and Joint Surgery (Am)* 81(5): 649–659.

193. Al-Qattan MM, and Clarke HM. 1994. A burn caused by the operating microscope light during brachial plexus reconstruction. *Journal of Hand Surgery (Br)* 19(5): 550–551.

194. Zalis OS, et al. 1965. Motor patterning following transitory sensory and motor deprivation. *Archives of Neurology* 13(5): 487–494.

195. Brown T, et al. 2000. Developmental apraxia arising from neonatal brachial plexus palsy. *Neurology* 55(1): 24–30.

196. Noetzel M, et al. 1996. A prospective analysis of recovery following brachial plexus injury. *Annals of Neurology* 40(2): 321A.

197. Tachdijian MO. 1990. *Pediatric Orthopedics*, vol. 3, 2nd ed. Philadelphia: Saunders, 2009.

198. Terzis JK, and Papakonstantinou KC. 2002. Outcomes of scapula stabilization in obstetrical brachial plexus palsy: A novel dynamic procedure for correction of the winged scapula. *Plastic and Reconstructive Surgery* 109(2): 548–561.

Notes

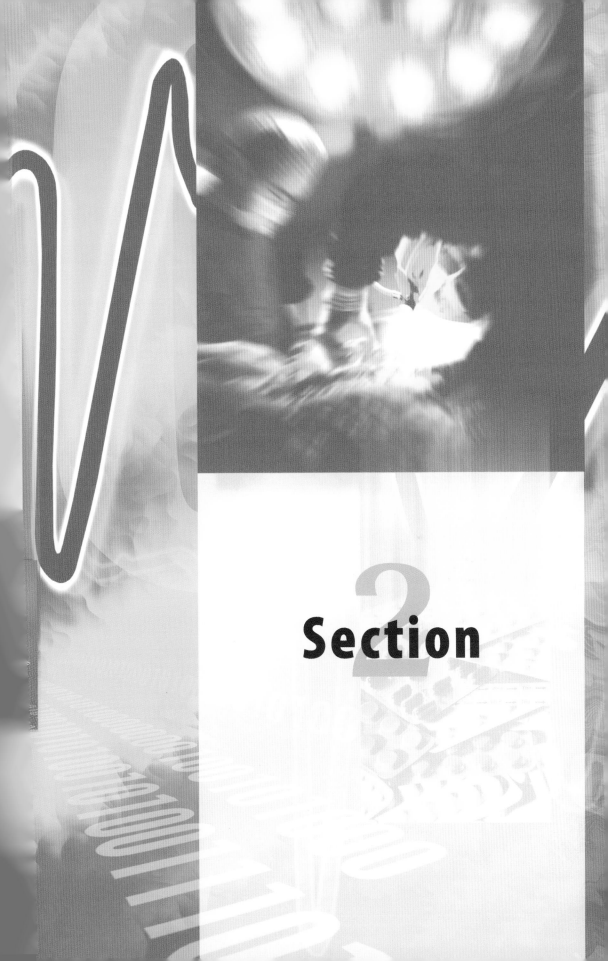

Section 2

Fluid, Electrolyte, and Nutritional Management of the Postsurgical Neonate

Cheryl A. Carlson, RNC, MS, NNP

Fluid and electrolyte management is a critical component in the care of the surgical neonate. It is based on knowledge of normal physiologic processes as well as an understanding of how both disease and surgical intervention can affect these processes. The gestation of the infant, in addition to the specific surgical procedure involved, guide administration of maintenance and replacement of fluids and electrolytes. Disease processes, such as patent ductus arteriosus, sepsis, and chronic lung disease, can complicate management. Excellent nursing assessment is imperative throughout the perioperative period.

This chapter begins with a review of general physiologic principles of fluid management in the body and homeostasis in the neonate. Disturbances in acid-base and fluid and electrolyte balances are then addressed. Fluid management of the surgical neonate from the preoperative period until postsurgery is outlined. The administration of total parenteral nutrition (TPN) and the transition to enteral feedings completes the material.

General Principles

BODY WATER COMPOSITION
A. Intracellular water
   1. This is the total amount of water in all body cells.
   2. It contains potassium, magnesium, and phosphate.
   3. The volume of intracellular water is maintained by potassium salts and regulated by the sodium-potassium pump: The mechanism that provides for active transport of sodium out of and potassium into the cell.
B. Extracellular water
   1. This is the total amount of water outside the cells, comprising both intravascular and interstitial fluids.

---

2. It contains sodium, potassium, magnesium, chloride, protein, and bicarbonate.
3. The volume of extracellular water is maintained by sodium salts and regulated by the kidneys.
4. The regulation between intravascular and interstitial volume is maintained by the colloid osmotic pressure of the plasma proteins.

BODY WATER CHANGES

A. The amounts of intracellular and extracellular water change throughout gestation and with growth. These changes affect not only body water composition, but also serum electrolytes (Figure 9-1).
B. Changes throughout gestation include the following.
   1. In the first trimester, the total body water of the fetus accounts for approximately 90 percent of body weight.
   2. Intracellular water increases from approximately 25 percent during the second trimester to 33 percent at term.[1]
   3. At term, the following occurs.
      a. Total body water decreases to approximately 75 percent.
      b. Thirty-five to 45 percent of the total body water is extracellular.
C. Weight loss in the immediate postnatal period occurs because of contraction of extracellular water, which is due to increased renal blood flow and function.
D. Differences in body water composition between full-term and preterm infants at birth are important when discussing fluid management.
   1. A premature infant born at 25–26 weeks gestation has 85 percent of the body weight as water, with 45–50 percent being extracellular.
   2. Premature infants have an increased proportion of extracellular water at birth and can lose 10–20 percent of their birth weight in the immediate postnatal period.[1,2]

RENAL PHYSIOLOGY

A. Renal function
   1. Increases with gestational and postnatal age
   2. Affected by disease processes and medications
   3. Renal tubules
      a. **Reabsorption** is the movement of substances from the peritubular capillaries across the tubular epithelium into the renal tubules.
      b. **Secretion** is the movement of substances from the peritubular capillaries across the tubular epithelium into the renal tubules.
B. Glomerular filtration rate (GFR)
   1. The amount of glomerular filtrate formed each minute in all the nephrons of both kidneys
   2. Low *in utero*
   3. Rises postnatally with the increase in renal blood flow
   4. Slower increase in GFR in infants born at <34 weeks gestation due to incomplete nephrogenesis[3]
   5. Increased tubular function after 34 weeks gestation[4]
C. Aldosterone
   1. This mineralocorticoid is produced by the adrenal cortex.
   2. It regulates extracellular water volume through its action on the renal tubules.
   3. It is released in response to adrenocorticotrophic hormone.

4. It acts on the renal tubules to reabsorb sodium and secrete potassium.
5. With increased sodium reabsorption, water will be absorbed, thereby increasing intravascular volume.

D. Antidiuretic hormone (ADH) vasopressin
   1. This regulates water balance by its effect on the collecting ducts.
   2. Vasopressin is produced by the hypothalamus, stored in the posterior pituitary, and released in response to an increase in plasma osmolarity.
   3. When vasopressin is present, the collecting ducts become more permeable to water, which increases water reabsorption into the peritubular capillaries, resulting in the formation of concentrated urine.
   4. Without vasopressin, the collecting ducts remain impermeable to water, less water is reabsorbed, and dilute urine is produced.

E. Acid-base balance
   1. The kidney plays an important role in acid-base balance through the reabsorption and excretion of bicarbonate and hydrogen ions.
   2. The level of bicarbonate in the serum is controlled by renal reabsorption.
   3. Up to a certain "threshold," all bicarbonate is reabsorbed; above that level, bicarbonate is excreted in the urine.[2]
      a. Renal threshold
         1) It is low in newborn infants, especially low birth weight (LBW) infants, when compared to children and adults.
         2) This low renal threshold results in the following.
            a) Low serum bicarbonate concentration
            b) Reduced buffering capacity
   4. The presence of acidosis causes the following.
      a. Increase in reabsorption of bicarbonate ions in the proximal tubule
      b. Increase in secretion of hydrogen ions in the distal tubule
   5. In the immediate newborn period, the following conditions prevail.
      a. Decreased ability of the collecting ducts to secrete hydrogen ions
      b. Limited capacity for excretion of hydrogen ions in the urine due to a decreased availability of buffers, especially phosphate and ammonium
      c. Decreased renal excretion of hydrogen ions due to decreased availability of buffers
   6. The presence of alkalosis causes the following.
      a. Excretion of bicarbonate
      b. Decrease in the secretion of hydrogen ions

FIGURE 9-1 ■ **Changes in body water during gestation and infancy.**

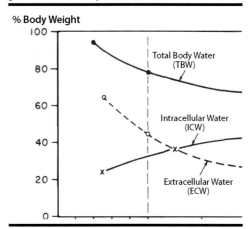

% Body Weight

From: Bell EF, and Oh W. 2005. Fluid and electrolyte management. In *Neonatology: Pathophysiology and Management of the Newborn*, 6th ed., MacDonald MG, Mullett MD, and Seshia MMK, eds. Philadelphia: Lippincott Williams & Wilkins, 363. Reprinted by permission.

F. Minerals reabsorbed or secreted by the renal tubules as needed to maintain homeostasis
   1. Calcium
   2. Magnesium
   3. Phosphorous

Assessment of Renal Function

A. Via urine
   1. Urine output
   2. Urine osmolality
   3. Urine specific gravity
   4. Creatinine level
   5. Urine electrolytes
      a. Useful in the evaluation of electrolyte abnormalities
   6. Urine pH
      a. An alkaline pH is suggestive of increased bicarbonate ion loss via the kidney.
B. Via blood
   1. Serum electrolytes
   2. Blood urea nitrogen (BUN)
C. General parameters
   1. Weight
   2. Fluid intake
   3. Vital signs

Electrolyte and Acid-Base Homeostasis

A. Factors affecting serum sodium, potassium, chloride, calcium, and bicarbonate levels
   1. The gestational age of the infant
   2. The rapid physiologic changes in the first week of life
   3. Disease state
      a. Illness (e.g., respiratory distress syndrome [RDS], intracranial hemorrhage)
      b. Infection
      c. Surgery
B. Sodium—the main extracellular cation
   1. Physiology
      a. Newborns have a large sodium reserve in the extracellular space.
      b. Sodium is absorbed in the gastrointestinal (GI) tract through the small intestines and colon.
      c. It is filtered by the glomerulus of the kidney and reabsorbed throughout the tubules.
      d. Approximately 90–95 percent of all sodium is reabsorbed because of the effects of oncotic and hydrostatic pressures in the peritubular capillaries.
      e. Aldosterone increases sodium absorption in exchange for potassium and hydrogen ions.
         1) The premature infant has a decreased ability to conserve sodium because the distal tubules have a limited response to aldosterone.[1]
   2. Maintenance and replacement therapy
      a. Sodium can be given as chloride, acetate, lactate, or phosphate salts.

    b. Sodium is not generally administered on the first day of life unless volume expansion is needed.

      1) Volume expansion is given as normal saline boluses (10 ml/kg).

    c. Administration of the maintenance sodium requirement of 2–4 mEq/kg/day may be started on the second day of life (depending on sodium balance).[1]

      1) Maintenance requirements are based on evaluation of the following.

        a) Serum electrolytes

        b) Body weight

        c) Urine sodium losses

      2) There is often a need for increased administration of sodium in premature infants during the second and third weeks of life because of their inability to conserve sodium.[1]

3. Hyponatremia

    a. Dilutional (extracellular fluid volume excess)

      1) This is defined as early hyponatremia that presents within the first week of life and is caused by excess water administration or fluid retention secondary to decreased renal function at birth.

      2) Infants at risk for dilutional hyponatremia include those with the following conditions.

        a) Congestive heart failure

        b) Renal failure

        c) Sepsis

        d) Necrotizing enterocolitis (NEC)

        e) Treated with neuromuscular paralysis

      3) Management consists of the following.

        a) Treatment of the underlying cause

        b) Fluid restriction

    b. Negative sodium balance

      1) Generally presents after the first week of life

      2) Caused by decreased intake or increased losses

        a) Extracellular volume deficit

- Increased renal or extrarenal losses:
  - Administration of diuretics
  - Severe renal immaturity due to prematurity
  - Renal tubular acidosis
  - Osmotic diuresis from glycosuria
- GI losses:
  - Gastric suction
  - Diarrhea
  - Surgical fistulas
  - Intestinal obstruction
  - Peritonitis
- Third space losses:
  - Skin sloughing
  - NEC
- Other losses:
  - Chest tube drainage
  - Cerebrospinal fluid (CSF)

    3) Management once etiology is determined
      a) Replace sodium deficit.
- If serum sodium is <120 mEq/liter, replace the calculated deficit over 24 hours.[1]
  - Na^+ deficit = (0.67 × birth weight [kg]) × (Na^+ desired – Na^+ actual)[5]
- Increase the sodium level no more than 1 mEq/hour.[6]

      b) Adjust maintenance fluids to include ongoing losses.

  c. Hyponatremia with normal extracellular volume[7]
    1) Overhydration (Table 9-1)
      a) Excess fluid administration
      b) Increased urine output and a low urine specific gravity

  d. Syndrome of inappropriate antidiuretic hormone (SIADH)
    1) Pathophysiology
      a) Increased secretion of antidiuretic hormone (vasopressin) *(In normal circumstances, vasopressin is released in response to an increase in serum osmolality or a drop in blood volume. In SIADH, vasopressin release occurs in the absence of these stimuli.[5])*
      b) Hyponatremia
      c) Low potassium, chloride, and calcium levels
      d) Decreased urine output and increased urine specific gravity
      e) Increased weight gain
      f) Increased urine osmolality, greater than plasma osmolality
      g) Urine sodium loss
      h) Normal adrenal and renal function

    2) Possible etiologies[8]
      a) Pain
      b) Opioid administration
      c) Intraventricular hemorrhage (IVH)
      d) Meningitis
      e) Asphyxia
      f) Pneumothorax
      g) Pneumonia
      h) Anesthesia
      i) Hypotension
      j) Positive pressure ventilation
      k) Surgery

    3) Components of differential diagnosis of overhydration vs SIADH
      a) Renal failure
      b) SIADH
      c) Overhydration
      d) Hyperaldosteronism

    4) Diagnosis
      a) Clinical assessment
- Evaluate for overhydration.
- Ensure accurate measurement of intake and output.
- Monitor sodium losses.
- Monitor weight.

      b) Diuretic therapy
      c) Laboratory studies
- Serum electrolytes

- Serum osmolarity
- Urine electrolytes
- Urine specific gravity

5) Management

   a) Fluid restriction for SIADH

   b) Appropriate fluid maintenance for treatment of overhydration

4. Hypernatremia

  a. Extracellular fluid volume normal or with deficit

   1) Increased insensible or renal water losses

    a) Very low birth weight (VLBW) infants are especially at risk for increased renal and insensible water losses.

    b) Increased water losses are also seen with the following.

- Vomiting
- Diarrhea
- Osmotic diuresis
- Other compartment losses via
  - Drains
  - Chest tubes

   2) Management

    a) Increase fluid administration slowly.

    b) Correct sodium administration slowly.

    c) Monitor electrolytes frequently.

    d) Monitor glucose.

  b. Extracellular fluid volume excess

   1) Excess fluid administration

   2) Reduced cardiac output

   3) Management

    a) Sodium restriction

C. Potassium—the main intracellular cation

  1. Physiology

   a. The concentration is maintained by the sodium-potassium pump.

   b. Potassium is important in regulating cell membrane potentials; Its most prominent effect is on myocardial cells.

   c. It is absorbed by the jejunum.

   d. It is actively secreted in the colon.

   e. In the kidney, the majority of filtered potassium is reabsorbed by the proximal tubules.

   f. Potassium is excreted in the urine.

    1) It is secreted almost entirely in the collecting ducts and distal tubules in response to aldosterone.

     a) The limited ability of the distal tubules to secrete potassium in premature infants may be because of the decreased responsiveness of the renal tubules to aldosterone.[3]

   g. Serum potassium levels have the following characteristics.

    1) Do not necessarily reflect total body potassium because potassium is an intracellular cation

TABLE 9-1 ■ Overhydration Compared to SIADH at a Glance

Overhydration	SIADH
Hyponatremia	Hyponatremia
Increased weight gain	Increased weight gain
Increased urine output	Decreased urine output
Low urine specific gravity	High urine specific gravity

        2) Are affected by the pH of the body compartments due to intracellular shifts of hydrogen and potassium ions (e.g., low pH, high potassium)

2. Maintenance and replacement therapy
   a. Potassium can be given as chloride, acetate, or phosphate salts.
   b. Potassium is not usually given in the first 24 hours of life.
   c. Assessments of renal function and urine output are critical prior to beginning potassium supplementation.
   d. Initially, 1–2 mEq/kg/day is appropriate maintenance therapy.[1,2]
      1) There may be an increased requirement for potassium during the following.
         a) Active growth
         b) Cellular repair

3. Hypokalemia
   a. Causes
      1) Inadequate intake
      2) Increased GI losses
         a) Vomiting
         b) Diarrhea
         c) Gastric suction
         d) Ileostomy drainage
      3) Increased renal losses
      4) Relative hypokalemia (Worsening hypokalemia can be seen with severe metabolic alkalosis.)
   b. Clinical effects:
      1) These are related to the effect of inadequate potassium on muscle cells.
         a) A possibly paralytic ileus
         b) Cardiac arrhythmia
      2) Concurrent increased loss of chloride can lead to a contraction alkalosis and hypokalemia.
   c. Treatment
      1) Determinants
         a) Serum level
         b) Clinical manifestations
      2) Increase in maintenance potassium in intravenous (IV) fluids
      3) Potassium chloride replacement
         a) Because of the risks of cardiac arrhythmia with rapid administration, potassium should be given over several hours, never as a bolus.
            • With a large deficit, the potassium should be replaced over 48–72 hours in order to monitor renal function and avoid cardiac complications.[1]

4. Hyperkalemia
   a. Infants at risk include those with the following conditions.[6]
      1) Critical illness
      2) Oliguria or clinical signs of renal failure
      3) VLBW (because of immature renal function)
      4) Disseminated intravascular coagulation
      5) Tissue destruction due to trauma leading to release of potassium from damaged cells
      6) Intracranial bleeding
      7) GI bleeding

        8) Metabolic acidosis
    b. The clinical effects of concern are cardiac.
    c. Treatment consists of the following.
        1) Basis
            a) The clinical condition of the infant
            b) The electrocardiogram
                • Presence of peak T waves
                • SST depression
                • Widening of the QRS complex
                • Prolonged PR interval
            c) The serum potassium level
        2) Goals
            a) A lower serum potassium level
            b) Decreased or no effects of hyperkalemia on the myocardium
        3) Procedure
            a) Stop all potassium administration.
            b) Furosemide (Lasix) may be given to increase potassium excretion.
            c) Calcium gluconate may be administered to act as an antagonist to the effect of potassium on the myocardium.
            d) Glucose and insulin administration will work to increase cellular uptake of potassium.
            e) Correction with sodium bicarbonate is appropriate if the infant is acidotic because alkalemia will promote increased cellular uptake of potassium ions in exchange for hydrogen ions.

D. Chloride
   1. Physiology
     a. Chloride losses lead to decreased secretion of bicarbonate ions and metabolic alkalosis.
       1) Hypokalemia will often accompany metabolic alkalosis because of
           a) Intracellular shifts of hydrogen and potassium ions
           b) Renal compensation to conserve hydrogen ions in place of potassium
   2. Causes of chloride losses
     a. Ileostomy drainage
     b. Gastric suction
     c. Vomiting
     d. Diarrhea
     e. Renal losses from defects in tubular reabsorption
     f. Renal losses from diuretic therapy
   3. Causes of chloride retention
     a. Premature infants may have a hyperchloremic metabolic acidosis caused by
       1) Renal immaturity
       2) Increased renal bicarbonate losses

E. Treatment of metabolic imbalance
   1. Depends on the underlying condition
   2. Metabolic alkalosis[6]
     a. Replacement therapy with sodium chloride and potassium chloride
     b. Increased fluid administration
     c. Removing acetate from TPN or IV fluids
   3. Metabolic acidosis
     a. A form of alkali may be administered.

      1) Sodium bicarbonate

      2) Tromethamine (THAM)

      3) Increased acetate in the TPN solution

    b. With correction of an acidosis, hypokalemia may be seen and will require correction.

CALCIUM, PHOSPHOROUS, AND MAGNESIUM HOMEOSTASIS

A. Physiology

    1. Calcium, magnesium, and phosphorous homeostasis is regulated through the actions of the following.

      a. Parathyroid hormone

      b. Vitamin D

      c. Calcitonin

    2. In the fetus, the majority of calcium and phosphorous is stored during the third trimester.

    3. Treatment of calcium, phosphorous, and magnesium disorders depends on serum levels, clinical manifestations, and underlying etiology.

    4. The ratio of calcium and phosphorous needs to be carefully maintained when increasing the amounts of calcium and phosphorous in IV fluids to accomplish the following.

      a. Prevent precipitation

      b. Maximize absorption

B. Calcium

    1. Maintenance of the following.

      a. Muscle contractility—smooth and skeletal

      b. Normal cardiac function

      c. Normal neuromuscular function

      d. A functional coagulation pathway

      e. Neural energy transmission in the peripheral and central nervous systems

    2. Hypocalcemia

      a. Causes

        1) Prematurity, because of lower calcium stores

        2) Stress

        3) Hypothermia

        4) Infection

        5) RDS

        6) Asphyxia

        7) Infant of a diabetic mother (IDM)

        8) Renal failure

        9) Hypomagnesemia

      b. Management

        1) Administer calcium gluconate, slowly, as a bolus.

        2) Additionally, increase the amount of calcium in the maintenance fluids.

        3) Lack of response to calcium administration can be a sign of hypomagnesemia.

    3. Hypercalcemia

      a. Causes

        1) Most commonly, excess administration of calcium and vitamin D

        2) Hyperparathyroidism

        3) Thiazide diuretics

        4) Hypophosphatemia

    b. Management

        1) Treat the underlying condition.

        2) Increase renal excretion of calcium.

          a) Administer furosemide.

          b) Restrict calcium intake.

          c) In severe cases, glucocorticoids may be used to decrease intestinal absorption and increase renal excretion of calcium.

        3) Treat associated hypophosphatemia.

C. Phosphorous

  1. Functions in the body

    a. Gene transmission as part of nucleic acids

    b. Cellular energy as adenosine triphosphate

    c. Component of lipoprotein that forms cell membranes

    d. Contributor to bone mineralization and matrix formation in premature infants

  2. Hypophosphatemia

    a. Risks

        1) Prematurity

        2) Lack of absorption

        3) Inadequate calcium/phosphorus ratio

    b. Management

        1) Maintain adequate calcium/phosphorous ratio to do the following.

          a) Prevent precipitation.

          b) Maximize absorption.

        2) Administer phosphorous as sodium or potassium phosphate.

        3) Consider vitamin D supplementation.

        4) Increase maintenance phosphorous.

  3. Hyperphosphatemia

    a. Causes

        1) Impaired renal excretion of phosphorous

        2) Hypoparathyroidism

        3) Excessive phosphorous administration

    b. Management

        1) Treat the underlying condition.

        2) Restrict phosphorous intake.

        3) If the condition is severe, dialysis may be required.

D. Magnesium

  1. Functions in the body

    a. Regulates DNA synthesis, cell growth, and reproduction

    b. Transfers, stores, and utilizes intracellular energy

    c. Maintains normal cell membrane formation

    d. Transmits neuromuscular, cardiac, and smooth muscle impulses

  2. Hypomagnesemia

    a. Causes

        1) Low serum levels in premature infants

        2) In the critically ill infant, possibly accompanies hypocalcemia

    b. Management

        1) Replacement therapy with magnesium sulfate

        2) Careful administration by IV to avoid complications

    a) Systemic hypotension
    b) Central nervous system (CNS) depression
    c) Metabolic bone disease
  3. Hypermagnesemia
    a. Causes
      1) Renal failure
      2) Prematurity
      3) Magnesium-containing antacids
    b. Management
      1) Loop diuretics to facilitate renal excretion
      2) Exchange transfusion if condition is severe
      3) IV calcium administration to reverse CNS effects of hypermagnesemia

GLUCOSE HOMEOSTASIS

A. Physiology[9]
  1. Glucose homeostasis in the newborn is regulated by insulin and glucagon, through the processes of glycogenolysis and gluconeogenesis.
  2. The presence of hepatic glycogen, gluconeogenic precursors, and normal endocrine functions are required for the maintenance of a normal glucose level.[9]
    a. Premature infants have the following.
      1) Limited glycogen stores
      2) An immature response to endogenous insulin
    b. Both hypoglycemia and hyperglycemia can result.
B. Hypoglycemia
  1. Not generally seen in the perioperative period without
    a. Inadequate calorie intake
    b. Underlying condition
      1) Hyperinsulinemia
        a) IDM
        b) Pancreatic islet cell tumor
      2) Endocrine or metabolic disease
      3) Large-for-gestational-age infant
  2. Management
    a. Treat the underlying condition.
    b. Increase the glucose infusion rate to maintain blood glucose >50 mg/dl.[10]
C. Hyperglycemia
  1. More common than hypoglycemia in the postoperative period[4]
    a. Close monitoring of glucose levels, to avoid complications, is important in all critically ill and premature infants.
    b. Close monitoring is especially important in the VLBW infant, who is at most risk for developing hyperglycemia related to surgery.
  2. Causes
    a. Administration of high volumes of a dextrose solution
    b. Metabolic response to operative stress
      1) Differences in response are based on gestational age and severity of the injury.[11]
      2) An increase in catabolic hormones, such as catecholamines, glucagon, and corticosteroids, and decreases in both the secretion and end organ response to insulin promote the following.

        a) Hepatic release of glucose

        b) Breakdown of protein and fat stores, which are the precursors for gluconeogenesis[12]

        c) Resultant release of glucose (causing hyperglycemia), which is important in supplying energy to the tissues

        d) Initially beneficial response (release of glucose) (However, ongoing stress in a critically ill or premature infant with decreased reserves can be detrimental.)

    c. Fentanyl used with inhalation anesthesia (attenuates the hyperglycemic response to surgery)[13]

  3. Complications[4,11]

    a. Hyperosmolarity

    b. Osmotic diuresis

    c. IVH

  4. Management

    a. Decrease the glucose concentration.

    b. Decrease the rate of glucose administration.

    c. Administer insulin.

NEONATAL FLUID REQUIREMENTS

A. Maintain homeostatic fluid balance.

  1. Water and electrolytes are normally lost through the following.

    a. Urine

    b. Skin

    c. Stool

    d. Respiratory tract

  2. To determine initial fluid requirements, consider the following.

    a. Gestational age

      1) Generally, the fluid requirement of a premature infant is higher than that of a term infant due to increased insensible water loss through the skin.

    b. Environment (including the use of humidity)

      1) There are further losses with the use of radiant warmers and nonhumidified incubators.

      2) Water loss from the respiratory tract will be increased in an infant who is tachypneic or with inadequate humidification of the ventilator circuit.

      3) Phototherapy also increases insensible water loss.

      4) The use of the following will help decrease insensible water loss.

        a) Self-adhering hydrogel dressings when needed

        b) A plastic blanket

        c) A heat shield

      5) With the use of incubators and high humidity, the daily fluid requirement of a premature infant can be decreased by up to 30 percent.[2]

  3. Increases in daily fluid administration will depend on the following.

    a. Body weight changes

    b. Serum electrolytes

    c. Cardiovascular status

    d. Urine output

    e. Abnormal losses

  4. Maintenance fluid administration begins when the infant is in fluid balance, often at the end of the first week of life, depending on the infant's clinical status.

B. Replace abnormal losses generated via the following.

  1. Gastric suction

  2. Loss of saliva

  3. Chest tube

  4. Ostomy

  5. Vomiting

  6. Diarrhea

  7. Surgical drains

  8. Ventriculostomy

  9. Lumbar puncture

  10. Wounds

  11. Third spacing of fluid

  12. Immature renal function

C. It is critical to to manage fluids precisely to avoid the risks of both fluid restriction and fluid overload.

  1. Fluid restriction can cause the following.

   a. Dehydration

   b. Hypoglycemia

   c. Hyperbilirubinemia

   d. Hypernatremia

  2. Fluid overload can cause the following.

   a. Patent ductus arteriosus

   b. Chronic lung disease

   c. IVH

   d. Dilutional hyponatremia

  3. Decrease total fluid in infants with these conditions.

   a. Renal failure

   b. Inappropriate ADH secretion

   c. Congestive heart failure

  4. Fluid restriction is considered in an infant with asphyxia.

  5. Fluid management is more difficult in critically ill infants who require the following.

   a. Blood pressure support with dopamine or dobutamine

   b. Antibiotics (Many penicillins contain large amounts of sodium and may result in an excessive sodium load in immature infants.)

   c. Blood products

  6. Medications and the flush solutions administered to clear lines for frequent blood sampling can increase the total fluid administered daily by 20–30 percent.

Fluid and Electrolyte Disturbances in Infants with Specific Conditions (Table 9-2)

CARDIOVASCULAR

A. Patent ductus arteriosus

  1. Electrolyte imbalances

TABLE 9-2 ■ Summary of Possible Fluid and Electrolyte Disturbances in Surgical Infants

Type of Surgery	Fluid	Sodium	Potassium	Calcium, Magnesium	Chloride	Phosphorus
Cardiovascular	Fluid overload	Hyponatremia	Hyperkalemia	Metabolic acidosis	Dehydration (fluid restriction, diuretic use)	
Gastrointestinal	Dehydration	Hyponatremia	Hypo/ hyperkalemia	Hypocalcemia	Hypochloremia, metabolic alkalosis	Metabolic acidosis
Genitourinary	Fluid overload	Hypo/ hypernatremia	Hyperkalemia	Hypocalcemia	Metabolic acidosis	Hyperphosphatemia
Central nervous system	Dehydration	Hyponatremia	Hyperkalemia	Respiratory acidosis or alkalosis		

Adapted from: John E, Klavdianou M, and Vidyasagar D. 1989. Electrolyte problems in neonatal surgical patients. *Clinics in Perinatology* 16(1): 219–232.

   a. Can be associated with decreased renal function
   b. Hyponatremia caused by fluid overload
  2. Indomethacin treatment
   a. May cause hyperkalemia because of decreased renal blood flow
   b. Hyponatremia, secondary to fluid retention
 B. Other cardiac disorders
  1. Electrolyte imbalances
   a. Hyponatremia caused by fluid overload
   b. Hyperkalemia (and azotemia) (These may occur postoperatively due to acute renal failure from intraoperative clamping of the aorta.)[6]
  2. Metabolic acidosis
  3. Fluid overload caused by
   a. Congestive heart failure
   b. Renal dysfunction

GASTROINTESTINAL

 A. General postoperative complications may be related to fluid and electrolyte imbalances with GI surgeries.
  1. Increased losses of saliva and intestinal secretions containing hydrogen, chloride, and potassium ions can cause the following.
   a. Dehydration
   b. Hyponatremia
   c. Hypokalemia
   d. Metabolic alkalosis
  2. Hypocalcemia may be seen if there is inadequate intake.
 B. With surgery, the infant may experience third space losses.

GENITOURINARY

 A. Postoperative complications related to fluid and electrolyte imbalances with genitourinary (GU) surgeries
  1. Complications are generally associated with fluid overload and hyponatremia.
  2. Hypernatremia may be seen if there is secondary nephrogenic diabetes insipidus.

3. Renal tubular acidosis may result in the following.
   a. Hyperkalemia
   b. Metabolic acidosis
   c. Hypocalcemia
4. Renal failure associated with hyperphosphatemia, fluid overload, hyperkalemia, and metabolic acidosis may be seen.
5. With postoperative diuresis and natriuresis, third space losses, and loss of urinary bicarbonate ions, there is an increased risk of the following.[6]
   a. Dehydration
   b. Hyponatremia
   c. Metabolic acidosis

CENTRAL NERVOUS SYSTEM

A. Hydrocephalus
   1. Electrolyte imbalance may occur.
      a. Dehydration and hyponatremia caused by excessive loss of CSF with external drainage
      b. Hyperkalemia in the presence of intracranial bleeding
   2. With changes in CNS control of respiration, there is a risk of respiratory alkalosis or acidosis.
B. Myelomeningocele
   1. If the lesion is open, dehydration and hyponatremia can occur with excess loss of CSF.
C. SIADH
   See SIADH, page 418.

TABLE 9-3 ■ Evaluation of Hydration Status

Marker	In Dehydration
Skin color	Pale
Skin turgor	Poor
Capillary refill	3–4 seconds
Heart rate	Tachycardia
Blood pressure	Hypotension
Weight	Weight loss
Anterior fontanel	Depressed
Tear production	Decreases
Serum Values	In dehydration
Sodium	Depends on type, see Table 9-4
Osmolarity	Depends on type, see Table 9-4
BUN	Increasing
Creatinine	Increased
Calcium	Increased
Acid-base status	Metabolic acidosis
Urine Values	In Dehydration
Output	Decreased
Electrolytes	
Specific gravity	

Fluid and Electrolyte Management

PREOPERATIVE

A. Goals
   1. Maintain fluid and electrolyte balance.
   2. Maintain homeostatic intravascular volume.
   3. Correct anemia or coagulopathy.
B. Evaluation of fluid and electrolyte balance
   1. Evaluate hydration status (Table 9-3).
      a. History
         1) Presence of preexisting and ongoing losses
            a) GI
            b) GU
            c) CNS

   b. Physical examination
     1) Cardiovascular status
        a) Skin and mucous
           membrane color, turgor,
           dryness
        b) Capillary refill
        c) Heart rate
        d) Blood pressure
     2) Weight gain or loss
     3) Presence/absence of tissue edema
     4) Palpation of anterior fontanel
   c. Assessment of intake and output adequacy
     1) Calculate intake as ml/kg/day.
     2) Calculate urine output as ml/kg/hour.
   d. Laboratory studies
     1) Serum
        a) Electrolytes
        b) BUN
        c) Creatinine
        d) Calcium
        e) Acid-base status
        f) Osmolarity
        g) Hematocrit
     2) Urine
        a) Electrolytes
        b) Specific gravity

TABLE 9-4 ■ Markers for Dehydration

Type of Dehydration	Isotonic	Hypotonic	Hypertonic
Serum sodium	130–150	<130	>150
Serum osmolarity	270–300	<270	>310

C. Deficit replacement
   1. Treat hypovolemia.
      a. Normal saline boluses may be used to treat hypotension.
      b. Hypovolemic shock requires immediate treatment with fluids (albumin, plasma, or packed red blood cells) to restore and maintain cardiovascular function, peripheral perfusion, urine output, and to correct lactic acidosis.[14]
D. Correction of dehydration[15] (Table 9-4)
   1. Critical in preventing anesthetic complications
      a. Anesthetic agents can decrease systemic vascular resistance and depress myocardial contractility, leading to bradycardia, decreased cardiac output, and hypotension.[16]
   2. Possible results of uncorrected dehydration
      a. Decreased circulating volume
      b. Acute renal failure
      c. Cardiovascular collapse
   3. Isotonic dehydration (serum sodium concentration 130–150 mEq/liter)
      a. Adjust maintenance administration to account for ongoing losses.
         1) Administer 150 ml/kg/day of a glucose and 0.2 percent sodium chloride solution.[14]
         2) If weight loss is greater than 10 percent and the infant has clinical manifestations of poor cardiac function, IV infusions of normal saline or 5 percent albumin may be indicated.[7]

4. Hypotonic dehydration (serum sodium concentration <130 mEq/liter)
   a. This is corrected with a glucose and 0.45 percent saline solution.[16]
   b. Additional sodium replacement may be required to correct the sodium deficit, depending on the severity of the CNS and cardiovascular symptoms.[6]
      1) Normal saline
      2) Three percent saline
   c. Increase the sodium level no more than 1 mEq/hour.[6]
5. Hypertonic dehydration (serum sodium concentration >150 mEq/liter)
   a. This requires careful attention to correct hypovolemia as needed.
   b. Replace the deficit with a glucose and 0.2 percent saline solution at 100 ml/kg/day.[14]
   c. Rapid correction of hyperosmolarity may lead to CNS complications such as seizures.

TABLE 9-5 ■ Electrolyte Content of Body Fluids

Fluid Source	Sodium (mEq/liter)	Potassium (mEq/liter)	Chloride (mEq/liter)
Stomach	20–80	5–20	100–150
Small intestine	100–140	5–15	90–120
Bile	120–140	5–15	90–120
Ileostomy	45–135	3–15	20–120
Diarrheal stool	10–90	10–80	10–110
Cerebrospinal fluid	130–150	2–5	100–130

From: Bell EF, and Oh W. 2005. Fluid and electrolyte management. In *Neonatology: Pathophysiology and Management of the Newborn*, 6th ed., MacDonald MG, Seshia MMK, and Mullet MD, eds. Philadelphia: Lippincott Williams & Wilkins, 370. Reprinted by permission.

E. Hypervolemia treatment
   1. Observe for clinical signs.
      a. Weight gain
      b. Edema
   2. Determine the etiology.
   3. Restrict fluids as necessary.
   4. Administer diuretics as ordered and appropriate.
   5. Administer electrolytes to correct imbalances if appropriate.
F. Homeostatic intravascular volume maintenance
   1. Maintenance fluids are determined after careful consideration of the neonate's hydration status and electrolyte needs.
      a. A dextrose solution with electrolytes added based on serum levels and replacement of any urinary losses is generally used.
      b. Consider the need for fluid restriction (e.g., with patent ductus arteriosus, hypoxic insult, or renal failure).
   2. Replace ongoing, abnormal losses.
      a. Ongoing fluid losses from the following can lead to dehydration.
         1) GI suction
         2) GU losses
         3) Open wounds
         4) Third space losses
            a) Caused by the shift of fluid out of the intravascular compartment because of changes in cell wall permeability as well as hydrostatic and oncotic pressure changes[16]
            b) May be seen as
               • Edema
               • Ascites

- Fluid in the pleural cavity
        c) Occur frequently in infants with inflammatory abdominal processes, such as NEC
   b. Replace ongoing fluid losses in addition to maintenance fluids. Assessment and replacement should be done every four hours, at least initially.
        1) The ordered replacement fluid is given over the following four hours.[17]
        2) Calculate the amount of the losses and evaluate of serum electrolytes to determine the type and amount of replacement fluids to be administered.[17]
            a) Generally, replacement can be done with either a lactated Ringer's solution or a saline solution.
            b) Gastric losses are corrected with 0.45 percent saline solution with addition of potassium.
            c) High small intestinal losses are corrected with lactated Ringer's solution with potassium added.[17]
   c. Table 9-5 lists the electrolyte composition of body fluids, useful in determining replacement needs.
   d. Correct fluid overload.
G. Correction of anemia and coagulopathy
   1. Administer blood products to:
      a. Maintain the oxygen-carrying capacity of the blood
      b. Replace clotting factors in the presence of a coagulopathy
H. Assessment of acid-base status to identify respiratory or metabolic disturbances
   1. Imbalances in acid-base status
      a. These can affect serum levels of potassium, PCO_2, and ionized calcium.[14]
   2. Metabolic acidosis
      a. These are seen in conditions with poor perfusion.
         1) Shock
         2) Hypothermia
         3) Asphyxia
         4) Hypoxia
         5) Renal disease
      b. Treat the primary cause.
      c. In severe acidosis, correct with 4.2 percent sodium bicarbonate solution.[18]
   3. Metabolic alkalosis
      a. This is seen with gastric losses.
      b. Correct it by administering a sodium, potassium, and chloride solution.
   4. Respiratory acidosis and respiratory alkalosis
      a. Correct it with ventilator management.
   5. Treatment as ordered
I. Assessment of glucose status
   1. Monitor serum glucose and urine glucose levels.
   2. Administer the appropriate glucose concentration, thereby avoiding complications associated with hypoglycemia and hyperglycemia.
J. Nursing measures
   1. Accurately measure all fluid administered, including the following.
      a. Medication volumes
      b. Flush solution volumes

2. Accurately measure intake and output.
   a. Accurate assessment of urine output may require placement of a urinary catheter.
   b. Ongoing losses need to be closely monitored and recorded on the flow sheet. **(See F. Homeostatic intravascular volume maintenance, above.)**
3. Assess cardiovascular status on an ongoing basis.
   a. Heart rate
   b. Blood pressure
   c. Perfusion
4. Administer ordered medications.
5. Monitor serum electrolytes and acid-base status in a timely manner.
6. Discontinue enteral feedings and begin IV fluids two to four hours prior to the scheduled surgery for those neonates who have been feeding prior to an elective surgery.

INTRAOPERATIVE FLUID MANAGEMENT

A. Intraoperative fluid administration is generally managed by the anesthesiologist.
B. The continued goals of fluid management are to provide maintenance fluids and to continue to replace ongoing losses.[4]
   1. Provide maintenance fluids.
      a. Critically ill neonates will require dextrose replacement due to:
         1) Decreased glycogen stores
         2) The increased stress of surgery
   2. Continue the replacement of ongoing losses.
      a. The amount of fluids required to replace losses is variable and depends on the surgical procedure.
      b. In major surgical procedures, there are increased third space losses that need replacement, usually with a lactated Ringer's solution.[6]
      c. With renal failure, replacement should be a normal saline solution with bicarbonate.[6]
      d. The following applies to blood loss during surgery.[19–21]
         1) It is commonly replaced with crystalloid at three times the amount of blood lost.
         2) Up to five times the amount may be indicated with continued bleeding, hypoperfusion, and increased capillary permeability.[15]
         3) Packed red blood cell transfusion is indicated if the surgical blood loss exceeds 10–20 percent of the infant's blood volume.[4,14,20]
C. Anesthesia is administered.
   1. A general anesthetic agent is used for most neonatal surgery.
      a. Inhalation anesthetics such as halothane are used along with fentanyl or morphine.
      b. Use of fentanyl as an anesthetic agent or adjunct to nitric oxide can help the infant to avoid hemodynamic instability if his intravascular volume status is normalized prior to its use.[4]
   2. Spinal anesthesia may be used in nonintubated infants for inguinal hernia repair.[16]
   3. Possible complications of anesthesia include the following.[16]
      a. Decreased myocardial contractility
      b. Decreased heart rate
      c. Decreased systemic vascular resistance

D. Nursing measures include the following.

    1. Document the medications used during surgery.

    2. Monitor the amount and type of fluid administered during surgery.

POSTOPERATIVE FLUID MANAGEMENT

A. The following are goals of postoperative fluid management.[6]

    1. Maintain the following.

      a. Intravascular volume

        1) Hypovolemia can cause hypotension and oliguria in the postoperative period.

          a) These can be corrected by bolus fluid administration of 10–20 ml/kg of an isotonic solution, such as normal saline.

      b. Cardiovascular integrity

        1) Give packed red blood cells as needed to maintain adequate oxygen-carrying capacity.

      c. Urine output

        1) Maintain a urine output of 1–2 ml/kg/hour.[22,23]

B. Determine the infant's postoperative baseline.

    1. Body weight

    2. Arterial blood gases

    3. Blood/serum levels of:

      a. Electrolytes

      b. Glucose

      c. Calcium

      d. BUN

      e. Creatinine

C. Correct any deficits or excesses that have occurred during the surgery.

    1. Ventilated infants may have a decrease in GFR. Therefore, maintenance fluids may be restricted to 60 percent of estimated maintenance requirements.[8]

    2. Third space losses that occurred during the intraoperative/postoperative period will require replacement fluids postoperatively, in addition to the maintenance volume.

      a. Approaches to estimating the amount of third space losses that have occurred and determining the amount of fluid to be replaced:[14]

        1) Increase the maintenance fluid volume by 1.5–2 times the volume for the first 24 hours postoperatively.[14]

        2) Range of third space losses or from open wounds can be from 5–20 ml/kg/hour.[24]

        3) A quadrant scheme for estimating the fluid losses of an infant after abdominal surgery has been described by Filston and colleagues.[22]

          a) Additional one-quarter of maintenance for each abdominal quadrant involved with inflammatory or obstructive disease or traumatized by the surgical procedure

          b) One-quarter of maintenance volume for each quadrant of abdominal cavity[25]

          c) Monitor and adjust by urine output

    3. Ongoing GI losses or fluids lost through dressings should be replaced every two to four hours to prevent dehydration.[6]

      a. An isotonic fluid is generally used to replace ongoing losses in surgical patients with the following conditions.

      b. Measure the electrolyte content of the losses, evaluate, and replace accordingly.[14]

      c. Administer albumin or fresh frozen plasma for serous losses, such as from a chest tube.[14,26]

D. Recognize responses to surgical stress.

  1. To meet metabolic demands postoperatively, there is a breakdown of nutrient stores of the following.

      a. Carbohydrate

      b. Protein

      c. Fat

  2. Catecholamines, corticosteroids, and glucagon are released.

      a. Lipolysis and ketogenesis occur secondary to catecholamine stimulation and lead to increased ketone body formation.

      b. Glucagon stimulates glycogenolysis and increases blood glucose.[11,27]

        1) This provides an alternative source of energy for the tissues.

        2) Postoperative fat utilization may exceed the rate of free fatty acid mobilization.[11]

          a) Ketogenesis occurs secondary to catecholamine stimulation and leads to increased ketone body formation, which provides an alternative source of energy for tissues.[12]

  3. The metabolic response to operative stress seen in infants differs from that in adults and older children.[12]

      a. There are fewer changes in metabolic rate and oxygen consumption in infants than in adults.

      b. Careful monitoring of blood and urine glucose levels is critical in the postoperative period to prevent complications caused by hyperglycemia.

  4. Consider the infant's response to surgical stress as well as his gestational age when determining optimal nutritional support.

Nutritional Management

A. TPN is used for premature and critically ill infants at risk for inadequate nutrition.

  1. Nutritional supplementation in the form of additional calories and protein is given to surgical and critically ill infants to bring them from a catabolic state into an anabolic state so continued growth and healing can occur.

  2. Initiation of parenteral nutrition depends on the infant's nutritional status preoperatively and the type of surgery.

  3. Provision of calories and nutrients is indicated for the following.[28]

      a. Term infants who will be without adequate nutrition for more than three days

      b. Preterm infants beginning on the first day of life

  4. Infants who require extensive intestinal surgery are often started on parenteral nutrition prior to surgery because they will be given nothing by mouth postoperatively to rest the GI tract following surgery.

B. Parenteral nutrition solutions are composed of the following.

  1. Crystalline solution

      a. Dextrose

        1) Glucose is the major energy source for the following.[11]

          a) Central nervous system

          b) Erythrocytes

    c) Retina

    d) Renal medulla

    e) Intestinal mucosa

2) The endogenous production rate of glucose for a premature infant is 4.6–7.6 mg/kg/minute, double that of the full-term infant at 3–4 mg/kg/minute.[29]

3) Dextrose (d-glucose), a monohydrate used for IV administration of glucose, has 3.4 kcal/gm due to the incorporation of a water molecule in the dextrose molecule.[28]

4) Initial IV fluid is given as 5 or 10 percent dextrose in water, with an initial glucose delivery rate of 4–6 mg/kg/minute to match the basal glucose utilization rates.[30,31]

    a) Full-term and premature infants who are critically ill, hypothermic, or have respiratory distress may require higher glucose infusion rates to meet energy needs.[9]

    b) In spite of the fact that premature infants have higher energy needs because of their higher metabolic rates and increased brain to liver weight ratios, they are at increased risk for hyperglycemia.

        • Hyperglycemia is seen in response to exogenous glucose administration. It is caused by decreased insulin secretion and increased peripheral and hepatic resistance to insulin.[32,33]

        • Hyperglycemia can be further complicated by increases in catecholamine and cortisol levels, as seen with surgery, which promote tissue catabolism to provide amino acids for gluconeogenesis.[33,34]

        • Term infants are able to increase insulin production in response to hyperglycemia.

        • Premature infants have a limited ability to increase insulin production, putting them at risk for more prolonged hyperglycemia.[33]

    c) The glucose infusion rate is gradually increased by 1–2 mg/kg/minute daily, based on serum glucose levels and the presence of little or no glucose in the urine, to a maximum of 11–12 mg/kg/minute.[32]

    d) When glucose administration exceeds body needs, there is an increase in oxygen consumption, carbon dioxide production, and energy expenditure caused by the conversion of the excess glucose into fat.

        • The exact glucose infusion rate at which this occurs in the neonate is not known, but it is approximately 12–13 mg/kg/minute.[32]

        • With higher glucose infusion rates, monitor for increased serum carbon dioxide levels.

5) The concentration of dextrose used has several determinants.

    a) The concentration of dextrose that can be infused into a peripheral vein is limited by the osmolality of the dextrose solution.

    b) Dextrose solutions >5 percent are considered hypertonic.[11]

    c) Dextrose solutions up to 12.5 percent can be administered through a peripheral vein.[35]

    d) Generally, dextrose solutions up to 25 percent may be given via central access.[35]

    e) The concentration of dextrose delivered centrally may be increased >25 percent in infants who require severe fluid restriction.

  b. Electrolytes

   1) These are added to the parenteral nutrition solution based on serum electrolytes.

   2) Adequate amounts of calcium and phosphorous are important to maintain bone mineralization.

    a) Administration by a peripheral or central vein determines the amount and molar ratio of calcium and phosphorous that can be added.

     • Greater amounts of calcium and phosphorous can be added to central parenteral nutrition.

    b) Cysteine added to the parenteral nutrition solution increases its acidity and allows increased amounts of calcium and phosphorous to be added.

   3) Solutions containing trace elements and water- and fat-soluble vitamins are given to prevent deficiencies.

    a) Dose is based on the infant's weight.

    b) Infants with excessive ileostomy or colostomy drainage often require increased amounts of copper and zinc.[36]

  c. Amino acids

   1) Protein supplies 4 kcal/gm. The following are the goals of early protein administration in the first 48 hours of life.

    a) Prevent protein catabolism

    b) Achieve intrauterine accretion rates

   2) Several types of crystalline amino acid solutions contain both essential and nonessential amino acids.

    a) The pediatric solutions TrophAmine (Kendall McGaw) and Aminosyn PF (Abbott Laboratories) have increased amounts of the amino acids essential for infants, such as taurine, tyrosine, cysteine, and histidine.[28]

   3) There are recommendations to initiate parenteral protein administration to premature infants on the first day of life to prevent protein catabolism.[33,35]

    a) Premature infants tolerate 1–1.5 gm/kg/day of an amino acid solution, beginning on the first day of life.[32]

    b) Daily incremental increases of 0.5–1 gm/kg/day to a maximum of 3 gm/kg/day in full-term infants, and up to 4 gm/kg/day in premature infants by four to five days of life, are well tolerated in most infants.[32,37]

    c) Term infants can receive 2.5 gm/kg of protein on postoperative day 1, with a positive effect on nitrogen balance.[38]

   4) With the addition of protein, another 2–3 mg/kg/minute of glucose are required to support protein deposition.[32]

    a) To allow for protein deposition, it is important to provide an adequate ratio of nonprotein to protein calories.

    b) Provide 24–32 nonprotein calories per gram of protein.[28,32]

 2. Fat emulsion

  a. Fat supplies 9 kcal/gm, providing a concentrated source of calories.

  b. Fat emulsions are available in 10 percent and 20 percent solutions.

   1) A 10 percent solution

    a) Has a higher phospholipid/triglyceride content

    b) Results in higher plasma triglyceride levels

        c) Results in higher plasma cholesterol concentrations than 20 percent solutions

    2) A 20 percent solution

        a) Is recommended for LBW infants[35]

        b) Allows for adequate intravenous fat emulsion intake at reduced volume

  c. An initial delivery rate of 0.5–1 gm/kg/day is started one to two days after the glucose/protein solution is initiated.[29]

    1) It is administered over a 16- to 24-hour period.[31]

    2) It increases by 0.5–1 gm/kg/day to a maximum of 3 gm/kg/day.

    3) The ability to increase fat administration is dependent on the infant's ability to metabolize fat, which is affected by the following.[32]

        a) Prematurity

        b) Medical conditions

          • Sepsis

          • Surgery

          • Malnutrition

  d. Essential fatty acid deficiency can be prevented with the administration of 0.5–1 gm/kg/day of an IV lipid solution.[32]

  e. Heparin is given in both peripheral and central solutions because it improves lipid utilization through release of lipoprotein lipase.[35,39]

    1) Lipoprotein lipase hydrolyzes fat particles to free fatty acids, improving utilization and decreasing serum triglyceride levels.

  f. Complications may be associated with IV fat administration.

    1) Fat embolism

    2) Impaired gas exchange

    3) Cholestatic jaundice

    4) Hypertriglyceridemia

        a) Lipid clearance is assessed by monitoring plasma triglyceride and cholesterol levels.

        b) The recommendations for a maximum triglyceride level range from 150–200 mg/dl.[32,37]

    5) Increased ventilation/perfusion mismatching, affecting oxygenation and pulmonary vascular resistance by producing vasoactive metabolites[32,34]

        a) This is related to excessive rates of lipid administration.

        b) Administration of lipids at 0.2 gm/kg/hour or less appears to be safe.[32]

C. Parenteral nutrition is administered to accomplish the following.

  1. Use of nonprotein energy sources such as glucose and fat allows amino acids to be used for tissue growth and repair.

  2. Use of a balance of carbohydrates and fat to can accomplish the following.

    a. Meet resting energy expenditure

    b. Decrease catabolism

    c. Improve protein retention

  3. The maintenance energy requirement for an infant receiving parenteral nutrition is 85–100 kcal/kg/day.[36,38] Calories needed per day is dependent on gestational age, use of warmer versus incubator for temperature control, and disease state.

    a. Increased calories are needed for infants with some medical conditions.[26,36,38]

      1) Acute stage of sepsis

      2) Chronic lung disease

      3) Congenital heart disease

      4) Postoperative healing

    b. Consider other factors, such as the postoperative use of narcotics for pain control, when planning an infant's caloric requirements.

D. There may be complications of parenteral nutrition.

   1. Electrolyte abnormalities

   2. Hypoglycemia

   3. Hyperglycemia

   4. Metabolic acidosis

   5. Hyperlipidemia

   6. Disturbances in pulmonary function

   7. Trace element deficiencies

   8. Essential fatty acid deficiency

   9. Increased risk of catheter complications such as thrombus formation, vein perforations, and bacteremia and septicemia with central administration

   10. Phlebitis, infiltrations, and skin sloughing (most commonly seen with peripheral administration)

E. Employ the following nursing measures.

   1. Monitor parenteral nutrition.

    a. Serum electrolytes

    b. Glucose

    c. Calcium

    d. Phosphorous

    e. Magnesium

    f. BUN

    g. Creatinine

   2. Daily monitoring of above while advancing nutritional support is recommended to prevent complications associated with TPN.[31]

   3. Liver function studies, including the following blood work, are indicated initially and at least monthly while the infant is on parenteral nutrition.

    a. Serum glutamic pyruvic transaminase

    b. Alkaline phosphatase

    c. Total and direct bilirubin

    d. Total protein

    e. Albumin

   4. Urine should be checked for glucose, protein, and specific gravity each shift.[31]

   5. Monitor triglyceride levels with the advancement of intravenous fat emulsion and then weekly.[35]

   6. Daily weights and weekly head circumferences are important measurements of growth when providing nutrition and calories to infants postoperatively.

ENTERAL NUTRITION

A. In critically ill infants or those with abdominal surgery, nasogastric suction or gravity drainage may be necessary until there is evidence of the following.

   1. Decreased gastric drainage and abdominal distention

   2. Increased bowel sounds

   3. Stool passage

B. These factors affect the initiation of enteral feedings.

    1. It is begun as soon as possible after surgery in infants who do not have any GI tract disturbances.

    2. The choice of formula used will depend on the following.

        a. Gestational age of the infant

        b. Type of surgery

        c. GI tract function

C. Loss of portions of the GI tract, anastomosis, or the creation of an ostomy may lead to decreased absorption of nutrients.

    1. Elemental formulas, which are more easily digested, may be needed.

    2. Initial feedings of a lactose-free formula can improve feeding tolerance because an infant who has had a bowel resection often will have lactose intolerance.

D. The following are recommendations for postoperative enteral nutrition.

    1. Enteral feedings should be done cautiously and individualized depending on the infant's gestational and postnatal age, clinical status, and degree of GI function.

    2. The gastrointestinal tract tolerates increases in feeding volume better than increases in the osmolarity of the feeding.

    3. Gastric feedings are preferred because they allow for normal digestive processes and hormonal responses.

    4. Continuous feedings, through gastric or transpyloric tube placement, can reduce the risk of vomiting and aspiration.

    5. Transpyloric feedings may be needed for infants with gastroesophageal reflux, delayed gastric emptying, or a depressed gag reflex.

    6. For long-term feeding tube management (tube in place longer than six to eight weeks), a surgically placed gastrostomy tube is more secure and easier to maintain.[39] **(See Appendix D: Gastrostomy Tube Placement.)**

E. Nursing measures include the following.

    1. Confirm feeding tube placement.

    2. Assess feeding tolerance by these steps.

        a. Monitoring residuals

        b. Assessing stooling patterns and ostomy output

    3. Prevent complications related to fluid, electrolyte, and nutritional management in the surgical neonate by understanding the following.

        a. The impact of the infant's gestational age on his ability to take feedings enterally

        b. The limitations of the infant's disease or anomaly

        c. The surgical procedure

REFERENCES

1. Bell EF, and Oh W. 2005. Fluid and electrolyte management. In *Neonatology: Pathophysiology and Management of the Newborn*, 6th ed., MacDonald MG, Mullett MD, and Seshia MMK, eds. Philadelphia: Lippincott Williams & Wilkins, 362–379.

2. Dell KM, and Davis ID. 2006. Fluid, electrolyte, and acid-base homeostasis. In *Neonatal-Perinatal Medicine: Diseases of the Fetus and Infant*, 8th ed., Martin RJ, Fanaroff AA, and Walsh MC, eds. St. Louis: Mosby, 695–712.

3. Nafday SM, et al. 2005. Renal disease. In *Neonatology: Pathophysiology and Management of the Newborn*, 6th ed., MacDonald MG, Mullett MD, and Seshia MMK, eds. Philadelphia: Lippincott Williams & Wilkins, 981–1065.

4. Sukhani R. 1989. Anesthetic management of the newborn. *Clinics in Perinatology* 16(1): 43–60.

5. Seri I, Ramanathan R, and Evans JR. 2005. Acid-base, fluid, and electrolyte management. In *Avery's Diseases of the Newborn*, 8th ed., Taeusch HW, Ballard RA, and Gleason CA, eds. Philadelphia: Saunders, 372–397.

6. John E, Klavdianou M, and Vidyasagar D. 1989. Electrolyte problems in neonatal surgical patients. *Clinics in Perinatology* 16(1): 219–232.

7. Lin PW, and Simmons CF. 2004. Fluid and electrolyte management. In *Manual of Neonatal Care*, 5th ed., Cloherty JP, Eichenwald EC, and Stark AR, eds. Philadelphia: Lippincott Williams & Wilkins, 101–114.

8. Hartnoll G. 2003. Basic principles and practical steps in the management of fluid balance in the newborn. *Seminars in Neonatology* 8(4): 307–313.

9. Hay WW Jr. 1994. Nutritional requirements of extremely low birthweight infants. *Acta Paediatrica. Supplement.* 402: 94–99.

10. Wilker RE. 2004. Metabolic problems. In *Manual of Neonatal Care,* 5th ed., Cloherty JP, Eichenwald EC, and Stark AR, eds. Philadelphia: Lippincott Williams & Wilkins, 569–579.

11. Luck SR. 1992. Nutrition and metabolism. In *Swenson's Pediatric Surgery,* 5th ed., Raffensperger JG, ed. Norwalk, Connecticut: Appleton & Lange, 81–90.

12. Pierro A. 1999. Metabolic response to neonatal surgery. *Current Opinion in Pediatrics* 11(3): 230–236.

13. Anand KJS, Sippell WG, and Anysley-Green A. 1987. A randomized trial of fentanyl anesthesia in preterm babies undergoing surgery: Effect on the stress response. *Lancet* 1(8524): 62–66. (Published erratum appears in *Lancet,* 1987, 1[8526]: 234.)

14. Walker CJ, and Taylor J. 1990. Fluid and electrolyte management and nutritional support. In *Neonatal Surgery,* 3rd ed., Lister J, and Irving IM, eds. London: Butterworth-Heinemann, 37–49.

15. Rice HE, Caty MG, and Glick PL. 1998. Fluid therapy for the pediatric surgical patient. *Pediatric Clinics of North America* 45(4): 719–727.

16. Presson RG Jr, and Hillier SC. 1992. Perioperative fluid and transfusion management. *Seminars in Pediatric Surgery* 1(1): 22–31.

17. Raffensperger JG. 1992. Fluids and electrolytes. In *Swenson's Pediatric Surgery,* 5th ed., Raffensperger JG, ed. Norwalk, Connecticut: Appleton & Lange, 73–79.

18. Zenk KE, Sills JH, and Koeppel RM. 2003. *Neonatal Medications & Nutrition: A Comprehensive Guide,* 3rd ed. Santa Rosa, California: NICU Ink, 521.

19. Barcelona SL, Thompson AA, and Cote GJ. 2005. Intraoperative pediatric blood transfusion therapy: A review of common issues. Part II: Transfusion therapy, special considerations, and reduction of allogenic blood transfusion. *Paediatric Anaesthesia* 15(10): 814–830.

20. Rusy L, and Usaleva E. 1998. Paediatric anaesthesia review. *Update in Anaesthesia* 8: 2–14.

21. Wilson CM. 2005. Perioperative fluids in children. *Update in Anaesthesia* 19: 36–38.

22. Filston HC, et al. 1982. Estimation of postoperative fluid requirements in infants and children. *Annals of Surgery* 196(1): 76–81.

23. Warner BW. 2003. Pediatric surgery. In *Sabiston Textbook of Surgery: The Biological Basis of Modern Surgical Practice,* 17th ed. Philadelphia: Saunders, 2097–2098.

24. Leelanukrom R, and Cunliffe M. 2000. Intraoperative fluid and glucose management in children. *Paediatric Anaesthesia* 10(4): 353–359.

25. Chesney RW, and Zelikovic I. 1989. Pre- and postoperative fluid management in infancy. *Pediatrics in Review* 11(5): 153–158.

26. Albanese CT, and Sylvester KG. 2006. Pediatric surgery. In *Current Surgical Diagnosis and Treatment,* 12th ed., Doherty GM, and Way LW, eds. New York: McGraw-Hill, 1271–1328.

27. Stanley CA, and Pallotto EK. 2005. Disorders of carbohydrate metabolism. In *Avery's Diseases of the Newborn,* 8th ed., Taeusch HW, Ballard RA, and Gleason CA, eds. Philadelphia: Saunders, 1410–1422.

28. Teitelbaum DH, and Coran AG. 1998. Perioperative nutritional support in pediatrics. *Nutrition* 14(1): 130–142.

29 Sunehag A, et al. 1993. Glucose production rate in extremely immature neonates (<28 weeks) studied by use of deuterated glucose. *Pediatric Research* 33(2): 97–100.

30. McGowan JE. 1999. Neonatal hypoglycemia. *Pediatrics in Review* 20(7): e6–e15.

31. Georgieff MK. 2005. Nutrition. In *Neonatology: Pathophysiology and Management of the Newborn,* 6th ed., MacDonald MG, Mullett MD, and Seshia MMK, eds. Philadelphia: Lippincott Williams & Wilkins, 380–412.

32. Thureen PJ. 1999. Early aggressive nutrition in the neonate. *Pediatrics in Review* 20(9): e45–e55.

33. Hemachandra AH, and Cowett RM. 1999. Neonatal hyperglycemia. *Pediatrics in Review* 20(7): e16–e24.

34. Wesley JR, and Coran AG. 1992. Intravenous nutrition for the pediatric patient. *Seminars in Pediatric Surgery* 1(3): 212–230.

35. Sapsford AL. 2000. Parenteral nutrition: Energy, carbohydrate, protein, and fat. In *Nutritional Care for High-Risk Newborns,* 3rd ed., Groh-Wargo S, et al., eds. Chicago: Precept Press, 119–149.

36. Lloyd DA. 1998. Energy requirements of surgical newborn infants receiving parenteral nutrition. *Nutrition* 14(1): 101–104.

37. Denne SC, et al. 2002. Nutrition and metabolism in the high-risk neonate. In *Neonatal-Perinatal Medicine: Diseases of the Fetus and Infant,* 7th ed., Fanaroff AA, and Martin RJ, eds. St. Louis: Mosby, 578–617.

38. Premer DM, and Georgieff MK. 1999. Nutrition for ill neonates. *Pediatrics in Review* 20(9): e56–e62.

39. Pereira GR, and Ziegler MM. 1989. Nutritional care of the surgical neonate. *Clinics in Perinatology* 16(1): 233–253.

Notes

Assessment and Management of Postoperative Pain

Marlene Walden, PhD, RNC, CCNS, NNP

Providing effective pain relief is central to the mission of providing high-quality patient care. The goal of pain management is to minimize procedural, postoperative, and disease-related pain common in the population served in the NICU. All neonates should be assessed for pain using an appropriate multidimensional scale. After the pain score has been determined, nonpharmacologic and pharmacologic interventions can be initiated.

Incidence of Pain in the NICU

A. Newborn infants, particularly those born prematurely, are regularly subjected to painful diagnostic and therapeutic procedures that are a necessary part of their care in the NICU.
  1. Barker and Rutter in 1995 reported:[1]
     a. Smaller and sicker neonates are subjected to the greatest numbers of painful procedures.
     b. In this study, one 23-week gestational age, 560 gm infant had 488 painful procedures performed during her hospital stay.
  2. Stevens and colleagues in 1999 found:[2]
     a. Infants born at 27–31 weeks gestation received, on average, 134 painful procedures within the first two weeks of life.
     b. Approximately 10 percent of the youngest or sickest infants had more than 300 painful procedures.

The Clinical Significance of Pain Management

A. Many lines of evidence suggest that there are cumulative effects on the developing brain after repeated painful medical procedures.
  1. Increased clinical complications[3,4]
  2. Adverse neurologic outcomes[3,4]

TABLE 10-1 ■ Common Instruments Used to Assess Pain in Neonates[5,14,15]

Instrument	Indicators	Population Age in Postconceptional Weeks	Pain Stimulus	Intervention Score*	Unique Contribution
Premature Infant Pain Profile (PIPP)[26]	Heart rate Oxygen saturation Brow bulge Eye squeeze Nasolabial furrow Gestational age Behavioral state	<28–40	Handling Heelstick Circumcision	≤6 = minimal or no pain 7–12 = mild pain Consider nonpharmacologic measures. >12 = moderate/severe pain Consider pharmacologic intervention in conjunction with nonpharmacologic measures.	Most extensively validated tool for use in extremely preterm infants Only instrument that incorporates contextual factors that may modify the pain response
CRIES[71]	Crying Requires oxygen to maintain saturation >95% Increased vital signs Expression Sleepless	32–56	Postoperative pain	≤4 = mild pain Consider nonpharmacologic measures. ≥5 = moderate/severe pain Consider pharmacologic intervention in conjunction with nonpharmacologic measures.	Useful in older, physiologically stable preterm neonates and infants up to 56 weeks postconceptional age
Neonatal Infant Pain Scale (NIPS)[28]	Facial expression Cry Arms Legs State of arousal Breathing pattern	28–38	Capillary, venous, or arterial puncture	Not reported	Particularly useful in newborn nursery areas where infants are not routinely monitored with cardiorespiratory equipment

* Scores must be interpreted in light of the pattern of how total scores change between pain and nonpain situations and whether risk factors for pain are present.

3. Increased mortality[4,5]
4. Increased demands on the cardiorespiratory system[6–9]
5. Elevation in intracranial pressure, increasing the risk for intraventricular hemorrhage and periventricular leukomalacia[8–10]

B. Adverse long-term developmental outcomes are also evident.[3,11–13]
   1. Decreased sensitivity to the commonplace pain of childhood
   2. Higher incidence of somatic complaints (physical complaints of unknown origin)
   3. Long-term structural changes in the brain and spinal cord

Standards of Practice

A. Need for standards[14,15]
   1. Pain is assessed and managed inadequately in a large proportion of neonates, despite the ready availability of assessment instruments and safe and effective pharmacologic and nonpharmacologic interventions.[16,17]
   2. Recognizing the widespread inadequacy of pain management, professional and accrediting organizations issued position statements and clinical recommendations in an effort to promote effective pain management in undertreated populations.
   3. There is a great deal of consistency among the recommendations set by these professional and accrediting organizations.

B. Core principles
  1. Use both nonpharmacologic and pharmacologic approaches to prevent and/or manage pain.[14,15]
  2. Policies and procedures should be established to provide consistency and quality of pain assessment and management practices.[15]
  3. Regular assessment and reassessment of pain must be done using a valid and reliable multidimensional pain assessment instrument.[14,15]
  4. New and regular employees must be educated in pain assessment and management.[14,15]
  5. Health care team members collaborate together and with the infant's family in developing an approach to pain assessment and management.[14,15,18]
  6. Documentation facilitates regular reassessment and follow-up intervention.[15]

Assessment of Pain

A. The following are general principles of pain assessment.
  1. Pain assessment has been advocated as the "fifth vital sign."[19]
  2. What is painful to an adult or child should be presumed painful to an infant, even in the absence of behavioral or physiologic signs.[5,20,21]
     a. Developmental maturity, health status, and environmental factors may all contribute to an inconsistent, less robust pattern of pain responses among preterm neonates and even in the same infant over time and different situations.[6,22,23]
  3. Pain assessment is an essential prerequisite to optimal pain management.[15,24]
     a. Pain should be assessed on admission and at regularly defined intervals throughout the infant's hospitalization.
        1) Frequency of assessment should be based on pain scores or clinical condition of the neonate.[5]
     b. Caregivers must employ a high index of suspicion in identifying infants who are in pain.[15]
  4. Multidimensional instruments with evidence of validity, reliability, and clinical utility should be used to assess pain in neonates.[5,15,25] The three multidimensional instruments most commonly used to assess pain in neonates are listed in Table 10-1. The scales are included in Appendix E.
     a. Premature Infant Pain Profile (PIPP)[26]
     b. CRIES[27]
     c. Neonatal Infant Pain Scale (NIPS)[28]
B. Use a multidimensional approach that incorporates both physiologic and behavioral parameters to assess pain.[15]
  1. Physiologic indicators of pain in the neonate include the following.
     a. Increases in heart rate[6-9,29]
     b. Decreases in oxygen saturation[6,8,9]
  2. Facial activity seems to offer the most specificity as an indicator of acute procedural pain.[9,29-31]
     a. Brow bulge
     b. Eye squeeze
     c. Nasolabial furrow
     d. Open mouth

3. Crying is an indicator of pain.
   a. Acoustic and temporal characteristics of pain cries have been demonstrated to be different than other cry types in both preterm and full-term infants.[9,30–35]
   b. Preterm infants may not cry in response to a noxious stimulus.[9,35–37] This absence of crying may only indicate the depletion of response capability and not lack of pain perception.[20]

C. Pain expression is altered by the contextual factors surrounding the painful event.[35,37,38]
   1. Behavioral state has been shown to act as a moderator of behavioral pain responses in both full-term and preterm infants.[26,30,35,37]
      a. Infants in awake or alert states demonstrate a more robust reaction to painful stimuli than infants in sleep states.
   2. Place infant behaviors within the context of the situation to accurately interpret the appropriateness of the infant's response.[39]
      a. Franck demonstrated that healthy full-term newborns use swiping motions by the unaffected leg to the lanced foot, as if trying to push away the noxious stimulus.[40]
   3. Research examining facial as well as bodily activity has demonstrated that the magnitude of infant response to painful stimuli has been observed to be less vigorous and robust with decreasing postconceptional age.[6,36,37,41]
      a. Craig and colleagues suggest that the less vigorous responses demonstrated by preterm infants "should be interpreted in the context of the energy resources available to respond and the relative immaturity of the musculoskeletal system" (p.296).[6]
   4. A study published in 1996 suggested that previous pain experience can affect pain responses to noxious stimuli. As the total number of invasive procedures that a preterm infant encounters increases with advancing postnatal age, a less mature behavioral response is seen.[38]
   5. Lack of response in preterm neonates to a heelstick procedure is influenced by the following.[37]
      a. Postnatal age at the time of the study
      b. Postconceptional age at birth
      c. Time since the last painful procedure
      d. Behavioral state
   6. Procedural techniques may modify pain expression in neonates.
      a. In comparing pain responses to a heelstick procedure versus venipuncture in full-term neonates, venipuncture was associated with less pain than the heelstick procedure.[42,43]
         1) Both crying and the total time required to obtain the blood sample were also reduced.
      b. Decreased bruising, fewer repeat punctures, and fewer behavioral and physiologic distress responses have been noted using spring-loaded mechanical lancets compared with heelstick procedures performed using manual lancets.[7,42]
         1) Use of a mechanical lancet was more effective than a eutectic mixture of local anesthetic (EMLA) cream or tactile and vocal stimulation in reducing infant pain response to the heelstick procedure.[7]

c. Preparatory handling and immobilization may increase infant responses to painful clinical procedures such as newborn circumcision or lumbar puncture by causing heightened activity in nociceptive pathways.[18,44,45]

Nonpharmacologic Approaches to Pain Management

A. Nonpharmacologic approaches
1. These should be used for minor to moderately stressful procedures to help minimize pain and stress.
2. They can maximize the infant's ability to cope with and recover from the painful procedure.
3. They can be useful in providing additive or synergistic benefits to pharmacologic therapy.[21,46]

B. Preventive measures
1. Reduce as much as possible the total number of painful procedures to which the infant is exposed.[15,46]
   a. Evaluate all aspects of caregiving.
   b. Evaluate the number and grouping of laboratory and diagnostic procedures.
   c. Schedule clinical procedures based on medical necessity versus a routine timetable.
2. Use environmental interventions such as reduced lighting and noise levels to minimize overall stress.[5,15,46]

C. Behavioral measures
1. Hand swaddling (facilitated tucking [holding the infant's extremities flexed and contained close to the trunk])
   a. Implemented prior to the heelstick procedure, this reduces pain responses in preterm neonates as young as 25 weeks gestational age.[47]
   b. Preterm infants in the postheelstick recovery phase demonstrated significantly reduced heart rates and crying and more stability in sleep-wake cycles in the hand swaddled position.[47]
2. Blanket swaddling
   a. Following a painful procedure, blanket swaddling can help reduce infant physiologic and behavioral distress in the post-heelstick recovery phase for older preterm infants (postconceptional age ≥31 weeks).[48]
3. Pacifiers and nonnutritive sucking (NNS)
   a. These are ranked by NICU nurses as the first choice for pain intervention.[49]
   b. NNS is thought to modulate the transmission or processing of nociception through mediation by the endogenous nonopioid system.[50,51]
   c. The efficacy of NNS is immediate, but it appears to terminate rapidly upon cessation of sucking.
   d. NNS has been shown to reduce pain responses in preterm infants during heel lances.[2]
   e. NNS reduced the duration of crying and soothed infants more rapidly during painful procedures than either blanket swaddling[52] or rocking.[53]
   f. Pain relief is greater in infants who receive both NNS and sucrose.[2,41]

D. Sucrose administration
1. A meta-analysis of 21 randomized clinical trials demonstrates that a single dose of 0.012–0.12 gm (e.g., 0.05–0.50 ml of 24 percent) sucrose given orally approximately two minutes before a painful stimulus is associated with

statistically and clinically significant reductions in heart rate, crying, facial expressions of pain, and pain scores after the painful stimulus.[54]

    a. Interval coincides with endogenous opioid release triggered by the sweet taste of sucrose.[2]

2. The safety of implementing repeated doses of sucrose in very low birth weight infants has not been confirmed. Therefore, caution should be used when repeated doses of sucrose are ordered to be given to preterm and critically ill neonates.[2,15,54]

    a. In a study published in 1999, no immediate adverse effects were noted when administering a 24 percent sucrose-dipped pacifier during four random, consecutively administered routine heelstick procedures.[2]

Pharmacologic Approaches to Pain Management

A. Indications

  1. Opioid analgesics should be used when moderate, severe, or prolonged pain is assessed or anticipated.[15]

  2. Nonopioids analgesics should be considered when mild to moderate pain is assessed or anticipated.

B. Types of therapy

  1. Systemic analgesic therapy

    a. Opioid analgesics

    b. Nonopioid analgesics

  2. Sedatives

  3. Regional anesthesia and analgesia

C. Opioid analgesics

  1. General principles

    a. Opioid analgesia should be used when moderate, severe, or prolonged pain is assessed or anticipated.[15]

    b. Longer dosing intervals are often required in neonates less than one month of age because of longer elimination half-lives and delayed clearance of opioids when compared with adults or children greater than one year of age.[55]

    c. Neonates should be monitored closely during opioid therapy and for several hours after opioids have been discontinued because enterohepatic recirculation in preterm and full-term neonates can result in higher plasma concentrations of opioids for longer periods of time when compared to older children.[55]

    d. Because of the immaturity of their descending pain pathways, preterm infants may require significantly higher opioid concentrations to achieve adequate analgesia when compared to older children.[13,55]

    e. Increased magnitude and prolonged duration of pain are observed in preterm neonates. Mechanisms supporting increased pain sensitivity in neonates include:[13]

      1) Nerve sprouting

      2) Hyperinnervation of the area surrounding the skin injury

      3) Widespread increases in neural excitability within the spinal cord

      4) A pain threshold 30–50 percent lower in the presence of repeated stimulation than that of adults

    f. Efficacy of opioid therapy should be assessed using an appropriate neonatal pain instrument.

    g. Opioid-induced cardiorespiratory side effects in neonates are uncommon.[55–58]

        1) Side effects can be minimized if bolus doses are administered slowly to neonates who are well hydrated.[55]

2. Intravenous (IV) opioids most commonly administered in the NICU[55]

    a. Morphine sulfate

        1) Intermittent dose: 0.05–0.1 mg/kg/dose IV given over four to five minutes every four hours as needed[59]

        2) Continuous infusion dose: IV loading dose of 0.1 mg/kg/dose infused over 1½ hours, followed by a maintenance infusion of 15–20 mcg/kg/hour (0.015–0.020 mg/kg/hour)[59]

        3) Adverse effects[5]

            a) Respiratory depression

            b) Decreased gastrointestinal motility

            c) Hypotension

            d) Urinary retention

    b. Fentanyl citrate

        1) Intermittent dose: 1–4 mcg/kg/dose IV given over at least one to two minutes every two to four hours[59]

        2) Continuous infusion dose: IV bolus of 1 mcg/kg/dose over at least one to two minutes followed by a maintenance infusion of 0.5–4 mcg/kg/hour[59]

        3) Adverse effects[5]

            a) Respiratory depression

            b) Hypotension

            c) Muscle rigidity

            d) Hypothermia

3. Result of prolonged use

    a. Pain relief decreases with the same dosage over time.[60,61]

    b. The development of analgesic tolerance is seen as increased wakefulness.

        1) Increased sympathetic responses such as[61]

            a) High-pitched crying

            b) Tremors when handled or disturbed

    c. Continued treatment with opioids to manage pain increases the possibility of tolerance and may require dose escalation to maintain analgesia.[14,60,61]

4. Weaning from opioid therapy

    a. Neonates who require opioid therapy for an extended period of time (more than one week) should be weaned slowly, usually by a dose reduction of 10–20 percent/day, depending on the duration of therapy and the presence of clinical symptoms of withdrawal.[60,61]

    b. Opioid withdrawal symptoms are most effectively managed by treatment with an opioid.[60–62]

    c. Rapid weaning of opioids may lead to withdrawal symptoms.[61]

        1) Neurologic excitability

        2) Gastrointestinal dysfunction

        3) Autonomic signs

            a) Sweating

            b) Low-grade fever

            c) Nasal stuffiness

FIGURE 10-1 ■ Neonatal withdrawal score sheet.

The Neonatal Withdrawal Score Sheet is used to assess the severity of withdrawal and to assist in determining if treatment is needed for:

- Infants born to drug-dependent mothers or those with a history of drug use
- Mothers or infants with a positive urine drug screen
- Infants having withdrawal symptoms
- Infants being weaned from long-term (>2 weeks) treatment with drugs that cause physiologic dependency, such as fentanyl or midazolam

The original scoring system by Finnegan was designed for infants withdrawing from narcotics.[1] It may, however, be used as a guide for identifying infants in withdrawal from other drugs and substances such as barbiturates and benzodiazepines.

INSTRUCTIONS:

- Score the infant every 3–4 hours, corresponding to the frequency of feedings. Behaviors should be assessed throughout the 3- to 4-hour interval, and the form should be completed at the time of feeding. Score all that apply.
- Try nonpharmacologic measures first: Comfort the infant by swaddling, provide a pacifier, and decrease visual and auditory stimulation.
- Consider treatment of withdrawal in babies scoring 8 or above.
  - Maintain effective dose for 3–5 days before tapering begins.
  - Decrease daily dose by about 10 percent every 1–2 days as tolerated using the withdrawal score as a guide.
  - Usually, 50 percent of babies will require 10–20 days of therapy (25 percent more, 25 percent less).
  - If a dose taper fails (score again is 8 or above), resume the previously effective dose for 3–5 days as tolerated; then begin taper again.

Signs and symptoms of other neonatal problems—for example, sepsis, hypoglycemia, and electrolyte imbalance—may mimic some of the signs of neonatal withdrawal. These other problems need to be ruled out or corrected.[2,3]

Signs and Symptoms	Date						
	Time						
	Initials						
Cry	**Score**						
• Excessive high-pitched (or other) crying	2						
• Continuous high-pitched (or other) crying	3						
• If intubated, continuous crying behavior	3						
Hours of Sleep after Feeding							
• Less than 1 hour	3						
• Less than 2 hours	2						
• Less than 3 hours	1						
Moro Reflex (wake the baby for this test)							
• Hyperactive	2						
• Markedly hyperactive	3						
Tremors—When Disturbed							
• Mild tremors	1						
• Marked tremors	2						
Increased Muscle Tone	2						

(continued on next page)

Signs and Symptoms	Date						
	Time						
	Initials						
Generalized Seizures	Score						
	5						
Gastrointestinal Symptoms							
• Frantic sucking of fists	1						
• Poor feeding	2						
• Regurgitation	2						
• Projectile vomiting	3						
Stools							
• Loose	2						
• Watery	3						
Dehydration	2						
Frequent Yawning (3–4 times/interval)	1						
Frequent Sneezing (3–4 times/interval)	1						
Nasal Stuffiness	1						
Sweating	1						
Mottling	1						
Fever							
• <38.3°C (37.3°C–38.3°C)	1						
• >38.3°C (38.4°C and higher)	2						
Respirations							
• More than 60/minute	1						
• More than 60/minute with retractions	2						
Excoriations of:							
• Nose							
• Knees	1						
• Toes							
4-Hour Total							

Use this form to document what interventions seemed to help calm the infant and what was tried and not helpful.

Date	Nursing Comments/Observations

Adapted from: Finnegan LP. 1985. Neonatal abstinence. In *Current Therapy in Neonatal-Perinatal Medicine,* Nelson N, ed. Philadelphia: Mosby, 262–270. Reprinted by permission.

REFERENCES

1. Finnegan LP. 1985. Neonatal abstinence. In *Current Therapy in Neonatal-Perinatal Medicine,* Nelson N, ed. Philadelphia: Mosby-Year Book, 262–270.
2. Zaichkin J, and Houston RF. 1993. The drug-exposed mother and infant: A regional center experience. *Neonatal Network* 12(3): 41–49.
3. Levy M, and Spino M. 1993. Neonatal withdrawal syndrome: Associated drugs and pharmacologic management. *Pharmacotherapy* 13(3): 202–211.

          d) Sneezing

          e) Yawning

          f) Skin mottling

       4) Poor weight gain

       5) Skin excoriation due to excessive rubbing

     d. If withdrawal symptoms develop, discontinue or reduce weaning rate for at least 24 hours; then slowly resume weaning. If withdrawal symptoms continue, consider adding benzodiazepine therapy.[62]

     e. An opioid weaning scale such as the Finnegan scoring system should be used to manage opioid withdrawal in neonates exposed to prolonged opioid therapy (Figure 10-1).[62]

D. Nonopioid analgesics

   1. Acetaminophen is a non-narcotic analgesic and antipyretic commonly used in the short-term for mild to moderate pain in neonates.

     a. Oral Loading dose: 20 to 25 mg/kg. Maintenance: 12 to 15 mg/kg per dose

     b. Rectal Loading dose: 30 mg/kg. Maintenance: 12 to 18 mg/kg per dose

     c. Maintenance intervals:

       1) Term infants: every 6 hours

       2) Preterm infants ≥32 weeks GA: every 8 hours

       3) Preterm infants <32 weeks GA: every 12 hours

     d. Peak serum concentration: reached approximately one hour after an oral dose[63]

     e. Peak analgesic effect: seen in one to two hours

E. Adjunctive drugs—sedatives

   1. General principles

     a. Sedatives blunt behavioral responses to noxious stimuli.[62]

       1) Promote calming

       2) Reduce stress in infants requiring long-term ventilation

       3) Reduce stress in older infants with severe chronic lung disease and reactive pulmonary hypertension

     b. Sedatives, including benzodiazepines and barbiturates, do not provide pain relief and should be used only when pain has been ruled out.[65]

   2. Most commonly administered sedatives in the NICU

     a. Midazolam

       1) Intermittent dose: 0.05–0.1 mg/kg/dose IV every two to four hours as needed[59]

       2) Continuous infusion dose:

         a) Loading dose of 0.05–0.2 mg/kg IV, *followed by*

         b) Maintenance dose of 0.2 mcg/kg/minute, with a maximum dose of 0.6 mcg/kg/minute[59]

       3) Safety: has been questioned because adverse neurologic effects have been reported:[10,66]

         a) Intraventricular hemorrhage

         b) Periventricular leukomalacia

     b. Chloral hydrate

       1) Intermittent dose to maintain sedation: 20–40 mg/kg/dose every four to six hours as needed, by oral or rectal route[59]

       2) Single dose for procedural sedation: 30–75 mg/kg/dose, 15–45 minutes before the procedure by oral or rectal route[59]

    3) Cautions:
        a) Use with caution with:
            • Infants with hepatic or renal disease
            • Low birth weight infants with immature renal and liver function
        b) Avoid large doses in infants with severe cardiac disease.
        c) Avoid repetitive dosing, which can cause accumulation of metabolites.
    4) Adverse effects:
        a) Gastric irritation
        b) Paradoxical excitation
        c) In large doses
            • Vasodilation
            • Hypotension
            • Respiratory depression
            • Cardiac arrhythmias
            • Myocardial depression

F. Regional anesthesia and analgesia
  1. Subcutaneous ring block involves subcutaneous injection of local anesthetic in a circumferential ring on the midshaft of the penis.[67]
  2. Dorsal penile nerve block involves subcutaneous injection of local anesthetic below Buck's fascia at the ten and two o'clock positions at the base of the penis.[67]
  3. EMLA cream (eutectic mixture of local anesthetics, lidocaine, and prilocaine) can be used.
    a. This is approved for use in children at birth with an age of 37 weeks gestation or greater.
    b. The local/topical dose is 0.5–2 gm under an occlusive dressing at least one hour prior to the procedure.[5]
    c. EMLA cream is not effective for the management of pain associated with heelsticks, but will reduce pain caused by the following.[68]
      1) Venipuncture
      2) Arterial puncture
      3) Percutaneous venous catheter placement
      4) Circumcision
        a) Studies suggest that EMLA cream diminishes pain associated with circumcision in male newborns as evidenced by:[69]
            • Reduced crying time
            • Reduced increases in heart rate
            • Less facial activity
        b) A subcutaneous ring block or dorsal penile nerve block remains the preferred choice for pain management for circumcision, but EMLA cream can be used when these anesthetic methods cannot be employed.[18]
    d. Adverse effects include the following.[5]
      1) Methemoglobinemia
        a) No complications from methemoglobinemia were noted in single-dose prospective studies in neonates >26 weeks.[68] However, additional research is needed before EMLA cream can be recommended for repeated administration.
      2) Redness
      3) Blistering
      4) Petechial rash

TABLE 10-2 ■ Suggested Management of Procedural Pain in Neonates

Procedures	Pacifier	Sucrose	Swaddling, Containment, or Facilitated Tucking	EMLA Cream	Subcutaneous Infiltration of Lidocaine	Opioids	Other
Heel lance	•	•	•				Consider venipuncture. Use skin-to-skin contact with mother. Use mechanical spring-loaded lance.
Percutaneous venous catheter insertion	•	•	•	•		•	Consider an approach similar to this for venipuncture.
Percutaneous arterial catheter insertion	•	•	•	•	•		Consider similar approach for arterial puncture.
Peripheral arterial or venous cutdown	•	•	•	•	•	•	
Central venous line placement	•	•	•	•	•	•	Consider general anesthesia.
Umbilical arterial/ venous catheter insertion	•	•	•				Avoid placement of sutures or hemostat clamps on skin around umbilicus.
Peripherally inserted central catheter placement	•	•	•	•		•	
Lumbar puncture	•	•		•	•		Use careful physical handling.
Subcutaneous or intramuscular injection	•	•	•	•			Give drugs intravenously whenever possible.
Endotracheal intubation						•	Various combinations of drugs are often used, including: atropine, ketamine, thiopental sodium, succinylcholine chloride, morphine, fentanyl, nondepolarizing muscle relaxant. Consider topical lidocaine spray.
Endotracheal suction	•	+/−	•			•	
Nasogastric-orogastric tube insertion	•	•			•	•	Use a gentle technique and appropriate lubrication.
Chest tube insertion	•	•			•	•	Anticipate need for intubation and ventilation in neonates spontaneously breathing. Consider short-acting anesthetic agents. Avoid midazolam.
Circumcision	•	•			•		Mogen clamp is preferred over Gomco clamp. Use dorsal penile nerve block or subcutaneous ring block using plain or buffered lidocaine. Consider acetaminophen for postoperative pain.
Ongoing analgesia for routine NICU care and procedures	•	+/−	•			•	Avoid long-term sedation. Avoid midazolam. Consider acetaminophen therapy. Reduce acoustic, thermal, and other environmental stresses.

Adapted from: Anand KJS. 2001. Consensus statement for the prevention and management of pain in the newborn. *Archives of Pediatrics and Adolescent Medicine* 155(2): 173–180.

4. Epidural anesthesia and analgesia can be administered.
   a. Epidural analgesia is an alternative pain management strategy that can be used to successfully manage postoperative pain in hospitalized neonates.
   b. Pain relief is achieved by the injection of a single-dose, intermittent, or continuous administration of local anesthetics and/or an opioid drug into the epidural space.[67,70]
   c. Indications for use are as follows.[70]
      1) Major abdominal or thoracic surgery
         a) Omphalocele or gastroschisis repair
         b) Tracheoesophageal repair
         c) Small congenital diaphragmatic hernia repair in a stable patient
         d) Inguinal hernia repair
         e) Takedown of colostomy/ileostomy
         f) Bladder exstrophy repair
      2) Lower extremity or hip surgery
      3) Surgery in an extubated infant with chronic lung disease who previously required prolonged intubation and is still at risk for postoperative apnea
   d. The following are contraindications.[70]
      1) Sepsis or local infection at the catheter insertion site
      2) Thrombocytopenia or other known coagulopathy
      3) Increased intracranial pressure
      4) Suspected neurologic disease
      5) Malformations of the vertebral column
      6) Infants who cannot tolerate a decrease in systemic vascular resistance because of, for example, tetralogy of Fallot
   e. Nursing care includes the following.[70]
      1) Ensure correct infusate, dose, and rate of infusion
      2) Keep area clean and dry and reinforce with a bio-occlusive dressing as necessary
      3) Inspect the catheter for kinking, and ensure the catheter connections are tight
      4) Regularly inspect the insertion site for:
         a) Leakage
         b) Drainage
         c) Hematoma
         d) Erythema
      5) Regularly assess for side effects.[70]
         a) Catheter related
            • Migration of catheter into blood vessel or cerebrospinal fluid (CSF)
            • Infection
            • Occlusion
            • Neural injury/paresthesia
            • Breaking of catheter upon removal
            • Hematoma formation at the insertion site
         b) Anesthetic related[70]
            • Injection into CSF resulting in a high block with muscle paralysis
            • Injection into a blood vessel resulting in:
               • Seizures
               • Hypotension
               • Dysrhythmia

- Cardiac arrest
  c) Opioid related[70]
     - Respiratory depression (Decreased depth and rate of respiration are always preceded by a decreased level of consciousness.)
     - Pruritus
     - Nausea/vomiting
     - Urinary retention
     - Myoclonic movements
6) Assess vital signs every 1–4 hours according to your unit's postoperative protocol, with assessment of respiratory rate every hour for at least 24 hours.
7) All infants should have continuous cardiorespiratory monitoring. Keep a bag, mask, and naloxone at the infant's bedside in case of respiratory depression.
8) Using an appropriate multidimensional neonatal scale, regularly assess the infant for pain according to unit protocol.
9) Assess for sensory/motor block. Notify anesthesia service if a motor block is present.

Pain Management for Procedures

A. A prospective study, published in 1996, of analgesic and sedation practices in 109 NICUs including 1,068 preterm neonates demonstrated that procedural pain was not routinely treated with either pharmacologic or nonpharmacologic interventions.[16]
B. Table 10-2 summarizes evidence-based strategies for management of procedural pain in neonates.

Parent Education

A. Health care professionals must talk openly and honestly with parents about acute and chronic pain associated with medical diseases as well as pain associated with operative, diagnostic, and therapeutic procedures.
B. Parents should be informed that effective pain relief is an important part of their infant's care in the NICU.[15] Parents should be provided information about:
   1. Physiologic and behavioral pain cues
   2. Pain versus irritability
   3. Comfort measures
   4. Signs that pain has been relieved
   5. The pain management plan for their infant
   6. Analgesic options and effects of pain medications
   7. Opioid dependency
      a. Physical dependence and tolerance may develop from prolonged opioid therapy.
      b. Infants do not become psychologically addicted.
   8. Pain control
      a. Pain cannot always be completely eliminated.

REFERENCES

1. Barker DP, and Rutter N. 1995. Exposure to invasive procedures in neonatal intensive care unit admissions. *Archives of Disease in Childhood. Fetal & Neonatal Edition* 72(1): F47–F48.

2. Stevens B, et al. 1999. The efficacy of developmentally sensitive interventions and sucrose for relieving procedural pain in very low birth weight neonates. *Nursing Research* 48(1): 35–43.

3. Porter FL, Grunau RE, and Anand KJ. 1999. Long-term effects of pain in infants. *Journal of Developmental and Behavioral Pediatrics* 20(4): 253–261.

4. Anand KJ. 1998. Clinical importance of pain and stress in preterm neonates. *Biology of the Neonate* 73(1): 1–9.

5. Anand KJ. 2001. Consensus statement for the prevention and management of pain in the newborn. *Archives of Pediatrics and Adolescent Medicine* 155(2): 173–180.

6. Craig KD, et al. 1993. Pain in the preterm neonate: Behavioural and physiological indices. *Pain* 52(3): 287–299.

7. McIntosh N, van Veen L, and Brameyer H. 1994. Alleviation of the pain of heel prick in preterm infants. *Archives of Disease in Childhood. Fetal & Neonatal Edition* 70(3): F177–F181.

8. Stevens BJ, and CC Johnston. 1994. Physiological responses of premature infants to a painful stimulus. *Nursing Research* 43(4): 226–231.

9. Stevens BJ, Johnston CC, and Horton L. 1993. Multidimensional pain assessment in premature neonates: A pilot study. *Journal of Obstetric, Gynecologic, and Neonatal Nursing* 22(6): 531–541.

10. Anand KJ, et al. 1999. Analgesia and sedation in preterm neonates who require ventilatory support: Results from the NOPAIN trial. Neonatal Outcome and Prolonged Analgesia in Neonates. *Archives of Pediatrics and Adolescent Medicine* 153(4): 331–338. (Published erratum appears in *Archives of Pediatrics and Adolescent Medicine*, 1999, 153[8]: 895.)

11. Grunau RV, Whitfield MF, and Petrie JH. 1994. Pain sensitivity and temperament in extremely low-birth-weight premature toddlers and preterm and full-term controls. *Pain* 58(3): 341–346.

12. Grunau RV, et al. 1994. Early pain experience, child and family factors, as precursors of somatization: A prospective study of extremely premature and fullterm children. *Pain* 56(3): 353–359.

13. Evans J. 2001. Physiology of acute pain in preterm infants. *Newborn and Infant Nursing Reviews* 1(2): 75–84.

14. American Academy of Pediatrics and Canadian Paediatric Society. 2000. Prevention and management of pain and stress in the neonate. *Pediatrics* 105(2): 454–461.

15. Walden M. 2001. *Pain Assessment and Management: Guideline for Practice.* Glenview, Illinois: National Association of Neonatal Nurses.

16. Anand K, Selanikio J, and SOPAIN Study Group. 1996. Routine analgesic practices in 109 neonatal intensive care units (NICUs). *Pediatric Research* 39(4): 192A.

17. Bauchner H, May A, and Coates E. 1992. Use of analgesic agents for invasive medical procedures in pediatric and neonatal intensive care units. *Journal of Pediatrics* 121(4): 647–649.

18. American Academy of Pediatrics, Task Force on Circumcision. 1999. Circumcision policy statement. *Pediatrics* 103(3): 686–693.

19. American Pain Society. 1995. *Pain: The Fifth Vital Sign.* Accessed October 12, 2006, from http://www.ampainsoc.org/advocacy/fifth.htm.

20. Walden M, and Franck LS. 2003. Identification, management, and prevention of newborn/infant pain. In *Comprehensive Neonatal Nursing: A Physiologic Perspective*, 3rd ed., Kenner C, and Lott JW, eds. Philadelphia: Saunders, 844–856.

21. Franck LS, and Lawhon G. 1998. Environmental and behavioral strategies to prevent and manage neonatal pain. *Seminars in Perinatology* 22(5): 434–443.

22. Johnston CC, et al. 1993. Developmental changes in pain expression in premature, full-term, two- and four-month-old infants. *Pain* 52(2): 201–208.

23. Shapiro CR. 1993. Nurses' judgments of pain in term and preterm newborns. *Journal of Obstetric, Gynecologic, and Neonatal Nursing* 22(1): 41–47.

24. Bell SG. 1994. The national pain management guideline: Implications for neonatal intensive care. *Neonatal Network* 13(3): 9–17.

25. Agency for Health Care Policy and Research. 1992. *Acute Pain Management in Infants, Children, and Adolescents: Operative and Medical Procedures: Quick Reference Guide for Clinicians.* Rockville, Maryland: U.S. Department of Health and Human Services.

26. Stevens B, et al. 1996. Premature infant pain profile: Development and initial validation. *Clinical Journal of Pain* 12(1): 13–22.

27. Krechel SW, and Bildner J. 1995. CRIES: A new neonatal postoperative pain measurement score. Initial testing of validity and reliability. *Paediatric Anaesthesia* 5(1): 53–61.

28. Lawrence J, et al. 1993. The development of a tool to assess neonatal pain. *Neonatal Network* 12(6): 59–66.

29. Bozzette M. 1993. Observation of pain behavior in the NICU: An exploratory study. *Journal of Perinatal and Neonatal Nursing* 7(1): 76–87.

30. Grunau RV, and Craig KD. 1987. Pain expression in neonates: Facial action and cry. *Pain* 28(3): 395–410.

31. Grunau RV, Johnston CC, and Craig KD. 1990. Neonatal facial and cry responses to invasive and noninvasive procedures. *Pain* 42(3): 295–305.

32. Fuller B. 1991. Acoustic discrimination of three types of infant cries. *Nursing Research* 40(3): 156–160.

33. Levine JD, and Gordon NC. 1982. Pain in prelingual children and its evaluation by pain-induced vocalization. *Pain* 14(2): 85–93.

34. Porter FL, Miller RH, and Marshall RE. 1986. Neonatal pain cries: Effect of circumcision on acoustic features and perceived urgency. *Child Development* 57(3): 790–802.

35. Stevens BJ, Johnston CC, and Horton L. 1994. Factors that influence the behavioral pain responses of premature infants. *Pain* 59(1): 101–109.

36. Johnston CC, et al. 1995. Differential response to pain by very premature neonates. *Pain* 61(3): 471–479.

37. Johnston CC, et al. 1999. Factors explaining lack of response to heel stick in preterm newborns. *Journal of Obstetric, Gynecologic, and Neonatal Nursing* 28(6): 587–594.

38. Johnston CC, and Stevens BJ. 1996. Experience in a neonatal intensive care unit affects pain response. *Pediatrics* 98(5): 925–930.

39. Walden M, Sudia-Robinson T, and Carrier C. 2001. Comfort care for infants in the neonatal intensive care unit at end of life. *Newborn and Infant Nursing Reviews* 1(2): 97–105.

40. Franck LS. 1986. A new method to quantitatively describe pain behavior in infants. *Nursing Research* 35(1): 28–31.

41. Gibbins S, and Stevens B. 2003. The influence of gestational age on the efficacy and short-term safety of sucrose for procedural pain relief. *Advances in Neonatal Care* 3(5): 241-249.

42. Shah VS, et al. 1997. Neonatal pain response to heel stick vs venepuncture for routine blood sampling. *Archives of Disease in Childhood. Fetal & Neonatal Edition* 77(2): F143–F144.

43. Larsson BA, et al. 1998. Venipuncture is more effective and less painful than heel lancing for blood tests in neonates. *Pediatrics* 101(5): 882–886.

44. Porter F, et al. 1991. A controlled clinical trial of local anesthesia for lumbar puncture in newborns. *Pediatrics* 88(4): 663–669.

45. Porter FL, Wolf CM, and Miller J. 1998. The effect of handling and immobilization on the response to acute pain in newborn infants. *Pediatrics* 102(6): 1383–1389.

46. Franck L, and Lawhon G. 2000. Environmental and behavioral strategies to prevent and manage neonatal pain. In *Pain in Neonates*, 2nd ed., Anand KJS, McGrath PJ, and Stevens BJ, eds. Amsterdam: Elsevier Science, 203–216.

47. Corff KE, et al. 1995. Facilitated tucking: A nonpharmacologic comfort measure for pain in preterm neonates. *Journal of Obstetric, Gynecologic, and Neonatal Nursing* 24(2): 143–147.

48. Fearon I, et al. 1997. Swaddling after heel lance: Age-specific effects on behavioral recovery in preterm infants. *Journal of Developmental and Behavioral Pediatrics* 18(4): 222–232.

49. Franck LS. 1987. A national survey of the assessment and treatment of pain and agitation in the neonatal intensive care unit. *Journal of Obstetric, Gynecologic, and Neonatal Nursing* 16(6): 387–393.

50. Blass E, Fitzgerald E, and Kehoe P. 1987. Interactions between sucrose, pain and isolation distress. *Pharmacology, Biochemistry, and Behavior* 26(3): 483–489.

51. Gunnar M, et al. 1988. Adrenocortical activity and behavioral distress in human newborns. *Developmental Psychobiology* 21(4): 297–310.

52. Campos RG. 1989. Soothing pain-elicited distress in infants with swaddling and pacifiers. *Child Development* 60(4): 781–792.

53. Campos RG. 1994. Rocking and pacifiers: Two comforting interventions for heelstick pain. *Research in Nursing and Health* 17(5): 321–331.

54. Stevens B, Yamada J, and Ohlsson A. 2004. Sucrose for analgesia in newborn infants undergoing painful procedures. Cochrane Database of Systematic Reviews (3): CD001069.

55. Franck LS, and Miaskowski C. 1998. The use of intravenous opioids to provide analgesia in critically ill, premature neonates: A research critique. *Journal of Pain and Symptom Management* 15(1): 41–69.

56. Purcell-Jones G, Dormon F, and Sumner E. 1987. The use of opioids in neonates: A retrospective study of 933 cases. *Anaesthesia* 42(12): 1316–1320.

57. Koren G, et al. 1985. Postoperative morphine infusion in newborn infants: Assessment of disposition characteristics and safety. *Journal of Pediatrics* 107(6): 963–967.

58. Farrington E, et al. 1993. Continuous intravenous morphine infusion in postoperative newborn infants. *American Journal of Perinatology* 10(1): 84–87.

59. Zenk KE, Sills JH, and Koeppel RM. 2003. *Neonatal Medications & Nutrition: A Comprehensive Guide*, 3rd ed. Santa Rosa, California: NICU Ink, 140–141, 240–242, 407–410, 411–414.

60. Franck L, and Vilardi J. 1995. Assessment and management of opioid withdrawal in ill neonates. *Neonatal Network* 14(2): 39–48.

61. Suresh S, and Anand K. 1998. Opioid tolerance in neonates: Mechanisms, diagnosis, assessment, and management. *Seminars in Perinatology* 22(5): 425–433.

62. Finnegan LP, et al. 1975. A scoring system for evaluation and treatment of the neonatal abstinence syndrome: A new clinical and research tool. In *Basic and Therapeutic Aspects of Perinatal Pharmacology*, Morselli P, Garanttini S, and Sereni F, eds. New York: Raven Press, 139–152.

63. Young TE, and Mangum OB. 2005. *NeoFax: A Manual of Drugs Used in Neonatal Care*, 18th ed. Raleigh, North Carolina: Acorn.

64. Anand KJS, et al. 2000. Systemic analgesic therapy. In *Pain in Neonates*, 2nd ed., Anand KJS, McGrath PJ, and Stevens BJ, eds. Amsterdam: Elsevier Science, 159–188.

65. Hartley S, Franck L, and Lundergan R. 1989. Maintenance sedation of agitated infants in the NICU with chloral hydrate: New concerns. *Journal of Perinatology* 9(2): 162–164.

66. Ng E, Taddio A, and Ohlsson A. 2003. Intravenous midazolam infusion for sedation of infants in the neonatal intensive care unit. *Cochrane Database of Systematic Reviews* (1): CD002052

67. Sethna N, and Koh J. 2000. Regional anesthesia and analgesia. In *Pain in Neonates*, 2nd ed., Anand KJS, McGrath PJ, and Stevens BJ, eds. Amsterdam: Elsevier Science, 189–201.

68. Taddio A, et al. 1998. A systematic review of lidocaine-prilocaine cream (EMLA) in the treatment of acute pain in neonates. *Pediatrics* 101(2): e1.

69. Taddio A, Ohlsson K, and Ohlsson A. 2000. Lidocaine-prilocaine cream for analgesia during circumcision in newborn boys. *Cochrane Database of Systematic Reviews* (2): CD000496.

70. Ochsenreither JM. 1997. Epidural analgesia in infants. *Neonatal Network* 16(6): 79–84.

71. Bildner J, and Krechel SW. 1996. Increasing staff nurse awareness of postoperative pain management in the NICU. *Neonatal Network* 15(1): 11–16.

Notes

Skin Care After Surgical Intervention

Sandra Young, RNC, MN, NNP
Barbara Bratton, RNC, MS, PNP
Judith West, RN, MN, DNS

This chapter addresses the embryology of the skin and wound and ostomy care issues of the neonate after surgical intervention. Information is limited to postoperative wound and skin care management of intestinal stomas and treatment of intravenous extravasation. This chapter does not address basic skin care of the premature neonate, management of the umbilical cord, skin cleansing, and bathing. For a comprehensive discussion of general skin care measures, the reader is referred to the Association of Women's Health, Obstetric and Neonatal Nurses (AWHONN) and the National Association of Neonatal Nurses (NANN) document on Neonatal Skin Care: Clinical Outcomes of the AWHONN/NANN Evidence-based Clinical Practice Guidelines.[1,2]

Anatomy and Embryology

ANATOMY

A. Figure 11-1 depicts the anatomy of the skin layers.[3–7]
B. The skin consists of three layers.
   1. Epidermis
   2. Dermis
   3. Hypodermis (subcutaneous fat)
C. The skin functions as a protective organ.
   1. It provides a mechanical barrier to substances, microorganisms, and ultraviolet light.
     a. Maturation of barrier function is accelerated at delivery, regardless of gestational age, compared with maturation *in utero*.
     b. Although the timetable of maturation varies with each individual, within two to three weeks postdelivery, barrier function matures dramatically.[8–11]
   2. It controls thermoregulation and transepidermal water loss.
   3. It performs sensory and immunologic functions.

FIGURE 11-1 ■ **Anatomy of the skin layers.**

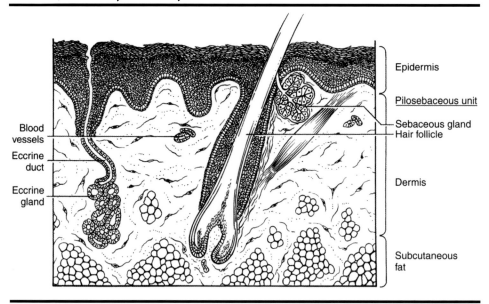

From: Mancini AJ. 2001. Structure and function of newborn skin. In *Textbook of Neonatal Dermatology*, Eichenfield LF, Frieden IJ, and Esterly NB, eds. Philadelphia: Saunders, 19. Reprinted by permission.

EMBRYOLOGY

A. Epidermis (Figure 11-2)
   1. It initially consists of a single layer of ectodermal cells.
   2. These cells start to proliferate at the beginning of the second month to form a layer of flattened cells, the periderm.
      a. Cells in the periderm are constantly replaced by cells generated by the basal layer (later the stratum germinativum).
      b. The periderm persists until approximately week 21 of gestation, when it disappears as the stratum corneum forms.
      c. Vernix caseosa, consisting of sebaceous gland secretions, shed lanugo hairs, and desquamated skin (partially exfoliated peridermal cells), is unique to the term infant.
   3. The epidermis contains four cell types.
      a. Keratinocytes, the predominant cell and structural support of the epidermis, cornify the outermost layer of the epidermis.
      b. Melanocytes are produced from melanoblasts.
         1) These are housed in the epidermis.
         2) They are responsible for pigmentation and ultraviolet protection.
         3) Melanin production and skin pigment are decreased in newborns, gradually reaching full production over several months.
      c. Langerhans cells are immunologically active.
      d. Merkel cells are touch sensitive and communicate with nerve endings.
   4. The epidermis is composed of many layers.
      a. The stratum corneum is one of the layers.
         1) It occupies the uppermost layer of the epidermis. It begins to form at about 21 weeks and achieves maturity by 34 weeks gestational age so

that transepidermal water loss approximates that of the adult.

2) Only several cell layers thick in the preterm infant, it matures in approximately two to three weeks after birth.

3) It controls transepidermal water loss; however, in the preterm infant, immaturity of the stratum corneum results in increased transepidermal water loss and increased energy loss through evaporative heat loss.

4) It serves as a physical barrier to the entry of organisms.

5) It is biologically sensitive, signaling damage to deeper layers of skin.

b. The stratum lucidum, lying just under the stratum corneum, is found only on the palms, fingertips, and soles of the feet.

c. The stratum granulosum, stratum spinosum, and stratum germinativum form the remaining layers.

1) Epidermal ridges are formed at about ten weeks from proliferation of cells in the stratum germinativum, which extend into the dermis. Ridges produce grooves on the palms of the hands and soles of the feet. These grooves are responsible for the patterns of fingerprints.[12–14]

2) The thick spinous layer contains fine tonofibrils.[14]

3) The granular layer cells contain small keratohyalin granules.[14]

FIGURE 11-2 ■ Successive stages of skin development.

A. Four weeks. B. Seven weeks. C. Eleven weeks. The cells of the periderm continually undergo keratinization and desquamation. Exfoliated peridermal cells form part of the vernix caseosa. D. Newborn infant. Note the position of the melanocytes in the basal layer of the epidermis and that their processes extend between the epidermal cells to supply them with melanin.

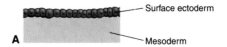
Surface ectoderm
A
Mesoderm

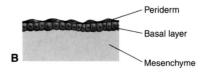
Periderm
Basal layer
B
Mesenchyme

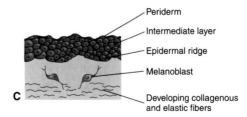
Periderm
Intermediate layer
Epidermal ridge
Melanoblast
C
Developing collagenous and elastic fibers

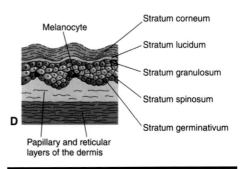
Melanocyte
Stratum corneum
Stratum lucidum
Stratum granulosum
Stratum spinosum
D
Stratum germinativum
Papillary and reticular layers of the dermis

From: Moore KL, and Persaud TVN. 2003. *Before We Are Born: Essentials of Embryology and Birth Defects,* 6th ed. Philadelphia: Saunders, 388. Reprinted by permission.

5. Immature barrier function and increased surface/absorptive area predispose the preterm infant to systemic absorption of topically applied products.

a. The skin of the preterm infant functions more like gastric mucosa than mature skin, putting infants in danger during routine use of topical agents.

B. Dermis
  1. The dermis is derived from the lateral plate mesoderm under the surface of the ectoderm.
  2. Mesenchymal cells form this layer and produce collagenous and elastic tissue fibers by 11 weeks gestation.
  3. During the third and fourth months of gestation, dermal papillae form. The dermis lies below the epidermis and is secured to it by the stratum germinativum, or basal layer of the epidermis.
    a. This interface has an undulating surface with projections called *rete ridges*.

FIGURE 11-3 ■ Schematic representation of wound healing.

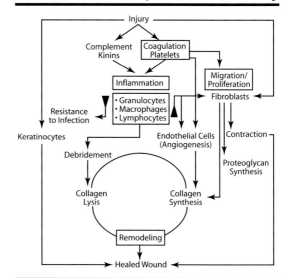

From: Hunt TK, Hopf H, and Hussain Z. 2000. Physiology of wound healing. *Advances in Skin & Wound Care* 13(2 supplement): S7. Reprinted by permission.

  b. The cohesion between these two layers increases with gestation. Therefore, care must be taken when removing adhesives from the skin of the less mature neonate.
  4. The dermis, like the epidermis, is thinner in the preterm infant than in the full-term infant.
  5. The dermis contains nerve endings, blood vessels, lymphocytes, hair follicles, as well as sebaceous, eccrine, and apocrine glands.
  6. The dermis is also composed of fibroblasts, collagen, protein, and elastin fibers.
  7. The dermis is responsible for production of collagen, elastin, growth substance, and proteins that form a tightly woven matrix; this provides strength and structure to the skin.
  8. Hair originates in the dermis and is evidence of skin maturation.[12–14]
    a. Hair begins to develop in weeks 9–12 of gestation.
    b. It is first recognizable on the eyebrows, upper lip, and chin areas.
    c. The stratum germinativum extends as a solid downgrowth of the epidermis into the dermis and forms a hair follicle.
    d. Hair bulbs are formed from hair buds and make up the germinal matrix, which later produces the hair.
    e. The hair follicle forms the epithelial root sheath.
    f. As cells in the germinal matrix develop, they are pushed to the surface and harden (keratinize) to form the hair shaft.
    g. Hair grows up through the epidermis and pierces the skin.
    h. Lanugo, the fine initial hairs, is shed near or shortly after birth and replaced by coarser hair from new hair follicles.
    i. Arrector muscles surround hair follicles. Contractions of these muscles depress skin over their attachment and cause skin around hair shafts to rise, causing "goose bumps." These are not well developed on the face and axilla.

j. Small buds in the epithelial walls of the hair follicles penetrate into the surrounding mesoderm.
   1) Sebaceous glands are formed from cells of these buds.
   2) A fatlike substance is secreted into the hair follicles as the cells from the gland degenerate.

k. Eccrine sweat glands are located throughout most of the body and begin as downgrowths from the epidermis to the mesenchyme.
   1) Buds elongate and form the secretory part of the gland.
   2) Cells function shortly after birth.

l. Apocrine sweat glands develop from the stratum germinativum that develops hair follicles. Ducts of these glands open into the upper part of hair follicles and secrete during puberty.

C. Subcutaneous tissue (hypodermis)
   1. This layer serves as a shock absorber and site of energy storage and helps maintain body heat.
   2. Brown fat, unique to the newborn, aids thermoregulation.
      a. Contributing up to 6 percent of total body weight, this substance is released by nonshivering thermogenesis.
      b. Brown fat is found in the scapula, mediastinum, kidneys, and adrenal glands.
      c. Over time, brown fat stores are depleted.

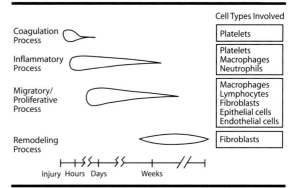

FIGURE 11-4 ■ Components of wound healing.

From: Hunt TK, Hopf H, and Hussain Z. 2000. Physiology of wound healing. *Advances in Skin & Wound Care* 13(supplement 2): S7. Reprinted by permission.

Healing of the Skin[3–5,15,16]

A. Wounds heal in three stages (Figures 11-3 and 11-4).
   1. Coagulation and hemostasis
      a. At the time of tissue injury, bleeding is controlled by the clotting cascade.
         1) Damaged blood vessels, constricted and inflamed, aid hemostasis.
      b. Platelets, activated by injury, convert thrombin to fibrinogen and then to fibrin, which interacts with platelets to form clots.
      c. Activated platelets release growth factors and cytokines that attract inflammatory cells (neutrophils and monocytes) and noninflammatory cells (fibroblasts and endothelial cells) to initiate the next phase of wound healing.
         1) This phase of inflammation helps the wound fight infection and sets the stage for repair.

    2) This stage begins very quickly after injury.

       a) Neutrophils are the first responders. They phagocytize bacteria and break down fibrin. These cells activate fibroblasts and keratinocytes and attract macrophages to the area of injury.

       b) Macrophages phagocytize pathogens, clean the wound, and secrete cytokines and growth factors.

       c) Cytokines and growth factors attract fibroblasts and endothelial cells, which convert oxygen to superoxide. This product serves as a natural antimicrobial agent, inhibiting infection in the wound bed.

2. Proliferation and cell migration

   a. Macrophages, fibroblasts, lymphocytes, and endothelial and epithelial cells move into the wound and begin the next phase of healing.

   b. Keratinocytes migrate into the wound bed to begin epithelialization.

   c. This, in turn, stimulates growth factor and cytokine activity and angiogenesis, or the formation of new blood vessels.

   d. Growth factors and cytokines stimulate fibroblast migration and the deposition of collagen in the wound bed.

     1) Collagen fills and strengthens the wound

   e. Fibroblasts release proteases, which digests dead tissue, and fibrin to clean the wound.

   f. During this phase, contraction of connective tissue brings wound edges closer together.

   g. Poor perfusion and tissue hypoxia can inhibit collagen deposition and angiogenesis and ultimately impair wound healing.

     1) Any stage of repair can be impaired by:

       a) Disease states

       b) Infection

       c) Hypoxia

       d) Poor nutrition

       e) Select medications, particularly immunosuppressive agents such as corticosteroids

3. Remodeling

   a. This phase of healing lasts the longest, up to a year.

   b. The collagen matrix remodels itself so that fibers thicken and are rearranged in an orderly pattern, along the stress lines of the wound.

   c. The remodeled wound does not recover the original organization pattern, impacting final function and strength.

   d. Healed wounds regain approximately 80 percent of their original strength.[16,17]

   e. Inadequate or excessive deposition of collagen will ultimately affect tensile strength and the final appearance of the scar.

B. Care plans that identify the hallmarks of each phase of wound healing assist nurses to provide interventions that are appropriate to that particular phase.

General Management

A. Pain management **(See also Chapter 10: Assessment and Management of Postoperative Pain.)**[18,19]

   1. This is an essential component of the wound care plan, particularly during dressing changes.

2. The presence or absence of pain must be noted. If present, pain must be treated before wound care is performed. Published pain assessment tools, such as the Premature Infant Pain Profile (PIPP),[20] CRIES: Neonatal postoperative pain assessment score, or Face, Legs, Activity, Cry and Consolability (FLACC),[21] are available for bedside use **(see Appendix E: Infant Pain Scales)**.

3. Pain control can be improved by combining analgesics and comfort measures.
   a. Analgesic orders should be written before wound care begins so medication can be obtained when needed.
   b. Comfort measures include the following.
      1) Positioning
      2) Bundling
      3) Offering a pacifier with sucrose[22]
      4) Maintaining warmth
      5) Minimizing ambient light, as appropriate
      6) Allowing family to participate in comfort measures, as appropriate

4. Documentation of the effectiveness of pain control measures is essential in guiding care during subsequent wound care interventions.[23]

B. Neonatal skin care goals
   1. To maintain skin integrity
   2. To promote epidermal maturation
   3. To protect skin from irritation and breakdown
   4. To optimize healing of open wounds
   5. To protect skin around intestinal stomas by:
      a. Securely attaching appliances
      b. Using protective pastes

C. Use of cleaning solutions[4,24–26]
   1. Use isotonic saline to gently cleanse wounds and periwound skin during dressing changes. Normal saline does the following.
      a. Reduces bacteria that may be present
      b. Supports a moist environment
      c. Does not harm healing tissue in the wound bed
   2. Some cleansing solutions damage tissue and impair healing.
      a. Hydrogen peroxide
      b. Sodium hypochlorite
      c. Povidone iodine
      d. Acetic acid
   3. Appropriate cleansing solutions may be used, but should be chosen carefully based on indications, risks, and the benefits to healing tissue.

D. Use of dressings
   1. Excellent guidelines for choosing a dressing are provided by Hess.[5]
      a. Does the dressing provide an effective barrier to bacteria?
      b. Does the dressing provide a moist wound-healing environment?
      c. Does the dressing provide thermal insulation?
      d. Can the dressing be removed without causing trauma to the wound?
      e. Does the dressing remove drainage and debris?
      f. Is the dressing free of toxins and particulates?
   2. There are many types of dressings.
      a. Gauze dressings[5,15,27]

1) Woven gauze is made from cotton strands and woven together like fabric.
2) Nonwoven gauze is made from synthetic material and is pressed together, not woven.
3) There are advantages to using gauze.
   a) Economy
   b) Absorbency
   c) Availability
   d) May be manufactured to contain agents such as antimicrobials
4) Gauze also has disadvantages.
   a) Rapid drying, requiring frequent replacement or rewetting
   b) Adherence to the wound, causing tissue injury when the gauze is removed
5) Dry gauze may be used as a dressing with significant exudate.
6) Moist gauze is used for wounds that are granulating to maintain a moist wound base to speed healing.
   a) "Wet to moist dressings" describes gauze that remains moist between changes.
   b) Dressings that have dried indicate that dressing changes should be done more frequently or that the primary dressing should be covered with a moisture-retentive secondary dressing.
   c) Gauze can remain in place for up to 24 hours between changes, if moist.
7) Gauze should not be placed so tightly into the wound that contraction is compromised.
8) The gauze can be used as a primary dressing with a secondary dressing required to hold the gauze in place.

b. Alginate dressings[5,15,27]
1) Alginates are composed of seaweed and packaged as ropes or pads.
   a) These dressings conform well to the wound shape, filling space within the wound bed.
2) Alginates are a good choice for wounds with significant drainage, absorbing 20 times their weight in wound exudate.
3) Used as a primary dressing, this product facilitates autolytic debridement. It is soft, easy to apply and remove, and generally requires a secondary dressing to secure.
4) Avoid using alginates in wounds with minimal drainage because they can dry the wound bed.

c. Foam dressings[5,15,27]
1) This absorptive material, often polyurethane, is manufactured in varying thicknesses as pads, sheets, and pillows.
2) Absorbent foam fosters a moist and warm environment, is nontraumatic to remove, and does not shed lint or debris into the wound.
3) It can be used with wounds that have minimal to moderate drainage.
4) It can be used as a primary or secondary dressing.
   a) Nonadhesive foam will require netting or tape to secure.
5) It conforms well to surgical appliances and tubes.

d. Hydrogel dressings[5,15,27]
1) These water- or glycerin-based products are packaged as sheets, gels, and gauzes.

        a) These dressings can contain as much as 95 percent water and are clear or translucent.

   2) They are available in three forms.

      a) Amorphous hydrogels packaged in tubes, packets, and spray bottles

      b) Impregnated gauze pads used to fill space in large wounds

      c) Sheet hydrogels, consisting of a thin layer of fiber mesh covered with hydrogel manufactured with and without adhesive borders

   3) They are used to maintain a moist wound environment in a granulating wound and facilitate autolytic debridement of devitalized tissue.

      a) Do not absorb wound drainage and are best used in wounds with minimal drainage; not useful in heavily draining wounds

      b) May be used as a primary dressing or secondary dressing if used in sheet form

      c) Easy to apply and atraumatic to remove

      d) Rehydrate a wound, fill in space in the wound bed, can be used in infected wounds

   4) These can dry if not covered.

  e. Transparent film dressings[5,27]

   1) These are sheets of polyurethane that are coated with adhesive.[5]

      a) Transparent

      b) Semiocclusive

      c) Impermeable to water and bacteria

      d) Permeable to moisture vapor

   2) They are a good choice for minimally draining wounds, lacerations, abrasions, or wounds with necrosis or that are sloughing.

   3) They allow for visualization of the wound field.

   4) They are not a good choice for highly exudative or draining wounds because film dressings are nonabsorbent.

   5) They may be used as a primary or secondary dressing.

   6) Film dressings will stay in place only if there is a border of dry and oil-free skin around the wound.

   7) Apply smoothly without wrinkles in order to seal the edges.

   8) Avoid stretching the film during application to prevent skin injury.

  f. Hydrocolloid dressings[5,27]

   1) They are composed of various materials.

      a) Pectin

      b) Gelatin

      c) Carboxymethylcellulose

   2) These dressings are available in three forms.

      a) Pastes

      b) Powders

      c) Sheets

   3) They may be translucent or opaque.

   4) Warm the dressing prior to application and hold in place to promote adherence.

   5) Hydrocolloid dressings have the following benefits.

      a) Absorptive, can be used with wounds that are draining moderately

      b) Occlusive, keeping water, oxygen, and organisms out of the wound

      c) Facilitate autolytic debridement by supporting a moist wound environment

- Can be placed on eschar or necrotic areas
    d) Flexibility to conform to various shapes and stay in place, even in areas of high friction
    e) Can be left in place for many days between changes
6) Limitations to use of this type of dressing include the following.
    a) Opacity obscures wound visibility.
        - Use of this dressing is not ideal when serial assessments of the site are required.
    b) Hydrocolloid dressings are very adhesive and may damage skin when removed.
7) Use hydrocolloid dressings as follows.
    a) Use a hydrocolloid sheet on periwound skin when repeated adhesive dressings will be applied and removed.
    b) Apply adhesive to the barrier, not to the skin, to avoid trauma to skin with removal.
    c) Apply around tracheostomy sites to prevent pressure injury from snug tracheostomy tubes.
    d) Apply a hydrocolloid sheet around gastrostomy tubes to protect from pressure injury around snug tubes and to protect skin from leaking.
    e) Hydrocolloid sheets are useful when anchoring devices in place.
        - The skin around thoracostomy tubes can be protected from tape by placing two strips of hydrocolloid on either side of the tube.
            - Place a small woven gauze around the thoracostomy tube to absorb drainage.
            - The gauze can be secured with adhesive tape to the hydrocolloid instead of directly to the skin.
        - Placing a hydrocolloid barrier over it can protect the upper lip of orally intubated patients.
            - Secure the endotracheal tube with tape placed on the barrier, not on the skin.
        - Indwelling orogastric or nasogastric tubes can be taped to the barrier, not to the skin.
        - Nasal cannula oxygen can be secured to hydrocolloid sheets on the cheeks.
8) Remove adhesive with alcohol-free adhesive removers to protect the skin from injury.[4]
    a) Cleanse to remove any product residue, and dry completely before a barrier is reapplied.[5]

Treatment of Injured Skin

A. Skin tearing or stripping of the epidermis (from friction, use of adhesives, or chemical agents)
1. Cleanse affected area with normal saline.
2. Apply a sheet of hydrogel, hydrocolloid, or a film dressing.
3. Remove the dressing when loose or, if using hydrogel, if dry.
4. Secure sheet hydrogel with an adhesive or netting.
B. Diaper dermatitis (a result of repeated exposure to urine or stool)[4,28]
1. Frequent diaper changes for all neonates are recommended.
    a. Moist skin is more easily damaged than dry skin.

   b. The pH of urine, coupled with the macerating effects of moisture, can rapidly result in diaper dermatitis.
2. Neonates are at highest risk of perianal skin injury following correction of anorectal malformations.
   a. Dermatitis can easily evolve into a deeper injury with time.
   b. Contributing factors to injury include the following.
      1) Increased frequency of stooling
      2) Changes in bowel flora or pH
      3) Antibiotic therapy, which often increases the frequency of stooling
3. Neonates at risk for skin breakdown caused by constant exposure to urine include those with the following conditions.
   a. Spina bifida
   b. Bladder exstrophy
   c. Neurogenic bladder
4. Nursing measures for prevention/treatment of diaper dermatitis include the following.
   a. Clean skin completely, once each day, in order to examine it thoroughly.
      1) Water or normal saline can be used to clean stool, urine, and products off of the skin.
      2) Products that are not water soluble can be removed with mineral oil.
   b. A skin sealant, such as Cavilon 3M No Sting Barrier Film, can be used alone or under other products.
   c. For severe cases of skin excoriation, take the following steps.
      1) Apply a barrier paste as indicated. Use continuously.
      2) When changing the infant's diaper after stooling, remove the stool from the paste, but do not remove the paste from the skin. This will prevent removal of the newly formed epithelium.
         a) Spray bottles are useful in cleaning perianal skin without trauma.
      3) Reapply more paste and rediaper.
      4) There are many useful commercial barrier pastes.
         a) Follow the manufacturer's instructions for use.
      5) Bedside barrier pastes can be made out of common ingredients.
5. Monitor for the presence of topical candidiasis in patients with diaper dermatis.
   a. Moisture promotes the growth of yeast.
   b. Apply antifungal powder or ointment as needed to treat topical candidiasis.
C. Intravenous extravasation
1. Prevention through close monitoring is critical.
   a. Note the pH and osmolarity of infusions. Avoid using peripheral sites for infusions or medication with a pH >8 or <5 or an osmolarity >500 mOsm/liter.[29,30]
   b. Select the site carefully, securing the needle or catheter in a manner that allows for visibility of the site at all times. If infiltration does occur, it is imperative to minimize the extent of extravasation.
   c. Diligent monitoring and recognizing any early signs of tissue infiltration are crucial for appropriate and timely intervention.
2. Nursing interventions include the following.
   a. Obtain an order to administer 2 percent Nitropaste or phentolamine mesylate (Regitine) for vasopressor extravasations.

      b. Consider hyaluronidase administration for extravasations other than blood products or vasoactive drugs.[31,32]

      c. Topical or systemic antibiotic therapy may be warranted to prevent infection when tissue is damaged.

      d. Consultation with a plastic surgeon may be required for deep tissue injury that has resulted from vessel damage and ischemia.[33]

D. Skin care following circumcision[3]

    1. Until healed, use a petroleum-based ointment or petroleum gauze.

    2. Routinely inspect the area for evidence of the following.

      a. Bleeding

      b. Inflammation

      c. Swelling that may obstruct the urethra

    3. Findings that require intervention include the following.

      a. Persistent bleeding (Treatment may include: application of Surgicel, silver nitrate cauterization, or placement of sutures.)

      b. Infection, which is rare (It will require antibiotic therapy.)

      c. Urinary obstruction (It will require catheterization.)

Care of Surgical Wounds
Healing by Primary Closure

A. Primary closure and dressings:[17]

    1. Provide a physical barrier to bacterial entry

    2. Prevent mechanical injury or trauma to the wound and surrounding skin

    3. Unimpeded epithelial resurfacing if the wound edges remain approximated

B. Dressings

    1. A protective, semipermeable film dressing may be used along with gauze or Telfa placed over the incision.

      a. The type of dressing will vary according to patient needs and clinical practice.

    2. Steri-Strips may directly cover the wound and can be left on until they loosen.

      a. These may be the only dressing or may be used under the film dressing/gauze or Telfa combination.

    3. Incisions closed with subcuticular, dissolvable sutures may have occlusive dressings that are removed before bathing, often as early as 48 hours postoperatively.

    4. Wounds closed with external sutures or staples should be kept dry and loosely covered until sutures or staples are removed.

    5. Document the appearance of the wound and dressing each shift. Monitor the incision for the following.[17]

      a. Approximation and epithelialization

      b. Drainage

      c. Evidence of infection (Notify the surgical team of any of the following.)

        1) Inflammation

        2) Erythema

        3) Induration

        4) Edema

    6. The optimal environment for intact skin is dryness. Dressings that are saturated with fluid should be changed as often as necessary to keep the periwound skin dry.

7. Dressings that have adhered to the wound should be moistened with saline or water to loosen them prior to removal. Dressings should be removed gently, to avoid causing trauma or bleeding.

Care of Open Surgical Wounds Healing by Secondary Intention

A. These are the goals of this type of care.
   1. Maintain a moist, warm wound environment to speed healing using the appropriate dressing.
   2. Keep the periwound skin dry to prevent maceration.
B. If maceration of the periwound skin occurs from wound exudate, take the following steps.
   1. Clean the skin with saline, and adjust the dressing to keep it dry.
   2. A water-soluble product, such as Aquaphor, can be applied to the periwound skin after cleansing to protect it from the macerating effects of chronic moisture.
   3. Alternatively, an alcohol-free skin sealant can be used on the periwound skin to protect it from moisture.
C. Open wounds and periwound skin should be gently irrigated with saline each dressing change.
D. Apply the dressing as follows.
   1. Loosely pack the primary wound dressing carefully into the wound to fill the contours of the cavity.
   2. Avoid overlap of the primary dressing onto the periwound skin to decrease skin maceration.
   3. The secondary dressing serves to support the function of the primary dressing and keep it intact.
E. Document the appearance of the wound each shift or dressing change.
   1. Measure the dimension and depth of the wound bed and document with drawings or photographs.
   2. Note the appearance of the following.
      a. The wound base (Is there granulation tissue or slough?)
      b. The wound edges
      c. The condition of the periwound skin (Is there erythema or edema? Is there drainage? Are there changes in the integrity of the tissue?)
F. Evaluate the dressing choice as the wound changes over time. Are current dressings still appropriate, or do new dressings need to be selected?

Ostomy Care in the Newborn

A. Small and large bowel stomas are created to divert stool away from the distal bowel in neonates who have disease or intestinal obstruction.
   1. The location and type of stoma created is determined by the surgeon at the time of the operation and is based on the diagnosis and findings during surgery.
   2. Common indications for ostomy creation include, but are not limited to the following.
      a. Cloacal malformations
      b. Necrotizing enterocolitis
      c. Hirschsprung's disease

FIGURE 11-5 ■ Cross-sectional view of end stoma.

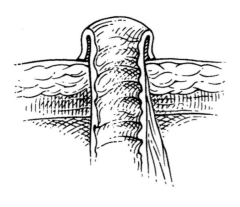

From: Hampton BG, and Bryant RA. 1992. *Ostomies and Continent Diversions*. St. Louis: Mosby, 355. Reprinted by permission.

FIGURE 11-6 ■ Cross-sectional view of end stoma with distal bowel oversewn and secured to anterior peritoneum at stoma site.

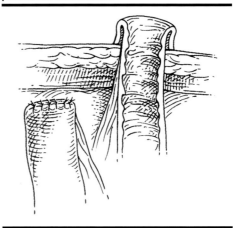

From: Hampton BG, and Bryant RA. 1992. *Ostomies and Continent Diversions*. St. Louis: Mosby, 355. Reprinted by permission.

       d. Imperforate anus
       e. Bowel atresia, stenosis, or obstruction
       f. Intestinal dysmotility disorders
   3. There are three stoma types.
       a. End (Figures 11-5–11-7)
          1) When an end stoma is created, the distal end of the bowel is oversewn and left within the abdomen. This is called a Hartmann's pouch.
       b. Loop (Figure 11-8)
       c. Double-barrel (Figure 11-9)
   4. Small bowel stomas are usually ileostomies, but may be jejunostomies or duodenostomies.
   5. Large bowel stomas are colostomies. A colostomy can be made at the ascending, transverse, descending, or sigmoid portions of the large intestine.

B. Effluent draining from a stoma can vary from thin to thick liquid.
   1. The more proximal the stoma, the more liquid the stool will be.
   2. The small bowel absorbs nutrients and produces fluid; stool draining from a stoma of the small bowel is very liquid.
   3. The large bowel absorbs fluid and stores stool, so a colostomy will produce thicker, pastier stool.

C. Stomas can be temporary or permanent.

FIGURE 11-7 ■ End stoma.

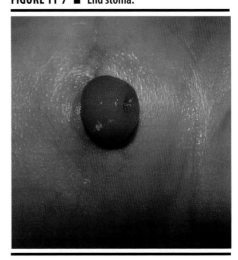

FIGURE 11-8 ■ Cross-sectional view of loop stoma.

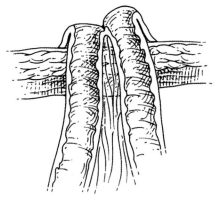

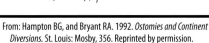

From: Hampton BG, and Bryant RA. 1992. *Ostomies and Continent Diversions*. St. Louis: Mosby, 356. Reprinted by permission.

FIGURE 11-9 ■ Cross-sectional view of double-barrel stoma.

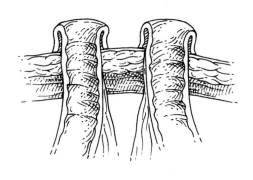

From: Hampton BG, and Bryant RA. 1992. *Ostomies and Continent Diversions*. St. Louis: Mosby, 356. Reprinted by permission.

D. Appliances may be used (Figures 11-10–11-13).[34]
   1. An appliance does not need to be used in the first few days following surgery.
      a. The stoma can be covered with petroleum gauze in the immediate postoperative period.
      b. When bowel function returns and stooling begins, an appliance choice can then be made.
   2. All small bowel stomas and proximal large bowel stomas should be dressed with an appliance when stooling begins.
      a. Principles of pouching:

FIGURE 11-10 ■ Neonatal pouch.

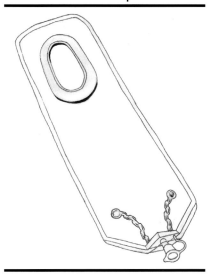

Illustration courtesy of Jon Lincoln.

FIGURE 11-11 ■ Neonatal wafer.

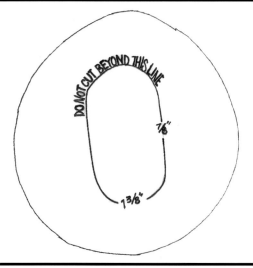

Illustration courtesy of Jon Lincoln.

FIGURE 11-12 ■ Newborn pouch.

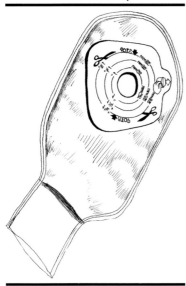

Illustration courtesy of Jon Lincoln.

FIGURE 11-13 ■ Tail closure.

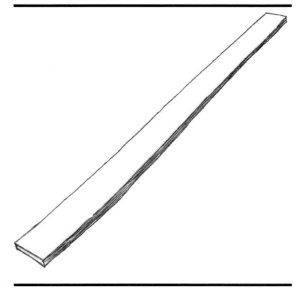

Illustration courtesy of Jon Lincoln.

1) Protect the skin from stool by using a securely sealed system (which is also odor proof).
2) Protect the stoma from trauma.
3) Protect the skin from trauma by using skin sealants.
4) Evaluate the skin and stoma with each pouch change.

3. Use of an appliance with a descending or sigmoid colostomy is optional because stool is often thick and easy to contain.

a. A discussion among the surgeon, neonatologist, family, and primary nurse will help identify the best method of care for the patient.

FIGURE 11-14 ■ Prolapsed stoma.

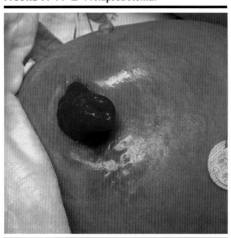

FIGURE 11-15 ■ Retracted stoma.

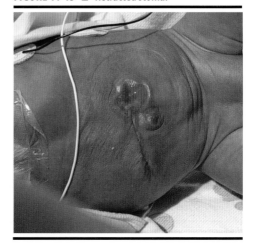

FIGURE 11-16 ■ Stoma measuring guide.

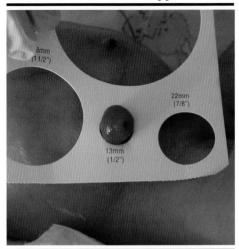

FIGURE 11-17 ■ Stoma measuring guide.

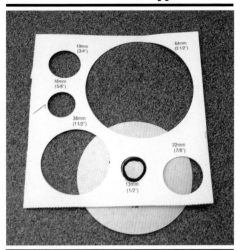

      b. Managing a stoma without an appliance requires use of a protective barrier paste applied to the skin around the stoma.

      c. Stool is collected in a diaper, instead of an appliance.

      d. At each diaper change, paste should be reapplied to the peristomal skin.

        1) Once a day, remove all paste and inspect the peristomal skin for injury.

        2) Skin injury may require cessation of barrier paste and use of an appliance.

E. Appliance removal.[34]

    1. Gently remove any existing appliance with water or adhesive remover. Clean the skin around the stoma carefully with water to remove any stool or product residue.

    2. Inspect the stoma and document the appearance.

      a. Healthy stomas are beefy red and shiny (see Figure 11-7).

      b. Stomas can prolapse (Figure 11-14), retract (Figure 11-15), or become ischemic, potentially leading to obstruction. Note any change in appearance.

      c. Note and record the volume and character of the effluent. Report any changes.

      d. Note trauma or bleeding.

        1) Stomas can be injured and bleed easily.

        2) If protected well, they will heal rapidly.

    3. Inspect the peristomal skin with each bag change.

      a. Peristomal skin should be smooth and intact, with the mucocutaneous junction approximated.

      b. Skin integrity is best maintained by ensuring the appliance fits correctly, with 1/8 inch or less exposed skin, adheres well, and the type of pouch is appropriate for the patient.

      c. Injured skin heals most quickly when protected from stool and covered securely.

F. Appliance application proceeds as follows (Figures 11-16–11-22).

    1. Cut a pattern to fit the stoma exactly where it joins the skin. This is called the mucocutaneous junction.

FIGURE 11-18 ■ **Stoma size traced from template onto neonatal wafer.**

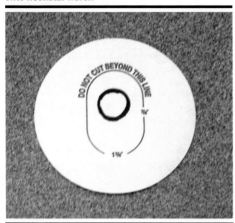

FIGURE 11-19 ■ **Wafer showing cut out opening for stoma.**

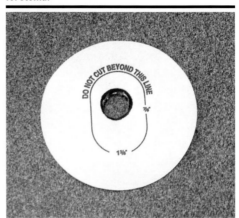

    a. No more than 1/8 inch of skin should be visible when the appliance is in place.

    b. For perfectly round stomas, measure the stoma with a precut pattern provided by the manufacturer.

        1) Create a template if one is not available. If the stoma is an irregular shape, make a custom template.

        2) Date the template and keep it at the bedside.

    c. Check the fit of the template before cutting the next appliance.

        1) Most stomas shrink steadily over the first several weeks, and the template will often become too large, unnecessarily exposing healthy skin to stool.

        2) Discard a template that fits poorly, and make a new one.

FIGURE 11-20 ■ **Skin barrier.**

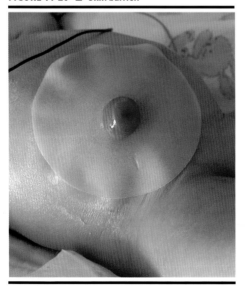

FIGURE 11-21 ■ **Appliance bag.**

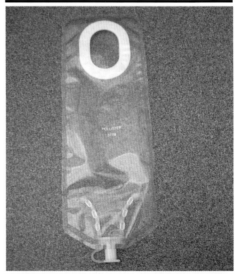

3) Date the template.

4) When you are certain the template is the correct size, trace the opening onto the back of the skin barrier portion of the appliance.

5) Adjust the location of the opening to allow the appliance to lay on the abdomen in the best possible position; many times this is not directly in the center, but off to one side.

6) Cut out the opening for the stoma without puncturing the stoma bag, if attached.

7) Smooth any rough edges with your fingers.

8) Make certain the skin surrounding the stoma is dry before application.

9) Warm the skin barrier in your hands well before removing the paper backing and applying the barrier to the skin. A warm barrier will be soft and conform well to the skin.

10) Once it is in place, run a finger around the stoma gently and press the barrier to the skin to remove any air pockets.

11) Attach the appliance bag to the skin barrier, if separate, and close the end with a tail closure device.

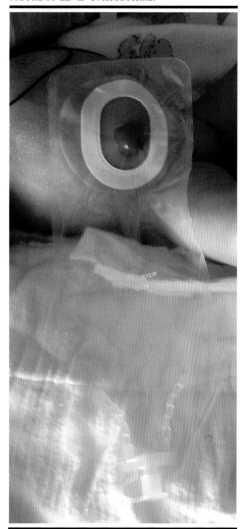

FIGURE 11-22 ■ Dressed stoma.

2. Use of stoma powder and paste are reserved for special circumstances and are not necessarily needed for routine use.

a. Stoma powder is used to dry out ulcerated or denuded skin and improve adherence of the appliance.

1) Take care to rub in any excess powder from surrounding intact skin, or the appliance may not adhere well.

b. Stoma paste can help prevent leakage of stool onto the skin.

1) Use it when stomas are flush with the skin or retracted.

2) Use it when the skin is uneven around the stoma (along a healing incision, for example) to maintain a level peristomal surface.

3) Use it to fill space in an area of breakdown at the mucocutaneous junction after stoma powder is applied.

       4) Paste is applied with a syringe to control the application.

       5) It is difficult to remove. Use a dry cloth to pull off excess.

       6) Residual paste can interfere with appliance adherence.

  3. For fungal rashes, dust the area with antifungal powder.

    a. Rub it in well to allow the bag to adhere.

    b. Alternatively, cover the powder with alcohol-free skin sealant, and then apply a skin barrier.

    c. Alcohol-free skin sealant can be used alone to prevent or treat damaged skin before placing the appliance.

  4. Bags can stay in place for many days and are changed when they loose adherence and are at risk of leaking.

    a. The skin barrier will appear to be pale yellow in color when exposed to moisture; this will grow slowly as a concentric ring around the stoma.

    b. If this area enlarges significantly or appears irregular in shape, it is suggestive of a leak of stool under the barrier.

    c. Barrier removal is best achieved with water or alcohol-free adhesive remover.

G. In preparation for discharge, teach family members and other caregivers how to do the following.

  1. Remove the appliance

  2. Inspect the area

  3. Clean the stoma and peristomal skin

  4. Cut the appliance to fit the stoma within 1/8 inch

  5. Warm and apply the barrier with attention to achieving a good seal

  6. Use paste, powder, and skin sealant appropriately

REFERENCES

1. Lund CH, et al. 2001. Neonatal skin care: Clinical outcomes of the AWHONN/NANN evidence-based clinical practice guideline. Association of Women's Health, Obstetric, Gynecologic, and Neonatal Nurses/National Association of Neonatal Nurses. *Journal of Obstetric, Gynecologic, and Neonatal Nursing* 30(1): 41–51.

2. Lund CH, et al. 2001. Neonatal skin care: Evaluation of the AWHONN/NANN research-based practice project on knowledge and skin care practices. Association of Women's Health, Obstetric and Neonatal Nurses/National Association of Neonatal Nurses. *Journal of Obstetric, Gynecologic, and Neonatal Nursing* 30(1): 30–40.

3. Witte MB, and Barbul A. 1997. General principles of wound healing. *Surgical Clinics of North America* 77(3): 509–528.

4. Lund C, et al. 1999. Neonatal skin care: The scientific basis for practice. *Neonatal Network* 18(4): 15–27.

5. Hess CT. 2005. *Clinical Guide: Wound Care,* 5th ed. Philadelphia: Lippincott Williams & Wilkins.

6. Fore-Pfliger J. 2004. The epidermal skin barrier: Implications for the wound care Practitioner. Part I. *Advances in Skin & Wound Care* 17(8): 417–425.

7. Fore-Pfliger J. 2004. The epidermal skin barrier: Implications for the wound care practitioner. Part II. *Advances in Skin & Wound Care* 17(9): 480–488.

8. Loomis CA, and Birge MB. 2001. Fetal skin development. In *Textbook of Neonatal Dermatology,* Eichenfield LF, Freiden IJ, and Esterly NB, eds. Philadelphia: Saunders, 1–17.

9. Mancini AJ. 2001. Structure and function of newborn skin. In *Textbook of Neonatal Dermatology,* Eichenfield LF, Freiden IJ, and Esterly NB, eds. Philadelphia: Saunders, 18–32.

10. Siegfried EC. 2001. Neonatal skin care and toxicology. In *Textbook of Neonatal Dermatology,* Eichenfield LF, Frieden IJ, and Esterly NB, eds. Philadelphia: Saunders, 62–72.

11. Williams ML. 2001. Skin of the premature infant. In *Textbook of Neonatal Dermatology,* Eichenfield LF, Frieden IJ, and Esterly NB, eds. Philadelphia: Saunders, 46–61.

12. Moore KL, and Persaud TVN. 2003. *Before We Are Born: Essentials of Embryology and Birth Defects,* 6th ed. Philadelphia: Saunders, 388–389.

13. Moore KL, and Persaud TVN. 2003. *The Developing Human: Clinically Oriented Embryology,* 7th ed. Philadelphia: Saunders, 486–487.

14. Sadler TW. 2004. *Langman's Medical Embryology,* 9th ed. Philadelphia: Lippincott Williams & Wilkins, 427–432.

15. Taquino LT. 2000. Promoting wound healing in the neonatal setting: Process versus protocol. *Journal of Perinatal & Neonatal Nursing* 14(1): 104–118.

16. Hunt TK, Hopf H, and Hussain Z. 2000. Physiology of wound healing. *Advances in Skin & Wound Care* 13(2 supplement): S6–S11.

17. Doughty DB. 2004. Wound assessment: Tips and techniques. *Advances in Skin & Wound Care* 17(7): 369–372.

18. Saniski D. 2005. Neonatal pain relief protocols in their infancy. *Nurseweek* February 14, 19–21.

19. Dallam LE, et al. 2004. Pain management and wounds. In *Wound Care Essentials: Practice Principles,* Baranoski S, and Ayello EA, eds. Springhouse, Philadelphia: Lippincott Williams & Wilkins, 217–238.

20. McNair C, et al. 2004. Postoperative pain assessment in the neonatal intensive care unit. *Archives of Diseases in Childhood. Fetal and Neonatal Edition* 89(6): F537–F541.

21. Merkel S, Voepel-Lewis T, and Malviya S. 2002. Pain assessment in infants and young children: The FLACC scale. *American Journal of Nursing* 102(10): 55–58.

22. Prince WL, et al. 2004. Treatment of neonatal pain without a gold standard: The case for caregiving interventions and sucrose administration. *Neonatal Network* 23(4): 33–45.

23. Senecal SJ. 1999. Pain management of wound care. *Nursing Clinics of North America* 34(4): 847–860.

24. Rodeheaver GT. 1997. Wound cleansing, wound irrigation, wound disinfection. In *Chronic Wound Care: A Clinical Source Book for Healthcare Professionals,* 2nd ed., Krasner D, et al., eds. Wayne, Pennsylvania: Health Management Publications, 97–108.

25. Linder N, et al. 1997. Topical iodine-containing antiseptics and subclinical hypothyroidism in preterm infants. *Journal of Pediatrics* 131(3): 434–439.

26. Pyati SP, et al. 1977. Absorption of iodine in the neonate following topical use of povidone iodine. *Journal of Pediatrics* 91(5): 825–828.

27. Ovington LG. 2001. Wound care products: How to choose. *Advances in Skin & Wound Care* 14(5): 259–264.

28. Visscher MO, et al. 2000. Development of diaper rash in the newborn. *Pediatric Dermatology* 17(1): 52–57.

29. Sharief N, and Goonasekera C. 1994. Soft tissue injury associated with intravenous phenytoin in a neonate. *Acta Paediatrica* 83(11): 1218–1219.

30. Robbins MS, Stromquist C, and Tan LH. 1993. Acyclovir pH—possible cause of extravasation tissue injury. *Annals of Pharmacotherapy* 27(2): 238.

31. Raszka WV Jr, et al. 1990. The use of hyaluronidase in the treatment of intravenous extravasation injuries. *Journal of Perinatology* 10(2): 146–149.

32. Subhani M, Sridhar S, and DeCristofaro JD. 2001. Phentolamine use in a neonate for the prevention of dermal necrosis caused by dopamine: A case report. *Journal of Perinatology* 21(5): 324–326.

33. Harris PA, Bradley S, and Moss AL. 2001. Limiting the damage of iatrogenic extravasation injury in neonates. *Plastic and Reconstructive Surgery* 107(3): 893–894.

34. Erwin-Toth P. 2003. Ostomy pearls: A concise guide to stoma siting, pouching systems, patient education and more. *Advances in Skin & Wound Care* 16(3): 146–152.

Notes

Notes

Transport of the Surgical Infant

Carol M. Johnson, RN, MSN, CNNP

In the early 1900s, infants born prematurely were exhibited as spectacles. Ironically, the vehicle that was used to transport babies to the World's Fair in Chicago for public display was subsequently donated to the Chicago Department of Health and became the first dedicated neonatal transport vehicle in the U.S.[1] Around the country, this vehicle was followed by others of increasing sophistication: fixed wing aircraft in the 1950s and helicopters in the 1960s. Over the last three decades, neonatal specialty care, along with tertiary centers, has evolved and is associated with reduced perinatal morbidity and mortality.[2-4] Although antenatal referral and delivery at a tertiary care center is considered optimal, unforeseen situations often preclude this option, and neonatal transport is necessary.

Transport services emanating from NICUs have proven invaluable in improving the outcome of infants referred for transport.[3] To successfully stabilize and transport the neonate, transport staff must understand the process of adaptation to extrauterine life, anticipate how that infant will respond to the physiologic challenges generated by the transport environment, and be aware of any surgical conditions that may be present.[5-8] Surgical candidates may often be small, fragile, and premature as well, adding an extra challenge.[9] This chapter presents information for transport team members caring for infants with surgical conditions. Although each entity—disease, adaptation, prematurity, and transport physiology—can be analyzed separately, it is the interaction of all these factors that challenges the neonatal patient in transport and must be managed by the transport team.

Transport Team Composition and Operation

A. Impact on outcome
   1. The outcome of transported infants is critically dependent on the effectiveness of stabilization following delivery or onset of illness and the quality of care given during transport.[10-12]
      a. Selecting a team with the necessary skills to deliver quality care is of vital importance.

TABLE 12-1 ■ Competency of Transport Team as Delineated by the National Association of Neonatal Nurses

Guideline II

C. Collectively, transport team members shall demonstrate competency in the following neonatal content areas, including, but not limited to:

1. American Heart Association and American Academy of Pediatrics' Neonatal Resuscitation Program (NRP) or Pediatric Advanced Life Support (PALS).
2. Maternal physiologic and pharmacologic factions affecting the neonate.
3. Neonatal assessment:
   a. Physical examination
   b. Gestational age assessment
   c. Interpretation of clinical laboratory and diagnostic data:
      1) Blood gases
      2) X-rays
      3) CBC
      4) Blood chemistries
      5) Cardiovascular monitoring
         a) EKG and basic arrhythmia interpretation
         b) Blood pressure monitoring
4. Thermoregulation
5. Oxygen monitoring
6. Fluid and electrolyte therapy
7. Pharmacology, including common drug calculations
8. Anatomy, physiology, assessment, and treatment of the following categories:
   a. Acute and chronic respiratory diseases
   b. Cardiovascular abnormalities
   c. Surgical problems
   d. Infectious diseases
   e. Musculoskeletal abnormalities
   f. Neurologic and spinal cord injuries
   g. Prematurity and postmaturity
   h. Gastrointestinal emergencies
   i. Genitourinary disorders
   j. Integumentary disruption
   k. Hematologic disorders
   l. Metabolic and endocrine disorders
   m. Genetic disorders
   n. Disorders of the head, eyes, ears, nose, and throat

9. Psychosocial and bereavement support and crisis intervention
10. Mechanical ventilation techniques on transport
11. Management of pain and agitation
12. Provision of developmentally supportive care
13. Transport relations and communication:
    a. With the referring hospital
    b. With the receiving hospital
    c. Within the hospital
    d. Within the team
    e. With the parents, siblings, and significant others
14. Problem solving and priority setting
15. Medical-legal concerns
    a. Scope of practice of all team members
    b. State and federal regulations regarding the transport and advanced practice
    c. Informed consent
16. Continuous quality improvement (CQI)
17. Advanced practice protocols, if applicable
18. Transport safety issues
19. Orientation to transport vehicle, if applicable
20. Transport equipment, including troubleshooting and back-up systems
21. Altitude physiology and flight safety as defined by the National Flight Nurses Association (NFNA) and Commission on Accreditation on Transport Medical Services (CATMS), if applicable, Department of Transportation (DOT), and Association of Air Medical Services (AAMS).

D. The transport team shall possess the combined expertise and legal scope of practice to perform the following neonatal procedures according to the established program guidelines and protocols, organizational policies and procedures, including, but not limited to:

1. Endotracheal intubation
2. Application of nasal CPAP
3. Oxygen administration
4. Needle aspiration of air or surgical placement of a chest tube
5. Initiate and maintain mechanical ventilation
6. Bag and mask ventilation

7. Intravenous and intra-arterial access, which may include:
   a. Peripheral venous cannulation
   b. Umbilical arterial and venous catheterization
   c. Percutaneous arterial line and puncture
   d. Intraosseous line
8. Venipuncture for laboratory specimen collection
9. Cardiopulmonary resuscitation
10. Medication administration

From: National Association of Neonatal Nurses. 1998. Education and competency of transport team members. In *Neonatal Nursing Transport Standards and Guidelines.* Glenview, Illinois: NANN, 268. Reprinted by permission.

   b. Improved care and fewer complications are associated with teams generated from Level III centers.

B. Factors in team selection

1. Consolidated Omnibus Reconciliation Act (COBRA) legislation requires that all medical facilities participating in Medicare programs choose qualified personnel and equipment for transported patients.[13]

2. Regional and local standards vary as to the discipline/licensure of the transport team.[14] Typically, the neonatal transport team is customized to meet the needs of the individual patient and consists of some combination of the following.[14-16]

   a. Neonatal staff nurses
   b. Respiratory therapists
   c. House staff
   d. Fellow
   e. Nurse practitioner
   f. Paramedic

3. There are published guidelines for neonatal team composition.

   a. The National Association of Neonatal Nurses (NANN)[17]
      1) Addresses the expertise of the team collectively rather than specifying the discipline or credentials of each participant
      2) Stipulates that the team shall possess the combined expertise to effectively assess actual and potential neonatal problems and to deliver appropriate interventions in transport (Table 12-1)

   b. The American Academy of Pediatrics[18]
      1) Emphasizes selection of team members with personal traits such as
         a) Independence
         b) Flexibility
         c) Stress tolerance
         d) Physical fitness
         e) Necessary licensure
         f) Clinical competence

C. Team orientation

1. In addition to formal degrees and licensure, team members must be oriented to deliver the care specific to their role and responsibilities in transport.[16,17]

   a. Clearly written learning objectives for each team member, which ultimately ensures more seamless delivery of care
   b. Information on equipment operation and troubleshooting[18]
   c. Information on documentation/paperwork specific to the institution[18]
   d. Information on team member roles and chain of command[18]
   e. Crash and survival information[18]
   f. Transport physiology[18]
   g. An overview of the safety and quality assurance (QA) issues specific to the patient population and other challenges encountered by each transport team

2. Team members may be required to take part in national learning programs that validate educational consistency at a national standard.[17]

   a. Neonatal Resuscitation Program (NRP)
   b. Pediatric Advanced Life Support Course (PALS)

3. New members of the team should obtain transport experience under the supervision of an experienced team member.[18]

D. Team member competency
1. Competency must be documented on an ongoing basis by the team coordinator or director through methods such as the following.[17,18]
   a. Written exams
   b. Skill laboratories
   c. Maintenance of national credentials
2. Competency must be maintained in all areas of neonatal care (see Table 12-1), including the following.
   a. Neonatal resuscitation
   b. Physical assessment
   c. Interpreting diagnostic studies
   d. Administering appropriate medications and therapies
   e. Use of transport equipment
   f. Family intervention
   g. Problem solving
   h. Safety issues
   i. QA
3. Certification in formal learning programs such as NRP and PALS is usually required because it provides standardized information and testing to determine competency.

E. Team leadership
1. A team leader, usually a physician or neonatal nurse practitioner (NNP), should accompany every transport to direct provision of patient care.[17] NNPs are often in this role because they possess the needed expertise,[18] are cost-effective,[19] and produce outcomes similar to physician-led transports.[20–23]
   a. Requirements[17]
      1) Demonstration of strong clinical skills
      2) Educational background in acute neonatal patient management
      3) Experience as a team leader[17]
   b. Responsibilities
      1) Directs the team in providing patient care, including code situations
      2) Reviews the plan of care (by phone) with the medical control physician (MCP)—the physician from either the receiving facility or the transport system who has accepted care of the infant
      3) Provides parents with essential information and may obtain informed consent[17]

TABLE 12-2 ■ Sample Standardized Transport Procedure

Endotracheal Intubation

Purpose

Insertion of endotracheal tube (ETT) to reverse hypoxia and provide ventilation in respiratory failure, to maintain patent airway, or to reverse apnea when indicated.

Eligibility

All NNPs in the SCV Health and Hospital system are eligible to perform this procedure, who are qualified according to the policy for NNP education and authorization.

Process

1. Assemble equipment:
   Laryngoscope with blade
   Suction equipment
   Resuscitation bag/pressure gauge
   ET tube/optional stylet
   Stethoscope
2. Prepare infant by washing and drying surrounding skin and place in neutral "sniffing" position.
3. Suction mouth/pharyngeal secretions and preoxygenate with bag respirations, if indicated.
4. Open infant's mouth and insert blade at right side and sweep to midline to sweep/control tongue.
5. Advance the blade to pass beneath the epiglottis and then lift the blade vertically to elevate the epiglottis and visualize the glottis. Request cricoid pressure if needed to move glottis into view.
6. Pass the ET tube through mouth into the glottis and advance appropriate distance.
7. Confirm tube placement by auscultation while providing respirations. Secure to upper lip with tape.
8. Confirm placement with chest x-ray.
9. Document procedure in note, including the size of tube and patient tolerance of procedure.

Physician Consultation

Physician consultation/notification will be done if the following occur:

1. There are any acute symptoms indicating tracheal perforation.
2. Respiratory failure is not reversed by ventilation.

Courtesy of C. Johnson. Manual of NP Protocols. Unpublished. Santa Clara, California: Valley Medical Center.

TABLE 12-3 ■ Sample Disease-Based Protocol for Neonatal Transport

Intestinal Obstruction

1. Obtain x-rays without contrast.
2. Keep head of bed (HOB) elevated if there is abdominal distention.
3. Place #10 Replogle tube to suction.
4. Increase fluids to 100–150 ml/kg/day.
5. Correct electrolyte abnormalities and acidosis.
6. Obtain cultures and begin antibiotics.

Intestinal Perforation

1. Elevate HOB.
2. Place #10 Replogle tube to suction—if severe abdominal distention despite NG suction, emergency abdominal paracentesis may be needed.
3. Intubate for respiratory support, as indicated.
4. Correct hypovolemia and shock.
5. May require dopamine to maintain blood pressure and increase abdominal perfusion.

Necrotizing Enterocolitis

1. Place #10 Replogle to suction.
2. Initiate vigorous IV hydration. May be as high as 100 ml/kg deficit.
3. Obtain cultures of stool, blood, and nasogastric drainage.
4. Start broad-spectrum antibiotics appropriate for coverage against *E. coli,* Klebsiella, and enterococci.
5. Give fluids as necessary to correct hypovolemic shock.

Esophageal Atresia

1. Obtain chest x-ray without contrast. Place OG tube into esophageal pouch and inject air. Air in abdomen with OG tube in blind pouch indicates TEF. 85% of esophageal atresias will present with fistula between the trachea and distal esophagus.
2. Place #10 Replogle tube to suction.
3. Elevate HOB.
4. Treat the complication of aspiration pneumonia, as indicated, with oxygen administration and antibiotic therapy.

Diaphragmatic Hernia

1. ET tube and paralyzation if assisted ventilation is required. Use minimal ventilatory pressures. Avoid mask ventilation.
2. Place #10 Replogle to suction.
3. Correct acidosis.
4. Intravenous line for rehydration, glucose, correction of metabolic acidosis, and drug administration.
5. Watch for pneumothorax.
6. Treat PPHN prn.

Courtesy of Jean Reimer-Brady. Manual of Transport Protocols. Unpublished. San Francisco: University of California. Reprinted by permission.

    4) Accepts primary responsibility to report QA issues

    5) Assures that the family is given follow-up information upon arrival at the receiving hospital[17]

    6) Selects the speed necessary in ground transports[16]

  2. A transport coordinator is essential to the day-to-day operations of the transport team.[18]

    a. Requirements

      1) Proficiency in neonatal nursing and the procedural skills of transport[20]

      2) Educational qualifications and clinical skills necessary to provide team education[20]

      3) Ability to assess the clinical competence of the team members[17]

    b. Responsibilities

      1) Scheduling needed personnel for transport[18]

      2) Providing team orientation, continuing education,[20] and documentation of competency[17]

      3) Participating in equipment purchase

      4) Assuring maintenance of equipment[18]

      5) Engaging transport vehicle services[18]

      6) Collecting transport data[18]

      7) Completing administrative work needed to keep the team operational[18,20]

F. Protocol and procedures
  1. Both must support transport nursing practice to maintain compliance with state nursing boards.
  2. Procedures include the following elements (Table 12-2).
    a. Indications for the procedure
    b. Specific steps to accomplish the procedure
    c. Findings/complications that mandate physician notification during the course of the procedure
  3. Disease-based protocol became prevalent in the 1980s and early 1990s (Table 12-3).
    a. Step-by-step directives to managing the treatment of various diseases and providing nursing care in transport
    b. Indications for procedures that will likely be needed for a given diagnosis
    c. Physician/unit preferences for various management styles to be integrated into policies
  4. Process-oriented protocols are becoming more common among teams led by NNPs who have advanced practice licenses (Table 12-4). Features that have resulted in increasing use of process protocols include the following.
    a. The process of data collection, assessment, intervention, and evaluation allows the practitioner to apply individual knowledge in practice.
    b. Greater flexibility exists to modify care for concurrent diagnosis or individual patient needs.
    c. Physician availability remains in place for consultation.

TABLE 12-4 ■ Sample Process-Based Protocol for Nurse Practitioners

Transport of Infants from Referring Facilities

Policy

The NNP is authorized to independently perform disease management, order diagnostic studies and infant medications, and perform procedures in the transport setting, according to the standardized NNP protocol/procedure manual.

Protocol

1. Following assessment and performance of any emergent procedures, the receiving physician will be contacted by telephone to collaborate on a plan of care.
2. All other applicable standardized procedures are followed during patient care management.
3. All general protocol regarding review, approval, setting, education, evaluation, patient records, supervision, and consultation are in force.

Courtesy of C. Johnson. Manual of NP Protocols. Unpublished. Santa Clara, California: Valley Medical Center.

Physiologic Stresses of Transport

A. The morbidity and mortality rates of infants transported to a facility are higher than those of inborn infants.[2,13,24]
B. Heat loss to the environment can be problematic for patients and staff.
  1. There are four mechanisms of heat loss.[6]
    a. **Conduction** of heat to objects in direct contact, such as the incubator mattress, stethoscope, and cold hands
    b. **Convection** of heat when cold air flows over a warmer object, such as cold drafts passing over the transport incubator
    c. **Radiation,** in which heat is lost to a cooler nearby object such as when heat is lost from the incubator to the aircraft frame (which cools as it ascends)
    d. **Evaporation**, which causes heat loss when moisture dissipates into cooler ambient air, as occurs with respiration
  2. Neonatal effects of heat loss and thermal management are discussed later in this chapter under **Care of the Neonate During Transport.**

3. Transport staff will endure heat loss in cold climates. Management techniques include the following.[18]
   a. Careful selection of layered clothing in fabrics that retain heat
   b. Completion of a survival training course specific to area climate
C. Motion sickness can be a problem.
   1. Occurrence
      a. Can occur in any moving vehicle
      b. Is most commonly associated with air travel
   2. Stimulation to the semicircular canals of the ear exacerbated by[7]
      a. Fear
      b. Stress
      c. Heat
      d. Odors
      e. Reactive hypoglycemia
   3. Motion sickness in infants
      a. Symptoms[8]
         1) Apnea
         2) Bradycardia
         3) Emesis
      b. Preventive care for neonates
         1) Removing the stomach contents prior to a flight
         2) Leaving an orogastric (OG) tube in place for transport
         3) Sedating the infant
   4. Motion sickness in transport personnel
      a. Serial progressing symptoms, which include[7,25]
         1) Headache
         2) Pallor
         3) Sweating
         4) Nausea
         5) Emesis
      b. Management of motion sickness in transport personnel[7]
         1) Inhaling supplemental oxygen
         2) Visual fixation on a stationary horizontal object
         3) Antiemetic medications such as meclizine or prochlorperazine (Compazine) in severe motion sickness (These medications can cause drowsiness and may impair judgment in some individuals.)[7]
D. Noise may be a stressor.
   1. It is a physiologic stressor to both patient and transport staff.
   2. The severity of this stressor is related to variables such as the type of transport vehicle or weather conditions as well as individual tolerance of the effects of noise.
   3. Like vibration, the primary noise source in most transport vehicles is the engine. This is most pronounced in helicopters.
   4. Neonates are exposed to noise that exceeds maximum recommended levels.[26] It is not mitigated by the transport incubators.[8] Lower frequency noise is reportedly amplified by the incubator.[8] The following are possible effects of noise exposure in neonates.[26]
      a. Cochlear damage and hearing impairment
      b. Sleep disturbances
      c. Blood pressure (BP) fluctuations

    5. Exposure to noise may also affect the transport staff.
       a. Potential for compromise in care due to difficulty with monitoring, auscultation, and staff communication[5]
       b. Headache[5,7]
       c. Auditory fatigue[7]
       d. General discomfort[5,7]
       e. Hearing loss with persistent exposure to excessive noise[5,7]
    6. Management strategies may help minimize noise exposure.
       a. Staff can wear snug-fitting head and ear protection during air transports.[5,7]
       b. Place earplugs on the neonate. Most transport teams do this, although the exact benefit is unknown.[8]
       c. Use acoustic matting beneath the incubator and the trolley. This has shown minimal success in dampening noise.[8]
       d. Change tires to all-season radials in ground vehicles. This produces a minor decrease in noise penetration.[26]

E. Vibration may occur.
    1. It is inherent in any transport vehicle.
    2. It is most problematic in helicopter transports.
    3. The primary source of vibration is the vehicle engine.[5] It has different effects at different frequencies.[27]
    4. Tolerable vibration levels are known to have a physiologic effect similar to mild exercise.
    5. The effects of vibration are different at different frequencies because each body tissue has its own natural frequency,[26] but 0.1–0.63 Hz is likely damaging to the human body.
    6. Six to 8 Hz (of vibration) is amplified by resonance within body organs and is associated with vasoconstriction, acute drop in BP, and bradycardia.
    7. The effects of vibration on the neonate are not well studied; however, reports in the literature suggest the following associated effects.
       a. Acute changes in vascular tone with associated BP fluctuations.[26,28] This is a grave concern in low birth weight infants because cerebral flow fluctuation appears to be the common pathologic factor in intraventricular hemorrhage.[29,30]
       b. Respiratory changes, including shortness of breath,[26] pulmonary edema,[28] and apnea[8]
       c. Recurrence of severe bleeding, either surgical or intracranial[26]
    8. Transport staff may suffer the following effects associated with vibration.
       a. Blurred vision[5]
       b. Increased metabolic rate[5]
       c. Interference with thermal regulation[5]
       d. Abdominal and chest pain[26]
       e. Muscle contractions[26]
       f. BP fluctuations[26]
    9. Vibration can be managed as follows.
       a. Directed toward minimizing the effects because there are no mechanisms to eliminate vibration.[5]
       b. Install padding on any surface in which personnel come into contact with the frame of the vehicle.[5]
       c. A gel mattress, used alone or with a foam mattress, is reported to least accentuate vibration to the infant.[31]

      d. Use of all-season radial tires (as opposed to snow tires) is reported to decrease noise and associated vibration.[26]

F. Gravitational force (G-force) may be a factor.

  1. The force that opposes inertia when there is a change in direction

      a. During any sudden or excessive change in direction or speed, such as aircraft ascent, an individual is subject to the effects of G-force.[5]

      b. On the neonate, the primary effect of G-force is theoretical and significant, albeit transient, redistribution of blood volume.

  2. Management of the neonate to decrease effects

      a. A neonate with cardiac disease should be positioned with his head toward the rear of the vehicle. Myocardial perfusion may then improve during acceleration.[5]

      b. A neonate with increased intracranial pressure should be positioned headfirst, which may help diminish fluctuations in intracranial blood flow.[5,25]

  3. Effects of G-force on transport staff[5]

      a. Vulnerable to being struck by an unrestrained object in an auto accident

      b. If not restrained, vulnerable to being ejected from a seat upon impact

  4. Measures to protect staff from negative effects of G-force

      a. Compliance with federal regulations that stipulate that items inside the cabin be restrained to withstand G-forces in three directions: Fore and aft, vertically, and side to side[32]

      b. Use of seatbelt and tie-down devices to prevent free objects from striking a cabin occupant[32]

      c. Use of a helmet in a rotary wing aircraft

G. Atmospheric changes related to altitude in flight affect the patient and transport team despite pressurized cabins. Each aircraft has a maximum differential or threshold altitude, after which atmospheric changes occur.[8]

  1. Gas expansion in flight

      a. The etiology of gas expansion is understood through Boyle's law, which states that, at a constant temperature, the volume of a given gas varies inversely to its pressure.[5,25]

      b. As the aircraft gains altitude and surrounding barometric pressure decreases, the volume of gas within an enclosed space, including body cavities, will expand.

        1) Effects on the neonate

          a) Compromised lung volume caused by gas expansion in the gastrointestinal (GI) tract either by placing pressure on the diaphragm[8] or directly, as in a diaphragmatic hernia

          b) Abdominal distention, discomfort, and an increased risk of perforation from GI gas expansion in patients with bowel obstruction or necrotizing enterocolitis

          c) Diminished lung volume due to expansion of gas with an air leak present, such as pneumothorax or pulmonary interstitial emphysema[8]

          d) Inner ear discomfort/pressure caused by gas expansion in the inner ear[8]

        2) Effects on transport team members

          a) GI discomfort accompanied by[8]

            • Belching

            • Nausea

            • Abdominal pain

            • Hyperventilation

 b) Barotitis or ear pain as a result of gas trapping in the middle ear or external ear[8]

 c) Sinus pain in the presence of an upper respiratory infection or cold[8]

 d) Tooth pain in the presence of recent dental work or dental caries[8]

c. Manage gas expansion at altitude as follows.

  1) In the neonate

   a) Place an OG tube prior to flight, either open to the air or attached to suction to decompress the stomach.[8]

   b) Evacuate all pneumothoraces by needle aspiration or chest tube placement as part of stabilization prior to flight.[8]

   c) Encourage pacifier use for those infants who are able to suck to relieve inner ear pressure through mandible manipulation.

   d) Maintain ready availability of a needle aspiration kit when transporting an infant with meconium aspiration syndrome, which predisposes the infant to air leak.

  2) In transport staff[8]

   a) Avoid heavy meals and gas-producing foods prior to flight.

   b) Wear loose, nonrestrictive clothing.

   c) Avoid flying shortly after dental work.

   d) Maintain good dental health.

   e) Use a vasoconstrictor nasal spray for sinus blockage pain.

   f) Avoid flying in the presence of upper respiratory congestion or infection.

2. Altitude-induced hypoxia

 a. The etiology of altitude-induced hypoxia is understood through knowledge of atmospheric changes explained by Dalton's Law and Henry's Law.

  1) Dalton's Law of partial pressures describes the pressure exerted by atmospheric gases at varying altitudes and states that the total pressure of a gaseous mixture is the sum of the partial pressures of all gas components.[5,25]

   a) As altitude increases and total barometric pressure declines, the partial pressures of the gaseous components of air reduce.

   b) Consequently, although oxygen is still a 0.21 fractional component of the atmosphere, the pressure gradient across the alveolar-capillary membrane is reduced, resulting in hypoxia.[5]

  2) Henry's Law states that the quantity of gas dissolved in a liquid is proportional to the amount of gas in the air surrounding the liquid.[5]

   a) This explains movement of gases from an area of higher concentration to an area of lower concentration (e.g., the transfer of oxygen from the alveoli to the blood).

   b) Thus, as the partial pressure of oxygen changes (Dalton's Law), gas-generated movement between blood and alveoli will be negatively affected.

 b. The following are effects of hypoxia.

  1) In neonates[8,25]

   a) Desaturation/decreased PaO_2/cyanosis

   b) Increased need for oxygen and possibly respiratory support

  2) In transport team members

   a) Visual problems[5,8]

   b) Disturbances in decision-making ability[5,8]

        c) Decreased acuity of fine motor skills[5]

  c. Manage altitude hypoxia as follows.

    1) In neonates

      a) Close monitoring with pulse oximetry

      b) Blood gases monitoring, if feasible

      c) Increased FiO_2 and respiratory support as indicated[8]

    2) In transport team members[5]

      a) Staff members should observe each other to identify signs of hypoxia.

      b) Supplemental oxygen should be administered to those affected.

Dispatch of the Transport Team

A. Consultation calls from referring physicians typically channel directly into the NICU to the consulting physician responsible for dispatch.

  1. In many institutions, this physician acts as the MCP throughout transport.[14]

  2. Information is collected and entered on a standard form for the transport team.[15]

B. Departure is coordinated through the dispatch center.

  1. Dedicated ground and helicopter teams can depart within 15 minutes.

  2. Fixed wing flights may take up to one hour to mobilize if the crew and pilot are not on call at the airport.[18]

  3. Many teams attempt to achieve a departure time of less than 30 minutes.

C. Documentation includes the following.[16,18]

  1. The consultation and dispatch transaction records are the responsibility of the accepting physician and the dispatch center.

  2. Records should include the call time and the time of dispatch, as well as any advice given to the referral center.[17]

Care of the Neonate During Transport

A. The goals are stabilization and care of the patient during transport.[33]

  1. To correct acute, life-threatening problems

  2. To achieve the maximum stability possible

  3. To protect the neonate against complications

B. The time in which stabilization and patient care are completed should be monitored by QA (Figure 12-1). Relevant factors regarding stabilization time include the following.

  1. The amount of time spent to stabilize the neonate is generally greater than the time needed to stabilize an adult for transport.

    a. Time is appropriately spent in essential activities designed to reduce the potential for adverse events.[33–36]

  2. Neonatal teams bring Level III care to the bedside.[33,34]

C. The steps in initial stabilization are as follows.

  1. Assess and manage the infant's airway.

    a. Signs of airway compromise

      1) Stridor

      2) Respiratory distress (i.e., increased work of breathing, retractions, grunting)

      3) Intermittent apnea

      4) Cyanosis/desaturation

      5) Hypercarbia/acidosis

FIGURE 12-1 ■ Duration of neonatal transports.

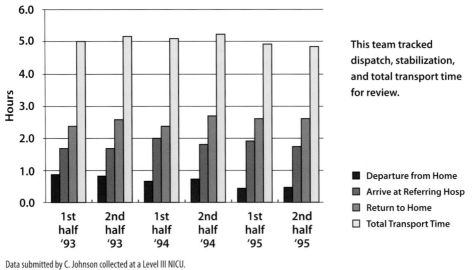

This team tracked dispatch, stabilization, and total transport time for review.

■ Departure from Home
■ Arrive at Referring Hosp
■ Return to Home
□ Total Transport Time

Data submitted by C. Johnson collected at a Level III NICU.

    b. The following conditions require airway management.
        1) Surgical lesions such as cystic hygroma or subglottic web that directly impinge on the airway
        2) Administration of medication, such as surfactant, via the tracheal route
        3) Hypoxia and acidosis
        4) Securing the infant's airway for transport (Intubation is the most effective means.)
            a) Vigorous term infants will need sedation for intubation.[35]
            b) Intubation should be done by the most experienced member of the transport staff.[15]
            c) The tube must be well secured to prevent accidental extubation en route.[15]
            d) Radiology confirmation of tube placement is advised, if available.[15,35]
  2. Assess and manage breathing at the same time the airway is assessed.[15]
    a. Surgical conditions such as cystic adenomatoid malformation and diaphragmatic hernia may directly interfere with lung volume and are often accompanied by pulmonary hypoplasia and/or pulmonary hypertension causing hypoxemia.[35]
    b. Management of patients in respiratory failure requires the transport team to act quickly and work together to accomplish the following.
        1) To give oxygen, intubate, and ventilate[35]
        2) To perform diagnostic activities, including:
            a) Physical examination
            b) Chest x-ray
            c) Transillumination to rule out pneumothorax
            d) Blood gases
            e) Complete blood count
            f) Hyperoxia test, if indicated, to rule out heart disease as the cause of cyanosis[37]

3) To place an arterial line and monitor blood gases[35]
4) To administer sedatives or paralyzing agents as needed to enhance oxygenation[35]
5) To consider nitric oxide (NO) to promote pulmonary vasodilation in infants who do not respond to conventional measures
   a) NO can also be used as a means of sustaining oxygenation during transfer to an extracorporeal membrane oxygenation (ECMO) center for this therapy.[38–40]
   b) Dosage and administration are as follows.
      • Improvement in oxygenation is reported in doses ranging from 20 to 80 parts per million.[38–40]
      • In transport, NO is blended into the inspiratory limb of the ventilator and monitored via NO portable monitoring systems.[41]
   c) Improvement in oxygenation may be transient because the disease underlying respiratory failure may be of a progressive nature (e.g., persistent pulmonary hypertension).
      • In these cases, withdrawal of NO for transport leads to acute deterioration.[41]
      • Availability of a team with the capability to deliver NO en route is vital for those facilities that administer NO to patients.[41]
   d) Because patients who qualify for this therapy are critically ill and labile, the MCP should be closely involved in any transport in which NO is administered.
6) To consider ECMO for patients with recalcitrant hypoxemia
   a) ECMO improves oxygenation by means of extrathoracic cannulation and is a supportive, not a therapeutic, intervention.[42] **(See Appendix B: Extracorporeal Membrane Oxygenation.)**
   b) It allows the opportunity for healing of respiratory disease or bridges the time until corrective surgery can be performed.[42,43]
   c) Transport of ECMO candidates includes the following.
      • Contact with the ECMO center must be made as soon as possible to determine if the patient is a candidate.
      • Selection and exclusion criteria are developed by ECMO centers to identify those patients who are most likely to benefit or who are most prone to complications of bypass.[43]
      • Patients with diaphragmatic hernia and correctable congenital heart lesions are usually referred directly to a center where ECMO is available.
      • The transport team plays an important role in assessing those patients referred for transport as possible ECMO candidates. It is imperative that infants identified as candidates be referred early enough to tolerate interhospital transport.[42,43]
      • Transport of ECMO candidates is challenging, requiring a team that is extremely well trained in ventilation strategy and possesses a thorough knowledge of disease pathology.[43]
      • The team must take appropriate measures to protect these fragile patients, who often respond adversely to noise, cold, stress, and vibration.[43]
      • The team must disclose the gravity of the situation to the parents, including the potential for deterioration or death.[43]

FIGURE 12-2 ■ The gastroschisis is protected in a normal saline–saturated sterile dressing and placed in a sterile plastic bag to minimize heat and evaporative losses in transport.

(Note that some variations in this practice may exist, according to the surgeon's preference.)

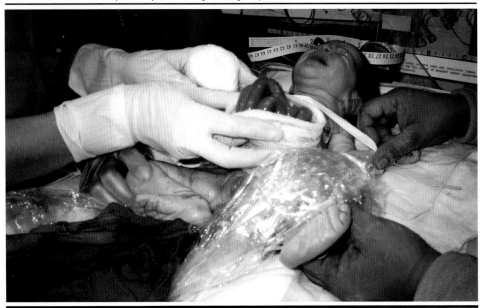

- The MCP should be closely involved in all clinical and interfacility communication issues regarding potential ECMO patients because these infants are gravely ill and all efforts must be made to expedite their transport.
- The proximity or availability of a service with ECMO on an aircraft should be known and considered for those patients whose instability precludes transport. Very few centers have this service because it requires considerable planning and resources.[44,45]

3. Assess and manage circulation to ensure adequate perfusion.
   a. Assessment parameters for circulation[15]
      1) Heart rate
      2) BP
      3) Urine output
      4) Level of hydration
         a) Skin turgor
         b) Mucous membranes
      5) Skin perfusion
         a) Capillary refill time
         b) Quality of central and peripheral pulses
         c) Color of skin
         d) Temperature of skin
      6) Level of consciousness
   b. Perfusion determinants
      1) Circulating blood volume
      2) Cardiac output

c. Factors that compromise circulating blood volume
  1) Evaporative losses, particularly in infants with open lesions
  2) Hypovolemia associated with birth events or trauma
  3) Septic shock and associated capillary leak syndrome
d. Management of compromised circulating volume
  1) Cover open lesions with saturated, prewarmed, saline dressings, and protect the dressed lesion with a sterile plastic bag to prevent further heat and fluid losses (Figure 12-2).[6]
  2) Replace fluids
    a) Place a venous line either peripherally or use umbilical/central access.[15]
    b) Give intravenous (IV) fluid boluses of 10 ml/kg over 30 minutes when signs of shock (hypotension, tachycardia, low urine flow) are present.[46]
    c) Assess and diagnose the etiology of the shock/perfusion compromise.
    d) Treat underlying pathology, such as infection.
e. Factors that compromise cardiac output
  1) Impaired cardiac muscle function, which can be caused by:
    a) Birth asphyxia
    b) An underlying metabolic disorder
  2) Congenital heart defects that impair flow, particularly those defects with left ventricular outflow tract obstruction
f. Management of patients with compromised cardiac output
  1) Administer oxygen, intubate, ventilate, and administer buffer agents to reverse hypoxia and acidosis.
  2) Perform diagnostic activities, including the following.
    a) Physical examination
    b) Chest x-ray
    c) Hyperoxia test
  3) Findings that distinguish congenital heart disease (CHD) from primary respiratory disease include the following.[47,48]
    a) A large heart on x-ray
    b) Presence of a murmur
    c) Failure to oxygenate when given 100 percent oxygen
  4) Administer prostaglandin E_1 (PGE$_1$ 0.05 mcg/kg/minute) to patients with findings of ductal-dependent CHD.[47–49]
    a) PGE$_1$ opens the ductus arteriosus, providing a pathway for blood flow to the lungs and the body.
    b) PGE$_1$ administration is indicated for the following.[49]
      • Right heart outflow obstruction:
        • Tricuspid atresia
        • Pulmonic stenosis
        • Pulmonary atresia
      • Left heart obstructive lesions:
        • Hypoplastic left heart syndrome
        • Aortic valve stenosis
        • Preductal coarctation of the aorta
        • Interrupted aortic arch

      c) Administer a trial dose of PGE_1 over 30 minutes, and evaluate blood gas results for improvement.[49]
- Referral hospitals usually do not have echocardiography, so the transport team will likely not know the specific heart lesion of the affected patient.
- PGE_1 is contraindicated in certain conditions.
  - Persistent pulmonary hypertension of the newborn with dominant left-to-right shunt
  - Truncus arteriosus
  - Ventricular septal defect

      d) Intubate patients who are receiving PGE_1 prior to transport because PGE_1 causes apnea.

  5) Administer dopamine to enhance systemic return and promote perfusion in patients with cardiogenic shock or CHD.

      a) The actions of dopamine are dose-dependent. A moderate dose of 5–10 mcg/kg/minute is indicated to improve cardiac output.[49]

4. Evaluate the infant's neurologic status and treat as necessary.

  a. Seizures should be managed with oxygen and measures to protect the airway.[50,51]

  b. Seizures should immediately be treated with anticonvulsants.

    1) Phenobarbital is the first choice of most practitioners for anticonvulsant therapy.

    2) The loading dose is 20 mg/kg IV, over 10–15 minutes. Additionally, 5 mg/kg can be given, up to a total of 40 mg/kg.[49,50]

  c. Perform diagnostic activities.

    1) Physical examination

    2) Review of relevant laboratory results and history

  d. Abnormal neurologic findings in neonates include the following.[50]

    1) Lethargy

    2) Hypotonia

    3) Irritability

    4) Seizures

  e. Identify the underlying cause of seizures, and treat to the extent that treatment is practical during transport. Possible underlying causes are listed in Table 12-5.

  f. Patients with known or suspected increased intracranial pressure should be positioned with head up, midline, and positioned toward the front of the vehicle to mitigate any secondary neuronal injury from G-force.[26]

D. The following are included in care of the infant after stabilization.

  1. Provide a neutral thermal environment.

    a. An infant's larger surface area, decreased adipose tissue, and immature nervous system make him prone to cold stress during transport.[6]

    b. These measures will ensure thermal stability.

      1) Transport the infant in an appropriately designed transport incubator with a circulating heat system and temperature monitoring.[15]

      2) Cover any open lesions, such as meningocele, with clear plastic to minimize heat loss through evaporation (see Figure 12-2).[6]

      3) Protect the baby with a blanket and a hat; maintain visibility of the infant.

      4) Use a space/mylar blanket over the transport incubator to reduce heat loss to the environment in cold climates.[6]

2. Maintain hydration.

a. This is vitally important to neonates for whom surgery is imminent because they are prone to fluid shifts and evaporative losses.[9]

b. Fluid calculations must be precise because there is a very narrow margin for error in neonates due to the relative inability of their kidneys to conserve or excrete sodium and fluids.[9]

c. Hydration can be maintained through the following measures.

1) Provide IV access for fluids and medication.

a) Place a peripheral IV or umbilical line.

b) Cover the site of IV access with a transparent dressing to maintain visibility of the site, and secure it well prior to departure.

2) Provide fluids.

a) Begin with $D_{10}W$ at 60–90 ml/kg/day, which delivers 4–6 mg/kg/minute of glucose to infants on the first day of life.[6]

TABLE 12-5 ■ Possible Causes of Neonatal Seizures

Trauma	**Drug withdrawal**
Subdural hematoma	Barbiturate
Subarachnoid hemorrhage	Heroin
Intraparenchymal hemorrhage	Methadone
Cerebral contusion	Alcohol
Cortical vein thrombosis	**Pyridoxine dependency**
Asphyxia	**Amino and organic acid**
Watershed infarction	**disturbances**
Basal ganglia infarction	Maple syrup urine disease
Periventricular leukomalacia	Nonketotic hyperglycinemia
Intraventricular hemorrhage	Methylmalonic aciduria
Subarachnoid hemorrhage	Propionic aciduria
Congenital anomalies (cerebral	**Urea cycle abnormalities**
dysgenesis)	**Kernicterus**
Metabolic disorders	**Toxins**
Hypocalcemia	Local anesthetics
Hypoglycemia	Isoniazid
Electrolyte imbalance (hyper-	**Familial seizures**
and hyponatremia)	Phakomatoses
Infections	Genetic syndrome with
Bacterial meningitis	mental retardation
Cerebral abscess	Benign familial epilepsy
Herpes encephalitis	
Coxsackie virus	
meningoencephalitis	
Cytomegalovirus	
Rubella	
Toxoplasmosis	
Syphilis	

From: Pope BA, and Painter MJ. 2002. Neonatal neurologic problems. In *Pediatric and Neonatal Transport Medicine*, 2nd ed., Jaimovich DG, and Vidyasagar D, eds. Philadelphia: Hanley & Belfus, 268. Reprinted by permission.

b) Increase fluid therapy by approximately 20–30 ml/kg/day with each advancing day of age.

c) Calculate the rate of administration using the following equation.[6]

$$\frac{(ml/kg/day) \times (weight\ in\ kg)}{24} = ml/hour$$

d) Increase fluids as needed to mitigate high evaporative water losses in neonates with open lesions.

• Most practitioners add 20 ml/kg to the maintenance fluid to compensate for open lesions.

e) Increase fluid provision for very low birth weight (VLBW) infants, who have high insensible water loss.

• Start fluids at 110–120 ml/kg/day, and advance 20–40 ml/kg/day over the next two to four days of life.

• VLBW infants under radiant warmers or phototherapy may have fluid requirements as high as 175–200 ml/kg/day until the end of the first week of life.[52]

- VLBW infants may develop hyperglycemia with administration of 10 percent dextrose and may need the glucose load reduced by infusing D_5W or $D_{7.5}W$.
  d. To determine the adequacy of fluid therapy, monitor the following.[52]
  1) Weight changes
  2) Intake and output
  3) Serum sodium concentration
  e. Provide maintenance IV electrolytes (Na, K).
  1) Administer Na and K 2–4 mEq/kg/day only for those infants who are over one day of age.
  2) Potassium should never be added to IV fluid until urine flow and renal function have been assessed.[52]
  f. Provide maintenance intravenous calcium (calcium gluconate).
  1) The maintenance dose is 200–800 mg/day.[53]
  2) The maximum recommended concentration for peripheral lines is 3 mg/ml (to reduce the risk of extravasation injury).[53]
  3) Lines with calcium infusion must be observed closely because of the risk of tissue damage with infiltrate.[53]

3. Maintain glucose homeostasis.
   a. Peripheral glucose utilization varies with the metabolic demands placed on the neonate.
   b. Balance is threatened by the demands of illness.
   c. Monitor blood glucose.
   d. Administer glucose.
   1) Use a starting rate of 6–8 mg/kg/day or 6 mg/kg/minute.
   2) Adjust as needed to maintain a normal serum glucose level.[54]
   3) The daily glucose load can be calculated using the following equations.
      a) Number of ml/hour × glucose load in decimal form* = glucose load
      *The glucose load is in decimal form (i.e., $D_{10}W$ = 0.1, $D_{12.5}W$ = 0.125, and so on).
      b) To calculate glucose loads on a per minute basis
      - Divide the number of milliliters per hour by 60 for the rate per minute.
      - Divide the result by the infant's weight in kilograms.
      - Multiply this result by the glucose concentration in milligrams per liter.**
      **$D_{7.5}$ = 75, $D_{10}W$ = 100, and so on
   e. Address hypoglycemia.[54]
   1) It is defined as blood glucose <40–45 mg/dl (2.2–2.5 mmol/liter).
   2) Verify the whole blood value obtained at the bedside with a serum glucose.
   3) Treat with an IV glucose infusion of 6 mg/kg/minute.
   4) Follow up.[54]
      a) Check the serum glucose level in 30–60 minutes.
      b) Adjust the glucose infusion as needed.
   f. Address hyperglycemia.
   1) It is usually defined as a serum glucose of >125 mg/dl (6.9 mmol/liter) in the term infant or >150 mg/dl (8.3 mmol/liter) in the preterm infant.[55]
   2) Decrease the glucose infusion until the serum glucose normalizes.[56]

3) Do not use a solution that is less than $D_{4.7}W$ percent without electrolytes being added because this solution is hypo-osmolar.

4) If the transport is of several hours duration, start an insulin infusion for persistent hyperglycemia.

   a) The loading dose of insulin is 0.05–0.1 unit/kg/dose over 15–20 minutes.[53]

   b) It is followed with a maintenance dose of 0.02–0.1 unit/kg/hour to titrate to the blood glucose level.[49]

4. Provide antimicrobial therapy.

   a. This is essential for infants with open lesions, infectious disease, or as surgical prophylaxis.

   b. Antibiotics must be administered before surgery for peak tissue levels to be reached by the time of operative contamination.[9] Hence, they are often first given by the transport team.

   c. Ampicillin and gentamycin are commonly administered because they provide broad-spectrum coverage.

      1) Aminoglycosides should be used with caution in neonates with compromised or uncertain renal statues.

   d. The surgeon accepting the case may have a preferred antibiotic regimen that will be used.

5. Provide pain relief for infants experiencing pain from illness or procedures. **(See Chapter 10: Assessment and Management of Postoperative Pain and Appendix E: Infant Pain Scales.)**

   a. Assessment of pain is challenging.

      1) Neonates cannot verbalize pain.

      2) Premature infants are limited in autonomic and self-regulatory abilities to deal with pain and stress, which decline with declining gestational age.[57]

      3) Observe for pain indicators during the physical examination. Although a variety of neonatal pain assessment tools is available, the time required to use them is not usually considered appropriate for transport.

      4) Pain parameters to observe include the following.

         a) Tachycardia

         b) Tachypnea

         c) Decreased oxygenation

         d) Apnea

         e) Mottling

         f) Vomiting

   b. Opioids are most often used to relieve pain in neonates.[57]

      1) Morphine is an effective analgesic. It should be used with discretion because it can cause hypotension in dehydrated patients.

         a) The dose is 50–200 mcg/kg/dose or continuous administration of 10–40 mcg/kg/hour. Its effect lasts two to four hours for full-term infants, and six to eight hours for preterm infants.[49]

      2) Fentanyl is also an effective analgesic.

         a) It requires the nurse to closely observe the infant because it can cause chest wall rigidity.[49,57]

         b) The intermittent dose is 1–4 mcg/kg/dose IV given over at least one to two minutes every two to four hours.[53]

       3) The continuous infusion dose is an IV bolus of 1 mcg/kg/dose over at least one to two minutes followed by a maintenance infusion of 0.5–4 mcg/kg/hour.[53]

    c. Provide nonpharmacologic comfort measures, such as positioning for body containment, which do not clearly relieve pain, but may reduce agitation.

       1) Employ these measures as often as possible in the transport process.

  6. Perform initial and ongoing assessments.

    a. Do a head-to-toe examination with particular attention to the system requiring potential surgery.

    b. Take vital signs every 15–30 minutes.[16]

    c. Observe the infant for any changes in condition, including his response to procedures or the stress of transport.[16]

  7. Provide family support.

    a. The need for information[32]

       1) Information is needed regarding the diagnosis and possible outcome.[35]

       2) To the extent that is feasible, the family needs to understand the reason for transport and what to expect in the transport process, including time, vehicle used, and so on.[35]

       3) If imminent surgery is anticipated, the transport team should act as a liaison in coordinating contact between the surgeon and parents to obtain consent.[35]

       4) Information should be given to the family in terms that are understandable by laypeople.[56]

       5) The family should be given information about the receiving physician and hospital, including directions, phone numbers, and visiting hours.[35]

    b. The need for emotional support, which is one of the more difficult tasks of the transport team

       1) Parents will experience feelings of shock, disbelief, and helplessness.

         a) Respond to crying or verbal outbursts with acceptance and reassurance that the infant is being cared for.[56]

         b) Parents may react strongly to seeing their infant with tubes, lines, and bandages.

           • It is important to provide brief, simple explanations of each device in understandable language.[56]

       2) Provide the parents with information about the infant's diagnosis and the anticipated outcome of intervention, which can help restore their feelings of control.[56]

       3) Communicate with parents in a way that reflects your awareness of the grief they are experiencing.[16]

         a) Encourage the mother to touch her infant prior to departure.

         b) Provide photos of the infant prior to departure.

Additional Transport Team Responsibilities

A. Gather information.[17]

  1. Maternal history

  2. Details of delivery

  3. Neonatal course to date

  4. Diagnostic tests

  5. Diagnostic imaging studies

FIGURE 12-3 ■ Neonatal transport record.

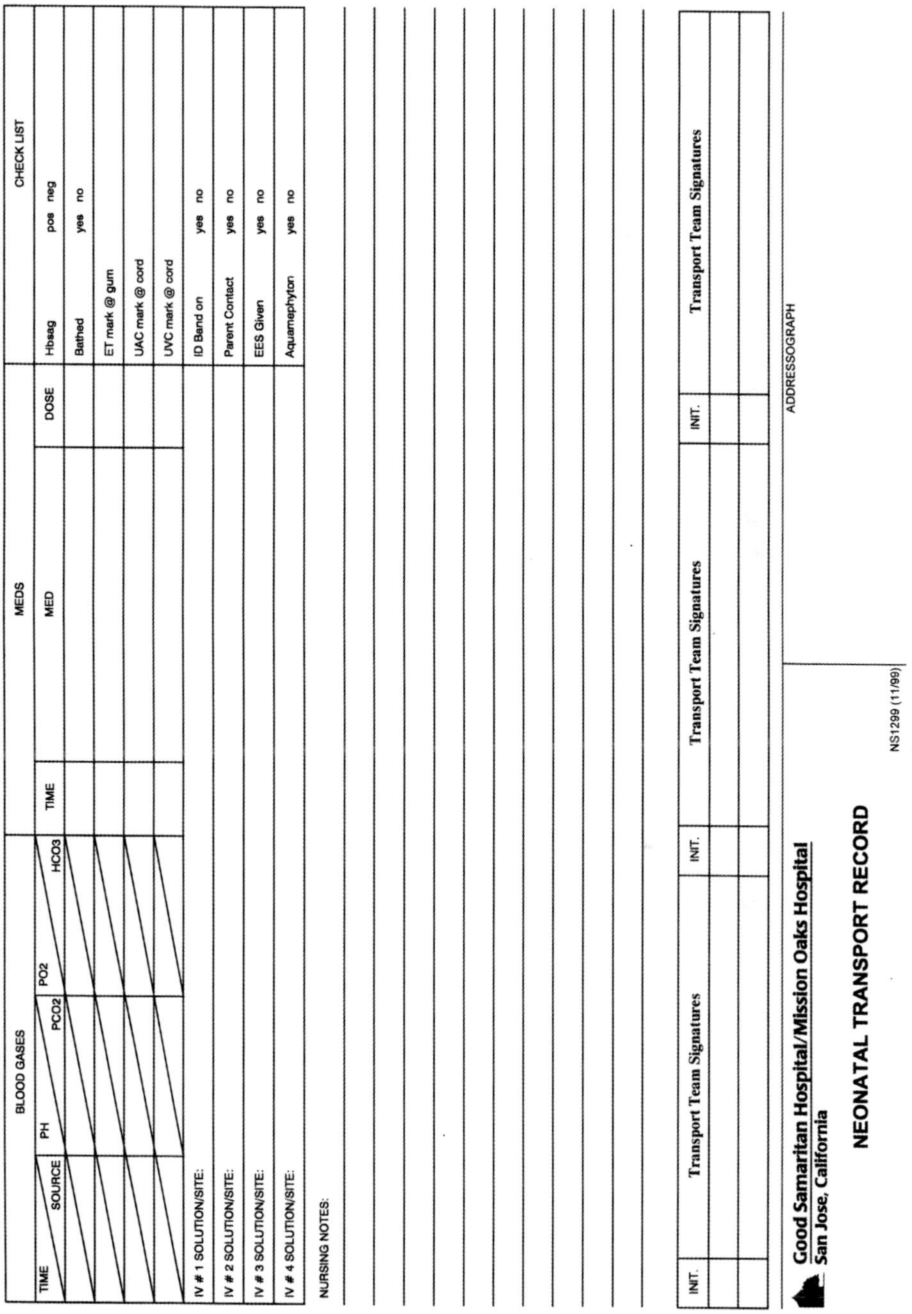

BLOOD GASES						MEDS			CHECK LIST	
TIME	SOURCE	PH	PCO2	PO2	HCO3	TIME	MED	DOSE	Hbsag	pos neg
									Bathed	yes no
									ET mark @ gum	
									UAC mark @ cord	
									UVC mark @ cord	
IV # 1 SOLUTION/SITE:									ID Band on	yes no
IV # 2 SOLUTION/SITE:									Parent Contact	yes no
IV # 3 SOLUTION/SITE:									EES Given	yes no
IV # 4 SOLUTION/SITE:									Aquamephyton	yes no

NURSING NOTES:

INIT.	Transport Team Signatures	INIT.	Transport Team Signatures	INIT.	Transport Team Signatures

Good Samaritan Hospital/Mission Oaks Hospital
San Jose, California

NEONATAL TRANSPORT RECORD

NS1299 (11/99)

ADDRESSOGRAPH

Courtesy of Good Samaritan Hospital..

FIGURE 12-3 ■ Neonatal transport record.

Good Samaritan Hospital/Mission Oaks Hospital
San Jose, California

ADDRESSOGRAPH

NEONATAL TRANSPORT RECORD

NS1299 (11/99)

	VITAL SIGNS				INTAKE		INTAKE		OUTPUT		VENTILATION				COMMENTS	
TIME	TEMP ISOL	HR RR	BP	MEAN	IV #1	IV #2	IV #3	IV #4	URINE	OTHER	MODE FIO2	PIP PEEP	RATE	O2 SAT	ASSUMED CARE OF PT @ -	INIT.
TOTAL IN/OUT:																

NURSING NOTES:

INIT.	Transport Team Signatures	INIT.	Transport Team Signatures	INIT.	Transport Team Signatures

Courtesy of Good Samaritan Hospital..

6. Laboratory data
7. Social and disease-based information

B. Obtain parental consent for the transport.
1. The consent form should include medical care given during the transport procedure.[14]
2. Explain any procedure and its inherent risks.
3. Follow the written institutional policy in the process of obtaining parental consent.[14]
4. Obtain consent in writing except in the following cases.
   a. Implied consent is allowed by law for emergency situations when the parents are unavailable.
      1) Emergency conditions are those in which there is a threat to life, limb, or the health of the patient, which will worsen without immediate treatment.[14]
   b. Implied consent exists when actions of the parents sufficiently imply that consent is granted.[14]

C. Document the following.
1. An admission note that is an overview of the transport, composed by the team leader.[17]
   a. Maternal and neonatal history and an overview of the transport
   b. List of actual and potential clinical problems
   c. Interventions and the patient's clinical responses
   d. Consultation with the controlling (receiving) medical physician and any orders or changes in the plan of care
2. Recorded vital signs taken every 15–30 minutes and intake and output
   a. Most institutions have a flow sheet to track this data (Figure 12-3).
3. Any exceptions in the transport process for QA review
   a. Injuries
   b. Delays
   c. Patient adverse effects

Transport Equipment and Medications

A. Appropriate equipment for each patient being transported (a requirement for transport teams from a Medicare-approved facility)[13]
B. Large equipment
1. Transport incubator
   a. This should be used for nearly all infants being transported.
   b. Exceptions can be made for term infants who can maintain body temperature and are stable without oxygen, who can be monitored in a car seat.
2. Ventilator
   a. It must be capable of delivering the small pressures or volumes needed for infant ventilation or for providing continuous positive airway pressure (CPAP).
3. Oxygen and air tanks
   a. It is necessary to be able to provide an FiO_2 of <1.0.
4. Monitors
   a. Cardiac
   b. Respiratory

      c. Internal and external BP monitoring capability

      d. Pulse oximetry

   5. Suction device and suction catheters

   6. IV pumps

      a. These are often mounted on the incubator for access and stability.

C. Small equipment

   1. Peripheral IV access

      a. IV catheters

      b. Tubings

      c. T-connectors

      d. Tape

      e. Armboards

      f. Syringes

      g. Flush solution

      h. Transparent dressings

   2. Umbilical line placement

      a. Umbilical single- and double-lumen catheters

      b. Sterile instruments for insertion of catheter(s)

      c. Stopcock

      d. Syringes

      e. Transducer

   3. Oxygen delivery and intubation

      a. Endotracheal tubes

      b. Laryngoscope and blades

      c. Suction catheters

      d. CPAP bag/anesthesia bag

      e. Nasal cannula

      f. Self-inflating bag

   4. Warming

      a. Blankets

      b. Hat

      c. Thermal gel mattress

      d. Plastic wrap

   5. Blood and urine collection and analysis

      a. Blood gas syringes

      b. Blood culture tubes

      c. Urine bags or syringes for suprapubic tap

      d. Point of care testing equipment for glucose and blood gases

      e. Lancet, capillary tubes, or other device to collect body fluids for analysis

   6. Chest tube insertion

      a. Trocars of various sizes

      b. Instruments for insertion

      c. Heimlich valve

      d. Petroleum jelly gauze

      e. Underwater seal suction system (optional as alternative to Heimlich valve)

      f. Suture material

      g. Dressings

   7. External lesion dressing

      a. Sterile saline

      b. Sterile dressings

  c. Plastic wrap
  d. Plastic sterile bowel bag
8. Monitoring
  a. BP cuffs
  b. Monitor leads
  c. Pulse oximetry probes
  d. Temperature probes
  e. BP transducer
D. Medications
  1. Volume expanders
    a. Normal saline
    b. Albumin
  2. Antibiotics
    a. Ampicillin
    b. Gentamycin
    c. Vancomycin
    d. Cefotaxime
    e. Cephalexin
  3. Cardiogenic/vasoactive medications
    a. Dopamine
    b. Digitalis
    c. Dobutamine
    d. Sodium nitroprusside
    e. PGE_1
  4. Parenteral solutions to administer glucose and fluid
    a. D_5W
    b. $D_{10}W$
    c. $D_{12.5}W$
    d. Normal saline (NS)
    e. D_5 1/2 NS
  5. Resuscitation medications
    a. Epinephrine
    b. $NaHCO_3$
  6. Analgesia and sedation medications
    a. Fentanyl
    b. Morphine
    c. Lorazepam
  7. Paralytics and reversal agents
    a. Pancuronium
    b. Vecuronium
    c. Neostigmine
  8. Anticonvulsants
    a. Phenobarbital
    b. Phenytoin
  9. Electrolyte and mineral additives
    a. NaCl
    b. KCl
    c. Calcium gluconate
  10. The pulmonary vasodilator, nitric oxide, if the ventilator circuit has the capability to deliver it

Transport Team Communication

A. Referral center access for phone consultation must be available at all times.
  1. Consultation calls[16]
    a. Should be received by a neonatologist, nurse practitioner, or fellow who is responsible to respond to them, can provide consultation to the referring facility or physician, and has direct access to the transport team.
    b. May result in a collaborative decision to continue care at the outlying facility, or may result in dispatch of the neonatal team.
    c. Should serve as an opportunity to collect pertinent information to give to the transport team in the event of its dispatch. Most tertiary care centers have a form to facilitate collection of information, which serves as a record of the phone consultation.
B. Channels for communication during transport include the following.
  1. Mobile phone for transport team access to the referring facility and the tertiary care center, available at all times[16]
    a. This allows the team to contact the referring facility as needed and to contact the referral center regarding any admission information or changes in patient condition.
    b. It provides an additional communication safety net, over and above the dispatch center, if the team should encounter any untoward weather or other delays.
  2. Interactive dispatch center through which emergency medical communication is channeled[17]
    a. This center facilitates communication for the following.
      1) The referring hospital
      2) The accepting physician
      3) The neonatal transport team members
      4) The operator of the vehicle selected
    b. The dispatch center must have an emergency medical communications system that is continuously monitored by trained staff.[18]
  3. Access to the MCP, who is available for phone contact by the transport team at all times
    a. The MCP assumes responsibility for dispatch and team composition and directs the clinical care given in transport.[14]
    b. This role is usually filled by the attending physician or fellow.[14]

Transport Safety

A. The increased use of transport systems has led to a growing number of accidents, making safety a primary concern of transport programs.[58]
B. The following safety principles apply to all vehicles.
  1. Personnel must be trained not only in the care of neonates, but also in emergency procedures.[18]
    a. Use of fire extinguishers
    b. Emergency exit protocol
    c. Location and operation of shutoff valves
    d. Use of emergency locator transmitter
  2. The infant, transport personnel, and all equipment must be secured with appropriate restraints to withstand G forces and acceleration.[18]

3. The need for transport shall not outweigh safety considerations of the transport personnel and infant.[17]

   a. For example, if weather is such that the transport presents danger to the team, it should be delayed or canceled, regardless of the patient's condition.[18]

4. A communication system must be available so that the transport team can communicate with each other and the dispatch center en route.[16]

C. These safety issues are specific to ground vehicles.[58]

   1. Appropriate use of the emergency flashing lights and siren

   a. Use of lights and siren does not give the vehicle absolute right of way.

   b. In some states, the laws allow emergency vehicles to proceed through red lights after giving other motorists ample time to clear the intersection.

   c. Use of emergency lights can increase the likelihood of motor vehicle accidents and should be reserved for true emergencies.

   2. Vulnerability to unpredictable road and traffic conditions

   a. Accidents and other road hazards can detain ground transports.

D. These safety issues are specific to fixed wing vehicles.[58]

   1. A safe distance must be maintained away from the engines and exhaust system to avoid toxic fumes and potential burns.

   2. The crew must be willing to follow the directions of the pilot (or other designated safety officer), who has ultimate responsibility for the safety of the medical crew and passengers.

   3. The staff must be knowledgeable about the vulnerability of the infant to atmospheric changes caused by altitude.

E. These safety issues are specific to helicopters.

   1. Proper procedure must be followed in approaching the aircraft to avoid injury from the following.[58]

   a. Blades

   b. Noise

   c. Wind

   2. Staff must follow the pilot's (or other designated safety officer's) direction in loading and unloading the patient.[58]

   a. In most cases, this is done when the engine is off and the blades are not turning.

   3. Use of protective eye- and headgear by the transport staff is encouraged (Figure 12-4).

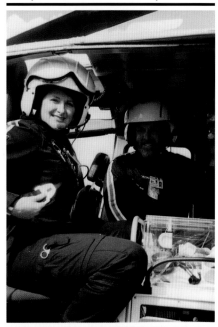

FIGURE 12-4 ■ Rotary wing aircraft neonatal team is appropriately dressed in flame-retardant suits, protective helmets, and headphones.

Courtesy of C. Johnson, Good Samaritan Hospital, San Jose, California. Reprinted by permission.

FIGURE 12-5 ■ Analysis of dispatch delay factors in neonatal transport.

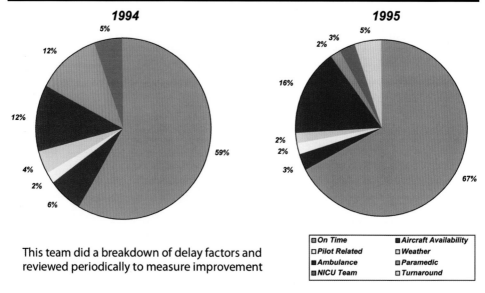

1994

5%
12%
12%
4%
2%
6%
5%
59%

1995

5%
3%
2%
16%
2%
2%
3%
67%

This team did a breakdown of delay factors and reviewed periodically to measure improvement

▣ On Time	■ Aircraft Availability
□ Pilot Related	□ Weather
■ Ambulance	▣ Paramedic
▣ NICU Team	□ Turnaround

Data submitted by C. Johnson collected at Presbyterian Health Center NICU, Albuquerque, New Mexico.

4. Flame- and heat-retardant clothing and footwear are recommended by the National Safety Board for staff protection (see Figure 12-4).[17]
5. A safe landing zone must be provided with adequate clearance.[20]
6. Ear protection and mattress or seat padding should be used to attenuate the effects of noise and vibration for patient and staff.

Quality Assurance for Transport

A. Purpose of a QA program for neonatal transport
  1. To systematically monitor the quality and appropriateness of patient care[17,56,59,60]
B. Topics relevant for a QA review
  1. Safety
    a. Equipment
    b. Policies
  2. Expediency in responding to transport requests
  3. Resource allocation
  4. Triage of transport requests
  5. Appropriateness of patient care
  6. Interface with referring facilities
  7. Equipment malfunction
  8. Personnel injury and related circumstances
  9. Patient morbidity and mortality
C. Process of QA
  1. The QA process helps the team to identify opportunities for improvement through examination of compiled information.[18]
  2. The process consists of the following.
    a. Compilation of a database containing objective and numeric information[61]

    b. Review of the data by the QA team to identify an area of needed improvement

3. A threshold or predetermined level of acceptable performance is set by the QA team.[14]

    a. Dispatch time is frequently an indicator, with the most common threshold level being a 30-minute dispatch objective.

4. The transport team assesses factors related to the need for improvement and designs activities to improve performance (Figure 12-5).

5. Transport data are periodically reviewed by the QA team in a time frame (such as monthly or quarterly) in which sufficient data are available.

6. Measured improvement over a period of time reflects the success of the QA activities (see Figure 12-5).

REFERENCES

1. Butterfield LJ. 1993. Historical perspectives of neonatal transport. *Pediatric Clinics of North America* 40(2): 221–239.

2. Phibbs CS, et al. 1996. The effects of patient volume and level of care at the hospital of birth on neonatal mortality. *JAMA* 276(13): 1054–1059.

3. Shenai JP, et al. 1991. A successful decade of regionalized perinatal care in Tennessee: The neonatal experience. *Journal of Perinatology* 11(2): 137–143.

4. Yeast JD, et al. 1998. Changing patterns in regionalization of perinatal care and the impact on neonatal mortality. *American Journal of Obstetrics and Gynecology* 178(1 part 1): 131–135.

5. Blumen IJ, and Rinnert KJ. 1995. Altitude physiology and the stresses of flight. *Air Medical Journal* 14(2): 87–100.

6. Gaylord MS, and Michaluk CA. 2002. General neonatal physiologic considerations. In *Handbook of Pediatric and Neonatal Transport Medicine*, 2nd ed., Jaimovich DG, and Vidyasagar D, eds. Philadelphia: Hanley & Belfus, 55–71.

7. Hubner L, and Dunn N. 1982. Aeromedical physiology: Implications for neonatal nurses. *Neonatal Network* 1(2): 10–18.

8. Miller C. 1994. The physiologic effects of air transport on the neonate. *Neonatal Network* 13(7): 7–10.

9. Katz AL, and Wolfson P. 2005. General surgical considerations. In *Intensive Care of the Fetus and Neonate*, 2nd ed., Spitzer AR, ed. St. Louis: Mosby, 1353–1368.

10. Chance GW, et al. 1978. Neonatal transport: A controlled study of skilled assistance. *Journal of Pediatrics* 93(4): 662–666.

11. Jain L, and Vidyasager D. 1993. Cardiopulmonary resuscitation of newborns. Its application to transport medicine. *Pediatric Clinics of North America* 40(2): 287–302.

12. Yoder BA. 1992. Long distance perinatal transport. *American Journal of Perinatology* 9(2): 75–79.

13. Boyko SM. 1994. Interfacility transfer guidelines: An easy reference to help hospitals decide on appropriate vehicles and staffing for transfers. *Journal of Emergency Nursing* 20(1): 18–23.

14. Reimer-Brady JM. 1996. Legal issues related to stabilization and transport of the critically ill neonate. *Journal of Perinatal & Neonatal Nursing* 10(3): 59–69.

15. Hawkins HS. 2002. Transport management considerations. In *Handbook of Pediatric and Neonatal Transport Medicine*, 2nd ed., Jaimovich DG, and Vidyasagar D, eds. Philadelphia: Hanley & Belfus, 15–26.

16. Majors CW. 2002. Organization of a neonatal transport program. In *Handbook of Pediatric and Neonatal Transport Medicine*, 2nd ed., Jaimovich DG, and Vidyasagar D, eds. Philadelphia: Hanley & Belfus, 27–42.

17. National Association of Neonatal Nurses. 1998. *Neonatal Nursing Transport Standards*. Glenview, Illinois: NANN, 1–4.

18. Macdonald MG, and Ginzberg HM, and American Academy of Pediatrics Task Force on Interhospital Transport. 1999. *Guidelines for Air and Ground Transport of Neonatal and Pediatric Patients*. Elk Grove Village, Illinois: American Academy of Pediatrics.

19. Mele PC, and Herbert CC. 2002. Nurse practitioners in the neonatal intensive care unit. In *Intensive Care of the Fetus and Neonate*, 2nd ed., Spitzer AR, ed. St. Louis: Mosby, 515–519.

20. Shenai JP. 1993. Neonatal transport: Outreach educational program. *Pediatric Clinics of North America* 40(2): 275–285.

21. Thompson TR. 1980. Neonatal transport nurses: An analysis of their role in the transport of newborn infants. *Pediatrics* 65(5): 887–892.

22. Zaritsky A, and Beyer AJ. 1992. MD or not MD: Is that the question? *Critical Care Medicine* 20(12): 1633–1635.

23. Beyer AJ, Land G, and Zaritsky A. 1992. Nonphysician transport of intubated pediatric patients: A system evaluation. *Critical Care Medicine* 20(7): 961–966.

24. Harding JE, and Morton SM. 1993. Adverse affects of neonatal transport between Level III centres. *Journal of Paediatrics and Child Health* 29(2): 146–149.

25. Woodward GA, and Vernon DD. 2002. Aviation physiology in pediatric transport. In *Handbook of Pediatric and Neonatal Transport Medicine*, 2nd ed., Jaimovich DG, and Vidyasagar D, eds. Philadelphia: Hanley & Belfus, 43–54.

26. Macnab A, et al. 1995. Vibration and noise in pediatric emergency transport vehicles: A potential cause of morbidity. *Aviation, Space, and Environmental Medicine* 66(3): 212–219.

27. Shenai JP, Johnson GE, and Varney RV. 1981. Mechanical vibration in neonatal transport. *Pediatrics* 68(1): 55–57.

28. Clark JG, et al. 1967. Initial cardiovascular response to low frequency whole body vibration in humans and animals. *Aerospace Medicine* 38(5): 464–467.

29. Paige PL, and Carney PR. 2002. Neurologic disorders. In *Handbook of Neonatal Intensive Care*, 5th ed., Merenstein GB, and Gardner SL, eds. St. Louis: Mosby, 644–678.

30. Volpe JJ. 1989. Intraventricular hemorrhage and brain injury in the premature infant: Neuropathology and pathogenesis. *Clinics of Perinatology* 16(2): 361–386.

31. Gajendragadkar G, et al. 2000. Mechanical vibration in neonatal transport: A randomized study of different mattresses. *Journal of Perinatology* 20(5): 307–310.

32. Office of the Federal Register, National Archives and Records Administration. 2005. *Code of Federal Regulations. Aeronautics and Space*, Title 14, parts 1–59. Washington, DC: Federal Aviation Administration.

33. Whitfield JM, and Buser MK. 1993. Transport stabilization times for neonatal and pediatric patients prior to interfacility transfer. *Pediatric Emergency Care* 9(2): 69–71.

34. Pon S, and Notterman DA. 1993. The organization of a pediatric critical care transport program. *Pediatric Clinics of North America* 40(2): 241–261.

35. Iyer RS, and Vidyasagar D. 2002. Transport issues in neonates with respiratory problems. In *Handbook of Pediatric and Neonatal Transport Medicine,* 2nd ed., Jaimovich DG, and Vidyasagar D, eds. Philadelphia: Hanley & Belfus, 211–232.

36. The Victorian Infant Collaborative Study Group. 1993. Improving the quality of survival for infants of birthweight <1,000 g born in non-Level-III centres in Victoria. *Medical Journal of Australia* 158(1): 24–27.

37. Javois AJ. 2002. Pediatric cardiology in transport medicine. In *Handbook of Pediatric and Neonatal Transport Medicine,* 2nd ed., Jaimovich DG, and Vidyasagar D, eds. Philadelphia: Hanley & Belfus, 93–124.

38. Day RW, et al. 1996. Acute response to inhaled nitric oxide in newborns with respiratory failure and pulmonary hypertension. *Pediatrics* 98(4 part 1): 698–705.

39. Karamanoukian HL, et al. 1994. Inhaled nitric oxide in congenital hypoplasia of the lungs due to diaphragmatic hernia or oligohydramnios. *Pediatrics* 94(5): 715–718.

40. Kinsella JP, et al. 1993. Clinical responses to prolonged treatment of persistent pulmonary hypertension of the newborn with low doses of inhaled nitric oxide. *Journal of Pediatrics* 123(1): 103–108.

41. Kinsella JP, et al. 1995. Inhaled nitric oxide treatment for stabilization and emergency medical transport of critically ill newborns and infants. *Pediatrics* 95(5): 773–776.

42. Bartlett RH, et al. 1986. Extracorporeal membrane oxygenation in neonatal respiratory failure. 100 cases. *Annals of Surgery* 204(3): 236–245. (Published erratum in *Annals of Surgery,* 1987, 205[1]: 11.)

43. Sahhar HS, Ostrowski D, and Jaimovich DG. 2002. Transport of neonatal and pediatric patients requiring extracorporeal life support. In *Handbook of Pediatric and Neonatal Transport Medicine,* 2nd ed., Jaimovich DG, and Vidyasagar D, eds. Philadelphia: Hanley & Belfus, 248–259.

44. Cornish JD, et al. 1986. Inflight use of extracorporeal membrane oxygenation for severe neonatal respiratory failure. *Perfusion* 1: 281–287.

45. Faulkner SC, et al. 1993. Mobile extracorporeal membrane oxygenation. *Annals of Thoracic Surgery* 55(5): 1244–1246.

46. Nunez JS. 2004. Hypotension and shock. In *Neonatology: Management, Procedures, On-Call Problems, Diseases, and Drugs,* 5th ed., Gomella TL, et al., eds. New York: McGraw-Hill, 273–277.

47. Nunez JS. 2004. Cyanosis. In *Neonatology: Management, Procedures, On-Call Problems, Diseases, and Drugs,* 5th ed., Gomella TL, et al., eds. New York: McGraw-Hill, 226–229.

48. Cottrill CM. 2004. Cardiac abnormalities. In *Neonatology: Management, Procedures, On-Call Problems, Diseases, and Drugs,* 5th ed., Gomella TL, et al., eds. New York: McGraw-Hill, 354–372.

49. Zenk KE. 2004. Commonly used medications. In *Neonatology: Management, Procedures, On-Call Problems, Diseases, and Drugs,* 5th ed., Gomella TL, et al., eds. Stamford, Connecticut: Appleton & Lange, 590–643.

50. Pope BA, and Painter MJ. 2002. Neonatal neurologic problems. In *Handbook of Pediatric and Neonatal Transport Medicine,* 2nd ed., Jaimovich DG, and Vidyasagar D, eds. Philadelphia: Hanley & Belfus, 267–276.

51. Goetting MC. 2002. Transportation of the child with seizures. In *Handbook of Pediatric and Neonatal Transport Medicine,* 2nd ed., Jaimovich DG, and Vidyasagar D, eds. Philadelphia: Hanley & Belfus, 277–293.

52. Berry DD, Adcock EW, and Starbuck A. 2002. Fluid and electrolyte management. In *Handbook of Neonatal Intensive Care,* Merenstein GB, and Gardner SL, eds. St. Louis: Mosby-Year Book, 283–297.

53. Zenk KE, Sills JH, and Koeppel RM. 2003. *Neonatal Medications & Nutrition: A Comprehensive Guide,* 3rd ed. Santa Rosa, California: NICU Ink, 140–141, 240–242, 327–331, 407–410, 411–414.

54. Gilmore MM. 2004. Hypoglycemia. In *Neonatology: Management, Procedures, On-Call Problems, Diseases, and Drugs,* 5th ed., Gomella TL, et al., eds. Stamford, Connecticut: Appleton & Lange, 262–266.

55. McGowan JE, Hagedorn MIE, and Hay WW. 2002. Glucose homeostasis. In *Handbook of Neonatal Intensive Care,* Merenstein GB, and Gardner SL, eds. St. Louis: Mosby, 298–313.

56. Westergaard F, and Gostisha ML. 2002. Administrative pearls. In *Handbook of Pediatric and Neonatal Transport Medicine,* 2nd ed., Jaimovich DG, and Vidyasagar D, eds. Philadelphia: Hanley & Belfus, 83–92.

57. Argawal R, Hagedorn MIE, and Gardner SL. 2002. Pain and pain relief. In *Handbook of Neonatal Intensive Care,* Merenstein GB, and Gardner SL, eds. St. Louis: Mosby-Year Book, 191–218.

58. Reyes G, and Wesolowski R. 2002. Transport safety. In *Handbook of Pediatric and Neonatal Transport Medicine,* 2nd ed., Jaimovich DG, and Vidyasagar D, eds. Philadelphia: Hanley & Belfus, 72–82.

59. Association of Air Medical Services Quality Assurance Committee. 1990. AANS resource document for air medical quality assurance programs. *Journal of Air Medical Transport* 9(8): 23–26.

60. Joint Commission on Accreditation of Healthcare Organizations. 2006. *Comprehensive Accreditation Manual for Hospitals: The Official Handbook.* Chicago: Joint Commission Resources.

61. Donn SM, Gates MR, and Kiska DJ. 1993. User-friendly computerized quality assurance program for regionalized neonatal care. *Journal of Perinatology* 13(3): 190–196.

Notes

13

Support for the Family of the Surgical Infant

Jeanette Zaichkin, RNC, MN
Brenda Lykins, RNC, BSN

A baby's birth is usually a much-anticipated and joyful event for parents. The birth of a baby with special needs requiring surgery changes this perspective, however. Coping mechanisms are unique to each family. The working partnership between parents and the health care team influences parental adaptation and, ultimately, the child's growth and development. The goal for health care professionals is to establish the kind of partnership that promotes the best outcome for the surgical neonate.

This chapter provides information on two aspects of this partnership. First, it assists the neonatal nurse in understanding concepts and strategies for implementing culturally competent, family-centered care. Second, it reviews strategies for assisting parents who must deal with grief and loss in the neonatal period.

Implementing Culturally Competent, Family-Centered Care

FAMILY-CENTERED CARE

Definition

A. Family-centered care is a philosophy of care "grounded in the belief that the family has the greatest influence in the health and well-being of infants and children and that the most important role of health care professionals is to foster parents' confidence and competence in the caregiving and decision-making roles (p. 401)."[1]

B. Family-centered care is a consumer-oriented approach for the "delivery of safe, adaptable care that focuses on the physical, psychologic, and cultural needs of the client, family, and newborn (p. 4)."[2]

Components[1]

A. Collaboration between parents and health care professionals

B. Recognition that both the infant's family members and health care professionals lend expertise to the infant's care

---

C. Sharing of information in an appropriate form and to a degree acceptable to the family
D. Empowering parents to meet their infant's needs with confidence and competence
E. Adaptation and flexibility in meeting the unique needs of the family and the infant
F. Recognition that "family" encompasses all individuals with an interest in the infant's care and outcome

CULTURALLY COMPETENT CARE

Definition

A. The goal of culturally competent care is to provide the best care possible while achieving congruence between the family's cultural belief system and the health care team's proposed interventions.[2]
 1. Culture refers not only to ethnic diversity, but to any characteristics of a particular community of people, including those unique to nontraditional family cultures such as adolescent, gay and lesbian, and adoptive families.
 2. In some cases, to provide culturally competent care, it is the health care professional, not the family, who must adapt.[3]
 3. Culturally appropriate care is essential for effective nursing intervention.[4]
B. Family-centered care must integrate culturally competent care.

Cross-Cultural Knowledge

A. It is unrealistic to expect health care professionals to know the details of every culture; however, they should know the basics of the cultures in their service area.
 1. An effective way to learn about the customs and traditions of clients is to contact a representative of each cultural/ethnic group in the region and ask for assistance.
B. Cultural variations exist even within cultures, and it is important to avoid stereotyping.
C. Respect for and willingness to learn about cultural differences are keys to successful interactions.

Cultural Assessment

A. In newborn care, the cultural assessment includes such practices as:[5]
 1. Feeding
 2. Bathing
 3. Swaddling
 4. Comforting
 5. Positioning for sleep
 6. Caring for the umbilical stump
 7. Expressing attachment behaviors
 8. Practicing spirituality, especially regarding death and dying in the newborn period

COMMUNICATION AND CULTURALLY COMPETENT, FAMILY-CENTERED CARE

Guidelines for Effective Communication

A. Effective communication is essential to providing culturally competent, family-centered care.[6]

B. Use an interpreter who is bilingual and bicultural and of appropriate age, gender, and social class.
  1. Ensure that the client is comfortable using the chosen interpreter.
    a. In some cases, the interpreter may be part of the client's community and know the family, making it difficult for the client to divulge sensitive information, such as family history of birth defects or family dysfunction. In this case, consider using an interpreter from outside the community, such as those available through major telephone companies.
C. Be aware of acceptable and unacceptable nonverbal communication cues, such as eye contact and touching.
D. Explain the purpose of interventions.
E. Attempt to combine Western and folk treatments if possible.
F. Determine who in the family is the designated decision maker. Obtain her or his support and approval of interventions.
G. Ask about fears and concerns regarding the hospitalization experience.
H. Use language-appropriate education materials.
I. Ask open-ended questions to assess understanding of what has been communicated.
  1. Do not ask, "Do you understand?" or "Is this okay?"
  2. Instead ask, "Please tell me what you know so far about your baby's health problem" or "Tell me what you understand about how this surgery will help your baby."

Individualized Information

A. Parents differ in the amount and type of information they desire.
  1. Ongoing assessment of the amount and type of information parents want is necessary because parental information needs change as the infant's hospitalization progresses.
B. Parents may initially be in crisis and be unable to process information.
  1. Repeat information as often as necessary.
  2. Provide written information if appropriate.
  3. Deliver important information to the mother and the support person at the same time whenever possible.

Parental Orientation to the Unit[7]

The orientation checklist for NICU parents appears in Table 13-1.

Answering Questions about the Infant's Surgical Procedure[8]

Table 13-2 lists common questions parents ask about surgery.

Facilitating Communication

A. Provide means for routine communication with parents of intensive care infants.
  1. Scheduled phone calls that suit the parents' schedule
  2. Postcards to parents who are parenting long-distance and can't visit often
  3. Photographs for parents of milestone events to record their infant's progress
  4. Care conferences, initiated by the health care team or the parent, to deliver important information regarding the changing plan of care

FAMILY ASSESSMENT

Assessment of Parental Knowledge

A. Assess parental knowledge of the infant's problem.
  1. Ask what the parents know about the following.

TABLE 13-1 ■ **Orientation Checklist for NICU Parents**

General Information for Parents

Nursery telephone number

Visiting policy for parents, siblings, grandparents

Location of cafeteria, restrooms, public telephone, family waiting area

Scrub and gown policy

Infant security policy

Safekeeping place for purses, coats, briefcases, and so on, while visiting in nursery

Breast pump use; milk pumping and storing policies

Feeding schedules; how to communicate wish to perform bathing, feeding, other baby care

How to arrange a consistent daily call from nursery to parent (especially if parent is far from NICU)

Policy regarding parent access to baby's chart

People Parents Need to Know

Primary nurse

Parent contact person (nurse manager, clinical nurse specialist, case manager)

Physician managing baby's care: how to contact, who covers when managing physician is unavailable

Lactation specialist or resource person for lactation support

Social worker assigned to baby

Other caregivers (physical therapist, development therapist, and so on): when they visit, how parents can participate

Other Useful Information for Parents

Classes and support groups for parents, siblings, grandparents

Discharge criteria

Discharge planning options (rooming-in, day pass to go home briefly before discharge)

Telephone numbers for medical records, financial counselor, business office

Information the Nursery Needs About Parents

Telephone numbers (best daytime phone, nighttime phone; who else to call in an emergency)

Special needs of parents (hearing or visual impairment, literacy or language barrier)

Cultural or spiritual values that will affect the baby's care or parents' involvement in caregiving

Social situation that might affect protection of baby, staff, or other NICU patients (restraining order against partner or others, child custody problems, history of unstable or violent behavior on part of significant other or family members, and so on)

From: Kearns SM. 2002. Getting acquainted. In *Newborn Intensive Care: What Every Parent Needs to Know,* 2nd ed., Zaichkin J, ed. Santa Rosa, California: NICU INK, 52. Reprinted by permission.

    a. The immediate situation

    b. The plan of care

    c. Their infant's prognosis

  2. Listen for cues that will influence care of the infant and family.

    a. Misinformation

    b. Parental priorities

    c. Cultural and spiritual beliefs

Assessment of Parental Social Support

A. Assess parental social support and family functioning.

  1. Assess family composition (traditional or nontraditional).

    a. Try to determine who is the leader and which members want to be included in decision making.

  2. Poor communication and misconceptions can increase tension between partners, especially when other stressors, such as financial problems and existing marital strain, are also present.

  3. Grandparents can be a source of support to the parents, although most are themselves stressed by this birth crisis.[9]

TABLE 13-2 ■ Questions Parents Ask About Surgery

About the Procedure

Why does my baby need surgery? What will happen if he doesn't have this surgery? When must the decision be made?

What is the outlook for my baby after surgery? (Will he walk, talk, see, hear, have bowel and bladder control?)

What type of procedure will be done?

What are the risks of this surgery?

Are there alternative treatments for this problem?

What is necessary to prepare the baby for surgery (diagnostics and tests, drawing blood, additional tubes and monitors, medications)?

Will my baby need more than one surgery?

How long will the operation take?

Who will perform the surgery?

How many times has the surgeon done this procedure?

When will I meet the surgeon?

Where will I be allowed to say good-bye to my baby when he goes to the operating room (in the NICU, outside the operating room)?

About the Anesthesia

What type of anesthesia will my baby receive?

Will my baby be intubated (on a ventilator) before, during, and/or after the surgery?

How long will the anesthesia last?

When will my baby wake up?

Who is the anesthesiologist?

When will I meet the anesthesiologist?

During the Surgery

Where do parents wait during the surgery?

Who will keep us informed during and immediately after the surgery? How often should we expect to hear news about our baby?

About the Postoperative Course

Where will my baby recover immediately after surgery?

How soon will I see my baby after surgery?

Where will my baby recuperate: in the NICU or in a different unit?

How will my baby look after surgery (for example, will he have an incision, tubes, bandages, or swelling)?

Will my baby be given pain medication? If so, what type?

Will my baby be given any other medications, such as antibiotics?

How long will the stitches (drains, tubes, and other medical equipment) stay in place?

How can I participate in my baby's recovery?

What special procedures will I need to learn in order to care for the baby at home?

How long will my baby need to stay in the hospital following the surgery?

When will we see the surgeon again for follow-up care?

What other members of the team will be involved in follow-up care?

Adapted from: Green KA. 2002. Neonatal surgery. In *Newborn Intensive Care: What Every Parent Needs to Know,* 2nd ed., Zaichkin J, ed. Santa Rosa, California: NICU Ink, 211–212. Reprinted by permission.

    a. Grandparents may find it difficult to see their own child in crisis.

    b. Grandparents often don't know how to support the family.

       1) They benefit from guidance and suggestions of supportive activities, such as making phone calls, running errands, and providing child care.

    c. Grandparents may relive their own birth experiences during this crisis.

    d. Grandparents benefit from NICU visitation and education, especially if they will be involved in the infant's home care.

  4. Siblings experience disruption in family routine.[9]

    a. Siblings may feel displaced while left with a babysitter.

    b. Parents have less time to spend with their older children during this crisis.

    c. Siblings may act out and demonstrate regressive behaviors.

    d. Siblings benefit from NICU visitation and age-appropriate education.

B. Recognize that men and women react and cope with crises differently.

    1. Men may become quiet and seemingly strong, become engrossed in work, and shield the mother from painful news.

    2. Mothers may be openly upset and view the man's stoicism as insensitive.

        a. Postpartum blues may make the mother even more sensitive, and even she may be surprised by the intensity of her feelings.

    3. Both parents need to detach from the image of the expected perfect baby and attach to their sick baby.

        a. This process takes time.

        b. The quality of nursing support has a major influence on the family's chances for a successful resolution of the crisis.

PARENT INVOLVEMENT IN CARE

Readiness

A. Assess parental readiness for involvement in care as soon after the infant's birth as possible.

    1. Encourage involvement in care while balancing the infant's needs for parent contact with the mother's needs for pain control, food, and rest.

    2. Promote involvement in simple activities first: touching, temperature taking, and so on.

Learning Style

A. Assess the parental learning style.

    1. Visual

    2. Auditory

    3. Hands-on

B. Customize teaching to optimize learning.

Teaching Infant Development

A. Provide parents with information on newborn behavioral capabilities as a basis for planning developmentally supportive care.

    1. Consider using the Newborn Individualized Developmental Care and Assessment Program (NIDCAP) observation instrument to document the infant's responses.[10]

        a. Autonomic

        b. Motor

        c. State system

    2. Consider using the Neonatal Behavioral Assessment Scale (NBAS) to formulate a plan of care for high-risk infants.[11]

B. Use infant cues to guide activities.

    1. Tailor parent activities to match the baby's developmental needs and growing tolerance for handling and interaction.[12,13]

    2. Teach parents nonstressful ways in which to interact with their fragile infant.

        a. Positioning

        b. Containment

       c. Soothing talk

    3. Teach parents about their infant's cues.

        a. Engagement

        b. Disengagement

    4. Offer kangaroo care or holding as appropriate.

5. Encourage parents to help during basic caregiving activities such as diapering and feeding.
6. Teach special skills, such as tracheostomy care.
7. Involve parents in discharge planning.

The Plan for Parental Visitation

A. Determine this early in the hospitalization.[14]
B. Positive considerations include the following.
   1. Visitation promotes attachment.
   2. Visitation provides an opportunity for parents to learn caregiving skills.
   3. The goal of the visitation schedule is to balance the staff's needs with the parents' needs.[15]
C. Assess factors that may make visitation difficult.
   1. Transportation
   2. Cost of child care for siblings left at home
   3. Financial implications of time lost from work
   4. An unstable social situation that makes daily personal survival a priority
   5. The parents' perception that parental presence is unimportant or unwelcome
   6. The parents not knowing what is expected during visitation
D. Assess reasons why some parents visit "too much."[15]
   1. They are concerned about the infant's well-being.
   2. They believe that it is their responsibility to keep a vigil at the bedside.
   3. If the parents prefer to stay at their baby's bedside, their wishes should be respected.
      a. Parents need accurate information stated in understandable language. They also need reassurance that they will be informed of changes in a stable baby's status.

THE RELATIONSHIP BETWEEN THE HEALTH CARE TEAM AND FAMILY

Mutual Respect

A. Communicate respectfully.
   1. Recognize that both the parents and health care professionals bring expertise to the infant's plan of care.
   2. Listen to what the parent tells you.
   3. Negotiate tactfully.
   4. Adapt when possible.
B. Recognize that parents may prefer to communicate directly with health care professionals, but make them aware of other useful sources of information as well.[16]
   1. Some parents of preterm infants spend 10–20 hours a week gathering information in the first month of the baby's hospitalization.
   2. Parent support groups may be helpful.
   3. Internet information on many topics is plentiful, but it is not always accurate. Encourage parents to clarify information they find on the Internet with a member of the health care team, especially when it conflicts with information they receive on the unit.
C. Promote effective interactions between parents and their preterm infant.
   1. Teach parents interventions that maximize the infant's periods of alertness.
   2. Coach parents during specific parent-infant interactions.

D. Facilitate network building to connect parents with social and community support systems.

DISCHARGE ISSUES

Return Transport[17]

A. Parents may be reluctant to see their infant leave the security of the NICU to convalesce in a community hospital.

B. Prepare parents for their infant's pending transfer well before the transport date.
   1. Do not surprise parents with an imminent transport date or with the news that their baby has been transferred to a different unit or hospital.
   2. Promote the community hospital as a competent and appropriate setting for continued convalescence.
   3. Prepare parents for differences in staffing levels and feeding protocols between the two facilities.
   4. Encourage parents to tour the community hospital nursery before their infant is transferred.

Homecoming

A. Recognize that homecoming can be as stressful for parents as the initial birth crisis.

B. Suggest rooming-in as a way to help reduce the stress of homecoming.

C. Help parents use home care equipment during baby care before discharge.

D. Set up home care and follow-up appointments before discharge.

E. Provide parents with resources for questions and help, especially in the first few days after discharge.

Understanding Grief and Loss in the Perinatal/Neonatal Period

BIRTH CRISIS

Parental Expectations

A. Expectant parents believe that pregnancy and birth are associated with joy and happiness for the future.
   1. Unfortunately, not all births have a happy ending.
   2. When a pregnancy does not fulfill the parents' expectations, they may be overwhelmed by grief.

B. Birth crisis may be the first exposure a young adult has to grief and loss.[9,18,19]
   1. Birth crisis is often sudden and unexpected.
   2. Birth crisis means loss of the opportunity to parent the child as the parents had fantasized throughout pregnancy.
   3. Grief is associated not only with perinatal loss, but also with unmet expectations about the baby.
   4. Crisis means loss of the anticipated "perfect" infant and the parents' associated hopes and dreams for the child's life.

Types of Grief and Loss

A. Anticipatory grief: Grieving that occurs before the actual loss[20]

B. Chronic grief: Unresolved grief that is often seen in parents of a child who requires continuing care[20]

C. Loss following a stillbirth:[18]
   1. Stillbirth is the nonlive birth of a previously viable fetus after 20 weeks gestation.
   2. In 50 percent of stillbirths, death is sudden, without warning, and cannot be explained.
   3. Stillbirth is accompanied by feelings of shock, denial, and anxiety.
   4. Labor involves both hope and fear: hope that the infant may be alive and dread of the realization of the baby's death.
D. Birth of a special care newborn[18]
   1. Parents react with grief and mourning for loss of the fantasized perfect child while also beginning to adapt to their child's reality.
   2. It is important not to try to hurry the parents' internal process of grief and acceptance, although the processes can be facilitated and supported.
   3. Feelings of guilt and inadequacy often accompany the grief process.
E. Birth of a premature newborn[18]
   1. Preterm birth interrupts the normal adaptations and attachments of pregnancy.
   2. Parents grieve the loss of a term pregnancy and birth.
   3. Preterm birth imposes premature parenting on parents who may not be ready for the experience.
F. Birth of an infant with illness, anomalies, or physical deformity[18]
   1. This occurrence is often considered a catastrophe because our society highly values physical beauty and intelligence.
   2. When the anomaly or illness is diagnosed or suspected *in utero,* the parents may begin anticipatory grief with shock, anger, guilt, and hope.
   3. Parents who know of the fetus's condition may approach labor and birth with feelings of hope and dread.
      a. Hope that the prenatal diagnosis was incorrect
      b. Dread of the realization of the illness, deformity, or anomaly
   4. Feelings of loss may be combined with feelings of guilt and self-blame as parents search for a reason for what has happened to their child.
   5. The parents and their family and friends may not celebrate the birth with announcements, gifts, and visits, and the parents may feel isolated.
   6. Parents may interpret the severity of the illness or anomaly differently from health care professionals.
      a. Parents have limited experience with medical terminology, and they may not know how to interpret the adjectives common and minor.
      b. Professionals may discount parents' feelings as "overreactions."
      c. If health care professionals do not show concern, the parents may distrust and discount their own feelings and experience a sense of isolation.
   7. Parents can become overwhelmed by the following, which can delay attachment to the infant.
      a. Daily crisis management (of procedures, surgery, recovery, and fear that their infant may die)
      b. Their realization that they have an infant who is ill or was born with a birth defect
      c. The grief and loss associated with the loss of their perfect infant
   8. In encouraging parents to attach to their sick or deformed infant, staff must recognize that parents must begin to resolve their grief before they can fully attach to their infant.

G. Neonatal death[18]

1. The liveborn child who is critically ill or who presents with a severe anomaly forces the parents to deal with the uncertainty of whether their child will live, continue to need extensive care, or die.

2. More deaths occur in the first 24 hours after birth than in any other period of life.

   a. Prematurity accounts for 80–90 percent of newborn deaths, and congenital anomalies account for 15–20 percent.

   b. Parents of preterm newborns experience grief because of their prenatal attachment and bonding with the newborn.

3. With multiple births, when one or more of the newborns die and there is at least one survivor, parents feel grief and loss, as well as love and anxiety for the surviving infant.

   a. These intense emotions are often draining and may slow attachment to the surviving infant.

   b. Supportive care involves recognizing the neonatal death as significant. The parents should not be told to be "thankful" for the surviving infant.

   c. Involve the parents in life-support decisions. They will live with the ramifications of those decisions.

GRIEF PROCESS

The Pinwheel Model of Bereavement

A. This is one of many current models of grief that recognizes the grief process as individual, dynamic, and unique for each person.[21]

B. This model views grief in the context of a person's history and experiences in life and is based on the following characteristics.

1. Being stopped: The interruption in the bereaved person's life

2. Hurting: Intense, painful emotions that can also manifest as physical symptoms

3. Missing: Awareness of all that has been lost, including past and future

4. Holding: Keeping all things that provide evidence of the deceased person's existence

5. Seeking: A search for help to find comfort and meaning

6. Valuing: Acknowledgment that the loss is cherished

7. Surrendering: Occurs when the person reaches out to rejoin life, with the knowledge that life will be different due to the loss

C. Grief is a lifelong experience, and revisiting the loss is normal and to be expected.

INTERVENTIONS FOR FAMILIES EXPERIENCING A LOSS

Helpful Interventions to Facilitate the Grief Process[18–21]

A. Listen to parents; allow them to express their feelings without judging them.

B. Allow parents the following.

1. Time alone with their baby

2. Time and private space for physical touch if at all possible

C. Show interest in parents' feelings; acknowledge their feelings of loss with comments such as these.

1. "Many parents feel overwhelmed and sad when their baby is sick."

2. "Many parents wonder if they may be to blame for what is happening."

D. Convey a helpful and accepting attitude toward the family.
   1. Help parents understand the grieving process.
   2. Provide information and referrals to support groups and grief counselors.
   3. Stress to family members that individuals process grief differently.
      a. Differences can cause misconceptions or communication difficulties between parents and within families.

TABLE 13-3 ■ Nonsupportive Comments That Parents May Hear

1. Well, you're young. You can have more babies.
2. Just have another baby right away.
3. Well, at least you have others at home.
4. It's better to lose her now when she's a baby than when she's 4 years old.
5. He never would have been totally normal anyway.
6. It's God's will.

Adapted from: Gardner SL, Hauser P, and Merenstein GB. 2002. Grief and perinatal loss. In *Handbook of Neonatal Intensive Care,* 5th ed., Merenstein GB, and Gardner SL, eds. St. Louis: Mosby, 765. Reprinted by permission.

E. Be sensitive to individual and cultural differences in attachment behaviors.
   1. Provide photographs, locks of hair, blankets, and footprints to parents, in response to the wishes of the family.
   2. Encourage the parents to name their infant.
   3. Help parents recognize their baby's physical features with such comments as "she has her father's nose" or "he has his mom's dark hair."
   4. Offer to arrange for the infant's baptism or another ritual that is culturally significant to the family.
F. Others will also respond and provide support.
   1. Talk with parents about ways in which those supporting them may respond to this loss.
      a. Others may minimize the loss in a misguided attempt to offer comfort (Table 13-3).
   2. Discuss the reaction of children to grief and loss.
      a. Provide developmentally appropriate resources for siblings.
   3. Discuss the feelings of grandparents who experience the loss of a grandchild.
      a. Explain that they often experience "double" grief.
         1) Grief for their grandchild's illness, anomaly, or death
         2) The helpless feeling of not being able to comfort their own child
   4. Connect grieving parents with another supportive parent who has gone through a similar experience.

REFERENCES

1. Gordin P, and Johnson BH. 1999. Technology and family-centered care: Conflict or synergy? *Journal of Obstetric, Gynecologic, and Neonatal Nursing* 28(4): 401–408.

2. Palmer DG. 1997. Family-centered care: Controversies and complexities. *Journal of Perinatal & Neonatal Nursing* 10(4): 4–8.

3. Mattson S. 2000. Providing care for the changing face of the U.S. *AWHONN Lifelines* 4(3): 48–52.

4. Willis WO. 1999. Culturally competent nursing care during the perinatal period. *Journal of Perinatal & Neonatal Nursing* 13(3): 45–49.

5. Mattson S. 2000. Working toward cultural competence: Making the first steps through cultural assessment. *AWHONN Lifelines* 4(4): 41–43.

6. Mattson S. 2000. Providing culturally competent care: Strategies and approaches for perinatal clients. *AWHONN Lifelines* 4(5): 37–39.

7. Kearns SM. 2002. Getting acquainted. In *Newborn Intensive Care: What Every Parent Needs to Know,* 2nd ed., Zaichkin J, ed. Santa Rosa, California: NICU Ink, 46–64.

8. Green KA. 2002. Neonatal surgery. In *Newborn Intensive Care: What Every Parent Needs to Know,* 2nd ed., Zaichkin J, ed. Santa Rosa, California: NICU Ink, 210–221.

9. McGrath JM. 2003. Family-centered care. In *Comprehensive Neonatal Nursing: A Physiologic Perspective,* 3rd ed., Kenner C, and Lott JW, eds. Philadelphia: Saunders, 92, 94, 96, 103–105.

10. Als H, and Gilkerson K. 1995. Developmentally supportive care in the neonatal intensive care unit. *Zero to Three* 15(6): 1–10.

11. Cole JG. 1995. Using the NBAS with high-risk infants. In *Neonatal Behavioral Assessment Scale,* 3rd ed., Brazelton TB, and Nugent JK, eds. London: MacKeith Press, 126–133.

12. Gretebeck RJ, Shaffer D, and Bishop-Kurylo D. 1998. Clinical pathways for family-oriented developmental care in the intensive care nursery. *Journal of Perinatal & Neonatal Nursing* 12(1): 70–80.

13. Krebs TL. 1998. Clinical pathway for enhanced parent and preterm infant interaction through parent education. *Journal of Perinatal & Neonatal Nursing* 12(2): 38–49.

14. Griffin T. 1999. Visitation patterns: Parents who visit "too little." *Neonatal Network* 18(6): 75–76.

15. Griffin T. 1998. Visitation patterns: The parents who visit "too much." *Neonatal Network* 17(7): 67–68.

16. Brazy JE, et al. 2001. How parents of premature infants gather information and obtain support. *Neonatal Network* 20(2): 41–48.

17. Dodds-Azzopardi SE, and Chapman JS. 1995. Parents' perceptions of stress associated with premature infant transfer among hospital environments. *Journal of Perinatal & Neonatal Nursing* 8(4): 39–46.

18. Gardner SL, Hauser P, and Merenstein GB. 2002. Grief and perinatal loss. In *Handbook of Neonatal Intensive Care*, 5th ed., Merenstein GB, and Gardner SL, eds. St. Louis: Mosby, 755–758, 765.

19. Woods J, and Esposito Woods J, eds. 1997. *Loss during Pregnancy or in the Newborn Period: Principles of Care with Clinical Cases and Analysis*. Pitman, New Jersey: AJ Jannetti.

20. Kenner C. 2004. Families in crisis. In *Core Curriculum for Neonatal Intensive Care Nursing*, 3rd ed., Verklan MT, and Waldron M, eds. Philadelphia: Saunders, 392–409.

21. Solari-Twadell PA, et al. 1995. The pinwheel model of bereavement. *Image: The Journal of Nursing Scholarship* 27(4): 323–326.

Notes

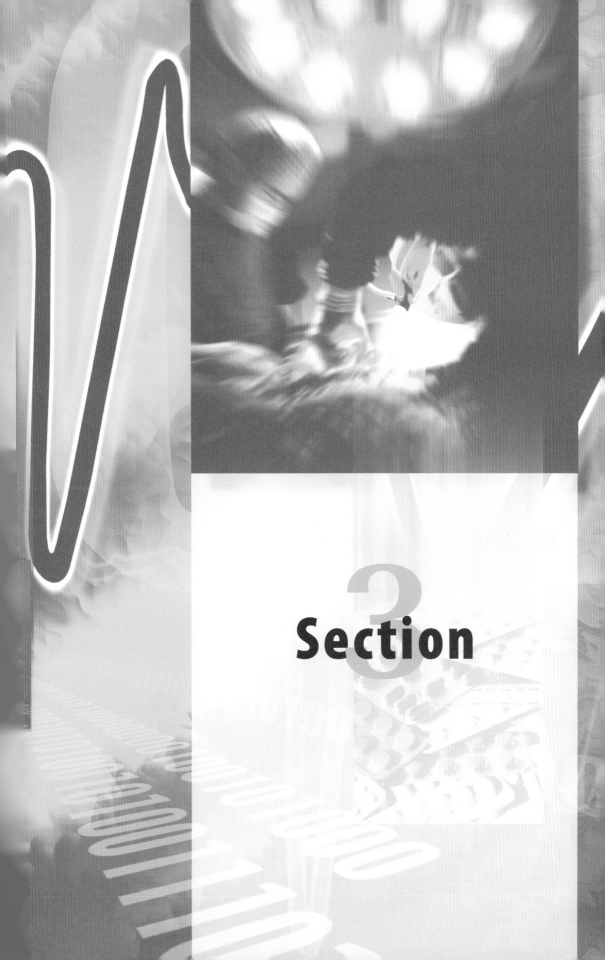

Section 3

Fetal Surgery

Lori J. Howell, RN, MS
Tracy M. Widmer, CRNP, MS

This chapter describes those fetal diagnoses that can be considered for prenatal surgery, the selection process, and patient preparation for surgery. In most pregnancies, detection of a fetal anomaly leads to a change in the timing, mode, and/or location of delivery to improve both maternal and infant outcomes.

Each of the anatomic malformations presented here shows a spectrum of severity, and only those fetuses with life-threatening or severely debilitating anomalies are considered candidates for fetal surgery (Table 14-1). Preparation for surgery of both the mother and fetus; pre-, intra-, and postoperative care; and long-term follow-up are discussed here. The role of a center for fetal diagnosis and treatment is also presented.

Patient Selection for Fetal Intervention

A. When a fetal abnormality amenable to fetal intervention is diagnosed, the prospective parents have three choices.
   1. Terminate the pregnancy if the gestation is prior to 24 weeks.
   2. Continue the pregnancy and plan for the best postnatal care if the diagnosis is after 24 weeks gestation.
   3. Intervene before birth.
B. An evaluation for fetal surgery consists of outpatient diagnostic tests and a review of the results by a multidisciplinary team.
   1. The detailed sonographic survey is performed to accomplish the following.
      a. To confirm the diagnosis
      b. To detect any additional fetal abnormalities
      c. To assess for the presence and severity of hydrops
   2. A fetal echocardiogram is done to accomplish the following.
      a. To detect any structural abnormalities of the heart
      b. In certain diagnoses, such as sacrococcygeal teratomas (SCT), to assess for subtle hemodynamic changes
   3. Ultrafast fetal MRI is a newer modality that provides striking anatomic detail and is particularly useful for the following purposes.
      a. To resolve diagnostic dilemmas such as the differential diagnosis of:

1) CCAM versus chronic lobar emphysema
2) Isolated CNS anomalies versus additional findings in the brain
  b. To confirm the position of the liver in CDH fetuses
4. If genetic karyotyping was not done at the referring institution, one of the following procedures is done to rule out chromosomal abnormalities associated with some fetal diseases.
  a. Amniocentesis
  b. Chorionic villus sampling
  c. Percutaneous blood sampling
  d. Rapid karyotyping for emergent problems by fluorescent *in situ* hybridization, which provides information about chromosomes 13, 18, and 21 and gender

C. An informed consent conference is held.
  1. At this time, test results are reviewed, and the available options for the pregnancy are explained. Participants should include the following.
    a. Family
    b. Fetal/pediatric surgeon
    c. Obstetric specialists
    d. Fetal and obstetric anesthesiologists
    e. Nurse coordinator
    f. Social worker
  2. All of these services should be coordinated so that the family can learn of their fetus' anomaly and their options in an unhurried, comprehensive manner.
  3. The informed consent conference provides the parents with the following.
    a. An in-depth description of the fetal surgery procedure
    b. Results from the procedure
    c. Maternal risks versus fetal benefits
    d. Alternatives such as termination of the pregnancy or standard postnatal treatment
  4. If the family opts for planned delivery and postnatal surgery, the following occurs.
    a. The surgeon counsels the parents regarding the anomaly, the surgical repair, and the anticipated neonatal course.
    b. Arrangements are made for maternal transport and planned delivery at a tertiary care center.
  5. If the fetus has a fatal defect not amenable to fetal or postnatal surgery or if the parents opt to terminate the pregnancy, the parents receive counseling from the reproductive geneticist.

TABLE 14-1 ■ Conditions Amenable to Fetal Surgery

Congenital Anomaly	Fetal Surgical Procedure
Congenital diaphragmatic hernia	Tracheal occlusion*
Congenital cystic adenomatoid malformation	Thoracoamniotic shunt Thoracotomy and fetal lobectomy EXIT[†] procedure
Sacrococcygeal teratoma	Tumor debulking
Spina bifida	Repair of spina bifida[‡]
Urinary tract obstruction	Vesicoamniotic shunt; open vesicostomy; fetoscopic laser of valves
Neck masses	EXIT[†] procedure

* Currently performed only in Europe.

† *Ex utero* intrapartum therapy.

‡ Only performed under NIH grant #HD 041666-03S1 IRB #2000-11-2226 "A Randomized Trial of Prenatal versus Postnatal Repair of Myelomeningocele (Management of Meningocele Study—MOMS)."

  a. Follow-up telephone and written consultations are provided immediately to the referring physician.
  b. Parents need to be supported regardless of their decision to minimize later feelings of guilt.

Fetal Congenital Diaphragmatic Hernia (CDH)

DEFINITION

A. In congenital diaphragmatic hernia, the diaphragm fails to develop properly during gestation, leaving an opening through which the intestines, stomach, and liver herniate into the chest.
   1. Absence of the diaphragm can occur on the left or right side, but is more common on the left.
   2. Bilateral hernias also occur; they are usually associated with multiple anomalies.

PATHOPHYSIOLOGY

A. The heart and lungs are compressed by the herniated abdominal organs.
   1. The lungs do not develop.
B. The high morbidity and mortality associated with CDH are related to the following:
   1. Pulmonary hypoplasia
   2. Pulmonary hypertension
C. The severity of the diagnosis can be predicted by the amount of liver in the chest.[1]
   1. There has been little improvement in mortality rates among those infants with livers herniated into the chest, despite advances in neonatal therapy.[2]

ETIOLOGY

A. The exact cause of CDH is not known.
   1. Genetic factors may play a role, but as of yet, no single gene has been identified.[3]
B. CDH occurs because of a failure of the pleuroperitoneal folds to close, which results in herniation of abdominal organs into the left or right side of the chest through the defect in the diaphragm. A bilateral hernia may also occur.

INCIDENCE

A. The reported incidence is 1/2,000–5,000 live births, though inclusion of fetally diagnosed cases likely affects this rate.[4]

PRENATAL DIAGNOSIS AND EVALUATION

A. If a diaphragmatic hernia is suspected, the mother should be referred to a specialty care center for these tests.
   1. Level II, high-resolution ultrasound
      a. CDH can be diagnosed by prenatal ultrasound.
         1) There will be a shift of the mediastinum to the right or left, depending upon the side of the diaphragmatic defect.
            a) A right-sided CDH will always have liver herniated into the chest.
            b) A left-sided CDH will have bowel, stomach, and possibly liver herniation.

    b. In addition to confirming the diagnosis, a Level II ultrasound can provide a lung-to-head ratio (LHR).

        1) The LHR is the measurement obtained in centimeters (cm), between 24 and 26 weeks gestation of the area of the right lung at the level of the atria divided by the head circumference to correct for gestational age.

            a) The LHR is used to predict those fetuses with left-sided CDH who will be most severely affected.

            b) The prognostic value of the LHR has not been corroborated in right-sided CDH.[5]

  2. Fetal echocardiogram

    a. A fetal echocardiogram is done to rule out structural heart disease.

  3. Ultrafast fetal magnetic resonance image (MRI) study

    a. The ultrafast fetal MRI is used to:[6]

        1) Assess the liver position

        2) Confirm the diagnosis

        3) Measure lung volumes

        4) Rule out other anomalies

B. Fetal karyotype should be done to rule out chromosomal problems, which are present in 10–20 percent of CDH fetuses.

INDICATIONS FOR FETAL INTERVENTION

A. In the U.S., a National Institutes of Health trial was conducted at the University of California, San Francisco. It determined that the mortality of CDH fetuses undergoing fetal surgery was similar to that of those receiving postnatal care.[7]

B. Currently, fetal intervention is primarily offered in Europe.[8] However, UCSF is performing this method based upon the European experience in a limited manner.[9]

C. Fetuses considered for intervention include those with the following.

  1. No maternal risk factors

  2. No associated anomalies

  3. A normal karyotype

  4. Liver herniation into the fetal chest

  5. A normal echocardiogram

  6. LHR <1

D. The fetus must be between 26 and 28 weeks gestational age and a singleton pregnancy.

  1. Mothers who are diagnosed after 28 weeks gestation are not candidates for fetal surgery because of the lack of adequate lung growth observed after this time.[8]

E. The family must be committed to the necessary follow-up.

  1. Multidisciplinary evaluation and nondirective counseling of prospective fetal surgery patients are crucial.

  2. As with all fetal surgeries, the family should be committed to staying in the vicinity of the tertiary care center for frequent monitoring and following of the fetus.

  3. Close surveillance must be provided after surgery.

Fetal Intervention

A. The intended outcome of tracheal occlusion fetal therapy is to promote lung growth by occluding the trachea. Fetal lung fluid normally produced is forced to remain in the lungs, increasing pulmonary pressures and leading to accelerated lung growth.

B. Preparation of the mother.
1. Mothers undergoing fetal surgery are generally admitted the morning of surgery.
2. Electronic fetal monitoring is done for the following.
   a. Fetal heart rate
   b. Uterine irritability
3. Indomethacin is administered for uterine relaxation.
   a. A suppository is given the night before surgery.
   b. A suppository is given two hours preoperatively.
4. Spinal anesthesia with conscious sedation is used during the procedure.

C. Surgery proceeds as follows.
1. A minimally invasive approach is used to gain access to the fetus using a scope.
2. Maternal abdominal incisions are made to insert the scope into the uterus, carefully avoiding the placenta.
3. The fetal head is positioned, the bronchoscope inserted, and a balloon deployed into the trachea.
4. The balloon is inflated, occluding the trachea.
5. The trocar is withdrawn, and the abdominal incisions are sutured.
6. The mother is typically discharged on postoperative day 1 on nifedipine.

D. Removal of the balloon
1. This occurs about 32 weeks gestation (approximately 4 weeks after placement).
2. Epidural anesthesia with conscious sedation is used during the procedure.
3. The balloon is deflated and removed via fetal bronchoscopy.

Delivery of the Fetus

A. Delivery of the fetus is determined by the following.
1. The development of preterm labor
2. The development of fetal hydrops
3. Attainment of 36 weeks gestational age with documented lung maturity

B. Delivery can be by vaginal or cesarean route, depending on obstetric indications.

C. The fetus is then intubated and ventilation is assessed.
1. The airway is suctioned.
2. Exogenous surfactant may be administered.

D. Umbilical arterial and venous lines are placed.

E. Standard neonatal intensive care therapies must be available at delivery.
1. High-frequency ventilation
2. Nitric oxide therapy
3. Extracorporeal membrane oxygenation

F. Once the neonate is stable, usually over days to weeks, the diaphragmatic hernia is repaired.

Postnatal Care

See Congenital Diaphragmatic Hernia in Chapter 2: Neonatal Pulmonary Disorders.

Congenital Cystic Adenomatoid Malformation (CCAM)

DEFINITION
CCAM is a rare, benign growth of cystic lung tissue.

PATHOPHYSIOLOGY
A. A CCAM is almost always unilateral, involving a single lobe.

B. Three pathologic types of CCAM have been characterized by Stocker and colleagues.[10]
  1. Type I consists of multiple large or a single dominant cyst with thick, smooth muscle and elastic tissue walls.
  2. Type II consists of multiple small cysts <1 cm in diameter.
  3. Type III is primarily solid.

C. Whatever the type of CCAM, if hydrops does not develop, these fetuses have a favorable outcome.[11]

D. A large CCAM can cause esophageal compression, which may lead to decreased fetal swallowing of amniotic fluid, resulting in polyhydramnios.

E. Hydrops fetalis can also occur, caused by the mass compressing the great vessels and heart.[12]
  1. Fetal hydrops ultimately leads to fetal demise and is the sole indication for performing fetal surgery.
  2. Mothers of hydropic fetuses can also exhibit signs and symptoms of the "maternal-mirror" syndrome. This is a preeclamptic state that mirrors the sick fetus.
  3. A fetus >32 weeks gestation and hydropic should to be considered for early delivery so that the lesion can be resected immediately after birth.
  4. If the mass remains large, or for the hydropic fetus after 32 weeks gestation, an *ex utero* intrapartum treatment (EXIT) procedure is considered to allow resection of the affected lobe while on "placental bypass." An EXIT procedure allows the resection to be performed in an unhurried fashion, eliminating an emergency thoracotomy in the delivery room.[13]

F. Fetuses with CCAM who do not develop fetal hydrops have an excellent chance of survival as long as provisions are made to deliver at a tertiary care center that can offer immediate resuscitation and surgical resection.

ETIOLOGY
A. CCAM is thought to result from an overgrowth of terminal respiratory bronchioles that form cysts of various sizes and that lack normal alveoli.

INCIDENCE
A. The actual incidence of CCAM is not known. CCAM is thought to be rare, with fewer than 1,000 cases reported in the literature.[14] It affects an estimated 1/25,000–35,000 pregnancies.[15] This represents 25 percent of all congenital lung malformations.[16,17]

B. Prenatal diagnosis is causing an increase in the number of cases reported.

PRENATAL DIAGNOSIS AND EVALUATION
A. Diagnosis is made by ultrasound.
  1. Frequent ultrasound imaging may be needed to follow mass size, degree of mediastinal shift, and development of polyhydramnios and hydrops. If the mass begins to shrink, imaging may be done less frequently.

    a. These lesions are followed closely *in utero* because many of the fetal CCAMs and the majority of bronchopulmonary sequestration (BPS) lesions shrink dramatically before birth.[18]

B. Ultrafast MRI is helpful in differentiating between the types of lesions.[19]
    1. The three types of CCAM
    2. CDH
    3. BPS
    4. Hybrid lesion
    5. Bronchogenic cyst
    6. Foregut duplication
    7. Lobar emphysema
    8. Pulmonary agenesis
    9. Congenital high airway obstruction syndrome (CHAOS)

C. MRI can also be used to assist with delivery planning and postnatal management.

D. A prospective tool known as the CCAM volume ratio (CVR) has been used to predict those fetuses most likely to develop hydrops.[20]
    1. CVR is a measurement obtained in cm of CCAM volume (using ultrasound, the height, length, and width of the mass are measured and multiplied by 0.52) divided by the fetal head circumference to correct for gestational age.[20]
    2. A CVR of >1.6 indicates a fetus at higher risk for developing hydrops.

E. An amniocentesis may be done.
    1. For advanced maternal age, to determine normal karyotype
    2. If additional anomalies are found on ultrasound

F. A fetal echocardiogram is done to rule out structural abnormalities and assess cardiac function.

INDICATIONS FOR FETAL INTERVENTION

A. Maternal
    1. No maternal risk factors such as:
        a. Clotting disorders
        b. Allergy to nonsteroidal anti-inflammatory medications
    2. Absence of maternal-mirror syndrome

B. Fetal
    1. <32 weeks gestational age
    2. Hydrops fetalis
        a. Maternal polyhydramnios
        b. Placentomegaly
        c. Ascites
        d. Skin/scalp edema
    3. Normal echocardiogram
    4. Singleton pregnancy
    5. No associated anomalies
    6. Normal karyotype (if performed)

FETAL INTERVENTION

A. Lung resection may be performed.
    1. General anesthesia is administered to the mother.
        a. General anesthesia crosses the placenta, thus anesthetizing the fetus and providing complete uterine relaxation.

2. After the maternal laparotomy and hysterotomy are done, the affected side of the fetus is positioned so that the fetal hand can be exposed, and a pulse oximeter is placed for intraoperative monitoring.

3. Continuous fetal echocardiogram monitoring is done to provide crucial information as to volume status of the fetus.[21]

4. The fetal chest is then entered, typically at the fifth intercostal space. The appropriate lobe is resected, the thoracotomy is closed, and the fetus is returned to the uterus.

5. The maternal hysterotomy and laparotomy are then closed.

6. Operative time is usually quite short, and blood loss is minimal.

B. In the case of very large cysts within the mass, a fetal thoracoamniotic shunt may be placed percutaneously in the hydropic fetus.

DELIVERY OF THE FETUS

A. The infant who is delivered near term via cesarean section after open fetal surgery and vaginal or cesarean section for thoracoamniotic shunt placement for a CCAM usually requires minimal intervention.

B. The fetus undergoing shunt placement requires the following.

1. Ultrasound surveillance for shunt dislodgment continued through gestation

2. A delivery plan to ensure the shunt is clamped at delivery

3. A thoracotomy and resection of the mass, sometimes performed when the neonate is stable

POSTNATAL CARE

A. Respiratory effort is evaluated and a chest x-ray obtained.

B. The surgical incision site is inspected for adequate closure.

C. A cranial ultrasound is often obtained to rule out any hemorrhage that may be associated with the stress of fetal surgery.

D. If all diagnostic tests and the physical exam are within normal limits, the infant is discharged to home.

Sacrococcygeal Teratoma

DEFINITION

Sacrococcygeal teratoma is usually seen as a firm or, more commonly, a cystic mass that arises from the coccyx.

PATHOPHYSIOLOGY

A. SCTs are classified by the American Academy of Pediatrics, Surgical Section, into four types.

1. Type I is primarily external and has only a small presacral component.

2. Type II is predominantly external, but has a significant intrapelvic portion.

3. Type III is partially external, but is predominately intrapelvic with abdominal extension.

4. Type IV may go unrecognized for years because it is located entirely within the pelvis and abdomen.

B. Most SCT tumors are Type I or II.[22]

ETIOLOGY

A. The cause of SCT is unknown, but several theories exist as to why these tumors occur.
1. An SCT is derived from totipotent cells in Hensen's node.[23]
2. An SCT occurs as a result of primitive germ cells that migrate from the yolk sac to the genital ridge.[24]
3. An SCT may be the result of a twinning accident with incomplete separation.

INCIDENCE

A. SCT is the most common tumor of the newborn.
1. The incidence is 1/35,000–40,000 live births.[25]
2. Approximately 75 percent of these newborns are females.[26]

PRENATAL DIAGNOSIS AND EVALUATION

A. The tumor when diagnosed in the fetus and neonate is not likely to be malignant.
B. Women diagnosed prenatally with fetal SCT often present to the obstetrician's office with fundal height measuring larger than the fetal gestational age would indicate.
1. This larger measurement may be due to tumor size or polyhydramnios.
C. Alpha-fetoprotein (AFP) measurement may be diagnostic.
1. Occasionally, an increase in the AFP level may also indicate that a mass is present.
2. AFP is an important tumor marker that is elevated in mothers carrying an infant with with any of the following.
a. SCT
b. Myelomeningocele
c. Abdominal wall defect
3. AFP is also elevated in mothers carrying twins.
D. An increase in fundal height and an elevated AFP warrant an ultrasound.
1. In addition, widespread screening by ultrasonography at 16–18 weeks gestation has resulted in an increased number of SCTs being detected in otherwise asymptomatic mothers.
2. The sonographic appearance of the SCT may include bizarre echogenic patterns secondary to areas of tumor necrosis, cystic degeneration, or hemorrhage.
E. Severity criteria of these tumors include the following.
1. Solid tumor mass
2. Tumor size greater than the biparietal diameter of the fetus
3. Rapid tumor growth
4. Development of placentomegaly, polyhydramnios, and hydrops
F. The makeup of the tumor can be somewhat predictive of fetal outcome: A primarily cystic mass usually presents with fewer problems than one that is primarily solid.
1. High-output cardiac failure is unlikely in infants with predominantly cystic teratomas because of low blood flow to the tumor.
2. Fetuses with large, solid tumors can develop hydrops from high-output cardiac failure because of the extremely high blood flow through the tumor.
a. Fetal hydrops progresses rapidly to fetal death.
b. Frequent sonographic surveillance is needed to assess the following.
1) Tumor growth

       2) Fetal status

       3) Amniotic fluid volume

       4) Early signs of hydrops fetalis

   c. Serial fetal echocardiograms are necessary to detect increasing combined cardiac output, which may lead to hydrops fetalis.

   d. Fetal complications for SCT include the following.

       1) Hydrops fetalis

       2) Maternal-mirror syndrome—a preeclamptic state in the mother

       3) Vascular steal resulting in cardiac failure

       4) Anemia due to tumor rupture

       5) Hemorrhage of the tumor

       6) Premature labor because of tumor bulk

       7) Polyhydramnios

       8) Neonatal death resulting from prematurity and/or tumor rupture and hemorrhage

INDICATIONS FOR FETAL INTERVENTION

A. No maternal risk factors

B. Absence of maternal-mirror syndrome

C. High output state in the fetus evidenced by increased combined ventricular output and a dilated inferior vena cava caused by vascular steal by the teratoma

D. Development of hydrops fetalis (polyhydramnios, placentomegaly [early signs], skin and scalp edema [late signs])

E. Fetus <32 weeks gestational age

FETAL INTERVENTION

A. The goal of fetal surgery is to debulk the tumor, thereby reversing the high-output cardiac failure.

   1. The presumed cause of fetal hydrops is a vascular steal by the teratoma placing an increased workload on the fetal heart.[22]

   2. Fetal surgery has been shown to reverse the high-output cardiac failure; however, the mother remains at increased risk for premature labor.[27,28]

B. Procedure

   1. Care is taken to avoid tumor rupture.

   2. Exposure of the fetal buttocks and the attached tumor is obtained through the hysterotomy.

   3. The anus is identified.

   4. A sterile intraoperative ultrasound is used to evaluate fetal hemodynamics in the event the fetus requires volume resuscitation during the procedure.

   5. A tourniquet is then applied to the base of the tumor and cinched down gradually to the vascular pedicle.

   6. Tumor debulking is then performed with a stapler as a palliative measure to reduce the cardiac workload.

   7. The entire procedure typically takes <15 minutes, with minimal blood loss.[22]

   8. The fetus is then returned to the uterus, and the hysterotomy and laparotomy are closed.

DELIVERY OF THE FETUS

A. A cesarean delivery is performed by obstetricians in the high-risk setting.

POSTNATAL CARE

A. A cranial ultrasound should be done at birth to rule out complications such as intracranial hemorrhage related to the fetal surgery.

B. It is important to assess for the following.[22]
1. Intra-abdominal and pelvic components
2. Bowel or urinary obstruction
3. Lower extremity function
4. Integrity of the spine

C. Urologic complications can be associated with SCTs.
1. Caused by the tumor pressing on the bladder or ureters
2. Possibility of damage during surgery to:[29]
    a. Pelvic nerve plexus
    b. Sacral nerve roots
    c. Sphincter structure

D. Once the neonate is stabilized postdelivery, resection of the coccyx and any residual mass is done.

E. With early care consisting of surgical excision of the tumor, including the coccyx, recurrence is rare despite the large size of the tumor.
1. Every three months for the first year, then at 1.5, 2, and 3 years of age, an AFP level will need to be drawn.
    a. An increased level may indicate tumor regrowth, and a computed tomography scan should be done to rule out tumor recurrence and any metastasis.

Myelomeningocele

DEFINITION

Myelomeningocele (MMC) is a bony defect in the vertebral column resulting in protrusion of the meninges and spinal cord through an opening in the vertebral body.

PATHOPHYSIOLOGY

A. The spectrum of the disease includes:
1. Spinal cord dysfunction
2. Chiari II hindbrain herniation
3. Ventriculomegaly

ETIOLOGY

A. MMCs are thought to occur as a result of "nonfusion of the primordial halves of the vertebral arches" (p. 435).[30]

INCIDENCE

A. MMC is the most common birth defect involving the central nervous system (CNS).

B. The incidence of MMC is 4.5/10,000 live births.

PRENATAL DIAGNOSIS AND EVALUATION

A. The prenatal diagnosis of MMC is usually a result of maternal serum AFP screening.
1. With an elevated AFP serum level, the mother is referred for a Level II ultrasound and amniocentesis to assess chromosomes and amniotic fluid AFP.

INDICATIONS FOR FETAL INTERVENTION

A. The National Institutes of Child Health and Human Development has funded a five-year, multicenter, randomized clinical trial for the treatment of fetuses with MMC to evaluate the efficacy and safety of fetal surgical repair versus standard postnatal repair of the spinal defect.

   1. Two hundred women will be enrolled in the study, with 100 in each surgical group. Individuals qualifying for enrollment will be assigned to one of the three participating Management of Myelomeningocele Study (MOMS) Centers: Children's Hospital of Philadelphia; University of California, San Francisco; or Vanderbilt University.

   2. Prospective mothers carrying a baby with MMC or their doctors should contact the program manager at 1-866-ASK MOMS for information and preliminary screening for participation in the MOMS. No fetal surgery for MMC is offered outside the trial.

   3. Once referral to a participating MOMS Center is made, an evaluation consisting of a comprehensive obstetric ultrasound, psychological testing, and an echocardiogram and MRI of the fetus will be done. If the eligibility criteria are met, the mother will be offered randomization into the study.

   4. Inclusion and exclusion criteria for participation in MOMS are outlined in the web site: www.spinabifidamoms.com.

FETAL INTERVENTION

A. Early gestation repair may arrest the neural destruction process.[31] Thus far, it has reversed the Arnold-Chiari malformation, potentially obviating the need for a shunt.[32]

B. Preoperative care proceeds as follows if a mother is randomized to the fetal surgery arm for MMC repair.

   1. The mother is admitted the morning of surgery.

   2. Contractions and fetal well-being are monitored externally.

   3. She receives an indomethacin suppository to assist with uterine relaxation.

   4. An epidural catheter is placed to provide pain relief to the mother and fetus postoperatively.

C. The operation proceeds as follows.

   1. A deep-inhalation anesthetic is administered to the mother and crosses the placenta to anesthetize the fetus.

   2. A maternal laparotomy and hysterotomy are performed.

   3. The fetal back is then positioned at the hysterotomy site, where the pediatric neurosurgeon completes an MMC repair just as he/she would in the postnatal period.

      a. The placode and the defect are excised.

D. Maternal postoperative care includes the following.

   1. The mother is extubated and awakened from general anesthesia before returning to Labor and Delivery for postoperative care and monitoring.

      a. Per protocol, mothers having this procedure are discharged to the nearby Ronald McDonald House on postoperative day 4 and return once a week for follow-up ultrasound and prenatal care.

   2. At 36 weeks gestation, or before if labor cannot be controlled with tocolytics, a cesarean section for delivery is scheduled.

DELIVERY OF THE FETUS

A. The mother undergoes a standard cesarean delivery, and the baby is resuscitated by the neonatology team.

POSTNATAL CARE

A. Once stabilized, the infant is transferred to the NICU for further evaluation.
   1. The baby is seen by the spina bifida team to assess the following outcomes.
      a. Neurologic
      b. Musculoskeletal
      c. Urologic
      d. Orthopedic
   2. The babies and their families return to their respective MOMS Center for follow-up.
   3. Children born with myelomeningocele often face a life of chronic illness requiring multiple surgeries and hospitalizations, including difficulties with ambulation, ventriculoperitoneal shunting, and bowel and bladder difficulties.

Giant Neck Masses

DEFINITION

A. Giant neck masses in the fetus, which include the following, can result in profound hypoxia and even death because of the inability to obtain an airway after birth.
   1. Cervical teratomas
   2. Hygromas
   3. Hemangiomas
   4. Anomalies such as CHAOS

PATHOPHYSIOLOGY

See Cystic Hygroma in Chapter 1: Neonatal Surgical Disorders of the Head, Ears, Eyes, Nose and Throat.

ETIOLOGY

See Cystic Hygroma in Chapter 1: Neonatal Surgical Disorders of the Head, Ears, Eyes, Nose and Throat.

INCIDENCE

See Cystic Hygroma in Chapter 1: Neonatal Surgical Disorders of the Head, Ears, Eyes, Nose and Throat.

PRENATAL DIAGNOSIS AND EVALUATION

A. A complete obstetric history is obtained, and physical and genetic evaluations are done.
   1. Genetic abnormalities such as 69XXX or syndromes such as Fraser's can be associated with CHAOS and require further evaluation.[33]
B. To ensure appropriate preparation for a planned delivery in the infant with a giant neck mass, prenatal ultrasound and ultrafast fetal MRI are used to do the following.[19]
   1. Rule out anomalies
   2. Establish fetal growth
   3. Detail airway anatomy

C. A fetal echocardiogram is performed for the following reasons.
   1. To rule out structural abnormalities
   2. To identify impending hydrops

INDICATIONS FOR FETAL INTERVENTION

A. EXIT procedure
   1. Cervical teratoma
   2. Cystic hygroma
   3. CHAOS
   4. Large CCAM
   5. Cervical neuroblastoma
   6. Cervical hemangioma
   7. Pulmonary agenesis

FETAL INTERVENTION

A. Although fetuses with giant neck masses do not undergo fetal surgery in the classic sense (i.e., the fetus is not returned to the womb after the operation), they can undergo multiple procedures for up to an hour while still attached to the placental circulation.[34,35]

B. EXIT procedure consists of the following.
   1. First described for delivery of a fetus in which tracheal occlusion had been performed for a severe case of CDH[36]
   2. This delivery technique was adapted to allow time to obtain an airway in a near-term fetus with a giant neck mass.[34]
   3. Delivery
      a. General maternal-fetal anesthesia is provided to enhance uterine relaxation and preserve uteroplacental circulation.
      b. For patients with severe polyhydramnios, a maternal laparotomy and an amniotic fluid reduction are done through a uterine trocar.
      c. When possible, a lower uterine segment hysterotomy is performed to expose the fetal head, neck, and thorax.
         1) This type of hysterotomy may allow a vaginal delivery in future pregnancies.
         2) A classical cesarean is necessary when extension of the head and neck cannot be done because of tumor size.
      d. The head, neck, thorax, and one arm are then delivered.
         1) The fetal heart rate and hemoglobin saturation are monitored continuously.
      e. Many procedures can be performed for up to an hour before clamping of the cord and subsequent delivery. These procedures may include the following.
         1) Laryngoscopy
         2) Bronchoscopy
         3) Intubation
         4) Tracheostomy
         5) Exogenous surfactant instillation
         6) Placement of umbilical lines
         7) Possible tumor resection

C. The advantage of the EXIT procedure is that multiple procedures can be performed without anoxic insult because of maternal-placental "bypass" before delivery.[34]

DELIVERY OF THE FETUS

A. An EXIT procedure is a specialized delivery technique detailed under FETAL INTERVENTION, above.

POSTNATAL CARE

A. If the mass is not resected at the time of the EXIT procedure, plans are made to return to the operating room for a definitive resection or other needed surgery.

B. If the pathology of the mass is positive for a teratoma, the AFP will need to be monitored.

C. A swallow study needs to be done to assure that the infant is able to protect his airway.

D. Depending upon the anomaly, a tracheostomy and tracheal reconstruction may be necessary.

Obstructive Uropathy

DEFINITION

A. Fetal obstructive uropathy is caused by a diverse group of anomalies of the urinary tract.

B. Those fetuses with complete posterior urethral valves or urethral atresia in the presence of little to no amniotic fluid may benefit from fetal vesicoamniotic shunting.[37]

PATHOPHYSIOLOGY

A. Partial obstructive uropathy is associated with the following.
   1. Normal amniotic fluid volume
   2. Minimal renal involvement

B. Complete bladder outlet obstruction is associated with the following.
   1. Early-onset oligohydramnios
   2. Renal and pulmonary insufficiency

C. This latter group of fetuses represents the "hidden mortality" of obstructive uropathy, with an estimated fetal death rate of up to 95 percent.[38] It is to this group that prenatal intervention is offered.

D. The two most common causes of lower urinary tract obstruction in the male fetus are the following.
   1. Posterior urethral valves (PUV) with an estimated incidence as high as 1/4,000 pregnancies[39]
   2. Urethral atresia

E. Less common causes of obstructive uropathy include the following.
   1. Partial urethral valves
   2. Urethral stenosis
   3. Anomalies of the penal orifice, such as meatal stenosis or hypospadias

F. Fetal urine production begins as early as 8 weeks gestation; however, it becomes the primary component of amniotic fluid around 13 to 14 weeks gestation.
   1. As a consequence of a high-grade obstruction, the bladder becomes distended and hypertrophic, and the amniotic fluid volume begins to decrease.
   2. Prolonged decrease or absence of amniotic fluid during critical times for lung development (from approximately 18 to 24 weeks gestation) results in fetal pulmonary hypoplasia and postnatal respiratory insufficiency, the leading causes of death in this group of infants.

G. Urinary reflux may result in hydroureters and pathologic changes within the renal parenchyma causing cystic dysplasia and renal insufficiency.

H. Lower urinary tract obstruction (LUTO) may occur.
1. It results in oligohydramnios and secondary deformities such as:
   a. Contractures
   b. Clubfeet
   c. Flattened facies, known as "Potter's facies"
2. The natural history of LUTO depends upon the timing, degree, and duration of the obstruction. A complete obstruction associated with early-onset oligohydramnios carries a poor prognosis because of pulmonary hypoplasia and long-standing renal damage.

Etiology

A. Posterior urethral valves are thought to occur between the 7th and 11th week of gestation and form from cloacal remnants.

Incidence

A. The incidence of PUV is reported to be 1/4,000 births.[39]

Prenatal Diagnosis and Evaluation

A. The classic sonographic presentation of an early-onset LUTO at mid-trimester includes the following.
1. Distended fetal bladder
2. Bilateral hydronephrosis
3. Oligohydramnios

B. A "keyhole sign" is indicative of proximal urethral obstruction.

C. Echogenic renal parenchyma and the appearance of microcysts on ultrasound are evidence of cystic dysplasia and generally associated with a poor renal prognosis.

D. In addition to careful sonographic and echocardiographic assessment, the prenatal evaluation algorithm includes ultrasound-guided serial vesicocentesis.
1. Assess residual renal function in order to distinguish fetuses who can benefit from prenatal intervention from those who will not.
2. A series of sequential bladder taps can help determine the extent of underlying renal damage and the potential for renal salvage.[40]
   a. Urine is sent for analysis of electrolytes and β_2–microglobulins as indicators of renal function before placing a vesicoamniotic shunt.
3. Ultrafast fetal MRI may provide additional information for counseling purposes.
   a. Oligohydramnios can make ultrasonography difficult, and additional anomalies, such as those in the CNS, may not be detectable on ultrasound.

Indications for Fetal Intervention

A. Maternal
1. No maternal risk factors

B. Fetal
1. Singleton pregnancy
2. No associated anomalies
3. Decreased amniotic fluid of known duration
4. Normal male karyotype
5. Favorable electrolyte and β_2–microglobulin levels
   a. Electrolytes
      1) Na <100 mEq/liter (<100 mmol/liter)

   2) Cl <90 mEq/liter (<90 mmol/liter)
   3) Osm <210 mEq/liter (<210 mmol/liter)
   4) Ca <8 mg/dl (<2 mmol/liter)
   5) PO_4 <2 mmol/liter
  b. β_2–microglobulin <2 mg/liter
 6. No cortical cysts

FETAL INTERVENTION

A. The current standard for *in utero* intervention for LUTO is ultrasound-guided percutaneous placement of a double-pigtail vesicoamniotic shunt.

B. Although less invasive than an open approach, fetal shunting carries some risks.
 1. Infection
 2. Preterm labor and delivery
 3. Shunt occlusion
 4. Shunt displacement

C. Prenatal shunting is a temporizing measure to facilitate pulmonary survival. It is not a cure.
 1. Postnatal surgical management is still necessary in the majority of cases.
 2. Chronic long-term renal issues may arise, with a potential need for dialysis or transplant.

D. Family education is imperative to informed consent.
 1. To help families grasp the surgical and postnatal management options, involvement of a pediatric urologist/nephrologist familiar with the natural history of LUTO as well as long-term outcomes is essential.

DELIVERY OF THE FETUS

A. The type of delivery selected is dependent on obstetric indication.

B. Fetuses with obstructive uropathy may be delivered vaginally or by cesarean section. The presence and location of a vesicoamniotic shunt should be noted.

POSTNATAL CARE

A. Current outcome data suggest that prenatal intervention may enhance lung development, but its effect on renal function is less clear.
 1. Freedman and colleagues reported on 34 fetuses who were shunted *in utero* over a nine-year period.[41]
  a. Of the 34, 38 percent (13/34) died, and 41 percent (14/34) were above age two at the time of this study.
  b. None of the survivors had long-term respiratory compromise, although 43 percent (6/14) of those who died following shunting had pulmonary hypoplasia.
  c. Of the 14 survivors, 57 percent (8/14) had renal failure or insufficiency and needed transplantation or dialysis, and 43 percent (6/14) had normal renal function.
  d. The majority had small stature (12/14 below the 25th percentile), but were continent.
  e. All children needed medical as well as surgical care related to their renal status.
  f. All were cognitively normal at the time of follow-up.
 2. Although these results appear encouraging, this study clearly indicates that intervention is not curative, and there is room for improvement with respect to patient selection.

Maternal and Fetal Management

PREOPERATIVE CARE

A. The preoperative admission is arranged when the complete evaluation indicates that the mother and fetus are candidates for fetal surgery and the parents choose to proceed.

B. The mother undergoes further preoperative teaching and preparation with the nurse coordinator and obstetric nurse specialist, including a tour of the obstetric and neonatal units.

C. The mother has a preoperative history and physical completed by the obstetrician and the anesthesiologist, and any additional questions and concerns are addressed.

D. The mother may be admitted the night before surgery for a fetus with hydrops or the morning of surgery in the majority of cases.

PERIOPERATIVE CARE

A. On the morning of surgery, uterine contractions and fetal well-being are assessed via the electronic fetal monitor.

B. Compression stockings are placed to prevent embolism.

C. An intravenous line is started, and an indomethacin suppository is administered to provide uterine relaxation.

D. Epidural anesthesia is used for postoperative pain management for the mother.

E. The mother may receive a second indomethacin suppository.

F. The mother is taken to the operating room for anesthetic induction and intubation.
   1. An arterial line and an additional intravenous line are placed.
   2. A Foley catheter is inserted into the bladder.
   3. A sequential compression device to prevent embolic events is activated.

G. The mother is then prepped and draped for the fetal surgery.

H. After sonography confirms no change from the preoperative evaluation, a low transverse maternal laparotomy is done.
   1. Sterile sonography is then used to mark the placental edges.
   2. If the placenta is anterior, the uterus must be lifted up so that the hysterotomy can be made on the posterior aspect of the uterus.
   3. If the placenta is posterior, the hysterotomy is made on the anterior side of the uterus. The hysterotomy is performed using a specially devised stapler, which cuts and staples.[42]

I. Surgery proceeds as follows.
   1. The arm of the fetus is brought out, and a pulse oximeter is applied and secured with a transparent dressing and foil.
   2. The affected portion of the fetus is then exteriorized, and the fetal surgery is performed.

J. Closure proceeds as follows.
   1. The pulse oximeter is removed.
   2. Warmed, normal saline with an antibiotic added is infused into the uterus to substitute for previously lost amniotic fluid.
   3. The hysterotomy is closed.
   4. The maternal abdomen is closed.
   5. A transparent dressing is applied to allow for postoperative sonographic evaluations.

POSTOPERATIVE CARE

A. The mother is awakened and extubated in the operating room.

B. The mother is then transported to the maternal-fetal intensive care unit (MFICU) where intensive monitoring is provided for 48–72 hours.

  1. The MFICU is a devoted area where maternal-fetal intensive care is provided. This includes the following.

    a. Arterial access

    b. Hemodynamic monitoring and special fetal monitoring

      1) Careful fluid management to

        a) Avoid hypovolemia, which leads to poor uterine perfusion

        b) Avoid hypervolemia, which can induce pulmonary edema when magnesium sulfate and betamimetics are used for tocolysis

      2) Daily ultrasound surveillance for fetal well-being and monitoring of amniotic fluid levels

      3) A daily fetal echocardiogram while the mother is receiving indomethacin to assess ductal constriction and tricuspid regurgitation of the fetal heart

    c. Tocolysis and vasoactive drug administration

C. When preterm labor is controlled, the following occur.

  1. The monitoring lines are removed.

  2. Tocolysis is weaned to oral nifedipine or subcutaneous terbutaline as needed.

  3. The epidural catheter and the Foley catheter are then removed.

D. The mother typically remains in the hospital for four days.

E. Plans are made for the discharge of the mother to the nearby Ronald McDonald House.

  1. This requires preauthorization for home monitoring and tocolytic administration.

  2. The Ronald McDonald House has wheelchair accessibility and provides a pager for immediate patient access.

  3. The mother usually remains on modified bed rest for the duration of her pregnancy.

  4. In the majority of fetal surgery cases, the family remains near the hospital for frequent sonographic evaluations and obstetric care for the duration of their pregnancy.

The Fetal Diagnosis and Treatment Center

A. A center for fetal diagnosis and treatment provides a coordinated approach to the care of the mother and fetus with an anomaly, utilizing the many necessary specialists and state-of-the-art facilities required.[43] Because the center focuses on maternal-fetal problems, this model offers a systematic approach for diagnosing and providing treatment options. Thus, expert, coordinated, efficient, and compassionate care is offered to parents facing a decision about their unborn child.

B. The center must provide the following.

  1. The institutional setting for a center must be able to provide a combination of clinical and basic science research with complex antepartum, intrapartum, and postpartum clinical care available for the maternal-fetal patient.

  2. An active maternal transport system and high-risk obstetric and neonatal units are essential.

3. A neonatal resuscitation room adjacent to the operating suite must be available to provide immediate neonatal care and surgical intervention to critically ill newborns as necessary.

4. Numerous items have required miniaturization, adaptation, and sterilization, including the following.[42]
   a. Special surgical instruments
   b. Specially devised staplers
   c. Atraumatic retractors
   d. Level I intrauterine warming device
   e. Fetal medications
   f. Fetal intravenous access equipment

5. In addition to the necessary medical specialists, nurses trained in the management of high-risk obstetric patients are crucial.
   a. Education about fetal surgery should be provided on an ongoing basis to the nursing staff.

6. A center should provide state-of-the-art education to community practitioners so that they can provide the most current information related to prenatal diagnosis and treatment.
   a. Patient education detailing fetal anomalies and supporting literature such as that found at www.fetalsurgery.chop.edu (Children's Hospital of Philadelphia) should be available to provide further education.

7. A center must provide immediate phone consultation and review of sonographic materials.
   a. A toll-free number such as 1-800-IN-UTERO should be established for physicians and families seeking consultations about their unborn child.

C. Many additional resources are required by a center for fetal diagnosis and treatment.

1. A Ronald McDonald House or guesthouse catering to pregnant women on bed rest is crucial to provide a home away from home.

2. Staff inservice education is essential.

3. A program similar to the "Adopt a Mommy to Be" program to provide support for fetal surgery mothers on bed rest may be developed.[43]

4. Travel funds are necessary to provide for immediate transportation needs.

Future Directions

A. The future of fetal therapy is evolving to include prenatal interventions for congenital heart disease,[21,44] cellular transplantation for such diseases as severe combined immunodeficiency[45] and hemoglobinopathies, and gene therapy for diseases such as cystic fibrosis.[46]

B. Further evolution in fetal treatment will include minimally invasive approaches to reduce the risk to the mother and fetus and broaden the applications for fetal surgery.[47]

C. Ongoing assessment, evaluation, and outcome of all clinical experience must be reviewed, analyzed, and reported in the literature.[48]

1. Only then will the natural history of fetal anatomic abnormalities be clarified for obstetricians, neonatologists, pediatricians, and pediatric surgeons.

D. The mandate to the surgical nurse providing care to a fetal, neonatal, or pediatric surgery patient is to understand the natural history of the disease and the future effects on the child so that optimal care and anticipatory guidance can be provided to the family.

REFERENCES

1. Albanese CT, et al. 1998. Fetal liver position and perinatal outcome for congenital diaphragmatic hernia. *Prenatal Diagnosis* 18(11): 1138–1142.

2. Flake AW, et al. 2000. Treatment of severe congenital diaphragmatic hernia by fetal tracheal occlusion: Clinical experience with fifteen cases. *American Journal of Obstetrics and Gynecology* 183(5): 1059–1066.

3. Hedrick HL. 2001. Evaluation and management of congenital diaphragmatic hernia. *Pediatric Case Reviews* 1(1): 25–36.

4. Arensman RM, Bambini DA, and Chiu B. 2005. Congenital diaphragmatic hernia and eventration. In *Pediatric Surgery*, 4th ed., Ashcraft K, Holcomb GW, and Murphy JP, eds. Philadelphia: Saunders, 306–323.

5. Hedrick HL, et al. 2004. Right congenital diaphragmatic hernia: Prenatal assessment and outcome. *Journal of Pediatric Surgery* 39(3): 319–323.

6. Hubbard AM, et al. 1997. Left-sided congenital diaphragmatic hernia: Value of prenatal MR imaging in preparation for fetal surgery. *Radiology* 203(3): 636–640.

7. Harrison MR, et al. 2003. A randomized trial of fetal endoscopic tracheal occlusion for severe fetal congenital diaphragmatic hernia. *New England Journal of Medicine* 349(20): 1916–1924.

8. Deprest J, et al. 2006. Current consequences of prenatal diagnosis of congenital diaphragmatic hernia. *Journal of Pediatric Surgery* 41(2): 423–430.

9. Farrell J. 2007. Personal communication.

10. Stocker JT, Madewell JE, and Drake RM. 1977. Congenital cystic adenomatoid malformation of the lung. Classification and morphologic spectrum. *Human Pathology* 8(2): 155–171.

11. Adzick NS, et al. 1998. Fetal lung lesions: Management and outcome. *American Journal of Obstetrics and Gynecology* 179(4): 884–889.

12. Rice HE, et al. 1994. Congenital cystic adenomatoid malformation: A sheep model of fetal hydrops. *Journal of Pediatric Surgery* 29(5): 692–696.

13. Hedrick HL, et al. 2005. The *ex utero* intrapartum therapy procedure for high-risk fetal lung lesions. *Journal of Pediatric Surgery* 40(6): 1038–1043.

14. Bianchi DW, Crombleholme TM, and D'Alton ME. 2000. *Fetology: Diagnosis and Management of the Fetal Patient.* Columbus, Ohio: McGraw-Hill, 289–298.

15. Laberge J, et al. 2001. Outcome of the prenatally diagnosed congenital cystic adenomatoid lung malformation: A Canadian experience. *Fetal Diagnosis and Therapy* 16(3): 178A–186A.

16. Revillon Y, et al. l993. Congenital cystic adenomatoid malformation of the lung: Prenatal management and prognosis. *Journal of Pediatric Surgery* 28(8): 1009–1011.

17. Sittig S, and Asay G. 2000. Congenital cystic adenomatoid malformation in the newborn: Two case studies and review of the literature. *Respiratory Care* 45(10): 1188–1195.

18. Kitano Y, and Adzick NS. 1999. New developments in fetal lung surgery. *Current Opinion in Pediatrics* 11(3): 193–199.

19. Hubbard AM, Crombleholme TM, and Adzick NS. 1998. Prenatal MRI evaluation of giant neck masses in preparation for the fetal exit procedure. *American Journal of Perinatology* 15(4): 253–257.

20. Crombleholme TM, et al. 2002. Cystic adenomatoid malformation volume ratio predicts outcome in prenatally diagnosed cystic adenomatoid malformation of the lung. *Journal of Pediatric Surgery* 37(3): 331–338.

21. Rychik. 2006. Impact of anomalies other than congenital heart disease on the fetal cardiovascular system. *Progress in Pediatric Cardiology* 22(1): 109–119.

22. Flake AW. 1993. Fetal sacrococcygeal teratoma. *Seminars in Pediatric Surgery* 2(2): 113–120.

23. Gross SJ, et al. 1987. Sacrococcygeal teratoma: Prenatal diagnosis and management. *American Journal of Obstetrics and Gynecology* 156(2): 393–396.

24. Hirose S, and Farmer DL. 2003. Fetal surgery for sacrococcygeal teratoma. *Clinics in Perinatology* 30(3): 493–506.

25. Pantoja E, Llobet R, and Gonzalez-Flores B. 1976. Retroperitoneal teratoma: Historical review. *The Journal of Urology* 115(5): 520–523.

26. Altman RP, Randolph JG, and Lilly JR. 1974. Sacrococcygeal teratoma: American Academy of Pediatrics Surgical Section Survey—1973. *Journal of Pediatric Surgery* 9(3): 389–398.

27. Hedrick HL, et al. 2004. Sacrococcygeal teratoma: Prenatal assessment, fetal intervention, and outcome. *Journal of Pediatric Surgery* 39(3): 430–438.

28. Langer JC, et al. 1989. Fetal hydrops and death from sacrococcygeal teratoma: Rationale for fetal surgery. *American Journal of Obstetrics and Gynecology* 160(5 part 1): 1145–1150.

29. Boemers TML, et al. 1994. Lower urinary tract dysfunction in children with benign sacrococcygeal teratoma. *The Journal of Urology* 151(1): 174–176.

30. Moore KL, and Persaud TVN. 2003. *The Developing Human: Clinically Oriented Embryology,* 7th ed. Philadelphia: Saunders, 435.

31. Adzick NS, et al. 1998. Successful fetal surgery for spina bifida. *Lancet* 352(9141): 1675–1676.

32. Sutton LN, et al. 1999. Improvement in hindbrain herniation demonstrated by serial fetal magnetic resonance imaging following fetal surgery for myelomeningocele. *JAMA* 282(19): 1826–1831.

33. Hedrick MH, et al. 1994. Congenital high airway obstruction syndrome (CHAOS): A potential for perinatal intervention. *Journal of Pediatric Surgery* 29(2): 271–274.

34. Liechty KW, et al. 1997. Intrapartum airway management for giant fetal neck masses: The EXIT (*ex utero* intrapartum treatment) procedure. *American Journal of Obstetrics and Gynecology* 177(4): 870–874.

35. Skarsgard ED, et al. 1996. The OOPS procedure (operation on placental support): *In utero* airway management of the fetus with prenatally diagnosed tracheal obstruction. *Journal of Pediatric Surgery* 31(6): 826–828.

36. Bealer JF, et al. 1995. The "PLUG" odyssey: Adventures in experimental fetal tracheal occlusion. *Journal of Pediatric Surgery* 30(2): 361–365.

37. Biard JM, et al. 2005. Long-term outcomes in children treated by prenatal vesicoamniotic shunting for lower urinary tract obstruction. *Obstetrics and Gynecology* 106(3): 503–508.

38. Mahony BS, Callen PW, and Filly RA. 1985. Renal urethral obstruction: US evaluation. *Radiology* 157(1): 221–224.

39. Cuckow PM. 1998. Posterior urethral valves. In *Pediatric Surgery and Urology: Long-Term Outcomes,* Stringer MD, et al., eds. Philadelphia: Saunders, 487–500.

40. Johnson MP, et al. 1995. Sequential urinalysis improves evaluation of fetal renal function in obstructive uropathy. *American Journal of Obstetrics and Gynecology* 173(1): 59–65.

41. Freedman AL, et al. 1997. Use of urinary beta-2-microglobulin to predict severe renal damage in fetal obstructive uropathy. *Fetal Diagnosis and Therapy* 12(1): 1–6.

42. Harrison MR, and Adzick NS. 1993. Fetal surgical techniques. *Seminars in Pediatric Surgery* 2(2): 136–142.

43. Howell LJ, and Adzick NS. 2003. Establishing a fetal therapy center: Lessons learned. *Seminars in Pediatric Surgery* 12(3): 209–217.

44. Levine JC, and Tworetzky W. 2006. Intervention for severe aortic stenosis in the fetus: Altering the progression of left sided heart disease. *Progress in Pediatric Cardiology* 22(1): 71–78.

45. Flake AW, et al. 1996. Treatment of X-linked severe combined immunodeficiency by *in utero* transplantation of paternal bone marrow. *New England Journal of Medicine* 335(24): 1806–1810.

46. Sylvester KG, et al. 1997. Fetoscopic gene therapy for congenital lung disease. *Journal of Pediatric Surgery* 32(7): 964–969.

47. Yang EY, and Adzick NS. 1998. Fetoscopy. *Seminars in Laparoscopic Surgery* 5(1): 31–39.

48. Flake AW, and Howell LJ. 1998. Fetal surgery. In *Pediatric Surgery and Urology: Long-Term Outcomes,* Stringer MD, et al., eds. Philadelphia: Saunders, 797–805.

Notes

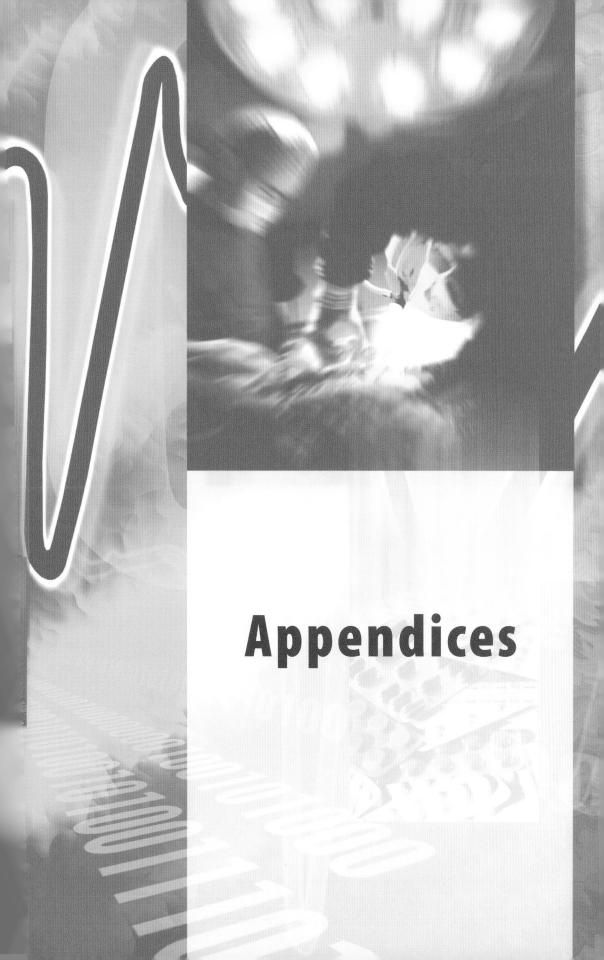

Appendices

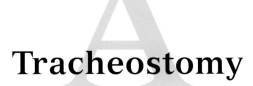

Tracheostomy

Valerie A. Ruth, RN, MS, NNP

INDICATIONS

A. A tracheostomy should be done when it is not possible or desirable to use an endotracheal tube (ETT) for anatomic or physiologic reasons.[1-4]
1. Congenital malformation
2. Advanced epiglottitis
3. Upper airway obstruction
4. Burns or trauma
5. Upper airway bypass
B. Tracheostomy should also be done when prolonged endotracheal intubation is anticipated or when long-term mechanical ventilation or control of airway is indicated due to a central nervous system disorder or failure to wean off the ETT

CONTRAINDICATIONS[2]

A. A tracheostomy is not indicated under the following conditions.
1. The infant has either of the following.
   a. Uncontrolled coagulopathy
   b. Known preexisting laryngeal pathology
2. The practitioner is not familiar with the procedure.
B. Emergency tracheostomy is usually not done. Instead, oro- or nasotracheal intubation or cricothyroidotomy should be attempted first. *It is important that a tracheostomy is performed only under controlled conditions.*

TRACHEOSTOMY PROCEDURE[1,2,4]

A. The following materials are needed.[4]
1. Tracheostomy tray
2. Variety of pediatric-sized tracheostomy tubes
3. Gowns, gloves, and masks for physicians
4. Suction
5. Headlight
6. Two percent lidocaine with epinephrine
7. Bovie electrocautery, if available

B. When appropriate equipment and personnel are available, an urgent tracheostomy can be performed in the emergency department, intensive care unit, or, most preferably, in the operating room.

C. Prepare the patient as follows.

    1. Connect him to a cardiorespiratory monitor. Obtain vital signs.

    2. Establish intravenous access.

    3. Administer general anesthesia.

    4. Introduce orotracheal intubation, if possible, and if not already present.

    5. Position the child supine with the shoulders elevated and the neck hyperextended.

    6. An assistant (either a respiratory therapist or anesthesiologist) aids the child's ventilation with the bag and mask, providing supplemental oxygen and positive pressure.

    7. Administer muscle relaxants as needed.

D. The following is a sample surgical procedure.[1-4]

    1. The larynx and trachea are palpated.

    2. The neck is prepared with povidone-iodine and infiltrated with lidocaine/epinephrine along a horizontal skin crease approximately one finger-breadth above the suprasternal notch.

    3. A horizontal skin incision about 2–3 cm long is placed down to the fascial layer beneath the subcutaneous fat below the cricoid and above the isthmus of thyroid gland. If available, Bovie electrocautery is useful in removing obstructing subcutaneous fat.

    4. Subcutaneous layers are separated, and strap muscles are spread to expose the tracheal rings.

    5. Tracheal cartilage is exposed by blunt dissection. Stay sutures of 4.0 or 5.0 silk or polypropylene are placed in the trachea 1–2 mm lateral to the midline on both sides of the proposed vertical tracheal cartilage incision. These sutures help position the trachea in the operative field and ease placement of the tracheostomy incision.

    6. Traction on the stay sutures elevates the trachea into the skin incision, and a vertical midline incision is made through the third or fourth tracheal rings with a No. 15 scalpel.

    7. Holding the trachea open, the ETT is withdrawn enough to insert an appropriate sized tracheostomy tube.

    8. Both of the infant's lung fields are ventilated and auscultated. Suction is used if necessary.

    9. After confirmation of adequate breath sounds, the tube is secured in place with either tracheostomy ties alone or a combination of ties and sutures placed through the tube flanges to the patient's skin. The skin incision is not sutured closed.

    10. The ETT is removed.

    11. The infant is connected to warm and humidified air or oxygen via the tracheostomy collar, T-piece, or ventilator.

COMPLICATIONS[1,2,4]

A. Aspiration

B. Completely severed trachea

C. Dysphagia

D. Hemorrhage

E. Placement of the tube into a "false passage"

F. Pneumothorax or pneumomediastinum

G. Pulmonary edema

H. Damage to the recurrent laryngeal nerve

I. Respiratory arrest

J. Sepsis

K. Subcutaneous emphysema

L. Tracheal stenosis

M. Tracheoesophageal fistula

N. Torn carotid arteries

POSTOPERATIVE NURSING CARE[1,3]

A. Obtain a chest x-ray postoperatively to ascertain the exact location of the tracheostomy tube tip in relation to the carina.

B. Monitor the infant closely in the NICU or PICU setting for 24 hours.

C. Monitor the infant closely for the following.
   1. Tube patency
   2. Tube position
   3. Any of the complications listed above

D. Ensure standby equipment is present at the bedside.
   1. Obturator
   2. Extra tracheostomy tubes
   3. ETT
   4. Small curved forceps
   5. Bag and mask
   6. Suction equipment
   7. Intubation equipment

E. Physicians and other health care providers should monitor for complications, especially during the nonacute postoperative period. They should be familiar with the equipment and techniques for handling tracheostomy-related emergencies.
   1. Obstructed tracheostomy tube
      a. An infant with a tracheostomy in respiratory distress should be assumed to have a partially or completely obstructed tracheostomy tube.
         1) The usual cause of obstruction is inspissated (thickened) mucus.
         2) Distal tracheal plugging can also occur.
      b. The infant should immediately be placed on high-flow humidified oxygen.
      c. Immediate suctioning should be attempted to clear the tracheostomy tube.
      d. If suctioning does not clear the obstruction, the tracheostomy tube should be removed and replaced with a new tube.
      e. If persistent respiratory distress occurs despite successful tracheostomy tube replacement, other etiologies should be considered (e.g., low tracheal stenosis, pneumonia, aspirated material).
      f. Oral endotracheal intubation should be considered if the physician is unable to replace the tracheostomy tube in a ventilator-dependent patient.
   2. False passage
      a. When a tracheostomy tube has been removed, the proper passage for easy insertion of a new tube may not be found. Simple extension of the neck will line up tissue planes and facilitate passage.
      b. False passages are easily created.

    c. Use of a catheter as a guide prior to removal of the old tube should prevent this complication.

    d. Insertion of a new tube into a false passage can be recognized by the following.

        1) Failure of positive-pressure ventilation to inflate the lungs

        2) Rapid development of subcutaneous emphysema

3. Hemorrhage

    a. After the immediate postoperative period, bleeding from a tracheostomy should be considered a life-threatening emergency until determined otherwise.

        1) Death is caused by exsanguination or asphyxiation from aspirated blood.

    b. A tracheoinnominate fistula has been reported and is most common between one and three weeks postoperatively.[5] The fistula is caused by the following.

        1) An improperly fitted or placed tube eroding tissue

        2) A low tracheotomy site

        3) A tight feeding tube

    c. If premonitory bleeding and hemoptysis occur, prompt bronchoscopy with the tube removed to inspect the tracheal mucosa and identify the bleeding site is necessary.

    d. When massive hemorrhage occurs and a tracheo-innominate fistula is suspected, a cuffed tube can be placed and overinflated to apply internal pressure to the trachea.

        1) If significant hemorrhage continues, digital pressure can be applied simultaneously over the skin of the suprasternal notch, or a gloved finger can be inserted through the skin incision and into the pretracheal soft tissues to compress the artery.

        2) Digital pressure is maintained until an emergency sternotomy can be done and the vessel ligated.

    e. Minor bleeding at the stoma may be due to minor trauma during tube insertion.

        1) If visual inspection clearly identifies a superficial bleeding site, it can be packed or cauterized.

4. Infection

    a. Bacterial contamination of the granulating stoma can occur, but infection is uncommon.

    b. Early peristomal cellulitis is treated with oral antibiotics and closely monitored.

    c. Paratracheal abscess requires prompt drainage and intravenous antibiotics to prevent mediastinitis.

    d. Necrotizing infections around the stoma are rare. Treatment consists of the following.

        1) Prompt removal of the tube

        2) Placement of an oral or nasal ETT

        3) Aggressive debridement of the area

        4) Administration of antibiotics

5. Tracheoesophageal fistula

    a. Tracheoesophageal fistula is rare in the postoperative period.

    b. If present, it is usually caused by the following.

1) Pressure on the membranous trachea by an overinflated tracheostomy tube cuff

2) A poorly positioned tube

c. Increased secretions and coughing after oral feeding are the common symptoms.

1) Aspiration of food or gastric contents may cause pneumonia or pneumonitis.

2) Gastric distention can also be a presenting symptom in ventilated patients.

3) Mediastinitis can also develop.

d. Treatment is surgical repair because this fistula does not spontaneously close.

1) Repair may be deferred until positive pressure ventilation is no longer required.

2) Usually a gastrostomy tube is necessary in these cases.

REFERENCES

1. Oakes D. 2000. *Neonatal/Pediatric Respiratory Care: A Critical Care Pocket Guide*. Oronon, Maine: Health Educator Publications.

2. Pfenninger JL, and Fowler GC. 2003. *Procedures for Primary Care*, 2nd ed. St. Louis: Mosby.

3. Roberts JR, and Hedges JR. 2003. *Clinical Procedures in Emergency Medicine*, 4th ed. Philadelphia: Saunders.

4. Taeusch HW, Christiansen RO, and Buescher ES. 1996. *Pediatric and Neonatal Tests and Procedures*. Philadelphia: Saunders.

5. Tintinalli JE, et al. 2004. *Emergency Medicine: A Comprehensive Study Guide,* 6th ed. McGraw-Hill.

Notes

Notes

Extracorporeal Membrane Oxygenation

Katherine M. Jorgensen, RNC, MSN/MBA, HonD

Extracorporeal membrane oxygenation (ECMO) therapy was first used successfully by Robert Bartlett in 1975.[1] There are a number of centers throughout the world today. The Extracorporeal Life Support Organization registry data set through 1995 reports 83 centers in the U.S. and 21 international centers.

A. There are differences between ECMO and cardiopulmonary bypass.
  1. ECMO uses many of the principles of cardiopulmonary bypass utilized in cardiac surgery, with some fundamental differences.
    a. Cardiopulmonary bypass is thoracic and used exclusively for operative procedures.
    b. ECMO is used as a rescue technique in infants with an 80 percent risk of death using conventional ventilatory modes of therapy.[2,3]
    c. ECMO cannulation is cervical.
    d. The average duration of ECMO is 5 days, with extremes reported of 10 to 21 days.[3–5]
B. The primary pulmonary pathology addressed by ECMO is pulmonary hypertension with significant right-to-left shunting.
  1. Persistent pulmonary hypertension of the newborn
  2. Pulmonary hypertension associated with other diagnoses[3,4,6]
    a. Meconium aspiration syndrome
    b. Sepsis
    c. Severe respiratory distress syndrome
    d. Pneumonia
    e. Congenital diaphragmatic hernia (CDH)
C. Criteria for the use of ECMO are based upon severity of illness and lack of success with conventional therapy.
  1. Conventional therapy is defined as maximal ventilatory support with the following.
    a. Conventional mechanical ventilation
    b. High-frequency oscillation
    c. Nitric oxide

2. To determine if the infant meets the criterion of 80 percent risk of death, several predictors are utilized.[1,3,6]

   a. Evaluation of alveolar/arterial oxygen gradient ($AaDO_2$) to measure ventilation-perfusion mismatch
      1) Criterion level: >600–624 mmHg for 4–12 hours at sea level
      2) Calculation:

      $$AaDO_2 = FiO_2 (760 - 47) - (PaCO_2/0.8)$$

      where: FiO_2 = fraction of inspired oxygen
      760 = barometric pressure (mmHg)
      47 = partial pressure of water vapor
      $PaCO_2$ = alveolar CO_2
      0.8 = respiratory quotient

   b. Evaluation of oxygenation index[1,3,6]
      1) Criterion level: >40 on three out of five blood samples done 30 to 60 minutes apart
      2) Calculation:[7]

      $$OI = \frac{MAP \times FiO_2 \times 100}{PaO_2}$$

   c. PaO_2 level <50 mmHg for four hours
   d. Acute deterioration
      1) PaO_2 level <40 mmHg in 100 percent oxygen for two hours

3. There are contraindications for use of this therapy.
   a. The infant is <34 weeks gestational age.
   b. The infant is <2 kg in weight.
      1) Because of their size, preterm infants and those <2 kg are at increased risk for
         a) Intraventricular hemorrhage (IVH)
         b) Difficulties in cannulation
   c. The infant has been treated for more than 10 days with mechanical ventilation.
   d. The infant has an irreversible cardiopulmonary condition.
      1) ECMO provides lung rest, but does not correct the underlying pulmonary pathology present in prolonged ventilation, such as barotrauma and oxygen toxicity.
      2) ECMO provides a reversal of pulmonary vasoconstriction with the avoidance of hypoxia, hypercarbia, and acidosis.
      3) Many institutions' ECMO criteria exclude congenital heart disease; however, ECMO is used in some postoperative cardiac situations as well as while awaiting transplant.
         a) Infants with severe CDH with significant lung hypoplasia and the absence of any effective oxygenation have very poor outcomes because this lung pathology is incompatible with life.[3]
   e. The infant has a bleeding disorder.
      1) Preexisting bleeding disorders will be exaggerated with the required anticoagulation needed for proper system function.
      2) The infant with IVH is disqualified because the anticoagulation state can cause extension of bleeding.
   f. The infant has major underlying neurologic abnormalities.[1,3,4,6]

4. There are further diagnostics once ECMO criteria are met.
   a. Cranial ultrasound to confirm the absence of an IVH
   b. Echocardiogram to rule out a major cardiac anomaly that could be present and responsible for the nonresponse to conventional treatment

D. The ECMO team performs the following tasks.
   1. The surgical team performs the cannulization.
   2. ECMO specialists are responsible for the ECMO circuit and patient care.
      a. One person is responsible for priming the pump prior to cannulization, accepting the infant, and beginning bypass.
      b. One person will remain responsible for maintaining the function of the pump and titrating gases and medication, while another person is responsible for monitoring the infant and providing patient care.

E. The ECMO circuit can be either venous/arterial or venous/venous.
   1. Venous/arterial circuit[5]
      a. The venous cannula is placed through the internal jugular vein and sits in the right atrium.
      b. The arterial cannula is inserted through the right carotid artery and is positioned with its tip at the aortic arch.
         1) Because of this cannula placement, the infant is at increased risk for neurologic compromise in the event of
            a) Any inadvertent introduction of clots or air emboli into the circulation
            b) Any abrupt alterations in flow
      c. The femoral vein and artery can also be used for placement.
      d. This mode provides both cardiac and pulmonary support.
      e. This is the most common circuit used in the neonatal population.
   2. Venous/venous circuit[5]
      a. The double-lumen cannula is placed most commonly in the internal jugular vein. Placement can also occur using single-lumen cannulae in the jugular and femoral veins.
      b. This mode provides pulmonary support exclusively and requires intrinsic cardiac function.
      c. Venous drainage can be more difficult with this mode, making it a less desirable option.
   3. Venous reservoir
      a. Venous blood is drained by gravity to the venous reservoir.
      b. This reservoir detects sufficient venous drainage and will shut off the pump if the volume is insufficient to proceed.
   4. Pump
      a. The blood flows from the reservoir to the membrane oxygenator with the assistance of a roller pump that provides a nonpulsatile flow.
   5. Membrane oxygenator
      a. The blood flows across the membrane of the oxygenator, where gas exchange occurs with the transfer of oxygen and carbon dioxide.
      b. The rate of flow and the blend of gases provided to the oxygenator membrane regulate the degree of gas exchange.
      c. The usual blood flow needed to achieve adequate gas exchange is 120–140 ml/kg/minute.
         1) This is 60–70 percent of the infant's cardiac output.[4]

    6. Heat exchanger
       a. The blood is rewarmed in the heat exchanger and returned to the infant via the arterial cannula.
F. ECMO is initiated as follows.
    1. The infant is medicated with fentanyl and pancuronium bromide for the procedure.
    2. The cannulae are placed by the surgical team.
       a. The right cervical area of the neck is prepped.
       b. The vessels are dissected.
       c. As the cannulae are placed, the following occurs.
          1) They are sufficiently flushed to displace air from the system, and the circuit is clamped.
          2) Between the venous and arterial circuits, a bridge is placed to allow passage of blood through the circuit until the infant is ready to be brought onto bypass.
       d. When the cannulae are stabilized, they are connected to the system.
          1) First, the arterial side is unclamped, the bridge is clamped, and finally the venous side is unclamped.
          2) The infant is now on bypass.
       e. The cannulae are secured in the cervical area with a sterile occlusive dressing.
    3. Slowly, the flow of the pump is increased to reach either of the following.
       a. The maximum flow of 120–140 ml/kg/minute[4]
       b. The appropriate flow for the infant as determined by blood gas and saturation values
G. Mechanical ventilation is adjusted.
    1. While the infant is on bypass, the ventilator settings are decreased to rest the lungs.
    2. The usual settings while on bypass are as follows.
       a. Fraction of inspired oxygen: (FiO_2) 0.21 (room air) to 0.30
       b. Peak inspiratory pressure: (PIP) 20–25 cm H_2O
       c. Positive end-expiratory pressure: (PEEP) 5–6 cm H_2O
       d. Rate: Ten breaths per minute[6]
    3. These minimal settings have three functions.
       a. Provide the lungs an opportunity to heal
       b. Help prevent atelectasis
       c. Minimize pulmonary edema
H. Indirect monitoring is carried out.
    1. The saturation of venous return is maintained at ≥80 percent.[6]
    2. Postoxygenator PO_2 is maintained between 150 and 400 mmHg to accomplish the following.
       a. Prevent excess oxygenation (>400 mmHg), which is associated with the formation of gas emboli[2]
       b. Provide a patient PO_2 of 50–80 mmHg
    3. Activated clotting time is monitored.
       a. It is checked every 30 to 60 minutes if it is stable.
       b. It is checked more frequently if it is abnormal due to systemic anticoagulation.

    c. The activated clotting time increases initially to a maximum of 400–600 seconds because of the bolus of heparin delivered at the time of cannulation and then decreases to the desired range of 200–220 seconds.[6]

    d. The heparin infusion is titrated to maintain the activated clotting time within this range.

    e. The circuit is periodically inspected for clot formation and air bubbles.

4. Platelet and hematocrit levels are obtained every 8–12 hours.[2] Replacement with platelets and packed red blood cells is provided as indicated.

5. Coagulation factors are assessed twice a week. Fresh frozen plasma is given for low fibrinogen levels.

I. Nursing care and monitoring encompass all of the usual parameters of care.

  1. Cardiovascular and hematologic

    a. Immediately after commencing bypass, a myocardial stun may occur.

      1) This is caused by relief of the cardiac systemic flow and the relatively low oxygen supply to the coronary arteries.

      2) Bradycardia and hypotension characterize this transient phenomenon.

      3) Increasing the circuit flow rate will compensate the infant.[6]

    b. After bypass has begun, arterial tracings will become dampened due to the nonpulsatile nature of flow.

    c. Mean arterial pressure is a reliable value to monitor and is maintained between 40 and 70 mmHg.[2]

    d. Alterations in cardiac output can be detected by changes in pulse pressure when on moderate flow. This allows for an increase in pulsatile flow.

    e. The infant can be weaned from the vasopressors used to maintain perfusion prior to ECMO initiation.

      1) The flow rate will maintain blood pressure while the infant is on ECMO.

    f. As the pulmonary hypertension resolves and volume is maintained, blood pressure stabilizes without the use of inotropic agents.

      1) Occasionally, transient, systemic hypertension can occur initially but rarely requires treatment.

    g. The infant is at great risk for blood loss because of ongoing heparin therapy.

      1) Platelets aggregate on the oxygenator membrane.

      2) Carefully assess bleeding indices in addition to the activated clotting time assessed within the circuit.

      3) Signs of bleeding must be addressed promptly.

  2. Respiratory

    a. Immediately after the initiation of bypass, the pulmonary field on chest x-ray is opaque with atelectasis and/or pulmonary edema.[6]

    b. This initial finding resolves with healing, and later films display clear fields and increased lung compliance that often correspond with readiness to wean off ECMO.

    c. Gentle vibratory chest physiotherapy and suctioning are performed as clinical need determines.

      1) The increased risk of bleeding requires extra care in these activities to decrease potential trauma.[8]

  3. Neurologic

    a. There is a high incidence of adverse neurologic events.[2]

      1) Prior hypoxic or ischemic insult

      2) Alteration in cerebral perfusion

        3) Intracranial hemorrhage due to abrupt shifts in blood pressure and anticoagulation therapy

   b. Assessment is ongoing.

   c. Observe for changes in the infant's behavior and movements.

   d. Seizure activity can be quite ominous in this infant because it can indicate the neurologic complications listed above.

   e. Ongoing monitoring by cranial ultrasounds and evaluation of pupil size and fontanels provide information regarding the presence of an IVH.

   f. Sedation is diminished over time, making infant behavior more meaningful when assessing response to care and interaction.

4. Skin

   a. Assessment of skin condition is necessary.

      1) Skin breakdown and pressure sores can develop with the following.

         a) Edema

         b) Inability to change position

   b. A soft mattress and bedding material will assist with this challenge.

5. Fluid and electrolyte balance

   a. Careful monitoring of all intake and losses is crucial in determining correct fluid balance.[8]

      1) Losses include the following.

         a) Urine output

         b) Blood sampling

         c) Drainage from chest tubes and wounds[2]

      2) The infant's weight will be unavailable if a bed scale is not utilized because the infant cannot be moved onto a freestanding scale.

   b. Fluid administration is initially decreased to 75–80 ml/kg/day, based on birth weight.[2]

   c. Capillary leak syndrome shifts fluids into the extravascular space.

      1) Diuretics may be employed in an attempt to mobilize this fluid.

      2) Hemofiltration can be added to the circuit if necessary to assist in removing excess fluid at a predetermined rate, which is set within the circuit.

   d. If additional fluids are required to maintain perfusion and renal function, albumin and fresh frozen plasma are administered to expand the intravascular space.

   e. As diuresis commences, fluids can be liberalized.

6. Nutrition

   a. To provide nutrition, hyperalimentation can be added to the ECMO circuit with the stabilization of electrolytes and glucose.

7. Prevention and treatment of infection

   a. Careful consideration must be given to aseptic technique.

   b. Antibiotic treatment may be used.

      1) It is administered via the venous side of the ECMO circuit as clinically indicated and ordered.

      2) Because of the volume and flow, the medication may have the following.

         a) A different distribution time than normal

         b) A delay in peak effect[9]

   c. Intramuscular injections and additional venipunctures are contraindicated because of the potential for bleeding caused by heparin therapy.[8]

8. Comfort and pain management

    a. The infant's movement is limited, and the usual comfort measures used with infants are unavailable.

    b. The nurse can promote comfort and decrease agitation with the following.

        1) Soft bedding

        2) Supportive and flexed positioning

        3) Control of the environment

    c. Analgesics such as morphine sulfate and fentanyl can be administered continuously to manage pain and provide sedation.

        1) Fentanyl doses required to obtain the desired effect will be increased because of the binding of fentanyl to the oxygenator membrane.[10]

        2) The infant receiving fentanyl over a number of days will do the following.

            a) Develop a tolerance to this opioid

            b) Require an increase of the dosage for continued desired effect

            c) Require weaning of the dosage prior to discontinuing fentanyl

        3) Sedation can be given concurrently as needed.

        4) Treatment for withdrawal after discontinuance may be necessary.[10]

J. The infant must be weaned off of ECMO.

  1. Weaning is done slowly by decreasing the flow rate.

  2. Periods off of ECMO are attempted prior to decannulation to assess readiness. Ventilatory support is increased to a modest level sufficient to provide physiologic support without causing an increased risk of barotrauma.

  3. When it is time to terminate the therapy, the following occurs.

    a. The circuit is clamped off in the reverse manner: First the venous side, then the arterial side, then unclamping of the bridge in between to permit circulation in the circuit without the infant.[6]

    b. The surgical team decannulates the infant.

        1) Current practice is to ligate the vessels used; however, reconstruction and reanastomosis are being attempted to restore normal circulatory routes.[6] These procedures are dependent on the case, the surgeon, and the institution. No long-term data are available at this time to determine the best potential practice.

  4. Ventilatory support is minimally increased right after decannulization, with many infants being extubated within a week.[6]

K. Parental support is provided.

  1. "Last resort" therapy looks very frightening.

  2. An infant on ECMO has a team of professionals with him at all times, and the parent has very little space at the bedside.

  3. Encourage the parent to provide positive touch that will assist in calming the infant as well as enhancing the parent's well-being and parenting role.

  4. Provide uncomplicated explanations.

  5. Discharge teaching should encompass all aspects of the infant's care as well as any sequelae experienced.

L. Outcomes are as follows.

  1. The reported survival rate is 80–86 percent.[1,3,5,6]

  2. Common long-term complications involve varying degrees of developmental delay.

    a. The question still to be answered in terms of neurologic morbidity is whether these findings are caused by the treatment or the severe conditions of the infants being treated.

REFERENCES

1. Cornish JD. 1993. Extracorporeal membrane oxygenation for severe cardiorespiratory failure. In *Neonatology for the Clinician*, Pomerance JJ, and Richardson CJ, eds. Norwalk, Connecticut: Appleton & Lange, 325–337.

2. Freitag-Koontz MJ, and Ryder S. 1992. Monitoring and evaluating the infant on venoarterial extracorporeal membrane oxygenation. *Journal of Perinatal & Neonatal Nursing* 5(4): 68–86.

3. Stork EK. 2006. Therapy for cardiorespiratory failure. In *Neonatal-Perinatal Medicine: Diseases of the Fetus and Infant*, 7th ed., Martin RJ, Fanaroff AA, and Walsh MC, eds. St. Louis: Mosby, 1168–1180.

4. Short BL. 1998. Physiology of extracorporeal membrane oxygenation. In *Fetal and Neonatal Physiology*, 2nd ed., Polin RA, and Fox WW, eds. Philadelphia: Saunders, 1243–1248.

5. Extracorporeal Life Support Organization. 1999. *Neonatal ECMO Specialist Training Manual*, 2nd ed. Ann Arbor, Michigan: ELSO.

6. Chandra S, and Baumgart S. 2005. Modern extracorporeal membrane oxygenation for the human newborn infant. In *Intensive Care of the Fetus and Neonate*, 2nd ed., Spitzer AR, ed. St. Louis: Mosby, 681–699.

7. Ortiz RM, Cilley RE, and Bartlett RH. 1987. Extracorporeal membrane oxygenation in pediatric respiratory failure. *Pediatric Clinics of North America* 34(1): 39–46.

8. Schwartz JE. 2003. New technologies applied to the management of the respiratory system. In *Comprehensive Neonatal Nursing: A Physiologic Perspective*, 3rd ed., Kenner C, and Lott JW, eds. Philadelphia: Saunders, 363–375.

9. Shields B. 2003. Principles of newborn and infant drug therapy. In *Comprehensive Neonatal Nursing: A Physiologic Perspective*, 3rd ed., Kenner C, Lott JW, eds. Philadelphia: Saunders, 857–867.

10. Caron E, and Maguire DP. 1990. Current management of pain sedation and narcotic physical dependency of the infant on ECMO. *Journal of Perinatal & Neonatal Nursing* 4(1): 63–74.

Notes

Broviac Insertion

Katherine M. Jorgensen, RNC, MSN/MBA, HonD

Central venous catheters are required for long-term venous access in infants with complex illnesses and a need for long-term parenteral nutrition.

A. Correct placement
1. The tip is in the superior vena cava near the right atrium.
2. Proper tip placement for saphenous access is in the inferior vena cava above or below the renal and mesenteric veins.[1]
B. Veins commonly used to place a Broviac catheter:
1. External and interior jugular
2. Facial
3. Axillary
C. Type of catheter
1. Silicone Broviac catheters with a Dacron cuff are available in single-, double-, and triple-lumen configurations and are generally used exclusively for hyperalimentation.
2. The silicone material is relatively nonthrombotic.
3. The Dacron cuff secures the placement of the line as well as deters ascending infection.[1]
D. Line placement
1. The catheter is placed surgically using a cut-down and tunneled approach.
2. The line is initially placed in a sterile manner, and maintenance of the line is a sterile procedure.
3. Dressing changes should be done according to unit protocol, using strict aseptic technique.
E. Complications
1. Infection
    a. The infection rate is reported to be 7–50 percent.[1]
    b. The most common bacterial agent identified was methicillin-resistant *Staphylococcus epidermidis* treated with vancomycin.[1]
    c. Any early signs of infection such as redness at the site or drainage must be noted immediately to ensure proper treatment.
    d. The antibiotic can be delivered via the Broviac line in an attempt to clear the line of the organism, which would eliminate the need for removal of the line.

2. Mechanical complications[1]
   a. Thrombi
   b. Emboli
   c. Dislodgement
   d. Extravascular delivery of fluid
   e. Breakage
   f. Occasionally, the cuff becomes lodged and will require surgical removal.

REFERENCE

1. Katz AL, and Wolfson P. 2005. Surgical management of the neonate. In *Intensive Care of the Fetus and Neonate*, 2nd ed., Spitzer AR, ed. St. Louis: Mosby, 1353–1368.

Notes

Gastrostomy Tube Placement

Diane B. Longobucco, RNC, MSN, APRN, NNP

DEFINITION

A gastrostomy tube (G-tube) is placed during a surgical procedure that creates a fistulous tract (opening or ostomy) between the stomach and abdominal wall.[1] A small, hollow tube is inserted through the abdominal wall and into the stomach. The stomach is then stitched closed around the tube, and the incision is closed. The tube can be used for feeding or drainage. This procedure is one of the oldest abdominal operations in continuous use.[1]

There are three components of the gastrostomy tube.[2] These are: 1) the portion within the stomach (retention tip), with either a balloon tip or a nonballoon tip; 2) the portion (body) on or outside of the skin. It may be a traditional tube or a skin-level device (button); and 3) the feeding port.

INDICATIONS[1,2]

A. A G-tube may be placed because an infant temporarily or permanently requires feeding directly into the stomach. The reasons may include:[2]
1. Congenital anomalies of the:
   a. Mouth
   b. Jaw
   c. Pharynx
   d. Esophagus
   e. Stomach
   f. Gastrointestinal (GI) tract and/or airway
      1) Problems sucking or swallowing
      2) Drainage or decompression of the stomach needed
      3) Severe neurologic impairment (cerebral palsy, encephalopathy)
      4) Additional nutrition for infants who cannot take enough food by mouth (either permanently or temporarily)

LOCATION

A. The preferred site of the G-tube is in the left upper quadrant below the left costal margin.

B. The following areas should be avoided.

    1. The costal margin—to reduce discomfort from tube migration with normal breathing efforts[3]

    2. The umbilicus

    3. The belt line—to reduce irritation at the edge of the diaper and pants with elastic as the infant gets older

    4. Any areas of folds, creases, or wrinkles[3]

PROCEDURES

A. An antireflux procedure such as Nissen, Thal, or Toupet fundoplication may be done in infants at high risk for gastroesophageal reflux.[2]

B. Surgically placed gastrostomy proceeds as follows.[2,3]

    1. The tube may be inserted laparoscopically or through an open incision under general anesthesia.

    2. A small incision is made on the left side of the abdomen, and then an incision is made through the stomach.

    3. The stomach is sutured to the abdominal wall to stabilize it.

    4. A small, flexible, hollow tube with a balloon or flared tip is inserted through the tract and into the stomach; it is then sutured into place.

    5. The stomach is sutured closed around the tube, and the incision is closed.

    6. The balloon is inflated to fit snugly against the abdominal wall.[2,3]

    7. Healing and maturation of the gastrostomy tube tract occurs four to six weeks following surgery.[4]

C. Percutaneous endoscopic gastrostomy (PEG) proceeds as follow.[2,3]

    1. It is done via endoscopy.

    2. Air is inserted to inflate the stomach.

    3. The stomach is transilluminated at the desired puncture spot.

    4. A small incision is made at the identified site.

    5. A needle is passed through the abdominal wall at the identified site.

    6. Suture wire is threaded through the needle into the stomach and grasped by the endoscopy snare.

    7. The other end of the suture wire is tied to the distal end of G-tube and pulled to the stomach through the abdominal wall.

    8. The tube is then stabilized with an internal "bumper" and an external attachment device.

    9. The endoscope is reinserted to verify correct positioning.

    10. Healing and maturation of the gastrostomy tract takes place in about 12 weeks.[4]

    11. This is a simple and safe way to place a G-tube.

        a. The infant does not require general anesthesia.

        b. This procedure holds a lower risk and complication rate than a surgically placed tube.

D. Radiologic placement

    1. This approach utilizes fluoroscopic guidance to place the gastrostomy tube into the correct position.

    2. A G-tube is introduced percutaneously to hold the gastric wall in opposition.[2]

ALTERNATE PROCEDURES

A. Gastrostomy button[2,3,5]

1. Gastrostomy buttons were developed in 1982 as a replacement for a gastrostomy tube.
2. The button is a skin-level device with a one-way valve.
3. It consists of a short silicone tube with:
   a. An internal and external anchor
   b. A one-way antireflux valve
   c. A connecting device
4. The adapter is passed through the one-way valve and connected to a feeding catheter.
5. There are two types of buttons: Those with a
   a. Mushroom or dome-style internal stabilizer
   b. Balloon tip as an internal stabilizer
6. The size of the button depends on
   a. The thickness of the abdominal wall
   b. The diameter of the prior gastrostomy tube
7. Care of the button is the same as that of a G-tube, with rotation of the button during daily cleaning to relieve skin pressure.[2]

POSTOPERATIVE PROCEDURAL CARE

A. Monitor
   1. Vital signs
   2. Gravity draining of the tube for first 24 hours
   3. The site at least once a shift for:
      a. Redness
      b. Drainage
      c. Induration
      d. Tube stability and fit: If the tube is too loose, leakage of gastric contents may cause skin irritation.
   4. Bowel sounds
      a. Begin feedings once bowel sounds are present.
      b. The gastrostomy tube can be flushed with sterile water postoperatively, prior to the initiation of feedings. (Institutional policies may vary.)
B. Document[2]
   1. Type of tube (mushroom or balloon tip)
   2. Balloon volume (measured daily)
   3. Tube length (insertion site to distal end of tube measured daily)
C. G-tube site care
   1. Healing takes place within two weeks.
   2. Skin care around the gastrostomy tube includes cleaning with a mild, pH-balanced soap and water.
      a. Half-strength peroxide for site care is no longer recommended because it is irritating and may be cytotoxic.[6,7]
   3. Use gauze or a cotton-tipped applicator to gently remove all crusty material (a small amount of clear drainage can be expected in the first few weeks following insertion).[8]
   4. Dry completely after cleaning.
   5. Maintain a dry dressing around the gastrostomy tube site, and change it once or twice a day as necessary to maintain dryness.

TABLE D-1 ■ **Sample of Products used to Stabilize G-tubes.**

Product	Advantages	Disadvantages
Baby bottle nipple, 4 × 4 gauze, tape	Inexpensive. Easy to apply.	Cannot be used by patients with adhesive or latex sensitivity.
Catheter tube holder	Easy to apply. G-tube can be repositioned.	Skin at insertion site is not protected. Cannot be used by patients with adhesive or latex sensitivity
Drain/tube attachment	Protective skin barrier. Self-Adhesive. Clamping mechanism used to keep tube in place. Hypoallergenic.	Cannot be used by patients with adhesive or latex sensitivities.
Semipermeable foam dressing, tape	Non-adherent. Very absorbent.	Cannot be used by patients with adhesive or latex sensitivity.

    a. Use this gauze until healing takes place.

    b. A dressing is not recommended after the incisional area has healed because it can keep the area moist and may cause skin breakdown.

  6. Rotate the external bumper or other retaining device 90 degrees once a day to prevent irritation and relieve skin pressure ulcers.[2,8]

  7. Assess the skin around the tube for necrosis.

    a. Very tight placement of the bumper at the skin level may result in pressure necrosis, leading to ulceration or migration of the tube into the abdominal wall.

D. Tube stabilization

  1. Ensure that the tube is secure so that excessive movement does not occur.

  2. If the tube is too large, it may need to be replaced with a thinner, softer one to decrease movement.

  3. Tubes can be stabilized using (Table D-1):

    a. Baby bottle nipples[7,8]

      1) Cut off the end of a nipple and slide the nipple over the tube until the base is against the infant's body. Secure the wide end of the nipple to the skin barrier and the tube to the nipple with tape.

      2) This type of stabilization is unsuitable for an infant with tape/latex sensitivities.

    b. Foam dressings

      1) Highly absorbent and nonadherent

      2) Unsuitable for infants with tape sensitivity

      3) Available in latex-free foam

    c. Drain/tube attachment device

      1) Provides a skin barrier

      2) Uses a clamping device to keep the tube stable

      3) Unsuitable for infants with tape/latex sensitivity

    d. Tube holder

      1) Easily applied

      2) Unsuitable for infants with tape sensitivity

  4. Taping techniques:[7]

    a. "H" or "goalpost" taping technique (Figure D-1)

    b. "Slit tape" taping method (Figure D-2)

  5. Secure the free end of the tube so that the infant cannot pull it:

    a. Tuck the tube inside a one-piece undershirt.

FIGURE D-1 ■ "H" or "goalpost" taping of G-tube.

A. Prepared tape with tabs. B. Prepared "T" tape. C. Completed securing method with slit 2×2 gauze sponge.

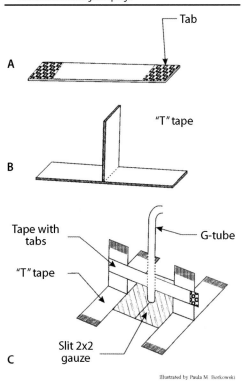

Illustrated by Paula M. Borkowski

Adapted from: Borkowski S. 2004. Similar gastrostomy peristomal skin irritations in three pediatric patients. *Journal of Wound, Ostomy, and Continence Nursing* 31(4): 202. Reprinted by permission.

FIGURE D-2 ■ "Slit tape" method of securing G-tube.

A. prepared tape with tab. B. Prepared tape in position on gastrostomy tube.

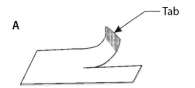

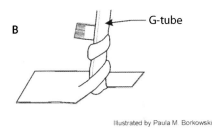

Illustrated by Paula M. Borkowski

Adapted from: Borkowski S. 2004. Similar gastrostomy peristomal skin irritations in three pediatric patients. *Journal of Wound, Ostomy, and Continence Nursing* 31(4): 203. Reprinted by permission.

    b. Wrap a piece of tape around the tubing, and secure it with a pin to the infant's diaper or clothing.

    c. Place the end of the tubing under the tabs of a disposable diaper.

E. Pain management **(See Chapter 10: Assessment and Management of Postoperative Pain.)**

FEEDING

A. Flush the gastrostomy tube with water after each feeding or medication given.

B. For bolus feedings, the infant should remain upright or on his right side (in seat or in arms) for 45 minutes following the feeding.

COMPLICATIONS

A. Increased risk with longer use

B. Infection at the incision site

    1. Usually limited to incision site, skin, and subcutaneous tissue, signs include the following.[1]

      a. Redness

      b. Discharge

      c. Swelling

      d. Soreness

      e. Odor

   2. Clean more frequently with mild soap and water.

   3. Use a gauze dressing if drainage occurs.

C. Bleeding

   1. Bleeding may occur in the postoperative period and is related to:[1]

      a. Inadequate hemostasis at the time of insertion *or*

      b. Difficulty with stapling or suturing

D. Granulation tissue

   1. Granulation tissue is overgrown epithelial tissue that is pink-red in color, inflamed, and may bleed easily.

   2. It can develop at the site as a result the body's reaction to a foreign body.

   3. Excessive G-tube movement may also cause or exacerbate the formation of granulation tissue.

   4. Topical application with silver nitrate ($AgNO_3$) sticks may be used to treat granulated tissue.[9]

      a. Applying petroleum ointment to the normal skin around the granulated tissue helps to prevent irritation from silver nitrate.[9]

E. Dislodgement

   1. Pulling on or applying tension to the tube can cause it to dislodge.

      a. Most tubes have internal (inside the stomach) and external (outside the stomach) anchors.

         1) The internal anchor keeps the tube from falling out.

         2) The external anchor keeps the tube from being pulled into the stomach.

   2. Dislodgement or accidental removal with subsequent reinsertion, especially in first two weeks after placement, may lead to peritonitis.

      a. During the attempt to replace tube, the stomach may be pushed away from the abdominal wall.[1]

      b. Because a fistula tract has not been established, the formula or gastric contents may leak into the peritoneal cavity.

   3. Replace the tube as quickly as possible.

      a. The tube needs to be replaced within four hours so that the tract does not close.

      b. Parents must be taught the following.

         1) How to avoid accidental removal

         2) How to replace the tube or to cover the site with gauze and notify the health care provider immediately for replacement

F. Leaking

   1. Leaking is a greater problem in infants and children than adults because of the following.

      a. Thinner abdominal wall

      b. More motion

      c. A proportionally larger tube

      d. Increased intra-abdominal pressure during crying[1]

   2. Less leakage is seen with PEG stomas

   3. Maintaining a sealed system created by the intragastric seal (balloon or mushroom) and the transabdominal seal (the portion of tissue between the stomach and the external abdominal wall) can alleviate leaking.

      a. Balloon inflation may need to be evaluated.[2,9]

4. Care of a leaking stoma includes the following.
   a. Clean fluid away with a wet gauze.
   b. For excessive exudates, use gauze around the site to absorb it.
      1) Gauze should not be left to soak the area, but should be changed frequently to keep moisture off of the skin.
   c. Occlusive dressings are not recommended.[1]
   d. A barrier cream or a foam dressing can be applied to protect the skin around the stoma.
   e. Stoma adhesive powder can be used at the site to help maintain dry skin but should be cleaned off each day to prevent buildup.[9]

G. Irritation
   1. The external anchor may be positioned too firmly against the skin and will irritate it.
   2. Irritation can be caused by leakage moistening the skin.
   3. Care includes the following.
      a. Clean the area more frequently.
      b. A barrier cream or another type of barrier can be applied to protect the skin around the stoma.

H. Blockage
   1. Prevent blockage by flushing the tube with sterile water before and after a feeding and/or medication administration to maintain patency of the tube.[9]
   2. If blockage occurs, a urethral catheter can be inserted into the plugged gastrostomy tube to dislodge the obstruction.[1]

I. Abdominal distention
   1. Gastric distention can cause acidic stomach contents to leak around the tube and result in skin irritation.
      a. A barrier ointment or skin barrier wipe can be used to protect the skin around the tube.
   2. Infants with fundoplication may require manual decompression before or after feedings in order to avoid abdominal distention.
      a. This is done by opening the tube to allow gas to escape the stomach.[4]

J. Separation of the stomach from the abdominal wall
   1. May occur on reinsertion of a displaced tube[10]
   2. Occurs with premature tube change before the gastrostomy tract has had time to heal and mature

K. Migration of the G-tube internally[1,7,9]
   1. To the esophagus, can cause:[7]
      a. Vomiting
      b. Potential aspiration
   2. To the pylorus, can cause:[7]
      a. Gastric outlet obstruction
      b. Vomiting
      c. Abdominal distention
      d. Discomfort
   3. To the small intestine, can cause:[7]
      a. Dumping syndrome
      b. Bloating, nausea, colic, and explosive diarrhea
      c. Diaphoresis, weakness, and pallor

L. Tube prolapse into duodenum[10]

M. Tube breakdown

N. Mechanical trauma from stripping of tape or other adhesive[8]

    1. Use adhesive removers to loosen adhesive.

O. Candidiasis (rash)

    1. Treat with a topical antifungal powder.

    2. Keep the area around tube dry.

P. GI symptoms related to multifactorial causes[1,11]

    1. High formula osmolality

    2. Rapid infusion of a large volume

    3. Lactose or feeding intolerance

    4. Cold feedings

    5. Nausea

    6. Vomiting

    7. Diarrhea

    8. Constipation

PARENT TEACHING

A. Skin care

B. Signs and symptoms of infection

C. What to do if tube is accidentally pulled out

D. Signs and symptoms of common complications

E. Feeding and medication administration

F. Assessing tube length (daily) and balloon volume (one to two times/week)[3]

G. Stabilizing and concealing the tube beneath clothing

REFERENCES

1. Gauderer ML, and Stellato TA 1986. Gastrostomies: Evolution, techniques, indications, and complications. *Current Problems in Surgery* 23(9): 661–719.

2. Burd A, and Burd R. 2003. The who, what, why and how-to guide for gastrostomy tube placement in infants. *Advances in Neonatal Care* 3(4): 197–205.

3. Young M, McClure E, and Thimsen-Whitaker K. 1992. Management of percutaneous tubes. In *Acute and Chronic Wounds. Nursing Management,* Bryant R, ed. St. Louis: Mosby, 213–247.

4. Rogers V. 2004. Commentary. *Journal of Wound, Ostomy, and Continence Nursing* 31(4): 205–206.

5. Gauderer MWL, et al. 1988. Feeding gastrostomy button: Experience and recommendations. *Journal of Pediatric Surgery* 23(1): 24–28.

6. Goette DK, and Odom RM. 1977. Skin blanching induced by hydrogen peroxide. *Southern Medical Journal* 70(5): 620–622.

7. Borkowski S. 2004. Similar gastrostomy peristomal skin irritations in three pediatric patients. *Journal of Wound, Ostomy, and Continence Nursing* 31(4): 201–205.

8. O'Brien B, Davis S, and Erwin-Toth P. 1999. G-tube site care: A practical guide. *RN* 62(2): 52–56.

9. Bordwewick AJ, Bildner JI, and Burd RS. 2001. An effective approach for preventing and treating gastrostomy tube complications in newborns. *Neonatal Network* 20(2): 37–40.

10. Thorne S, and Radford MJ. 1998. A comparative longitudinal study of gastrostomy devices in children. *Western Journal of Nursing Research* 20(2): 145–165.

11. Farley JM. 1988. Current trends in enteral feeding. *Critical Care Nurse* 8(4): 23–38.

Notes

Infant Pain Scales

FIGURE E-1 ■ Neonatal Infant Pain Scale (NIPS) operational definitions.

Facial expression	
0 - Relaxed Muscles	Restful face, neutral expression
1 - Grimace	Tight facial muscles, furrowed brow, chin, jaw (negative facial expression—nose, mouth, and brow)
Cry	
0 - No Cry	Quiet, not crying
1 - Whimper	Mild moaning, intermittent
2 - Vigorous Cry	Loud scream, rising, shrill, continuous (Note: Silent cry may be scored if baby is intubated, as evidenced by obvious mouth, facial movement.)
Breathing patterns	
0 - Relaxed	Usual pattern for this baby
1 - Change in Breathing	Indrawing, irregular, faster than usual, gagging, breath holding
Arms	
0 - Relaxed/Restrained	No muscular rigidity, occasional random movements of arms
1 - Flexed/Extended	Tence, straight arms, rigid and/or rapid extension, flexion
Legs	
0 - Relaxed/Restrained	No muscular rigidity, occasional random leg movement
1 - Flexed/Extended	Tense, straight legs, rigid and/or rapid extension, flexion
State of arousal	
0 - Sleeping/Awake	Quiet, peaceful, sleeping or alert and settled
1 - Fussy	Alert, restless, and thrashing

Copyright 1989, Children's Hospital of Eastern Ontario. Reprinted by permission.

FIGURE E-2 ■ CRIES: Neonatal postoperative pain assessment score.

	Scoring Criteria for Each Assessment			
	0	1	2	Infant's Score
Crying	No	High-pitched	Inconsolable	
Requires O$_2$ for saturation >95%	No	<30%	>30%	
Increased vital signs*	HR and BP within 10% of preoperative value	HR or BP 11–20% higher than preoperative value	HR or BP 21% or more above preoperative value	
Expression	None	Grimace	Grimace/grunt	
Sleepless	No	Wakes at frequent intervals	Constantly awake	
			Total score†	

* BP should be done last.

† Add scores for all assessments to calculate total score.

© S. Krechel, MD, and J. Bildner, RNC, CNS. Neonatal pain assessment tool developed at the University of Missouri–Columbia. Reprinted by permission.

FIGURE E-3 ■ FLACC behavioral pain scale.

Categories	Scoring		
	0	1	2
Face	No particular expression or smile	Occasional grimace or frown, withdrawn, disinterested	Frequent to constant frown, clenched jaw, quivering chin
Legs	Normal position or relaxed	Uneasy, restless, tense	Kicking, or legs drawn up
Activity	Lying quietly, normal position, moves easily	Squirming, shifting back and forth, tense	Arched, rigid, or jerking
Cry	No cry (awake or asleep)	Moans or whimpers, occasional complaint	Crying steadily, screams or sobs, frequent complaints
Consolability	Content, relaxed	Reassured by occasional touching, hugging, or being talked to, distractable	Difficult to console or comfort

Each of the five categories (F) Face; (L) Legs; (A) Activity; (C) Cry; (C) Consolability is scored from 0–2, which results in a total score between zero and ten.

© 2002, The Regents of the University of Michigan. All Rights Reserved. Reprinted by permission.

FIGURE E-4 ■ Premature Infant Pain Profile (PIPP).

Infant study number: _____
Date/time: _____
Event: _____

Process	Indicator	0	1	2	3	Score
Chart	Gestational age	36 weeks and more	32 weeks to 35 weeks, 6 days	28 weeks to 31 weeks, 6 days	28 weeks and less	
Observe infant 15 seconds Observe baseline Heart rate ____ Oxygen saturation ____	Behavioral state	Active/awake Eyes open Facial movements	Quiet/awake Eyes open No facial movements	Active/sleep Eyes closed Facial movements	Quiet/sleep Eyes closed No facial movements	
Observe infant 30 seconds	Heart rate maximum ____	0–4 beats/minute increase	5–14 beats/minute increase	15–24 beats/ minute increase	25 beats/minute or more increase	
	Oxygen saturation minimum ____	0–2.4% decrease	2.5–4.9% decrease	5.0–7.4% decrease	7.5% or more decrease	
	Brow bulge	None 0–9% of time	Minimum 10–39% of time	Moderate 49–69% of time	Maximum 70% of time or more	
			Minimum 10–39% of time	Moderate 49–69% of time	Maximum 70% of time or more	
			Minimum 10–39% of time	Moderate 49–69% of time	Maximum 70% of time or more	
					Total Score	

Adapted from: Stevens B, et al. 1996. Premature Infant Pain Profile: Development and initial validation. *The Clinical Journal of Pain* 12(1): 22. Reprinted by permission.

Notes

Notes

Glossary

Acholic stool: Without bile, as in pale stools.

Aerophagia: Abnormal swallowing of air.

Agenesis: Failure of formation or development.

Alae: A winglike structure or appendage.

Albumin: A simple protein found in blood that acts as a carrier molecule and helps to maintain blood pressure and volume.

Alginate: A wound dressing produced from brown seaweed. Used as a primary dressing.

Amblyopia: Poor vision caused by abnormal development of visual areas in the brain in response to abnormal visual stimulation in early development.

Amelia: Congenital absence of limb or limbs. Autosomal dominant, autosomal recessive, and X-linked forms have been reported, but most cases are sporadic.

Amorphous: Not crystallized, without definite shape or differentiation in structure that is visible.

Anechoic: Capable of transmitting, rather than reflecting, sound waves to an ultrasound transducer. Refers to fluid-filled structures (e.g., gallbladder, urinary bladder) that appear dark on ultrasound.

Anemia: Any condition in which the number of red blood cells, the amount of hemoglobin, and the volume of packed red blood cells in the blood are lower than normal levels. Symptoms include fatigue, lethargy, shortness of breath, pallor of the skin and mucous membranes, heart palpitations, and soft systolic murmurs.

Angiogenesis: The formation of new blood vessels.

Anions: An ion carrying a negative charge.

Anlage: The beginning of an organized tissue, organ, or part in an embryo.

Anoplasty: Reconstructive surgery of the anus.

Anorchid: Congenital absence of the testes.

Antegrade: Moving forward or in the same direction as the flow.

Anterior commissure: Bundle of white fibers connecting the cerebral hemispheres across the middle; contains fibers from olfactory tracts.

Anticipatory grief: Grief that occurs prior to the loss; for example, anticipatory grief is experienced when a family receives a prenatal diagnosis known to have a poor neonatal outcome.

Apocrine gland: A large sweat gland that produces fluid; found in select areas of the body such as the axilla and pubic region. It appears after puberty and has a characteristic odor.

Approximation: A placing or bringing closer together.

Aqueduct of Sylvius: The channel that connects the third ventricle to the fourth ventricle.

Ascites: Accumulation of serous fluid within the peritoneal cavity.

Asphyxia: Impaired oxygenation and perfusion resulting in acidosis, hypoxia, or hypercarbia.

Atelectasis: Airlessness; decreased or absent expansion of all or part of the lung resulting in volume loss.

Atresia: Congenital absence of a normal opening or patent lumen.

Autolytic: A self-dissolving that occurs in tissues or cells in some pathologic conditions or after death.

Avulsion: The ripping or tearing away of a part either accidentally or surgically.

Azotemia: Presence of nitrogenous bodies, especially urea in increased amounts, in the blood.

Balanoposthitis: Inflammation of the skin covering the glans penis.

Barotitis (Aerotitis): Inflammation of the ear, especially in the middle ear due to failure of the Eustachian tube to remain open during changes in pressure such as those that occur during flying.

Barotrauma: Stretch injury to pulmonary tissue, generally as a consequence of mechanical ventilation.

Bicornate: Having two projections or processes.

Bile: The yellowish brown or green fluid secreted by the liver into the duodenum where it assists in the emulsification of fats, increases peristalsis, and slows putrefaction.

Biliary atresia: A rare condition that is caused by the abnormal development of the bile ducts inside or outside the liver.

Biliary cirrhosis: Due to biliary obstruction, which may be a primary intrahepatic disease or secondary to obstruction of extrahepatic bile ducts. The latter may lead to cholestasis and proliferation in small bile ducts with fibrosis. Marked disturbance of the lobular pattern is infrequent.

Bilirubin: A pigment produced when the liver processes waste products. Excess bilirubin is associated with jaundice.

Bilirubinemia: The presence of bilirubin in the blood.

Biopsy: Process of removing tissue from patients for diagnostic examination.

Bossing: A bulge of the frontal areas of the skull.

Bronchoscopy: Technique of inspection of interior of the airway, utilizing a specialized device such as bronchoscope; may be either a diagnostic or therapeutic procedure.

Calyx: A cuplike extension of the renal pelvis that surrounds the papilla of a renal pyramid.

Cardioplegia: Intentional temporary arrest of cardiac function by medication, electrical stimuli, or hypothermia in order to reduce the need for oxygen.

Carina: Ridge separating the openings of the right and left mainstem bronchi as they join with the trachea.

Cations: Positively charged ions.

Caudal: Pertaining to any taillike structure.

Cecal: Pertaining to the cecum.

Cephalad: Toward the head.

Chemotaxis: The movement of white blood cells to an area of inflammation in response to the release of chemical mediators by neutrophils, monocytes, and injured tissue.

Chemotherapy: Treatment of disease by means of chemical substances or drugs; usually used in reference to neoplastic disease.

Chiari deformation: An abnormality in which the inferior poles of the cerebellar hemispheres and the medulla protrude through the foramen magnum into the spinal canal. It is one of the causes of hydrocephalus and is usually accompanied by spina bifida cystica and meningomyelocele.

Choanae: A funnel-shaped opening of the posterior nares.

Cholangitis: Inflammation of the bile duct.

Chondral: Pertaining to the cartilage.

Chordee: Painful downward curvature of the penis during an erection.

Choroid: The vascular layer of the eye between the retina and the sclera.

Choroid plexus: A capillary network located in each of the four ventricles of the brain (two lateral, the third, and the fourth) that produces cerebrospinal fluid by filtration and secretion.

Choroidal vessels: Network of vessels in the dark blue vascular layer of the eye between the sclera and retina.

Chronic grief: Unresolved and continuing grief, for example, when an infant continues to have special care needs.

Cicatricial: A scar that constricts.

Cicatricial retinal changes: Changes in a retinal scar.

Cicatrix: A scar left by a healed wound.

Cirrhosis: Chronic liver disease characterized by diffuse damage to hepatic parenchymal cells with ineffective regeneration, scarring, and disturbance of normal architecture.

Clinical utility: Psychometric measure of the ability to use the results of the instrument in a meaningful, useful way in the clinical setting.

Cloaca: A cavity lined with endoderm at the posterior end of the body that is a passageway for urinary, digestive, and reproductive ducts.

Clonic: Alternately contracting and relaxing the muscles.

Collagen: Fibrous, insoluble protein that is produced by fibroblasts. Comprises bone, cartilage, ligaments, connective tissue, and skin. In wounds, collagen fibers and granulation tissue help wounds heal.

Colloid: Aggregates of atoms or molecules in a finely divided state (submicroscopic), dispersed in a gaseous, liquid, or solid medium and resisting sedimentation, diffusion, and filtration, thus differing from precipitates.

Coloboma: Any defect, especially of the eye due to incomplete closure of the optic fissure.

Colostomy: Surgical creation of an opening from the abdominal wall into the colon.

Columella: A little column.

Commissure: A transverse band of nerve fibers that pass over the midline in the central nervous system.

Congenital: Existing at birth, referring to certain mental or physical traits, anomalies, malformations, and diseases that may be either hereditary or due to an influence occurring during prenatal development.

Conjugated bilirubin: Direct reacting bilirubin.

Contextual factors: Set of facts or circumstances that surround a situation or event.

Contraction alkalosis: Caused by the loss of bicarbonate-poor, chloride-rich extracellular fluid via thiazide or loop diuretic therapy or chloride diarrhea. Contraction of the extracellular fluid volume causes an increase in bicarbonate concentration.

Contralateral: On the opposite side of the body.

Conus (conus medullaris): The cone-shaped lower end of the spinal cord at the level of the upper lumbar vertebrae; also called c. terminalis and terminal cone of spinal cord.

Corneal button: Used in corneal transplantation. A circular section or button cut from the clear corneal tissue.

Cremaster: Fascia-like muscle that envelopes and suspends the testicles.

Cremasteric reflex: Retraction of the testis when the skin is stroked on the front inner side of the thigh.

Cryotherapy: The use of cold in the treatment of disease.

Cryptorchidism: Failure of the testes to descend into the scrotum.

Crystalloid: A substance capable of crystallization, which can diffuse through membranes, opposite a colloid.

Culturally competent care: A philosophy of care that strives to achieve congruence between the family's cultural belief system and the health care team's proposed interventions.

Cyanoacrylate: Any of a group of adhesives and cements containing cyanoacrylate; widely used in surgery and dentistry.

Cyanosis: Visible blue color of skin and/or mucus membranes; may represent significant percentage of desaturated hemoglobin.

Cystic: Abnormal sac containing gas, fluid, or semisolid material.

Cystic fibrosis: A recessive genetic disorder in which the body produces thick, sticky mucus that affects the lungs and pancreas. This leads to breathing problems, frequent lung infections, poor weight gain, and other problems.

Cystoureterogram: A radiograph of the bladder and ureter obtained after instillation of a contrast medium.

Cytokine: A protein that is released from a cell to trigger a specific interaction between cells. Cytokines function as intercellular mediators, such as interleukins and lymphokines.

Dandy Walker syndrome: A congenital abnormality of the fourth ventricle characterized by fourth ventricle (posterior fossa) cystic dilation, hydrocephalus, and improper formation of the cerebellar vermis.

Debridement: Removal of dead or damaged tissue or foreign material from a wound.

Decerebrate posturing: Lesion in midbrain or pons that results in posturing with extension of legs and extension and internal rotation of arms with flexed wrists.

Decorticate posturing: Posture of bilateral arm adduction, pronation, and flexion of elbows and wrists with extension, internal rotation, and plantar flexion of the legs; indicates lesion in central hemispheres.

Deformation (Deviation of form from the normal): Specifically, an alteration in shape and/or structure of a previously normally formed part. It occurs after organogenesis and often involves the musculoskeletal system. Abnormalities may be in shape, form, or positioning.

Degloving injuries: Forcible tearing away of the skin of the hand or foot, removing most or all of the skin and subcutaneous tissue.

Dehiscence: A separation of a wound, especially an abdominal surgical wound.

Dehydration: Removal of water from a substance.

Demarcation: A boundary.

Demyelination: Destruction or removal of the myelin sheath of nerve tissue, seen in many neurologic diseases.

Dependency: Physiologic phenomenon manifested by development of withdrawal symptoms when treatment is substantially decreased or discontinued abruptly.

Dermal sinus: A congenital dermal sinus is a tract lined by stratified squamous epithelium extending from the skin to deeper structures, especially the spinal cord.

Dermis: The layer of skin laying directly under the epidermis. Structures within the dermis include the eccrine and apocrine glands, nerves, blood vessels, and lymphatics.

Dermoid cyst: A tumor consisting of displaced ectodermal structures along lines of embryonic fusion, the wall being formed of epithelium-lined connective tissue, including skin appendages, and containing keratin, sebum, and hair.

Developmental: Act or state of developing.

Diastematomyelia: A congenital fissure of the spinal cord, frequently associated with spina bifida cystica.

Diencephalon: The region of the brain that includes the thalamus, hypothalamus, epithalamus, and subthalamus. It is derived from the prosencephalon. Located at the midline of the brain, above the mesencephalon of the brainstem.

Differential diagnosis: Prioritized list of alternate explanations (diagnoses) for clinical findings and symptoms.

Dislocatable hip: The femoral head can be easily manipulated outside of the acetabulum, causing complete loss of contact, but returns to the acetabulum once the stress ceases.

Dislocated hip: A condition in which the cartilage of the acetabulum and the femoral head are not in contact when at rest.

Dislocation: Displacement of one or more bones at a joint.

Disruption: Interruption of the normal course (e.g., an organ or body part is forming correctly, but is damaged before it has a chance to fully form).

Dolichocephaly: A skull with a long anteroposterior diameter.

Doll's eye maneuver: A test of the oculocephalic reflex that may be used to assess the integrity of the brainstem in neonates. During the evaluation of the newborn whose nervous system is immature, the irises normally remain in midline despite the rotation of the head.

Double barrel stoma: The proximal and distal ends of the bowel are brought to the surface as two separate stomas. The proximal stoma is the functional stoma, and the distal stoma, referred to as a mucous fistula, does not function. Usually there is a bridge of skin between the two stomas.

Duodenostomy: Surgical creation of an opening into the duodenum.

Dysphagia: Impaired speech or production of understandable speech.

Dysplasia: Abnormal growth or development of tissues, organs, or cells.

Dysreflexia, autonomic: An exaggerated response of the nervous system to a specific trigger, such as an overfull bladder, that occurs because the brain is no longer able to control the body's response to the trigger. A reflex action takes place, tightening blood vessels and causing blood pressure to rise. If the high blood pressure is not controlled, it may cause a stroke, seizure, or death.

Ecchymosis: Superficial bleeding under the skin or mucous membrane.

Eccrine gland: Sweat gland that functions to regulate body temperature. All eccrine glands are present at 28 weeks gestation and are fully functional at 36 weeks gestation.

Elastin: A protein that provides elasticity to structures including skin, blood vessels, heart, lungs, intestines, tendons, and ligaments.

Electrolytes: Minerals in blood and other body fluids that carry an electric charge. They include acids, bases, and salts (such as sodium, potassium, and chlorine).

End stoma: Proximal intestine brought to the skin as a single stoma.

Endoscopy: Technique of inspection of interior of hollow organ or canal utilizing a specialized device.

Enteral: Within, or by way of, the intestine or gastrointestinal tract, especially as distinguished from parenteral.

Enterohepatic: Pertaining to the liver and intestines.

Eosinophilic fibrillar material: An undifferentiated material found in the Homer-Wright pseudorosettes.

Epidermis: The outer, protective, nonvascular layer of the skin that covers the dermis.

Epididymo-orchitis: Inflammation of the epididymis with orchitis.

Epileptiform: Having the appearance of epilepsy, a disease marked by recurrent seizures.

Epispadius: A congenital condition in which the opening of the urethra is on the dorsum of the penis.

Eventration: Protrusion of the intestine through an opening in the abdominal wall.

Expectant management: Relief of symptoms as they arise.

Extracellular: Outside the cells.

Extracorporeal membrane oxygenation (ECMO): A method of cardiopulmonary bypass that maintains the functions of oxygen delivery and CO_2 removal, thus allowing time for cardiac or pulmonary dysfunctions to resolve.

Extravaginal: Outside the vagina.

Extravasation: Escape of fluid from its physiologic space into the surrounding tissue.

Extravascular: Outside a vessel.

Extrinsic: Coming from or originating outside; having relation to parts outside the organ or limb in which found.

Exudate: Fluid released by the cells that contains a high amount of protein, cells, or solid debris.

Family-centered care: A philosophy of care that promotes parental confidence and competence in caregiving and decision making and builds parent/professional partnerships.

Fiberoptic: The transmission of light through flexible glass or plastic fibers by reflections from the side walls of the fibers. This permits transmission of visual images around sharp curves and corners. Devices that employ fiberoptic materials are useful in endoscopic examinations.

Fiberoptic nasopharyngoscopy: Examination of the nasopharynx using a flexible fiberoptic scope.

Fibrin: A protein produced by the action of thrombin on fibrinogen. A component of the clotting cascade that forms the clot.

Fibrinogen: A protein that is converted to fibrin to promote clotting.

Fixed wing aircraft (FWA): A broad category of aircraft for which lift is principally generated by aerodynamic wings that are structured in a fixed position.

Flaccid: Flabby, weak, or no tone to muscles.

Foam dressing: Lint-free, absorbent dressing that serves as primary and secondary dressing.

Focal: A specific location.

Foramen of Monro: Point of communication between the third and lateral ventricles of the brain.

Foregut: Cephalic division of the primitive digestive tract of the embryo.

Fovea: A cuplike depression of the surface of the body.

Fraction of inspired oxygen (FiO2): Percentage of oxygen concentration in inspired gas; room air is 21 percent oxygen.

Gallbladder: A pear-shaped receptacle on the inferior surface of the liver, in a hollow between the right lobe and the quadrate lobe; it serves as a storage reservoir for bile.

Gastrostomy: Surgical creation of an opening from the abdominal wall into the stomach; a feeding tube may be inserted through the opening.

Gastrulation: Creation of the third layer of the brain known as the mesoderm.

Glioblasts: Cells that provide nutritive and structural support to the brain cells.

Gliosis: Overgrowth of the astrocytes in an area of damage in the brain or spinal cord.

Glomerulosclerosis: Scarring of the kidneys' tiny blood vessels (glomeruli), the functional units in the kidney that filter urine from the blood.

Glossopexy: Technique by which the tongue is sutured to the lower lip, thereby pulling the tongue forward, providing a larger airway.

Glossoptosis: Displacement of the tongue into the pharynx, causing partial or complete obstruction.

Gravitational force (G-force): Force or pull exerted on the human body or other object that is equal to the weight of the person or object. The force increases positively with acceleration and negatively with reversal or deceleration.

Hartmann's pouch: Oversewn distal bowel left in the abdomen.

Heimlich valve: A collapsible valve that permits air to exit and prohibits air entry.

Hematocele: An infusion of blood into a cavity.

Hematuria: Blood in the urine.

Hemoptysis: Spitting up of blood, as from lungs or bronchi.

Hemostasis: An arrest of bleeding or circulation.

Histologic: Relating to the minute structure of cells, tissues, and organs.

Holoprosencephaly: A primary failure of neural induction resulting in varying degrees of fusion of the forebrain.

Homer-Wright pseudorosettes: Clusters of neuroblasts surrounding areas of eosinophilic neuropil. They are diagnostic of neuroblastoma.

Homogenous: Uniform structure or composition.

Hydranencephaly: Absence of the forebrain secondary to vascular accident or severe infection with destruction and liquefaction of the cerebral hemispheres.

Hydrocolloid dressing: Occlusive and semiocclusive dressing composed of gelatin, pectin, and carboxymethylcellulose used as a primary or secondary dressing.

Hydrogel dressing: A water- or glycerin-based gel, gauze, or sheet that functions as a primary or secondary dressing.

Hydrops: Excess fluid within tissue or a body compartment.

Hydronephrosis: Stretching of the renal pelvis due to obstruction of urinary outflow.

Hyomandibulopexy: Procedure in which the larynx is anteriorly anchored.

Hypernatremic dehydration: Dehydration in which intravascular volume is preserved at the expense of intracellular water.

Hyperresonance: Greater than normal resonance on a percussion area, as in chest hyperresonance overlying an area of pulmonary overinflation.

Hypertrichosis: Excessive hairiness.

Hyponatremic dehydration: Dehydration with serum sodium <140 cellular overhydration from movement of fluid from serum into cells.

Hypophosphatasia: Signs and symptoms of rickets due to a deficiency of alkaline phosphatase.

Hypospadias: A congenital condition in which the urethral opening is on the undersurface of the penis.

Hysterotomy: Incision of the uterus.

Ileostomy: Surgical creation of an opening from the abdominal wall into the ileum.

Induration: An area of tissue that is hardened.

Insensible water loss: The continual loss of body water by evaporation from the respiratory tract and diffusion through the skin.

Inspissated: Thick or condensed.

Instability: Lack of resistance to sudden change.

Interstitial: Placed or lying between.

Intracellular: Within a cell.

Intravascular: Within a blood vessel.

Intraventricular: Within a ventricle.

Intrinsic: Innate; pertaining to inherent qualities.

Ipsilateral: On the same side.

Iridotomy: An incision of the iris, done to make a new aperture in the iris when the pupil is closed.

Isotonic: Having equal pressure; a solution that has the same osmotic pressure as a reference solution.

Isotonic dehydration: Loss of volume without electrolyte disturbance.

Jaundice: Yellowing of the skin and whites of the eyes by bilirubin, a bile pigment.

Jejunostomy: Surgical creation of an opening from the abdominal wall into the jejunum.

Keel: Hood Laryngeal White Umbrella Keels are designed for use following repair of anterior laryngeal stenosis. Indicated for use after hemilaryngectomy to prevent stenosis. It is designed so the keel can be held tightly enough to inhibit synchronous motion between the intralaryngeal keel insert and the vocal cords, thus preventing granulation formation and preserving phonation.

Keratinocytes: Predominant cell of the epidermis produces the protein keratin, the major structural protein of the epidermis.

Keyhole sign: The sonographic appearance of the fetal bladder, indicative of proximal urethral obstruction such as posterior urethral valves or urethral atresia.

Langerhans cells: Considered to be the dendritic cells of the epidermis, responsible for immunologic activity.

Leptomyelolipoma (Lumbosacral lipoma): A common soft-tissue tumor found in the trunk posterior to a spina bifida defect. Usually occurs in infants, but can be seen in adults.

Lipoma: A common soft-tissue tumor found under the skin, but also can appear in deeper tissues and even in various body organs, such as the heart, brain, and lung.

Lipomyelomeningocele: Myelomeningocele with an overlying lipoma.

Lithiasis: A condition characterized by the formation of stones in the hollow organs or ducts of the body, occurring most often in the gallbladder, kidneys, and lower urinary tract.

Localized: Restricted or limited to a definite part.

Loop stoma: A loop of bowel is brought to the skin, resulting in a single stoma with a proximal and distal opening.

Low birth weight: Birth weight <2,500 grams.

Lucency: Clarity; degree of radiographic transparency or blackness.

Maceration: Softening of the skin by soaking in a fluid.

Macrocephaly: Large head.

Macrophage: A type of white blood cell that ingests foreign matter and triggers stimulation of the immunologic system.

Macular region: An oval area of the sensory retina, 3 by 5 mm, temporal to the optic disc corresponding to the posterior pole of the eye; at its center is the central fovea, which contains only cones.

Malformation: Failure of proper or normal development; more specifically, a primary structural defect that results from a localized error of morphogenesis.

Mass effect: The displacement of normal structures by a mass-occupying lesion.

Maternal mirror syndrome: A phenomenon in which fetal distress is associated with severe preeclampsia in the mother.

Meatus: A passage or opening.

Median prosencephalic vein: A centrally located vessel that drains the choroid plexus. Also referred to as vein of Galen or vein of Markowski.

Mediastinum: Portion of the thoracic cavity not containing lungs; includes the heart, esophagus, trachea, mainstem bronchi, thymus, and major blood supply.

Medical control physician (MCP): The physician who accepts care of the transport patient and directs all facets of care throughout the transport process.

Melanocytes: Epidermal cells that produce melanin for pigmentation and ultraviolet protection.

Merkel cells: Touch cells that communicate with terminal nerve endings.

Meromelia: Partial absence of a free limb.

Mesencephalon: The midbrain. One of three primitive cerebral vesicles from which develop the corpora quadrigemina, the crura cerebri, and the aqueduct of Sylvius.

Mesoderm: The middle of the three primary germ layers of the embryo (the others being the ectoderm and endoderm). The mesoderm is the origin of connective tissues; myoblasts; the blood, cardiovascular, and lymphatic systems; most of the urogenital system; and the lining of the pericardial, pleural, and peritoneal cavities.

Metastasis: The spread of a disease process from one part of the body to another, as in the appearance of neoplasms in parts of the body remote from the site of the primary tumor; results from dissemination of tumor cells by the lymphatics or blood vessels or by direct extension through serous cavities or subarachnoid or other spaces.

Metencephalon: The anterior portion of the embryonic rhombencephalon, from which the cerebellum and pons arise.

Methemoglobinemia: A clinical condition in which more than 1 percent of hemoglobin in blood is oxidized to the ferric form and does not transport oxygen. Signs and symptoms include cyanosis, dizziness, drowsiness, headache, and neurologic symptoms.

Microcephaly: Small head.

Microcoil: Embolic agent, delivered by microcatheters, used to reduce blood flow.

Micrognathia: Abnormally small jaw or mandible.

Monozygotic: Resulting from a single fertilized ovum that becomes separated at an early stage into independent embryos of the same sex and identical genetic composition.

Myelencephalon: The most posterior portion of the embryonic hindbrain (rhombencephalon), which gives rise to the medulla oblongata.

Myelodysplasia: 1) A condition, present at birth, that can affect the development of the vertebrae, spinal cord, surrounding nerves, and the fluid-filled sac that surrounds the spinal cord. This neurologic condition can cause a portion of the spinal cord and the surrounding structures to develop outside, instead of inside, the body. The saclike lesion can occur anywhere along the spine. 2) Dysplasia of myelocytes and other cells in bone marrow; may cause suppression or abnormal proliferation.

Myelomeningocele: Hernial protrusion of the spinal cord and its meninges through a defect in the vertebral arch.

Myoclonic: Twitching or spasm of a muscle or group of muscles.

Myoelastic: Relating to elastic and muscle tissue.

Myopia: Nearsightedness.

Nasal alae: The wings of the nostrils.

Nasopharyngoscope: A device used to visualize the nasal passage and pharynx.

Neoumbilicus: A new belly button.

Neovascularization: Formation or proliferation of new of blood vessels.

Neurulation: Formation of the neural plate in the embryo and the development and closure of the neural tube.

Nitric oxide (NO): A relaxing factor derived from endothelium that is administered in a gas form to promote vascular relaxation/dilation in infants with hypoxic respiratory failure.

Nociception: The stimulus-response pain mechanism involving the stimulation of peripheral nerve fibers and the transmission of the impulse to the central nervous system, where the stimulus is perceived as pain.

Notochordal process: Precursor of the central nervous system.

Noxious: Harmful or injurious.

Obturator: Any structure that occludes an opening.

Oligohydramnios: An abnormally small amount of amniotic fluid.

Omphalitis: Inflammation of the umbilicus.

Opacity: Opaque or nontransparent; degree of radiographic density or whiteness.

Opioids: Pharmacologic agents derived from the poppy species Papaver somniferum, which is believed to relieve pain by interaction with specific body receptors.

Ora serrata: Notched anterior edge of the sensory portion of the retina.

Orchiopexy: The suturing of an undescended testicle to fix it in the scrotum.

Osmolarity: Concentration of osmotically active particles in a solution.

Ostomy: Surgical procedure creating an opening from the bowel or ureters to the abdomen, resulting in a stoma, for the purpose of eliminating waste (stool/urine). **(See Stoma.)**

Pain: An unpleasant sensation caused by noxious stimulation of the sensory nerve endings.

Paracentesis: Passage of an instrument (e.g., trocar and/or needle) into a body cavity with intention of removing fluid.

Paradoxical: Something that seems untrue, but is actually true.

Paraexstrophy flaps: Skin from the lower abdomen adjacent to the bladder neck and mucosa of the penile skin and glans that is used to lengthen or reconstruct the urethra in male infants with bladder exstrophy. The urethra does not usually need to be lengthened in females.

Paraphimosis: Strangulation of the glans penis due to retraction of a narrowed or inflamed foreskin.

Paraplegia: Paralysis of both lower extremities.

Parenchyma: Specific cellular components of an organ or gland contained within and supported by connective tissue.

Peak inspiratory pressure (PIP): Highest pressure reached during the inspiratory phase of mechanical ventilation; measured at proximal airway.

Permeability: The ability of allowing the passage of substances (e.g., liquid, gas, heat) through a membrane or other structure.

Permissive hypercarbia: Ventilatory strategy utilizing minimized pressure and/or rate, with tolerance of increased PCO_2 and decreased pH, to minimize barotraumas.

Phagocyte: A white blood cell that engulfs and destroys microorganisms, debris, and particles in the blood or tissues. Principle phagocytes include neutrophils and monocytes.

Phagocytosis: A process in which phagocytes engulf and destroy microorganisms and bacteria.

Phenotype: The entire physical, biochemical, and physiologic makeup of an individual as determined both genetically and environmentally.

Phimosis: Narrowing of the preputial orifice so that the foreskin cannot be pushed back over the glans penis.

Photocoagulation: A beam of electromagnetic energy is directed to specific tissue, resulting in coagulation from absorption of light energy.

Piriform aperture stenosis: A narrowing or blockage of the bony opening at the entrance of the nose.

Plagiocephaly: Generic term used to describe congenital asymmetry of the skull caused by irregular closure of the cranial sutures.

Plasticity: The ability of tissues to grow or integrate with others during development, after trauma, or after an illness.

Pneumatic craniotome: A device that forces air to perforate and divide a fetal skull in labor in order to allow labor to continue when a fetus has died *in utero*.

Polyhydramnios: A condition of pregnancy characterized by an excess of amniotic fluid.

Polymerization: The process of changing a simple chemical substance or substances into another compound having the same elements, usually in the same proportions, but with a higher molecular weight.

Polyuria: Excessive secretion and discharge of urine.

Pontine: Pertaining to the pons varolii.

Positive end expiratory pressure (PEEP): Pressure in the airway during the expiratory phase of mechanical ventilation.

Posthitis: Inflammation of the foreskin.

Pressurization: Maintenance of a sealed climate within an aircraft; usually in the range of sea level to 10,000 feet, to which the human body can easily adapt.

Prevesical space: Space in front of the bladder.

Priapism: An abnormal, painful, and continuous erection.

Prolabium: The isolated central soft tissue segment of the upper lip in the embryonic state and in an unrepaired bilateral cleft palate.

Prosencephalic: The forebrain in development, which develops into the telencephalon and diencephalon.

Proteases: Enzymes that hydrolyze or break down proteins into peptides and amino acids.

Prothrombin: A plasma protein coagulation factor that is converted into thrombin per the clotting cascade.

Pyelostomy: Creation of an opening into the renal pelvis.

Quality assurance (QA): A process of review and intervention with the intent of achieving or maintaining defined standards of service.

Radiotherapy: The treatment of disease with nonionizing or ionizing radiation.

Referral center: The facility, usually a hospital, that requests transfer for a patient presently in its care.

Reflux: A return or backward flow.

Reliability: The psychometric measure that refers to how reproducible the results of the instrument are under different conditions or by different raters.

Resonance: The quality of vibratory sound heard on percussion of a hollow structure such as the chest or abdomen.

Retrograde: Moving backward; degenerating from a better to a worse state.

Rhabdomyosarcoma: A malignant neoplasm derived from skeletal (striated) muscle, occurring in children or, less commonly, adults; classified as embryonal alveolar (composed of loose aggregates of small, round cells) or pleomorphic (containing rhabdomyoblasts).

Rhombencephalon: The hindbrain.

Rotary wing aircraft (RWA): A broad category of aircraft for which liftoff is principally generated by one or more wings that rotate at high speeds around a fixed point of the aircraft.

Rugae: A fold or crease.

Scaphocephaly: Deformed head, projecting like the keel of a boat.

Scleral support ring: Sutured to the sclera before the beginning of a corneal graft. It helps to prevent collapse of the globe, prolapse of the ocular contents, or distortion of the corneal rim. The ring is secured to the sclera anterior to the rectus insertion with at least four scleral sutures.

Sclerose: To become hardened or indurated.

Seminiferous: Producing or conducting semen.

Sequence: The order of a series of related events.

Short-bowel syndrome: Inadequate absorption of nutrients resulting from a surgical procedure that removes or bypasses a large portion of the intestinal tract.

Small for gestational age (SGA): Infant under the tenth percentile for weight, plotted on a standardized growth chart.

Somatic: Pertaining to nonreproductive cells of tissues.

Sphincter: A muscle that encircles a duct, tube, or orifice in such a way that its contraction constricts the lumen or orifice.

Spirometry: Inspiratory and/or expiratory pulmonary measurements made with a spirometer to determine air flow and volume.

Stasis: Stoppage of the normal flow of fluids, as of the blood, urine, or feces.

Stoma: Opening. When used in reference to ostomy care, it is a segment of bowel or (less often) ureter brought to the surface of the abdomen. It is formed of mucosal tissue and is red and moist in appearance. Ideally, it will protrude about 1.5–2.5 cm.

Stratum corneum: The outer layer of the epidermis, comprised of corneocytes and intercellular lipid lamellae that form a semipermeable barrier.

Stratum germinativum: The innermost layer of the epidermis that is in contact with the epidermis. Contains basal keratinocytes responsible for replacing cells that move to the skin surface and are lost.

Stratum granulosum: A thin layer of keratinocytes that lays below the stratum lucidum. Helps form the lipid barrier component of the epidermis.

Stratum lucidum: The layer of the epidermis, beneath the stratum corneum, consisting of two or three layers of flat, clear cells without nuclei; found only on palms, soles of feet, and fingertips.

Stratum spinosum: The thickest layer of epidermis, residing between the stratum spinosum and the stratum granulosum and housing Langerhans cells.

Stridor: High-pitched, adventitious, upper airway breath sound, suggesting obstructed air flow.

Subarachnoid space: The space between the pia mater and the arachnoid, containing the cerebrospinal fluid.

Subcutaneous: Beneath the skin.

Subdural space: The narrow space between the dura and the arachnoid.

Subgaleal area: The area beneath the galea aponeurotica (i.e., the epicranial aponeurosis).

Subluxable hip: At rest, the hip is in correct position. The joint has increased mobility and laxity. Manipulation of the hip allows partial dislocation with partial contact between the femoral head and acetabulum.

Subluxation: Incomplete dislocation of a bone in a joint.

Suprahyoid: Above the hyoid bone.

Suspension laryngoscopy: A technique required to establish the viewing space necessary to identify the epiglottis and ultimately the larynx.

Syndrome: A group of signs, symptoms, laboratory findings, and physiologic disturbances that are linked by a common anatomical, biochemical, or pathologic history.

Synergism: Two or more agents or organs working together.

Synostosis: Joining of separate bones by osseous tissue.

Telencephalon: Primitive forebrain (cerebral hemispheres).

Teratologic dislocation of the hip: Occurs before birth and is associated with other conditions such as spina bifida, arthrogryposis, and Larsen's syndrome.

Thoracentesis: Paracentesis of the pleural cavity.

Thoracostomy: Surgical creation of an opening into the chest wall.

Thoracotomy: Incision of the chest wall into the pleural space.

Thrombosis: Formation or presence of a thrombus; clotting within a blood vessel that may cause infarction of tissues supplied by the vessel.

Through transmission: Water density substances (e.g. bile, cerebrospinal fluid, or urine) pose no impedance to sound waves, and few echoes are reflected to the transducer while passing through them. Because these substances do not absorb as much sound as their surroundings, fluid-filled visci have increased sound transmission from the posterior wall and soft tissues (i.e., "through transmission")

Tolerance (drug): Process of the decreasing effectiveness of a drug over time.

Tortuous: Having many twists and turns.

Trabeculae: Supporting strands of connective tissue that project into an organ and become part of its framework.

Trabeculation: Having trabeculae.

Tracheoinnominate fistula: A fistula caused by erosion from an improperly fitted or placed tube, a low tracheotomy site, or a tight feeding tube.

Tracheostomy: Surgical creation of an opening into the trachea for the insertion of a tube or airway.

Transparent film: A flexible sheet of semipermeable polyurethane, coated with adhesive. Used as a primary or secondary dressing.

Transplant: To transfer from one part to another, as in grafting and transplantation.

Trigonocephaly: Triangular malformation of the skull due to premature synostosis of the cranial bones with compression of the cerebral hemispheres.

Unconjugated bilirubin: Free bilirubin that has not been attached to a glucuronide molecule. Also called indirect bilirubin.

Urachal: Related to the urachus.

Ureterostomy: Formation of a permanent fistula for drainage of a ureter.

Ureterovesical junction: Valve that prevents urine from flowing backward into the ureter; located where the ureter meets the bladder.

Urinoma: A cyst containing urine.

Validity: Psychometric measure of an instrument's ability to assess what it was intended to assess.

Vein of Galen: The vein running through the tela choroidea formed by the joining of the terminal and choroids veins that forms the great cerebral vein, which empties into the straight sinus of the brain.

Vein of Markowski: The embryologic precursor to the vein of Galen.

Velopharyngeal dysfunction: Pertaining to the dysfunction of the soft palate (velum palatinum) and the pharyngeal walls.

Ventriculitis: Inflammation of a ventricle.

Ventriculostomy: Surgery to establish communication between the floor of the third ventricle of the brain and the cisterna interpeduncularis; done to treat hydrocephalus.

Verumontanum: An elevation on the floor of the prostatic portion of the urethra where the seminal ducts enter.

Vesicostomy: Surgically produced opening into the bladder.

Vesicoureteral: Concerning the urinary bladder and a ureter.

Vitrectomy: The surgical removal of the vitreous of the eye.

Vomer: The bone that forms the lower and posterior portion of the nasal septum.

Vomer-plasty: Surgical repair of the flat, trapezoidal-shaped bone that forms the lower and posterior portion of the nasal septum.

Wheeze: Adventitious, high-pitched inspiratory or expiratory breath sound, suggesting airway narrowing and impeded airflow.

Bibliography

A to Z health and disease information. Penn State Milton S. Hershey Medical Center (http://www.hmc.psu.edu/healthinfo).

American Heritage Online Dictionary (www.bartelby.com/61/).

Dorland's Online Medical Dictionary (www.mercksource.com/pp/us/cns/cns_home.jsp).

Emedicine from WebMD (www.emedicine.com).

Gomella TL, et al. 2004. *Neonatology: Management, Procedures, On-call Problems, Diseases, and Drugs,* 5th ed. New York: McGraw-Hill.

Haynes R. 2001. Developmental dysplasia of the hip: Etiology, pathogenesis, and examination and physical findings in the newborn. AAOS Instructional Course Lectures 50: 535–540.

Medial College of Wisconsin. HealthLink (http://healthlink.mcw.edu/article/943054092.html).

Merriam-Webster Online Dictionary (www.m-w.com/home.htm).

Primary Care Electronic Library (PCEL). St. George's, University of London (www.pcel.info).

Stedman's Medical Dictionary, 27th ed. 2000. Philadelphia: Lippincott Williams & Wilkins.

Stedman's Online Medical Dictionary (www.stedman's.com).

Taber's Cyclopedic Medical Dictionary, 20th ed. 2005. Philadelphia: FA Davis.

Taber's Medical Encyclopedia Online (www.rxlist.com/cgi/Tabersearch.cgi).

Tappero EP, and Honeyfield ME. 2003. *Physical Assessment of the Newborn: A Comprehensive Approach to the Art of Physical Examination,* 3rd ed. Santa Rosa, California: NICU INK.

The Children's Hospital at Montefiore, Bronx, New York (www.montekids.org/healthlibrary/).

United Ostomy Association of Canada (www.ostomycanada.ca/definitions.htm).

University of Alabama at Birmingham. Spinal Cord Injury Information Network (www.spinalcord.uab.edu/show.asp?durki=19679).

Willis RB. 2001. Developmental dysplasia of the hip: Assessment and treatment before walking age. AAOS Instructional Course Lectures 50: 541–544.

Witt C. 2003. Detecting developmental dysplasia of the hip. *Advances in Neonatal Care* 3(2): 65–75.

Notes

Notes

• Table of Abbreviations •

AaDo$_2$:	Alveolar/arterial oxygen gradient		CSF:	Cerebrospinal fluid
AAMS:	Association of Air Medical Services		CT:	Computed tomography
			CVR:	CCAM volume ratio
ACTH:	Adrenocorticotropic hormone		CVR:	Cerebral vascular resistance
ADAM:	Amniotic deformity, adhesions, mutilations		DDH:	Developmental dysplasia of the hip
ADH:	Antidiuretic hormone		DOT:	Department of Transportation
AFP:	α-fetoprotein		DPNB:	Dorsal penile nerve block
AgNO$_3$:	Silver nitrate		EA:	Esophageal atresia
AP:	Anteroposterior		ECF:	Extracellular fluid
ASD:	Atrial septal defect		ECG:	Electrocardiogram
A-V:	Arteriovenous		ECMO:	Extracorporeal membrane oxygenation
AVM:	Arteriovenous malformation			
AVP:	Arginine vasopressin		EMLA:	Eutectic mixture of local anesthetic
BP:	Blood pressure		ERCP:	Endoscopic retrograde cholangiopancreatography
BPS:	Bronchopulmonary sequestration			
BUN:	Blood urea nitrogen		ETT:	Endotracheal tube
CATMS:	Commission on Accreditation on Transport Medical Services		EXIT:	Ex utero intrapartum treatment
			FiO$_2$:	Fraction of inspired oxygen
CBC:	Complete blood count		FENa:	Fractional excretion of sodium
CBF:	Cerebral blood flow		FSH:	Follicle-stimulating hormone
CCAM:	Congenital cystic adenomatoid malformation		G-force:	Gravitational force
			G-tube:	Gastrostomy tube
CCP:	Cerebral perfusion pressure		GER:	Gastroesophageal reflux
CDH:	Congenital diaphragmatic hernia		GERD:	Gastroesophageal reflux disease
CF:	Cystic fibrosis		GFR:	Glomerular filtration rate
CHAOS:	Congenital high airway obstruction		GI:	Gastrointestinal
			GMH:	Germinal matrix hemorrhage
CHARGE:	Acronym for coloboma, heart disease, choanal atresia, retarded growth and development, genital hypoplasia, ear anomalies with deafness		GnRH:	Gonadotropin-releasing hormone
			GU:	Genitourinary
			hCG:	Human chorionic gonadotropin
			HCO$_3$:	Hydrogen ions as bicarbonate
CHF:	Congestive heart failure		HFOV:	High-frequency oscillatory ventilation
CHILD:	Congenital hemidysplasia with ichthyosiform erythroderma and limb defects			
			HFV:	High-frequency ventilation
			HIDA:	Hepatobiliary iminodiacetic acid
CMV:	Cytomegalovirus		HOB:	Head of bed
CNS:	Central nervous system		Hox:	Homeobox
COBRA:	Consolidated Omnibus Reconciliation Act		HVA:	Homovanillic acid
			ICP:	Intracranial pressure
CPAP:	Continuous positive airway pressure		IDM:	Infant of a diabetic mother
			IICP:	Increased intracranial pressure
CQI:	Continuous quality improvement		IV:	Intravenous
CRIES:	Acronym for crying, requires oxygen to maintain saturation <95 percent, increased vital signs, expression, sleepless		IVH:	Intraventricular hemorrhage
			LBW:	Low birth weight

LDH:	Lactate dehydrogenase
LH:	Luteinizing hormone
LHR:	Lung-to-head ratio
LP:	Lumbar puncture
LUTO:	Lower urinary tract obstruction
MAP:	Mean arterial pressure
MCP:	Medical control physician
MCT:	Medium-chain triglycerides
MFICU:	Maternal-fetal intensive care unit
MIBG:	Methyliodobenzylguanadine
MIS:	Müllerian-inhibiting substance
MMC:	Myelomeningocele
MOMS:	Management of Myelomeningocele Study
MRI:	Magnetic resonance imaging
NaCl:	Sodium chloride
NaHCO$_3$:	Sodium bicarbonate
NBAS:	Neonatal Behavioral Assessment Scale
NCPAP:	Nasal continuous positive airway pressure
NEC:	Necrotizing enterocolitis
NFNA:	National Flight Nurses Association
NIDCAP:	Newborn Individualized Developmental Care and Assessment Program
NIPS:	Neonatal Infant Pain Scale
NIS:	Nationwide Inpatient Sample
NNS:	Nonnutritive sucking
NO:	Nitric oxide
NPO:	Nothing by mouth
NRP:	Neonatal Resuscitation program
NS:	Normal saline
NSE:	Neuron-specific enolase
OEIS:	Omphalocele-exstrophy-imperforate anus-spinal
OFC:	Occipitofrontal circumference
OG:	Orogastric
PALS:	Pediatric Advanced Life Support
PDA:	Patent ductus arteriosus
PEEP:	Positive end-expiratory pressure
PEG:	Percutaneous endoscopic gastrostomy
PHH:	Posthemorrhagic hydrocephalus
PIE:	Pulmonary interstitial emphysema
PIP:	Peak inspiratory pressure
PIPP:	Premature Infant Pain Profile
PMR:	Posteromedial release

PPHN:	Persistent pulmonary hypertension of the newborn
PRS:	Pierre Robin sequence
PT:	Prothrombin time
PTH:	Parathyroid hormone
PUV:	Posterior urethral valve
PVR:	Peripheral vascular resistance
QA:	Quality assurance
RBF:	Renal blood flow
ROP:	Retinopathy of prematurity
RVR:	Renal vascular resistance
SBS:	Short bowel syndrome
SCT:	Sacrococcygeal teratoma
SGA:	Small for gestational age
SIADH:	Syndrome of inappropriate antidiuretic hormone secretion
SIDS:	Sudden infant death syndrome
TAR:	Thrombocytopenia with absent radius
TEARS:	The early amnion rupture spectrum
TEF:	Tracheoesophageal fistula
TOF:	Tetralogy of Fallot
TORCH:	Acronym for toxoplasmosis, other viruses, rubella virus, cytomegalovirus, and herpes simplex virus
TPN:	Total parenteral nutrition
UTI:	Urinary tract infection
VACTERL:	Acronym for vertebral anomalies, anal atresia, cardiac defect (most often a ventricular septal defect), tracheoesophageal fistula, renal anomalies, and limb anomalies
VAD:	Ventricular access device
VATER:	Acronym for vertebral defects, anal atresia, tracheoesophageal fistula with esophageal atresia, and radial and renal anomalies
VCUG:	Voiding cystourethrogram
VDRL:	Venereal Disease Research Laboratory
VLBW:	Very low birth weight
VMA:	Vanillylmandelic acid
VPD:	Velopharyngeal dysfunction
VSD:	Ventricular septal defect
VURD:	Acronym for valves, unilateral reflux, dysplasia
WOB:	Work of breathing

• Index •

A

A-V. *See* arteriovenous gradient
AaDO₂. *See* alveolar/arterial oxygen gradient
AAP. *See* American Academy of Pediatrics
abdomen
  loops in. *See* bowel loops
  megaureter presentations in, 281
  neuroblastoma found in, 204–206
    imaging of, 208
  tenderness of, in necrotizing enterocolitis, 172
abdominal distention
  in biliary atresia, 193
  decompression of. *See* gastric decompression
  in esophageal atresia with fistula, 148, 150
  gastrostomy tube and, 569
  intestinal atresia/stenosis associated with, 162
  intestinal malrotation/volvulus causing, 166
  in neuroblastoma, 205
  ovarian cysts and, 304
  postoperative, in prune belly syndrome, 293
abdominal girth measurements, 174, 286
abdominal mass, 161, 205, 304–305
abdominal muscular deficiency syndrome, 287
abdominal pain, neuroblastoma causing, 205
abdominal pressure, increased
  gastroschisis repair and, 157
  in inguinal hernia, effect of, 183–184
abdominal quadrants, fluid loss estimates based
    on, 433
abdominal wall
  abnormal musculature of, 287–289. *See also*
    prune belly syndrome
    reconstruction of, 293
  defect
    in bladder exstrophy, 263
    in cloacal exstrophy, 271, 274
    in gastroschisis, 155
    in omphalocele, 158
    rectal prolapse and, 263
  stomach separation from, gastrostomy tube
    and, 569
abduction
  closed reduction for, 398
  in DDH, 398
  of foot, in talipes equinovarus casting, 388
  with Pavlik harness, 397–399, 397*f*
abduction bar, for talipes equinovarus, 388, 389*f*
ablation therapy, endoscopic, for posterior
    urethral valves, 246*f*, 247
  complications of, 249
  postoperative nursing care, 250
absent radius, 378–381
  associations of, 379
  clinical presentation of, 378*f*, 379
  complications of, 381

  definition of, 378
  diagnosis of, 379–380
  differential diagnosis of, 379
  etiology of, 378
  incidence of, 379
  outcomes of, 381
  pathophysiology of, 378
  treatment of
    conservative, 380–381
    postoperative nursing care, 371–372, 381
    surgical, 381
accidents
  during infant transport, 504–505
  skull fractures resulting from, 348
acetabular index on x-ray, in DHH, 395
acetabulum, dysplasia of, 391–399. *See also*
    developmental dysplasia of the hip
    (DDH)
acetaminophen, 450
  for circumcision, 310, 312
  for inguinal hernia, 186
Achilles tendon, in talipes equinovarus, 383, 388
acholic stool, 193, 575
acid-base balance
  in congenital diaphragmatic hernia, 90, 92–93
  in congenital heart disease, 126, 137
  in congenital lobar emphysema, 67
  in necrotizing enterocolitis, 173–174
  preoperative assessment of, 431
  in pulmonary disorders, 107
  renal regulation of, 233–237, 415–416, 421
acid salts, in renal physiology, 235–237
acidity effect, in laryngomalacia, 42
acidosis
  intestinal malrotation/volvulus causing, 166,
    168
  metabolic. *See* metabolic acidosis
  in pyloric stenosis, 161
  renal ammonium regulation role, 237
  renal effects of, 415
  respiratory, 431
acini(ae), embryology of, 62, 63*f*
acrobrachycephaly, synostotic, 50*f*, 51–52
acrosyndactyly, 374, 377
ACTH. *See* adrenocorticotropic hormone
Active Movement Scale, in brachial plexus
    injury, 404
active transport, in nephrons, 228
activity, of infant
  in congenital heart disease, 118
  limitation of. *See* immobilization; restraints
  in pain response, 442*t*, 443–444
  in utero, 367, 375
acyanotic lesions, in congenital heart disease,
    113

ADAM. *See* amniotic deformity, adhesions, mutilations
adaptation, in family-centered care, 510
adduction, of forefoot, 382, 382f–383f, 385
adductor tenotomy, percutaneous, for DDH, 398
adenocarcinoma, bladder exstrophy and, 271
adenomatoid malformation, congenital cystic, 70–76
    fetal surgery for, 524t, 528–530
ADH. *See* antidiuretic hormone
adhesions
    with circumcision, 313
    with ovarian cyst surgery, 308–309
adhesive removers, 466, 473, 476
adjunctive agents
    for bladder exstrophy repair, 270
    for pain management, 450–451
"Adopt a Mommy to Be," 542
adrenal glands, in reproductive physiology, 240
adrenal medulla, malignancies arising from, 203–204
adrenocorticotropic hormone (ACTH), 240, 414
Adzik classification, of congenital cystic adenomatoid malformation, 71
aerophagia, 575
aerotitis, 575
AFP. *See* alpha-fetoprotein
aganglionosis, in Hirschsprung's disease, 169–170
agenesis, 575
    anorectal, 175–181, 176f
    renal, contralateral, 281
agitation relief
    for congenital heart disease, 138
    during infant transport, 497–498
    postoperative, for pulmonary disorders, 109
air bubble
    in bowel wall, 172f, 173
    double, in stomach, 163
air embolism
    in spinal cord injury, 357
air extravasation, extrapulmonary, 101–109
air leak, pulmonary, 101–106. *See also* pulmonary air leak
air transport, gas expansion during, 487–488
aircraft
    fixed wing, 489, 505, 579
    for infant transport, 487–488, 492
    rotary wing, 505, 505f, 583
airway fluoroscopy, in tracheomalacia, 48
airway intubation. *See* endotracheal intubation; *specific anatomy*
airway management
    during infant transport, 489–490
    for pulmonary disorders
        immediate stabilization, 106–107
        postoperative, 108
        preoperative, 106–107
airway obstruction
    bronchial, 64–65
    choanal atresia and, 30–31
    cleft lip/palate and, 32
    congenital high, 535
    cystic hygroma and, 12, 14, 16
    giant neck masses causing, 524t, 535–537
    laryngeal web and, 43

laryngomalacia and, 39, 39f, 41
    postoperative, in cleft lip/palate repair, 35
    Robin sequence and, 38
    tracheomalacia and, 47–49
    vocal cord paralysis and, 45–46
alae, nasal, 575, 581
albumin, 429, 434, 575
alcohol, Robin sequence association with, 37
aldosterone
    in renal physiology, 229–230, 236, 414
    in water and electrolyte homeostasis, 414–416, 419
alert state, pain expression during, 444
alginate dressings, 464, 575
alkaline phosphatase, deficiency of, 580
alkalosis
    ammonium regulation role, 237
    contraction, 577
    metabolic, 421, 431
    renal effects of, 415
    respiratory, 428, 431
allantoic duct, 255
allantois, 220, 255–256
alpha-fetoprotein (AFP)
    in cloacal exstrophy, 274
    in fetal sacrococcygeal teratoma, 530
    giant neck masses and, 536
    in myelomeningocele, 533
    in omphalocele, 159
α_1-antitrypsin deficiency, biliary atresia *vs*, 194
altitude, threshold, for aircraft, 488
altitude hypoxia, during infant transport, 487–489, 505
alveolar/arterial oxygen gradient (AaDO$_2$), 554
alveolar ducts, embryology of, 62
alveoli
    embryology of, 62–63, 63f
    rupture of, 101
ambiguous genitalia, 178, 310
amblyopia, 575
amelia, 369, 575
American Academy of Pediatrics (AAP)
    sacrococcygeal teratoma classification by, 530
    transport team composition guidelines of, 481
amino acids
    in jaundice evaluation, 195, 195t
    in parenteral nutrition solutions, 436
    renal excretion of, 229, 237
aminoglycosides, 497
Aminosyn PF solution, 436
ammonium
    in immediate newborn period, 415
    renal production of, 236–237
amniocentesis, for fetal chromosome karyotyping, 524, 529, 533
amnion, tears in, limb defects associated with, 372f–373f, 373–378
amniotic band syndrome, 373–378
    associations of, 375
    classification of, 375–376
    clinical presentation of, 374
    complications of, 377
    definition of, 373
    diagnosis of, 375
    differential diagnosis of, 375
    etiology of, 373–374

incidence of, 374
intrinsic *vs* extrinsic causes of, 373
outcomes of, 378
pathophysiology of, 372f–373f, 373
treatment of, 375–378
  factors influencing, 375–376
  postoperative nursing care, 371–372, 377
  surgical, 376–377
amniotic fluid
  in fetal surgery, 540
  herniated bowel exposure to, 155
  in obstructive uropathy, 537–539
  posterior urethral valves effect on, 243
amniotic sheets, 375
amorphous, 575
  hydrogel dressing, 465
ampicillin, 497, 503
amputation, in amniotic band syndrome,
    376–377
anal canal, embryology of, 146
anal dimple, 177–178
anal membrane, 146
  in external genitalia, 226f
  persistent, 175, 176f, 177
anal sphincter
  in bladder exstrophy, 263
  dysfunction of. *See* bowel incontinence
analgesia
  administration during transport, 497, 503
  caudal. *See* caudal anesthesia/analgesia
  for congenital heart disease, 138
  epidural. *See* epidural anesthesia/analgesia
  for inguinal hernia, 186
  for limb reduction defects, 371
  nonopioid, 445, 450
  opioid. *See* opioid analgesics
  regional, 451
  for wound care, 463
anastomosis
  atrial, of total anomalous pulmonary venous
    connection, 135
  intestinal
    for atresia/stenosis, 164
    enteral nutrition absorption with, 439
    for Hirschsprung's disease, 170
    for meconium ileus, 165
    for necrotizing enterocolitis, 174
  in megaureter repair, 284–285
androgens, adrenal, in reproductive physiology,
    240
anechoic cysts, of ovaries, 306–307
anechoic structures, 575
anemia, 575
  brain hemorrhage resulting from, 353–355
  Fanconi's, absent radius associated with,
    379–380
  neuroblastoma causing, 205
  preoperative management of, 431
anesthesia
  caudal. *See* caudal anesthesia/analgesia
  for circumcision, 310–311
  complications of, 432
  dehydration risks and, 429
  epidural. *See* epidural anesthesia/analgesia
  fluid and electrolyte management during,
    432–433

inhalation, 432
local. *See* local anesthesia
maternal, for fetal surgery, 527, 540
regional, for pain management, 451
spinal, for inguinal hernia repair, 184, 432
  with conscious sedation, 527
anger, as parental reaction, 517
angiogenesis, 462, 575
angiography
  in arteriovenous malformation, 9–10
  in bronchopulmonary sequestration, 81–82
  in ureteropelvic junction obstruction, 299
angiotensin converting enzyme, in renal
    physiology, 230
angiotensin II, in renal physiology, 230–231, 237
angiotensinogen, in renal physiology, 230
angle of His, 151–152
anions, 575
  organic, renal excretion of, 238
anlage, 384, 392, 575
ankle
  equinovarus deformity of, 382–391. *See also*
    talipes equinovarus
  equinus deformity of, 382, 382f–383f, 385
  reduced plantar flexion of, 390
anomalies, 577. *See also* congenital
    malformations; *specific anatomy*
  grief and loss reactions to, 517
anoperineal fistula, 176f, 177
anoplasty, 278, 575
anorchid, 254–255, 575
anorectal canal, embryology of, 221, 226f
anorectal malformations, 175–181
  associations of, 177
  clinical presentation of, 176–177
  complications of, 180
  definition of, 175
  dermatitis risk with, 467
  diagnosis of, 177–178
  differential diagnosis of, 177
  etiology of, 175–176
  incidence of, 176
  male *vs* female, 178f, 179f
  outcomes of, 181
  pathophysiology of, 175
  treatment of, 178–180
    algorithms for, 178f, 179f
    postoperative nursing care, 180
    supportive, 178–179
    surgical, 179–180
  types of, 175, 176f
anorectoplasty, for anorectal malformations, 180
  male *vs* female, 178f, 179f
anorectovaginourethroplasty, posterior sagittal,
    180
antegrade, 247, 575
antenatal diagnosis. *See* prenatal diagnosis
antenatal referral, 479, 489, 583
antenatal surgery. *See* fetal surgery
antenatal ultrasound. *See* prenatal (fetal)
    ultrasound
anterior commissure, 575
  Keel placement for healing of, 44
anterior innominate osteotomy, for bladder
    exstrophy closure, 266f, 267

antibiotic therapy
    administration during transport, 497, 503
    for anorectal malformations, 180
    for bladder exstrophy, 264
    for bladder exstrophy closure, 270
    for bronchopulmonary sequestration, 82
    for choanal atresia, 30
    for cholangitis, 200
    for cleft lip/palate repair, 36
    for cloacal exstrophy, 275
    for craniosynostosis repair, 54
    for cystic hygroma, 14, 16
    for gastroschisis, 156
    for Hirschsprung's disease, 170
    for IV extravasation, 468
    for Kasai portoenterostomy, 201
    for laryngomalacia, 42
    for malrotation/volvulus, 168
    for meconium ileus, 165–166
    for megaureter, 282–284, 286
    for necrotizing enterocolitis, 174–175
    neonatal fluid requirements and, 426
    for omphalocele, 159
    for prune belly syndrome, 292
    for retinopathy of prematurity, 24
    for ureteropelvic junction obstruction, 300,
        302
anticholinergics, for posterior urethral valves,
    247
anticipatory grief, 516–517, 575
anticipatory guidance, 543
anticoagulation
    spinal cord injury and, 357
    for tetralogy of Fallot repair, 127–128
anticonvulsants, 494, 503
antidiuretic hormone (ADH)
    in renal physiology, 229–230, 238, 415
    syndrome of inappropriate, 418–419
        overhydration vs, 418, 419t
        skull fracture repair and, 351
antifungal powder, for stoma care, 476
antimicrobial ointments, for circumcision, 312
antineoplastic agents. See chemotherapy
antispasmodics, for bladder exstrophy closure,
    270
α_1-antitrypsin deficiency, biliary atresia vs, 194
anus
    anomalies of. See anorectal malformations
    in bladder exstrophy, 263
    dilations of, for anorectal malformations, 180
    embryology of, 221, 226f
    imperforate, 176, 181
    stricture of, 180
aorta
    coarctation of, 114t
    embryology of, 114t, 116
    overriding, 124, 124f, 126–127
    transposition of, 128–129, 129f
        surgical switch procedure for, 130, 130f
aortic arch
    double, 47–49, 114t
    embryology of, 114t, 116
aortic atresia, 114t
aortic stenosis, 114t
aorticopulmonary system
    defects of, 114t

embryology of, 114t, 116
    transposition of, 128–130, 129f
aortopexy, for tracheomalacia, 49
aphonia, laryngeal web and, 43
apnea
    brain hemorrhage causing, 354–355
    gastroesophageal reflux associated with, 152
    necrotizing enterocolitis causing, 172
    obstructive, 38, 41
    obstructive sleep, 40
    spinal cord injury causing, 360
apocrine gland, 460–461, 575
apoptosis
    in fetal lungs, 72
    of ureters, in ureteropelvic junction
        obstruction, 296
appendectomy, for intestinal malrotation/
        volvulus, 168
appendix, embryology of, 145
appliance bag, 474f, 475–476
appliances, for stomas
    application of, 473–476, 473f–475f
    discharge teaching on, 476
    optional use of, 472–473
    principles of use, 471–472
    removal of, 472f, 473
    types of, 471–472f
approximation, 575
apraxia, developmental, 406
aqueduct of Sylvius, 324, 575
    stenosis of, hydrocephalus related to, 327–328,
        332
arachnoid villi, CSF absorption in, 325–326
arginine vasopressin (AVP), in renal physiology,
    231
arms. See forearm; upper extremities
Arnold-Chiari malformation, 534. See also
        myelomeningocele (MMC)
arrector muscle, 460
arrhythmias. See cardiac arrhythmias
arterial blood gases, in congenital heart disease,
    126, 137
arterial embolization, for arteriovenous
        malformation, 9–10, 11f
arterial switch procedure, for D-transposition of
        the great arteries, 130, 130f
arteriopexy, for tracheomalacia, 49
arteriovenous (A-V) gradient, in pleural effusion,
    80
arteriovenous malformation (AVM), 8–11
    associations of, 9
    clinical presentation of, 8
    definition of, 8
    diagnosis of, 9
    differential diagnosis of, 9
    etiology of, 8
    incidence of, 8
    outcomes of, 11
    pathophysiology of, 8
    treatment of, 9–11
        medical, 9
        postoperative nursing care, 11
        surgical, 9–11, 11f
artery(ies)
    absence of, limb reduction defects associated
        with, 368–369

anomalous, in bronchopulmonary
    sequestration, 80–81, 84
in branchial arches, 24t, 25
cerebral, arteriovenous malformation in, 8–11
great, D-transposition of, 114t, 128–130
innominate, in tracheomalacia, 47–49
mesenteric
    inferior, 146
    occlusion of during embryogenesis, 146
    superior, 145
pulmonary. See pulmonary artery
rectal
    inferior, 146
    superior, 146
renal
    physiologic role, 227–228
    in ureteropelvic junction obstruction, 295
    in utero physiology of, 227
spermatic, 252
arthritis, 390, 399
arthrodesis. See fusion(s)
arytenoidectomy, for vocal cord paralysis, 46
arytenoids, embryology of, 61
ascending colon, embryology of, 144–145
ascites, 575
    in biliary atresia, 193
    ovarian cysts and, 304, 308
    post-Kasai portoenterostomy, 202
    urinary
        posterior urethral valves and, 242–243
        in prune belly syndrome, 288
ASD. See atrial septal defect
aseptic technique
    for cloacal exstrophy repair, 278
    for invasive devices, 109, 210, 283
    for suprapubic catheters, 270
asphyxia, 575
aspiration
    esophageal atresia with fistula and, 148
    therapeutic. See needle aspiration
    tracheostomy risk for, 551
    vocal cord paralysis associated with, 45–46
Association of Women's Health, Obstetric and
        Neonatal Nurses (AWHONN), 457
atelectasis, 293, 575
atmospheric changes, during infant transport,
        487–488, 505
atresia(s), 575
    anorectal, 175–181, 176f
    aortic, 114t
    biliary, 190–203, 576. See also biliary atresia
    choanal, 28–31. See also choanal atresia
    duodenal, 162–164
    esophageal, 146–151, 147f. See also esophageal
        atresia (EA)
    ileal, 162–163
    intestinal, 162–164. See also intestinal atresia
    jejunal, 162–163
    pulmonary, 114t
    urethral, fetal surgery for, 524t, 537–539
atria
    embryology of, 114t, 115, 115f
    in total anomalous pulmonary venous
        connection, 134, 134f
atrial natriuretic factor, in renal physiology, 231
atrial septal defect (ASD), 114t, 134

atrial septum, development of, 114t, 115–115f
atrioventricular (AV) canal, embryology of, 114t,
        115, 115f
atrophy
    of muscles, in talipes equinovarus, 383
    of testes, 252
attachment, parental-infant. See bonding
auricle (of the ear), embryology of, 6, 368
auscultation, in congenital heart disease, 118
autoamputation, of ovaries, 303
autolytic, 575
    debridement, 464–465
autonomic dysreflexia, in spinal cord injury,
        358–359
autosomal dominant disorders, absent radius
        associated with, 379–380
autosomal recessive disorders, absent radius
        associated with, 379–380
AV. See atrioventricular canal
avascular necrosis, in DDH, 398–399
AVM. See arteriovenous malformation
AVP. See arginine vasopressin
avulsion injury, 575
    of cervical nerve roots, 400, 401f, 404
    of spinal cord, 356
AWHONN. See Association of Women's Health,
        Obstetric and Neonatal Nurses
axial skeleton, embryology of, 364–365
azotemia, 575

B

β_2–microglobulins, urine, in obstructive
        uropathy, 538
Baby Jane Doe, 360
bacterial flora, intestinal, necrotizing
        enterocolitis associated with, 171
balanoposthitis, 575
balloon septostomy
    for congenital heart disease, 121
    for total anomalous pulmonary venous
        connection, 135
    for D-transposition of the great arteries, 130
bands, in utero
    fetal defects associated with, 373–378. See
        also amniotic band syndrome
    innocent, 375
barbiturates, 450
barium enema
    in diagnosis of Hirschsprung's disease, 170
    for meconium ileus, 165
barium swallow
    in bronchopulmonary sequestration, 81
    in tracheomalacia, 48
Barlow maneuver, for DDH diagnosis, 394, 395f
Barlow splint, for DDH, 397
barometric pressure, during infant transport,
        487–488
barotitis, 575
barotrauma, 90, 576
barrel chest, in congenital diaphragmatic
        hernia, 88
barrier function, of skin, 457, 459
    nursing measures for. See skin barriers
barrier paste
    for skin care, 467

for stomas, 473
basilar skull fractures, 348
behavior, developmental
  delay in. See developmental delay
  teaching to parents infant cues of, 514–515
behavioral measures, in pain management, 445
behavioral pain scale, FLACC, 463, 572f
behavioral parameters, in pain assessment, 442t,
      443–444, 571f–573f
beliefs, cultural, 510
benign tumors, neuroblastoma vs, 206
benzodiazepines, for pain management, 450
bereavement. See grief/grieving
bicarbonate (HCO$_3$)
  factors affecting level of, 416
  renal regulation of, 229–230, 235–237
    threshold for, 415–416
  therapeutic. See sodium bicarbonate
      (NaHCO$_3$)
bicornate, 576
bile, 190, 576
bile ducts
  congenital malformations of, 191
  embryology of, 143–145
  intra- vs extrahepatic, 190
  obstruction of, 190–191. See also biliary
      atresia
bile salts, intraluminal, 202
biliary apparatus
  embryology of, 143
biliary atresia, 190–203, 576
  associations of, 194
  bile flow in, 190, 193, 201
  clinical presentation of, 193–194
  complications of, 199–201
  definition of, 189–190, 576
  diagnosis of, 195–197, 195t
  differential diagnosis of, 194
  etiology of, 191–192t, 193
  incidence of, 193
  morphologic classification of, 190, 191f
  nursing care for, 197–198
  outcomes of, 203
  pathophysiology of, 190–191
  treatment of, 197–199
    postoperative nursing care, 201–203
    supportive, 197–198
    surgical, 198–199
biliary cirrhosis, 189, 191, 197, 576
bilingualism, in family-centered care, 511
bilirubin, 576
  conjugated, 577
  direct
    in biliary atresia, 193
    in jaundice evaluation, 195, 195t
  liver processing of, 189
  total, in jaundice evaluation, 195, 195t
  unconjugated, 584
bilirubinemia, 576
biliverdin, 193
biologic markers, of neuroblastoma, 207, 211
biopsy(ies), 576
  bone, in neuroblastoma, 208
  liver, in biliary atresia, 197
  rectal, in Hirschsprung's disease, 170
birth crisis

grief related to
  interventions for, 219t, 518–519
  process of, 518
  types of, 516–518
  parental expectations and, 516
birth trauma. See labor and delivery
birth weight
  inguinal hernia repair and, 185–186
  low, 580
    biliary atresia associated with, 193
    patent ductus arteriosus and, 122
    pulmonary air leak risk and, 101, 106
    necrotizing enterocolitis and, 171–172
    retinopathy of prematurity and, 18
  very low
    fluid therapy during transport, 495–496
    gastroesophageal reflux in, 152
bivalved casts, for talipes equinovarus, 388
bladder
  embryology of, 146, 221–222, 222f, 255
  in patent urachus, 255–256
  in prune belly syndrome, 287–288
    reconstruction of, 293
  urodynamic studies of, in posterior urethral
      valves, 244
bladder dysfunction. See urinary incontinence
bladder exstrophy, 260–271
  associations of, 262
  clinical presentation of, 262
  cloacal exstrophy vs, 261–262, 272
  complications of, 268–269
  definition of, 260
  diagnosis of, 263–264
  differential diagnosis of, 262
  etiology of, 261
  incidence of, 261–262
  outcomes of, 271
  pathophysiology of, 261
  rare variants of, 262
  treatment of, 264–271
    postoperative nursing care, 269–271
    preoperative goals for, 264
    surgical, 265–268, 266f
    timing of, 264–265
bladder neck
  in prune belly syndrome, 288
  reconstruction of, in bladder exstrophy, 265,
      267
bladder outlet obstruction, fetal surgery for,
      524t, 537–539
bladder spasms, 247, 270–271, 286
bladder taps, sequential, for obstructive
      uropathy, 538
Blalock-Taussig shunt
  for hypoplastic left heart syndrome, 132, 133f
  for tetralogy of Fallot, 126–127, 127f
blebs, lung, rupture of, 101
bleeding. See also hemorrhage
  of bronchogenic cyst, postoperative, 70
  with circumcision, 310–312
  gastrointestinal, portal hypertension and, 200
  with gastrostomy tube, 568
  nephrostomy tube and, 283
  urinary, in megaureter repair, 283, 285–286
bleeding disorders. See coagulopathy
bleomycin, for cystic hygroma, 14

blindness, in retinopathy of prematurity, 16, 18
blockage complications
    of Broviac catheter, 561–562
    of gastrostomy tube, 569
blood circulation/flow
    assessment parameters for, 492. *See also*
        hemodynamics
    cardiac development for, 114–117, 114*t*
    cerebral, 8, 324*f*, 325
    collapse of, in hypoplastic left heart
        syndrome, 131, 131*f*
    factors compromising, 493
    fetal (intrauterine)
        embryology of, 114–117, 114*t*
        transition to extrauterine, 115
    management during transport, 492–494
    renal, 227–231, 296
    in total anomalous pulmonary venous
        connection, 134, 134*f*
blood collection/sampling. *See also* heelsticks;
        venipuncture
    neonatal fluid requirements and, 426
    percutaneous, for fetal chromosome
        karyotyping, 524
blood pressure
    assessment of, in congenital heart disease, 119
    increased. *See* hypertension
    kidney regulation of, 227
    in tetralogy of Fallot, 126
blood transfusions
    brain hemorrhage and, 355
    for craniosynostosis repair, 53
    intraoperative indications for, 432
    for necrotizing enterocolitis, 174
    postoperative indications for, 433
blood type/typing, 195, 195*t*, 199
blood urea nitrogen (BUN), 137, 416
blood vessels. *See* artery(ies); vein(s)
blood volume
    arteriovenous malformation impact on, 8
    loss of. *See* hypovolemia
    patent ductus arteriosus and, 122–123
    in tetralogy of Fallot, 126
"blue" spells, with tetralogy of Fallot, 125–126
Bochdalek diaphragmatic hernia, 87–88
body brace, for brachial plexus injury, 405
body fluids, electrolyte content of, 430*t*, 431
body heat loss
    factors contributing to, 107
    during infant transport, 484–485, 492*f*,
        493–494
    maneuvers to limit, 107
    mechanisms of, 107, 484
    skin protection from, 457, 459, 461
body surface area, heat loss related to, 107, 494
body water composition
    changes during gestation and infancy, 414,
        415*f*
    extracellular, 413–414
    intracellular, 413
    renal physiology of, 239, 414–416
        functional assessment of, 416
bonding, parental-infant
    cultural differences in, 519
    death and, 518
    delayed, 517

    strategies for promoting, 514–515
bone(s)
    embryology of, 2, 367
    head and neck, origin of, 2*t*, 3, 7*f*
    limb reduction defects of, 368–372
    neuroblastoma metastasis to, 206
    ossification of, 367
bone biopsy, in neuroblastoma, 208
bone grafts/grafting, in cleft lip/palate repair, 36
bone-joint procedures
    for amniotic band syndrome, 377, 377*f*
    for limb reduction defects, 370
bone marrow aspirates, in neuroblastoma, 208
bone scan. *See* radionuclide scanning
bossing, frontal, 51*f*, 52, 576
botulinum toxin type A (BTXA, Botox)
    for brachial plexus injury, 405
    for talipes equinovarus, 388–389
bowel. *See* intestine(s); *specific anatomy*
"bowel bag"
    for cloacal exstrophy, 275
    for gastrointestinal anomalies, 156, 159
bowel incontinence
    in anorectal malformations, 180–181
    in Hirschsprung's disease, 171
    myelomeningocele and, 337, 340
    myelomeningocele impact on, 337, 340
    neuroblastoma causing, 205
    in spinal cord injury, 359–360
    spinal dimples/sinuses and, 343–345
    tethered cord causing, 340–342
bowel infarction, malrotation/volvulus causing,
        168
bowel loops
    in extraembryonic cavity, 145
    in inguinal hernia, 181, 182*f*, 184–185
    in intestinal atresia/stenosis, 163
    in necrotizing enterocolitis, 173–174, 173*f*
bowel obstruction
    anorectal malformations associated with, 177
    atresia/stenosis causing, 162–164
    gastroesophageal reflux associated with, 152
    in Hirschsprung's disease, 169
    inguinal hernia causing, 183
    malrotation/volvulus causing, 166–169
    meconium causing, 164–165
    pyloric stenosis causing, 161
bowel prep, for hepatic portoenterostomy, 197
bowel rest, post-Kasai portoenterostomy,
        202–203
bowel wall, air in, 173, 173*f*
Bowman's capsule, embryology of, 219*f*, 220
Boyle's law, of gas expansion, 487
BPD. *See* bronchopulmonary dysplasia
BPS. *See* bronchopulmonary sequestration
braces/bracing
    body, for brachial plexus injury, 405
    for DDH, 398
brachial arches, embryology of, 114*t*
brachial plexus, nerves of, 400, 401*f*
brachial plexus injury, 400–406
    associations of, 402
    clinical presentation of, 401–402, 403*f*
    complications of, 405
    definition of, 400
    diagnosis of, 402–404

differential diagnosis of, 402
etiology of, 400–401, 401f
incidence of, 401
lower, 400
motor function assessment for, 403–404
outcomes of, 405–406
pathophysiology of, 400
total, 400
treatment of, 404–406
    conservative, 404–405
    postoperative nursing care, 405
    surgical, 405
upper, 400
brachycephaly, synostotic, 50f, 51–52
bradycardia
    brain hemorrhage causing, 354–355
    necrotizing enterocolitis causing, 172
bradykinin, in renal physiology, 231, 237
brain
    arteriovenous malformation in, 8–11
    blood flow. See cerebral blood flow
    cytodifferentiation of, 323–324
    embryology of, 7f, 82, 322–323
    in encephalocele, 345–348
    hemorrhage in, extra- and intracranial, 350f, 351–356
    ischemic injury of, 9, 11
    painful procedures effects on, 441–442
brain stem dysfunction, hemorrhage causing, 354–355
branchial apparatus remnants, 25–28
    associations of, 26
    cleft lip and, 27, 27f
    complications of, 28
    definition of, 24t, 25
    diagnosis of, 27
    differential diagnosis of, 26–27
    etiology of, 25–26
    incidence of, 26
    outcomes of, 28
    pathophysiology of, 25
    surgical treatment of, 27–28
        postoperative nursing care, 28
branchial arches
    anomalies of, 25–28
    development of, 24t, 25
branchial clefts, 25
branchial cyst, 4f, 5, 26
branchial fistula, 26
branchial pouches, 25
branchial sinus, anomalies of, 26
    surgical treatment of, 27–28
breast milk, chylothorax and, 99
breath sounds
    in congenital diaphragmatic hernia, 88
    in congenital heart disease, 118
    in eventration of diaphragm, 95
breathing
    anomalies impact on. See airway obstruction
    assessment during transport, 490
breech delivery, spinal cord injury with, 357
bridges, dental, in cleft lip/palate repair, 35
British Medica Research Council, on brachial plexus injury, 404
bronchi, embryology of, 59, 61
bronchial intubation

for congenital lobar emphysema, 66
for pulmonary air leak, 104
bronchioles
    embryology of, 62–63, 63f
    terminal, overgrowth of, 528. See also congenital cystic adenomatoid malformation (CCAM)
bronchogenic cyst, 68–70
    associations of, 69
    clinical presentation of, 69
    definition of, 68
    diagnosis of, 69, 70f
    differential diagnosis of, 69
    etiology of, 68–69
    incidence of, 69
    outcomes of, 70
    pathophysiology of, 68
    surgical treatment of, 70
        postoperative nursing care, 70
bronchogram, in bronchopulmonary sequestration, 81
bronchomalacia, 48
bronchopulmonary dysplasia (BPD), 105
bronchopulmonary sequestration (BPS), 76–84
    associations of, 79, 529
    clinical presentation of, 78
    definition of, 76
    diagnosis of, 80–82, 81f
    differential diagnosis of, 80
    etiology of, 77–78
    incidence of, 78
    outcomes of, 84
    pathophysiology of, 76–77, 76f, 79f
    treatment of, 82–84
        immediate stabilization, 82
        postoperative nursing care, 83–84
        prenatal management, 82
        surgical, 82–83
bronchoscopy, 576
    in bronchopulmonary sequestration, 81
    in congenital lobar emphysema, 67
    in esophageal atresia with fistula, 150
    in tracheomalacia, 48–49
    in vocal cord paralysis, 46
Broviac catheter
    complications of, 561–562
    insertion of, 561
    types of, 561
brown fat, 107, 461
bruit, cranial, in arteriovenous malformation, 8
Bryant's traction, for bladder exstrophy closure, 269
Buck's traction, modified, for bladder exstrophy closure, 269
buffer agents, for congenital diaphragmatic hernia, 90
buffer system
    renal, in immediate newborn period, 415
Bugbee electrode, 247
bulbous cordis, embryology of, 114t, 115f, 116
bulboventricular loop, 114, 114t
bullectomy, for pulmonary interstitial emphysema, 105
BUN. See blood urea nitrogen
bupivacaine, for inguinal hernia, 186

C

C cells, embryology of, 3
calcaneocuboid joint, in talipes equinovarus, 383
calcaneus, in talipes equinovarus, 382–383
calcium
    in parenteral nutrition solutions, 436
    physiologic functions of, 422
    renal regulation of, 228–229, 233
    skeletal development and, 367
calcium gluconate, for hyperkalemia, 421
calcium level
    decreased, 422
    factors affecting, 416
    homeostasis physiology of, 422
    increased, 422–423
    ionized, 233
    management of
        postoperative, 108, 128
        during transport, 496, 503
    phosphorous ratio to, 422
calculi, urinary
    bladder exstrophy repair and, 268, 271
    megaureter and, 280t, 281, 284, 287
calf muscles, in talipes equinovarus, 383, 388–389, 391
calories
    daily requirement for, 437–438
    in parenteral nutrition solutions, 434–437
calvarial vault
    embryology of, 7, 7f
    remodeling of, for craniosynostosis, 54
calyx/calyces, 576
    major and minor, embryology of, 219f, 220
    renal, in ureteropelvic junction obstruction, 295
canalicular stage, of lung development, 62, 63f
cancer(s)
    bladder exstrophy and, 271
    choanal atresia vs, 30
    neuroblastoma as, 203–212
    of penis, circumcision and, 309
candidiasis, topical, 467
capillary(ies)
    cerebral
        arteriovenous malformation in, 8–11
        CSF flow through, 325
    pulmonary, embryology of, 62, 63f
    renal, embryology of, 219f, 221
    retinal, injury mechanisms of, 17
capillary leak syndrome, 137, 160
capillary refill, 108, 371
caput succedaneum, 350f, 351–352
carbohydrates
    in parenteral nutrition solutions, 434–435, 437. See also dextrose
    in renal physiology, 239
carbon dioxide, partial pressure of, 554
    in congenital diaphragmatic hernia, 90, 92
cardiac anomalies. See congenital heart disease
cardiac arrhythmias
    fetal, in congenital heart disease, 117
    potassium level and, 420–421
    tetralogy of Fallot repair and, 128

cardiac catheterization
    in bronchopulmonary sequestration, 82
    in congenital heart disease, 120–121
    for patent ductus arteriosus closure, 124
cardiac conduction, in congenital heart disease, 117–118, 120
cardiac development, fetal, 114–117, 114t
    embryology of, 2–3
cardiac failure, high-output, 531
cardiac output (CO)
    cerebral blood flow component, 325
    in congenital heart disease, 118, 120, 131
        stabilization of, 137
    factors compromising, 493
    management during transport, 493–494
    ovarian cyst hemorrhage and, 307
    in patent ductus arteriosus, 122
    in pulmonary disorders, 84, 88
        postoperative management, 108
    in renal physiology, 227–228
cardiac ventricle(s)
    embryology of, 114t, 115, 115f, 116
    left, hypoplasia of, 131–133, 131f
    right, hypertrophy of, 124, 124f, 126–129, 132
cardiogenic cords, 114
cardiogenic shock, management during transport, 494, 503
cardioplegia, 576
cardiopulmonary bypass
    extracorporeal membrane oxygenation vs, 553
    postoperative nursing care for, 136
    for tetralogy of Fallot repair, 127–128
    for D-transposition of the great arteries repair, 130, 130f
cardiotonics, for postoperative pulmonary stabilization, 109
cardiovascular system, 113–138
    brain hemorrhage and, 354
    bronchopulmonary sequestration and, 82, 84
    in cloacal exstrophy, 273, 275–276
    congenital lobar emphysema and, 67
    congenital malformations of, 117–138. See also congenital heart disease
    embryology of, 2–3, 114–117, 114t
    extracorporeal membrane oxygenation and, 557
    function of, 114
    management during transport, 492–494
    opioids effects on, 447, 454
    in pulmonary disorders, postoperative stabilization of, 109
    surgery for, fluid and electrolyte disturbances with, 426–427, 427t
    surgical conditions of, 113
care conferences, 511
carina, 576
carotid pulse, in arteriovenous malformation, 8
carpals/carpus, embryology of, 364f
Carpenter syndrome, 51
cartilage
    in branchial arches, 24t, 25
    chondral, 35, 576
    embryology of, 364f, 365, 367
    hip defects of, in DDH, 392–393
    nasal, development of, 6
    pulmonary, development of, 61, 72

of skull, 7, 7*f*
types of, 366–367
cartilage grafts, in cleft lip/palate repair, 35
casts/casting
    for absent radius, 380–381
    for brachial plexus injury, 405
    for DDH, 398–399
    for lower limb anomalies, 278
    for talipes equinovarus, 382
        bivalved, 388
        postoperative nursing care, 390
        removal of, 391
        serial, 387–388, 391
catabolism, prevention of, 436–437
catecholamines
    parenteral nutrition and, 435
    in pulmonary disorders, 108
    in surgical stress response, 434
    urinary, 207, 230
catheters/catheterization
    Broviac, 561–562
    cardiac. *See* cardiac catheterization
    central line. *See* central vascular catheter
    epidural
        maternal placement of, in fetal surgery, 540
        nursing care for, 453–454
    French indwelling
        infection control for, 109
        for tension pneumothorax, 105
    for infant transport, 502
        placement of, 493, 495
    percutaneous insertions of, pain management
        for, 451, 452*t*
    sump, for esophageal atresia with fistula, 150
    umbilical
        insertions during infant transport, 493,
            495, 502
        pain management for, 451, 452*t*
    ureteral, for bladder exstrophy closure, 266
    urethral. *See* urethral catheter
    urinary. *See* Foley catheter; suprapubic
        catheter
    ventriculostomy, for hydrocephalus, 331–332,
        331*f*
cations, 576
    organic, renal excretion of, 238
caudal, 322, 576
caudal anesthesia/analgesia
    for inguinal hernia repair, 184
    for megaureter repair, 286
    for ureteropelvic junction obstruction, 302
cautery, of bronchogenic cyst, 70
CBC. *See* complete blood count
CBF. *See* cerebral blood flow
CCAM. *See* congenital cystic adenomatoid
    malformation
CDH. *See* congenital diaphragmatic hernia
cecal diverticulum, embryology of, 145
cecum, 576
    embryology of, 144–145
    in intestinal malrotation/volvulus, 168
cell migration, in wound healing, 461*f*, 462
cellular transplant, future directions for, 542
cellulose products, for circumcision, 311
central nervous system (CNS)
    embryology of, 2, 321–324, 364

physiology of, 324*f*, 325–326
surgical conditions of, 325–361. *See also*
    neurosurgical disorders
vocal cord paralysis and, 45–46
central vascular catheter
    indications for, 157, 160
    infections with, 109, 210
    pain management during placement of, 452*t*
cephalad, 576
cephalhematoma, 350*f*, 351
cephalosporins, for cholangitis, 200
cerebellum, 323
cerebral arteries, arteriovenous malformation
    in, 8–11
cerebral blood flow (CBF)
    arteriovenous malformation impact on, 8
    hemodynamics of, 324*f*, 325–326
    pressure autoregulation in, 325
cerebral capillaries
    arteriovenous malformation in, 8–11
    CSF flow through, 325
cerebral hemispheres, 323, 584
cerebral hemorrhage, arteriovenous
    malformation associated with, 9, 11
cerebral infarction, 11, 352
cerebral metabolism, 326
cerebral perfusion pressure (CPP), 325–326
cerebral periosteum, hemorrhage in, 350*f*, 351
cerebral vascular resistance (CVR), 325
cerebral veins, 8, 328, 584
cerebral ventricles
    embryology of, 323–324, 324*f*
    enlargement of, 326
cerebrospinal fluid (CSF)
    in brain hemorrhage, 353
    diversion devices for. *See* CSF diversion
    in encephalocele, 345–348
    flow of, 324*f*, 325
    in hydrocephalus, 326–328
        medical management of, 330
        surgical management of, 330–335, 331*f*, 333*f*
    leaks of, in skull fractures, 349–351
    physiologic control of, 325–326
    production of, 325
certifications, for infant transport team, 481–482
cervical flexure, of brain, 323
cervical nerve roots, avulsive tears of, 400, 401*f*,
    404
cervical sinus, embryology of, 4*f*, 5–6
cervical spine, masses in, neuroblastoma as, 205
cervix, embryology of, 224, 224*f*
cesarean delivery
    in adult females born with bladder exstrophy,
        271
    for fetal ovarian cysts, 308
    for gastroschisis, 156
CF. *See* cystic fibrosis
Cha classification, of congenital cystic
    adenomatoid malformation, 71–72
CHAOS. *See* congenital high airway obstruction
CHARGE association, atresias associated with,
    31, 149
CHD. *See* congenital heart disease
chemotaxis, 576
chemotherapy, 576
    for choanal atresia, 30

for neuroblastoma, 208–210
chest assessment
    for air leak, 103
    in congenital diaphragmatic hernia, 525
    in congenital heart disease, 119
chest tube
    for chylothorax, 99
    for congenital cystic adenomatoid
        malformation, 76
    for congenital diaphragmatic hernia, 91
    for congenital lobar emphysema, 67–68
    insertion of
        during infant transport, 502
        pain management for, 452*t*
    nursing care for, 106
    for tension pneumothorax, 105
chest x-ray
    in arteriovenous malformation, 9
    in bronchogenic cyst, 69–70*f*
    in bronchopulmonary sequestration, 81, 81*f*
    in chylothorax, 98
    in congenital cystic adenomatoid
        malformation, 74, 75*f*
    in congenital diaphragmatic hernia, 89, 89*f*
    in congenital heart disease, 119, 123, 129, 135
    in congenital lobar emphysema, 66, 66*f*
    in eventration of diaphragm, 95, 95*f*
    in neuroblastoma, 208
    in prune belly syndrome, 291
    in pulmonary air leak, 103–104, 104*f*
    in pulmonary lymphangiectasia, 86, 86*f*
    for tracheostomy location, 549
CHF. *See* congestive heart failure
Chiari deformity, 327, 576
Child Abuse and Treatment Act (1984), 360, 361*t*
chloral hydrate, for pain management, 450–451
chloride
    body fluid content of, 430*t*, 431
    loss factors, 416, 421
    physiology of, 421
    renal regulation of, 230, 232–233, 238
    retention factors, 416, 421
choanae, nasal, 5, 29, 576
    congenital obstruction of, 28–31
choanal atresia, 28–31
    associations of, 29
    clinical presentation of, 29
    complications of, 31
    definition of, 28
    diagnosis of, 30
    differential diagnosis of, 29–30
    etiology of, 28
    incidence of, 29
    outcomes of, 31
    pathophysiology of, 28
    treatment of
        postoperative nursing care, 31
        surgical, 30
        symptomatic, 30
choking, in esophageal atresia with fistula,
        148–149
cholangitis, 576
    Kasai portoenterostomy and, 199–200
choleretics, 200–201
cholestasis, 189, 194, 196. *See also* biliary atresia
chondral cartilage, 576

graft, in cleft lip/palate repair, 36
chondrification centers, 365, 367
chondroblasts, 365
chondrocranium, embryology of, 7, 7*f*
chondrosarcoma, mesenchymal, neuroblastoma
        vs, 206
chordee, 576
chorion, separation of, limb defects associated
        with, 372*f*–373*f*, 373–378
chorionic villus sampling, 524
choroid layer, of eye, 576
choroid plexus, 323, 324*f*, 325, 576
    papilloma of, hydrocephalus related to, 328
choroidal vessels, 576
chromosomal analysis, in cloacal exstrophy,
        275–277
chromosome 1, abnormalities of, 205, 207
chromosome 2, myelomeningocele and, 335
chromosome 13, abnormalities of, 524
chromosome 15q, diaphragm development and,
        63
chromosome 18, abnormalities of, 524
chromosome 21, abnormalities of, 524
chromosome 22q11, deletion of, 43
chromosome disorders. *See also* trisomy *entries*
    absent radius associated with, 379–380
    branchial apparatus anomalies and, 27
    congenital heart disease associated with, 117
    congenital high airway obstruction associated
        with, 535
    hydrocephalus as, 328–329
    karyotyping of. *See* karyotypic analysis
    laryngeal web and, 43
    in myelomeningocele, 335
    myelomeningocele associated with, 335–337
    neuroblastoma as, 205, 207
    omphalocele associated with, 159
    prune belly syndrome associated with,
        289–290
    talipes equinovarus as, 384–385
chronic grief, 516, 576
chyle, 97
chylothorax, 97–100
    associations of, 98
    clinical presentation of, 98
    congenital *vs* acquired, 97–98
    definition of, 97
    diagnosis of, 98, 99*f*
    differential diagnosis of, 98
    etiology of, 97–98
    incidence of, 98
    outcomes of, 100
    pathophysiology of, 97
    treatment of
        conservative, 99
        postoperative nursing care, 100
        prenatal therapy in, 99
        surgical, 99–100
chylous fluid
    analysis of, 98
    volume of, 99–100
cicatricial retinal changes, 20, 25, 576
cicatricial scar, 576
cicatrix, 576
cilia, lower respiratory tract, 61–62
cimetidine, for gastroesophageal reflux, 153

circulation. *See* blood circulation/flow
circulation assessment, for limb reduction
      defects, 371–372
circumcision, newborn, 309–313
  complications of, 311
  contraindications to, 310
  definition of, 309
  incidence of, 309
  outcomes of, 313
  pain management for, 451, 452*t*
  possible indications for, 309
  posterior urethral valves and, 249–250
  potential medical benefits of, 309
  preprocedural assessment, 310
  skin care following, 312–313, 468
  surgical management, 310–311
    postoperative nursing care, 312–313
circumferential excision, for amniotic band
      syndrome, 376, 376*f*
cirrhosis, 576
  biliary, 189, 191, 197, 576
clavicle fracture, brachial plexus *vs*, 402–403
cleaning solutions, for wound care, 463
cleft(s)
  orofacial. *See* cleft lip; cleft palate
  pubovesical, 261
cleft lip, 31–37
  associations of, 32
  branchial apparatus remnants and, 27, 27*f*
  clinical presentation of, 32
  complications of, 35
  definition of, 31
  diagnosis of, 32
  differential diagnosis of, 32
  etiology of, 31
  incidence of, 31–32
  outcomes of, 36–37
  pathophysiology of, 31
  surgical treatment of, 33–37
    bone grafting, 35
    lip repair, 33–34
    nose reconstruction, 34–35
    palate repair, 34–34*f*
    pharyngeal flap/pharyngoplasty, 35
    postoperative nursing care, 35–36
    secondary procedures, 34, 35*f*
    timing of, 33
    types of, 32*f*, 33*f*
cleft lip/palate feeder, 32, 36
cleft palate, 6, 31–37
  associations of, 32
  clinical presentation of, 32
  complications of, 35
  definition of, 31
  diagnosis of, 32
  differential diagnosis of, 32
  etiology of, 31
  incidence of, 31–32
  outcomes of, 36–37
  pathophysiology of, 31
  primary *vs* secondary, 32*f*
  surgical treatment of, 33–37
    bone grafting, 35
    lip repair, 33–34
    nose reconstruction, 34–35
    palate repair, 34–34*f*

    pharyngeal flap/pharyngoplasty, 35
    postoperative nursing care, 35–36
    secondary procedures, 34, 35*f*
    timing of, 33
  types of, 32*f*–33*f*, 33*f*
  U-shaped soft, 32, 37
clicks, cardiac, in congenital heart disease, 118
clinical utility, of instruments, 443, 576
clitoris, 226*f*, 273
cloaca, 576
  embryology of, 146, 221
  persistent, 175, 176*f*, 180
  repair of, urinary incontinence with, 181
cloacal exstrophy, 271–279
  associations of, 274
  bladder exstrophy *vs*, 262, 272
  clinical presentation of, 272–273
  complications of, 278
  definition of, 271–272
  diagnosis of, 274–275
  differential diagnosis of, 274
  embryology of, 272
  etiology of, 272
  incidence of, 272
  nursing care for, 275–276
  outcomes of, 279
  pathophysiology of, 272
  treatment of, 275–279
    goals for, 276–277
    initial supportive, 275–276
    postoperative nursing care, 278–279
    surgical, 276–278
cloacal membrane, 146
  in bladder exstrophy, 261
  in cloacal exstrophy, 272
  in external genitalia, 226*f*
cloacal sphincter, 146
closed reduction, of DDH, 397–398
closed system drainage device(s)
  for chest. *See* chest tube
  postoperative, for cystic hygroma, 15–16
closed vitrectomy, for retinopathy of
      prematurity, 20*t*, 22–24
closure, surgical
  of bladder exstrophy, 264
  of cloacal exstrophy, 277
  of congenital diaphragmatic hernia, 91
  of foramen ovale, 115
  of gastroschisis, 157, 157*f*
  of omphalocele, 159, 159*f*
  of patent ductus arteriosus, 123–124
clot removal, for spinal cord injury, 358
clotting time, extracorporeal membrane
      oxygenation and, 556–557
clubbing, of fingers, 125
clubfoot, 382–391. *See also* talipes equinovarus
  congenital idiopathic, 384–385, 384*f*
  historical descriptions of, 382
  normal foot *vs*, 382–383, 383*f*
  tetralogic, 383, 385
clubhand, radial, 379, 381
CMV. *See* cytomegalovirus
CNS. *See* central nervous system
CO. *See* cardiac output
CO_2 laser vaporization
  of choanal atresia, 30

of cystic hygroma, 15
of laryngeal web, 44–45
coagulation factors, extracorporeal membrane oxygenation and, 557
coagulation stage, in wound healing, 461–462, 461f
coagulopathy
brain hemorrhage resulting from, 352–353
treatment of, 355–356
as circumcision contraindication, 310
postoperative, in tetralogy of Fallot repair, 127–128
preoperative management of, 431
spinal cord injury and, 358
coarctation, of aorta, 114t
COBRA. See Consolidated Omnibus Reconciliation Act
coccygeal dimple, 343, 343f
coccyx, sacrococcygeal teratoma arising from, 530–533
coelom, embryology of, 63
cognitive function, myelomeningocele impact on, 340
Cohen classification, of laryngeal webs, 42
cold stress, management during transport, 484–485, 492f, 493–494
colitis, necrotizing enterocolitis vs, 173
collaboration
in family-centered care, 509
during infant transport, 482t, 484, 501, 504
in pain assessment/management, 443
collagen, 576
in wound healing, 460f, 462
collagen fibers
in skin, 460
urogenital, in ureteropelvic junction obstruction, 295
collecting tubules, renal
cysts of, ovarian cysts vs, 305
duplex, 281
embryology of, 219f, 220–221
"pacemaker" sites in, 295
physiology of, 227, 229, 236, 414
water and electrolyte regulation in, 414–422.
See also specific electrolyte
colloids, 577
for pulmonary disorders, 100, 108
water regulation by, 414
coloboma, 577
colon
absence of ganglion cells in, 169–170
distal, short, 272
embryology of, 144–146
stricture of, in necrotizing enterocolitis, 174–175
colonic irrigation, for Hirschsprung's disease, 170
color, skin
in congenital heart disease, 117–118
in limb reduction defects, 371
colostomy, 470, 577
for anorectal malformations, 178–180
male vs female, 178f, 179f
appliances for, 472–473
for cloacal exstrophy, 277–279
for Hirschsprung's disease, 170

columella, 577
nasal, lengthening of, 34, 35f
comfort measures
for bladder exstrophy repair, 270
for congenital heart disease, 138
for esophageal atresia with fistula, 150
for extracorporeal membrane oxygenation, 558–559
for megaureter, 286
for neonatal death, grieving, 519–519t
for wound care, 463
commissure(s), 577
anterior, 575
labial, embryology of, 226f, 227
common bile ducts, obstruction of, 190–191, 191f
communicating hydrocele, 181, 182f
communication
in family-centered care
culturally-competent, 510–511
facilitating, 511
mutually respectful, 510, 515–516
with transport team, 492, 504–505
community hospital, return transport to, 516
compassionate care, for hydrocephalus, 330
competent care
culturally, 510–511, 519, 577
for infant transport, 480t, 482
complete blood count (CBC)
in jaundice evaluation, 195, 195t
in neuroblastoma evaluation, 207, 210
compression, fetal. See intrauterine environment
computed tomography (CT) scan
in arteriovenous malformation, 9
in biliary atresia, 196
in brain hemorrhage, 353
in bronchogenic cyst, 69
in bronchopulmonary sequestration, 81
in congenital cystic adenomatoid malformation, 74, 75f
in congenital lobar emphysema, 66, 67f
in craniosynostosis, 53
in cystic hygroma, 13
in encephalocele, 346
fiberoptic, in choanal atresia, 30
in hydrocephalus, 329
in myelomeningocele, 337
in neuroblastoma, 208
in patent urachus, 258
in pulmonary lymphangiectasia, 86
in spinal cord injury, 357
conchae, embryology of, 5
conduction
cardiac, in congenital heart disease, 117–118, 120
heat loss through, 107, 484
conductive hearing loss, middle ear surgery for, 28
conferences
care, 511
informed consent, for fetal surgery, 524
congenital cystic adenomatoid malformation (CCAM), 70–76
associations of, 73
clinical presentation of, 72–73
complications of, 75
definition of, 70

diagnosis, 73–74, 74f–75f
differential diagnosis, 73
etiology of, 72
fetal surgery for, 524t, 528–530
incidence of, 72
outcomes of, 76
pathophysiology of, 71–72
treatment of, 74–76
    immediate stabilization, 74–75
    postoperative nursing care, 75–76
    prenatal management in, 74
    surgical, 75
volume ratio (CVR), 529
congenital diaphragmatic hernia (CDH), 87–94
  associations of, 88–89
  clinical presentation of, 88
  definition of, 87
  diagnosis of, 89, 89f
  differential diagnosis of, 89
  etiology of, 87–88
  fetal surgery for, 524t, 525–527
  incidence of, 88
  outcomes of, 92–94
  pathophysiology of, 87
  treatment of, 90–92
    fetal therapy in, 90
    immediate stabilization, 90–91
    postoperative nursing care, 92
    surgical, 91–92
congenital heart disease (CHD), 117–121
  acyanotic vs cyanotic lesions, 113, 125, 129
  anorectal malformations association with, 177
  D-transposition of great arteries, 128–130
  developmental alterations in, 113, 114t
  diagnosis of, 113
    neonatal, 117–120
    prenatal, 117
  differential diagnosis of, 119–120
  ductal-dependent, 125, 128
    management during transport, 493–494
  esophageal atresia associated with, 149
  fetal surgery for, 542
  hypoplastic left heart syndrome, 131–133
  myelomeningocele associated with, 336–337
  omphalocele associated with, 159
  patent ductus arteriosus, 121–124
  postoperative nursing care for, 136–138
  preoperative stabilization of, 120–121
  primary respiratory disease vs, 493
  prune belly syndrome associated with, 290
  tetralogy of Fallot, 124–128
  total anomalous pulmonary venous
    connection, 134–136
  tracheomalacia associated with, 47–49
congenital high airway obstruction (CHAOS),
  535
congenital laryngeal stridor, 39
congenital lobar emphysema, 64–68
  associations of, 65
  clinical presentation of, 65
  definition of, 64
  diagnosis of, 66, 66f–67f
  differential diagnosis of, 65
  etiology of, 64–65
  incidence of, 65
  outcomes of, 68

pathophysiology of, 64
treatment of, 66–68
  immediate stabilization, 66–67
  postoperative nursing care, 67–68
  surgical, 67
congenital malformations, 577, 581. See also
    specific anomaly
  of cardiovascular system, 121–138
  congenital diaphragmatic hernia associated
    with, 88–89
  of extremities, 368–406
  fetal surgery for, 523–542
  of gastrointestinal tract, 146–186
  of genitourinary tract, 240–313
  grief and loss reactions to, 517
  of head, ears, eyes, nose, and throat, 8–55
  of liver, gallbladder, and biliary apparatus,
    190–212
  of lung, 64–109
  of neurologic system, 326–361
Congenital Malformations Registry of New York
    State, 288–289
congenital pulmonary airway malformation, 71
congenital ring constriction, of limbs, 373
congenital venolobar syndrome, 77
congestive heart failure (CHF)
  arteriovenous malformation associated with,
    8–11
  in congenital heart disease, 117, 128
    preoperative stabilization of, 120–121, 126
  in patent ductus arteriosus, 122
conjugated bilirubin, 577
conjunctival sac, embryology of, 6
connective tissue
  embryology of, 2, 365
  formation disorders of, inguinal hernia and,
    183
  gastrointestinal development of, 142–143
  pulmonary development of, 61–62
consent
  informed, for fetal surgery, 524
  parental, for infant transport, 501
    implied, 501
conservative management
  of brachial plexus injury, 404–405
  of brain hemorrhage, 354
  of chylothorax, 99
  of eventration of diaphragm, 96
  of ovarian cysts, 306–307
  of tethered cord, 342
  of ureteropelvic junction obstruction, 299–300
Consolidated Omnibus Reconciliation
    Act (COBRA), infant transport
    requirements, 481
constipation
  anorectal malformation repair and, 181
  in Hirschsprung's disease, 169, 171
  in prune belly syndrome, 292–293
constriction(s)
  in amniotic band syndrome, 373–378, 374f
  congenital ring, 373
constriction band syndrome, 373
  deep vs superficial, 376, 376f
consultation(s)
  for cleft lip/palate management, 33
  for fetal interventions, 525, 542

genetic. *See* genetic consultation
for myelomeningocele management, 338–340
orthopedic, for prune belly syndrome, 290–291
physician, during infant transport, 482*t*, 484, 501, 504
plastic surgery, for IV extravasation, 467
contextual factors, of pain response, 444, 577
continence, loss of. *See* incontinence
continuing education
on fetal surgery, 542
for transport team, 481, 485, 504
continuous positive airway pressure (CPAP)
nasal, 38, 41
pulmonary air leak risk and, 101–102
contraction alkalosis, 577
contracture(s)
shoulder, in brachial plexus injury, 405–406
soft tissue, in absent radius, 381
spinal cord injury and, 358–359
contralateral, 577
contrast studies
congenital diaphragmatic hernia contraindication for, 89
enema. *See* barium enema
esophageal
in bronchogenic cyst, 69
in esophageal atresia with fistula, 150
nasal, in choanal atresia, 30
in patent urachus, 258
swallow. *See* barium swallow
upper gastrointestinal
in gastroesophageal reflux, 153
in tracheomalacia, 49
conus (medullaris), 577
low, 340–342. *See also* tethered cord
convection, heat loss through, 107, 484
convoluted tubules, distal and proximal
embryology of, 219, 219*f*
physiology of, 228–229, 233
Coombs test, in jaundice evaluation, 195, 195*t*
coping mechanisms
gender differences in, 514
during painful procedures, 443–445
copper, in parenteral nutrition solutions, 436
cornea, embryology of, 6
corneal button, 577
coronal synostosis, 51–52
treatment of, 53–55
coronary arteries, arteriovenous malformation impact on, 9
corpus cavernosum, embryology of, 226*f*
corpus spongiosum, embryology of, 226*f*
cortex
ovarian, embryology of, 223*f*
renal, embryology of, 219*f*, 220–221, 223
corticosteroids
for cholangitis, 200–201
in surgical stress response, 434
cortisol level, parenteral nutrition and, 435
costodiaphragmatic recess, 64
CPAP. *See* continuous positive airway pressure
CPP. *See* cerebral perfusion pressure
cranial meningocele, 345
cranial nerve(s)

IX (glossopharyngeal nerve), pharyngeal arch origin of, 2*t*, 3
V (trigeminal nerve)
in brachial plexus injury, 400–406
pharyngeal arch origin of, 2*t*, 3
VI, in brachial plexus injury, 400–406
VII (facial nerve), pharyngeal arch origin of, 2*t*, 3
VIII, in brachial plexus injury, 400–406
X (vagus nerve), pharyngeal arch origin of, 2*t*, 3
embryology of, 2*t*, 3, 5
cranial sutures
in hydrocephalus, 328
ICP control and, 325
premature fusion of, 49–55. *See also* craniosynostosis
cranial ultrasound, in arteriovenous malformation, 9
craniectomy, suboccipital, for brain hemorrhage, 355
craniocaudal folding, 323
craniofacial reconstruction, for branchial arch anomalies, 28
craniosynostosis, 49–55
associations of, 52
categories of, 50*f*, 51
clinical presentation of, 51–52, 51*f*, 52*f*
complications of, 54, 54*t*
definition of, 49, 584
deformational, positional *vs* structural, 50, 52–53
diagnosis of, 52–53
differential diagnosis of, 52
etiology of, primary *vs* secondary, 51, 55
incidence of, 51
outcomes of, 55
pathophysiology of, 50–51
primary *vs* secondary, 50
simple *vs* complex (compound), 50
surgical treatment of
goals of, 53–54
postoperative nursing care, 54–55
timing of, 53
syndromic *vs* nonsyndromic classification, 51–52, 55
craniotome, pneumatic, 582
craniotomy, direct, for arteriovenous malformation, 10
cranium
craniosynostosis of, 49–55
embryology of, 6, 7*f*
cranium bifidum, 345
creatinine level
in congenital heart disease, 137
in renal function, 228, 247
urinary diversion indications, 247–249, 248*f*, 250
cremaster muscle, 577
cremasteric reflex, 253, 577
cricoid malformations, laryngeal web and, 43–44
cricothyroidotomy, emergency, 547
CRIES: Neonatal postoperative pain assessment score, 442*t*, 443, 572*f*
crisis management, daily, 517
cross-cultural knowledge, 510

croup, laryngeal web and, 43
crura, embryology of, 64
cry/crying
    in inguinal hernia, 183–184
    as pain response, 442t, 444
    vocal cord paralysis and, 45–47
cryotherapy, 577
    for retinopathy of prematurity, 20t, 21–22, 24
cryptorchidism, 289, 577
crystalline parenteral solutions, 434–436
crystalloid infusion, 108, 432, 577
CSF. See cerebrospinal fluid
CSF diversion
    for brain hemorrhage, 354–355
    for encephalocele, 347–348
    for hydrocephalus
        devices for, 330–332, 331f
        indications for, 330
        shunts for, 332–333, 333f
    for myelomeningocele, 339
CT scan. See computed tomography scan
cues, in infant behavior development, 514–515
cultural assessment, 510
cultural diversity, 510
culturally competent care, 510, 577
    communication in, 510–511
    for grief process, 519
culture(s)
    in jaundice evaluation, 195, 195t
    in posterior urethral valves assessment,
        244–245
customs, cultural, 510
CVR. See congenital cystic adenomatoid
        malformation
CVR. See cerebral vascular resistance
cyanoacrylate, 577
cyanosis, 577
cyanotic lesions
    in congenital heart disease, 113, 125, 129
    ductal-dependent, 125, 128
        management during transport, 493–494
cycloplegic agent, postoperative, for retinopathy
        of prematurity, 24
cyst(s)
    branchial, 26
    bronchogenic, 68–70
    cystic hygroma excision cautions with, 14
    inclusion, with circumcision, 313
    leptomeningeal, 350
    in obstructive uropathy, 538
    ovarian, 303–309. See also ovarian cysts
    sacrococcygeal teratoma as, 530–533
    subcutaneous, neuroblastoma vs, 206
    urachal, 256, 257f, 258–260
    urinary system, ovarian cysts vs, 305
cyst decompression, in utero, for ovarian cysts,
        307
cysteine, in parenteral nutrition solutions, 436
cystic adenomatoid malformation, congenital,
        70–76
    fetal surgery for, 524t, 528–530
cystic duct, 143
cystic fibrosis (CF), 577
    biliary atresia vs, 194, 196
    inguinal hernia and, 183
    meconium ileus associated with, 164–165

cystic hygroma, 11–16
    associations of, 13
    clinical presentation of, 12–13
    complications of, 15–16
    definition of, 11
    diagnosis of, 13
    differential diagnosis of, 13
    etiology of, 12
    incidence of, 12
    outcomes of, 16
    pathophysiology of, 12
    recurrent, 16
    treatment of, 13–15
        acute, 14
        alternative therapies, 14–15
        expectant, 14
        factors influencing, 13
        postoperative nursing care, 16
        surgical, 14–15
cystic sac, 577
cystostomy tube, suprapubic, for bladder
        exstrophy closure, 266, 268
    postoperative nursing care, 270–271
cystoureterogram, 577
cytokines, 577
    in wound healing, 461–462, 461f
cytomegalovirus (CMV), in biliary atresia, 191,
        192t, 193

D

D-bar (Denis Browne) splint, for talipes
        equinovarus, 388, 389f
daily weights, 438
Dalton's Law, of partial pressures, 487–488
Dandy Walker syndrome, 328, 332, 577
database, for infant transport quality assurance,
        506–507, 506f
DDH. See developmental dysplasia of the hip
death, neonatal
    grief and loss reactions to, 518
    statistics on. See mortality
debridement, 577
debulking procedure, intrauterine, for
        sacrococcygeal teratoma, 532
decerebrate posturing, 577
decision making, in family-centered care, 509,
        511, 518
decompression
    of ovarian cysts, in utero, 307
    of stomach. See gastric decompression
decorticate posturing, 577
deformity/deformation, congenital, 577. See also
        congenital malformations
    grief and loss reactions to, 517
degenerative joint disease, in DDH, 399
degloving injuries, 311, 577
dehiscence, 577
dehydration, 577
    fluid and electrolyte disturbances with, 427,
        427t
    hypernatremic vs hyponatremic, 580
    hypertonic vs hypotonic, 429t, 430
    isotonic, 429, 429t, 580
    markers for, 428–429, 429t
    post-vesicostomy, for PUV, 251

preoperative correction of, 429–430, 429t
in pyloric stenosis, 161
dehydrocholic acid, for cholangitis, 200
delayed treatment
of encephalocele, 347
of hydrocephalus, 330
of skull fractures, 349
delivery. See labor and delivery
demarcation, 577
demyelination, 577
Denis Browne. See D-bar splint
dental rehabilitation, in cleft lip/palate repair,
35–36
dependency, 578
depressed skull fractures, 348–349, 349f, 351
dermal papillae, 460
dermal sinus, 578
dermatitis, diaper, 180, 466–467
dermis, 578
anatomy of, 457, 458f
embryology of, 459f, 460–461
dermoid cyst, 206, 578
descending colon, embryology of, 146
detorsion technique, for testicular torsion, 253
development, infant, 578
teaching to parents, 514–515
developmental behavior, infant cues of, 514–515
developmental delay
arteriovenous malformation associated with,
11
encephalocele causing, 347–348
pulmonary disorders and, 93, 109
skull fractures causing, 350
developmental dysplasia of the hip (DDH),
391–399
associations of, 393
clinical presentation of, 393
complications of, 398–399
definition of, 391
diagnosis of, 394–396, 394f–396f
differential diagnosis of, 393–394
etiology of, 392–393
Graf classification of, 396, 396f, 397t
incidence of, 393
outcomes of, 399
pathophysiology of, 391–392
treatment of, 397–399
closed reduction, 398
goals of, 397
newborn to six months, 397–398, 397f
postoperative nursing care, 399
surgical, 398
developmental outcomes
cleft lip/palate impact on, 36
pain effects on, 442
of pulmonary disorders, 59
dextrocardia, 114t
dextrose infusions
for dehydration, 429–430
for homeostasis maintenance, 108, 430
during infant transport, 495–497
with insulin, for hyperkalemia, 421
intraoperative indications for, 432
in parenteral nutrition, 434–435
concentration determinants, 435–436
delivery rates, 435–436

diagnosis, differential, 578
diaper dermatitis, 180, 466–467
diaphragm, 87–97
congenital hernia of, 87–94
fetal, 524t, 525–527
embryology of, 63–64, 143
eventration of, 94–97, 579
paralysis of, in spinal cord injury, 359
diaphragmatic hernia, 87–94. See also congenital
diaphragmatic hernia (CDH)
diaphyses (shaft), ossification of, 367
diarrhea, intractable, 206, 210
diastematomyelia, 341, 578
diastole, arteriovenous malformation impact
on, 9
diencephalon, 323, 578
diet. See nutrition/nutritional support
differential diagnosis, 578
diffusion, in renal physiology, 229–230
DiGeorge syndrome, 3, 26
digital examination, rectal, for malformations,
177
digital ray, 364f, 365, 366f
digits. See fingers; toes
digoxin, for congenital heart disease, 120–121
dilation
of anus, for anorectal malformations, 180
of ureters. See megaureter
dilutional hyponatremia, 417
dimples/dimpling
coccygeal, 343, 343f
of extremity joints, in prune belly syndrome,
289
sacral, 343, 343f
spinal, 336, 342–345. See also spinal dimples
direct bilirubin
in biliary atresia, 193
in jaundice evaluation, 195, 195t
directed donor blood, for craniosynostosis
repair, 53
discharge criteria, post-Kasai portoenterostomy,
203
discharge planning/teaching, 516. See also
parent teaching
for congenital heart disease, 126, 138
for prune belly syndrome, 294
for pulmonary disorders, 109
on stoma care, 476
on ventriculoperitoneal shunts, 334
discipline, for transport team, 481
disease-based protocols, for infant transport,
483t, 484
dislocatable hip, 392, 578
dislocated hip, 392, 578
teratologic, 392, 584
dislocation, 578
of shoulder, brachial plexus vs, 402
dispatch center, for transport team, 489, 504
dispatch delay, of transport team, 506f, 507
dispatch time, threshold for, 507
disruption, 578
distal convoluted tubule
embryology of, 219–220, 219f
physiology of, 229
diuretic renal scan, in megaureter, 282–283
diuretics

for congenital heart disease, 123, 135, 137
for hydrocephalus, 330
for pulmonary disorders, postoperative, 108
diversion devices
CSF. *See* CSF diversion
fecal, 174, 179
urinary. *See* urinary diversion
DNA testing, for cystic fibrosis, 166
dobutamine, for tetralogy of Fallot, 126
documentation
of feeding problems, in gastroesophageal
reflux, 153
of infant transport, 499f–500f, 501
team dispatch, 489
of pain assessment/management, 443, 463
of stoma assessment/care, 473, 475
of wound healing, 468–469
dolichocephaly, 578
synostotic, 51–52
treatment of, 53–55
Doll's eye maneuver, 578
dopamine
administration during transport, 494, 503
low-dose, for congenital heart disease, 137
in renal physiology, 231
for tetralogy of Fallot, 126
urine/serum screening, in neuroblastoma, 207
Doppler flow study
in arteriovenous malformation, 9
in bronchopulmonary sequestration, 80
in congenital heart disease, 120
Doppler stethoscope, for testicular torsion
detection, 253
Doppler ultrasound
color, indications for, 9, 81, 120
in testicular torsion, 253
dorsal nerves, in brachial plexus injury, 400–406
dorsal penile nerve block (DPNB), 311, 451
dorsiflexion, of foot, in talipes equinovarus
casting, 388
double aortic arch, 47–49, 114t
double-barrel stoma, 470, 471f, 578
double bubble, of air, in stomach, 163
Doxycycline, for cystic hygroma, 14
DPNB. *See* dorsal penile nerve block
drain(s)
closed system devices
for chest. *See* chest tube
postoperative, for cystic hygroma, 15–16
Jackson Pratt, for cystic hygroma, 16
Penrose
for megaureter repair, 285–286
for ureteropelvic junction obstruction, 301
percutaneous peritoneal, for necrotizing
enterocolitis, 174
drainage
effluent, from stoma, 470, 473
excision and, of urachal cyst, 259–260
external ventricular, for hydrocephalus,
331–332, 331f
incision and, of cystic hygroma, 14
of thorax. *See* thoracostomy drainage
of urine. *See* urinary drainage
wound. *See* wound care/management
dressings
for bladder exstrophy, 264

changes, pain management for, 462–463
for circumcision, 312
for cloacal exstrophy, 275
fluid and electrolyte losses through, 427, 427t,
433
for gastroschisis, 156, 492f
for megaureter repair, 286
for omphalocele, 156, 492f
for open lesions. *See* open lesions
for primary closure wounds, 468–469
for closure by secondary intention wounds,
469
types of, 463–466, 579–580
for urinary diversion stomas, 250
use guidelines for, 463
drooling, esophageal atresia with fistula and,
148–149
drug tolerance, 584
ductus arteriosus
embryology of, 114t, 116
in hypoplastic left heart syndrome, 131, 131f
patent, 121–124. *See also* patent ductus
arteriosus (PDA)
prostaglandin E$_1$ indications for, 120, 125, 130,
132, 135
during infant transport, 493–494
ductus venosus, in total anomalous pulmonary
venous connection, 134, 134f
duodenal atresia, 162–164
duodenostomy, 470, 578
duodenum, embryology of, 143, 145
duplication cysts, bronchial, 68–69
dura mater, in spinal dimples/sinuses, 344
dynamic test, for DDH, 396
dysphagia, 45–46, 578
dysplasia, 578
of hip, 391–399. *See also* developmental
dysplasia of the hip (DDH)
of radius, 378–379
renal
posterior urethral valves causing, 242, 251
in prune belly syndrome, 288, 290
dysraphism, spinal, occult, 341
dysreflexia autonomic, 578
dystocia
ovarian cysts associated with, 308
of shoulder, brachial plexus injury associated
with, 405

E

EA. *See* esophageal atresia
Eagle-Barrett syndrome, 287
early amnion rupture spectrum, the, 372f, 373,
373f
ears
branchial arch development and, 26–27
embryology of, 3, 7f, 368
external, 3, 6
inflammation of, 575
inner, infections of, cleft lip/palate and, 32
middle, 3, 28
protection of, for transport team, 505–506,
505f
Ebstein anomaly, 9
ecchymosis, 578

eccrine gland, 460–461, 578
ECG. *See* electrocardiogram
echocardiography
    in bronchopulmonary sequestration, 82
    in congenital heart disease, 117, 120, 129, 135
    in congenital lobar emphysema, 67
    in fetal surgery, 523, 526, 529, 535, 538, 541
    in myelomeningocele, 337
    in prune belly syndrome, 291
    in tracheomalacia, 48
echogenic mass
    of lung, 80
    of ovaries, 306
    of renal parenchyma, 538
ECMO. *See* extracorporeal membrane
        oxygenation
ECMO specialists, 555
ectoderm, 1–3, 5, 25, 141
    in nerve development, 321–322, 364
    in reproductive tract, 222, 226f
    in skeletal development, 363, 364f, 365
    in skin, 458, 459f
    in spinal dimples, 342–343
ectopic tissue, in ears, 26–27
ectopic ureter, in megaureter, 280t, 281
edema
    extremity
        in limb reduction defects, 372
        neuroblastoma causing, 206
    pulmonary disorders and, 108
education
    continuing professional
        on fetal surgery, 542
        for transport team, 481, 485, 504
    for family caretakers. *See* parent teaching
education materials, in family-centered care, 511
educational degrees, for transport team, 481
effluent drainage, from stoma, 470, 473
ejaculatory ducts, embryology of, 224, 224f
ejection murmur, systolic, in tetralogy of Fallot,
        125
elastic cartilage, 368
elastic fibers, in skin, 460
elastin, 578
elbow
    in absent radius, 380
    embryology of, 364f, 365, 366f
    in limb reduction defects, 369
electric prosthetics, for absent radius, 381
electrical stimulation, slow-pulse, for brachial
        plexus injury, 405
electrocardiogram (ECG)
    in congenital heart disease, 120
    in hypoplastic left heart syndrome, 132
    in total anomalous pulmonary venous
        connection, 135
electrocautery, for circumcision, 310
electroencephalogram, in craniosynostosis, 53
electrolyte balance
    in congenital heart disease, 128, 137
    in extracorporeal membrane oxygenation, 558
    factors affecting, 416
    gestational changes in, 414, 415f
    in necrotizing enterocolitis, 173–174
    in pulmonary disorders

    immediate stabilization, 107
    postoperative management, 108
    in pyloric stenosis, 161
    renal regulation of, 231–235, 414–422
electrolyte management, 413–439
    general principles of, 413–426
    for homeostasis maintenance, 430–431
    during infant transport, 496–497, 503
    intraoperative, 432–433
    nursing measures for, 431–432
    in nutritional support, 434–439
    postoperative, 433–434
    preoperative, 428–432
    for specific conditions, 426–428, 427t
electrolytes, 578. *See also specific electrolyte*
    body fluid content of, 430t, 431
    in extracellular water, 413–414
    in intracellular water, 413
    in parenteral nutrition solutions, 436
    in renal physiology, 227, 229–230, 239, 416
    urine, in obstructive uropathy, 538–539
electromyography, in brachial plexus injury, 404
electron microscopy, of neuroblastoma, 204
elemental formulas, 439
ELS. *See* extralobar sequestration
embolism
    fat, 437
    in spinal cord injury, 357
embolization, for arteriovenous malformation,
        arterial *vs* venous, 9–10, 11f
embryoblasts, 321
embryology
    of cardiovascular system, 114–117, 114t
    of extremities
        lower, 365, 366f, 367
        upper, 364f, 365, 366f, 367
    of gastrointestinal tract, 141–146
    of genitourinary tract, 217–227
    of head, ears, eyes, nose, and throat, 1–8
        final development, 8
        overview of, 1
        week eight, 6–7
        week five, 4f, 5–6, 7f
        week four, 2–5, 2t
        week seven, 6
        week six, 6
        week three, 2
    of hepatobiliary system, 2, 59, 143–145, 190,
        579
    of neurologic system, 2, 321–324, 364
    of pulmonary system, 59–64
        stages of, 60f, 61–63
    of respiratory tract
        lower, 59–64
        upper, 1–8
    of skeletal extremities, 363–368
    of skin, 365, 458–461, 459f
embryonic disc, 1, 363
    incomplete folding of, 155, 158
embryonic stage, of lung development, 60f,
        61–62
embryonic theory
    of DDH, 392–393
    of talipes equinovarus, 384
emergencies
    implied consent for, 501

protocol/procedures for transport team, 504–505
emergency medical communication system, 504
emergency vehicles, safety issues of, 505
emesis
  bilious
    in gastrointestinal conditions, 162–163, 166, 169
    ovarian cysts and, 304
  gastroesophageal reflux associated with, 152
  in necrotizing enterocolitis, 172
  nonbilious, 161
  ovarian cysts causing, 304
  projectile, 161
EMLA cream. *See* eutectic mixture of local anesthetic cream
emollients, for circumcision, 312
emotional support, for family, 515–516
  with infant losses, 516–519, 519*t*
  during infant transport, 498
emphysema, congenital lobar, 64–68
empowerment, in family-centered care, 510
encephalocele, 345–348
  associations of, 346
  clinical presentation of, 346
  complications of, 347
  definition of, 345
  diagnosis of, 346
  differential diagnosis of, 346
  etiology of, 345
  incidence of, 346
  nursing care for, 347
  outcomes of, 348
  pathophysiology of, 345
  treatment of, 346–348
    delayed or palliative, 347
    immediate, 346–347
    postoperative nursing care, 347–348
    surgical, 347
encephalomeningocele, 345
encephalopathy, hypoxic-ischemic, 357
end-stage renal disease, posterior urethral valves causing, 251–252
end stoma, 470, 470*f*, 578
endocardial cushions, atrioventricular, 115, 115*f*, 116
endochondral bone, formation of, 367
endocrine gland(s), 3, 5, 27
endoderm, 1, 3, 25
  in gastrointestinal development, 141
  in nerve development, 321–322
  in pulmonary development, 59, 61
endoscopic ablation therapy, for posterior urethral valves, 247
  complications of, 249
  postoperative nursing care, 250–251
endoscopic retrograde cholangiopancreatography (ERCP), 197
endoscopy, 578
  for decompression, in congenital lobar emphysema, 67
  in esophageal atresia with fistula, 150
  for gastrostomy tube placement, 564
  rigid, in laryngomalacia, 40
  in tracheomalacia, 48

endothelial cells, in wound healing, 461–462, 461*f*
endothelin B, in renal physiology, 231
endotracheal intubation
  for choanal atresia, 30
  for congenital cystic adenomatoid malformation, 75
  for congenital diaphragmatic hernia, 90
  for cystic hygroma, 16
  during infant transport, 482*t*, 484, 490, 502
  for laryngeal web, 44
  pain management for, 452*t*
  for pulmonary disorders, 107
  tracheomalacia related to, 47
  tracheostomy *vs*, 547
endotracheal suctioning
  for bronchogenic cyst, 70
  for congenital cystic adenomatoid malformation, 76
  congenital heart disease and, 137
  for congenital lobar emphysema, 67
  for pulmonary disorders, 106–107
enema, barium contrast
  in Hirschsprung's disease, 170
  for meconium ileus, 165
energy expenditure
  glucose administration and, 435
  resting, 437
energy requirements
  daily, 437–438
  of premature infants, 435
energy sources
  for cerebral metabolism, 326
  in parenteral nutrition solutions, 434–437
enolase, neuron-specific, in neuroblastoma evaluation, 207
enteral, 578
enteral nutrition, 438–439
  for chylothorax, 99–100
  decreased absorption of, 439
  discontinuation for surgery, 432
  for gastroesophageal reflux, 154
  gastrointestinal status and, 438–439
  initiation factors for, 439
  for intestinal malrotation/volvulus, 168
  necrotizing enterocolitis associated with, 171
  nursing measures for, 439
  post-Kasai portoenterostomy, 202–203
  postoperative recommendations for, 439
enterocolitis, in Hirschsprung's disease, 169–170
enterohepatic, 578
environmental factors
  in congenital heart disease, 116–117
  in DDH, 392–393
  intrauterine. *See* intrauterine environment; prenatal conditions
  in neuroblastoma, 204
  in talipes equinovarus, 384
eosinophilic fibrillar material, 578
ependymal cells, 323
epiblast, 321
epidermis, 578
  anatomy of, 457, 458*f*
  embryology of, 458–459*f*
  injured, treatment of, 466
  layers of, 458–459

epididymis, embryology of, 224, 224f
epididymo-orchitis, 578
epidural anesthesia/analgesia
    contraindications for, 453
    indications for, 453
    for megaureter repair, 286
    nursing care for, 453–454
    for ureteropelvic junction obstruction, 302
epidural catheter
    maternal, in fetal surgery, 540
    nursing care for, 453–454
epidural hemorrhage, 351
epiglottis, embryology of, 61
epiglottoplasty, for laryngomalacia, 41
epileptiform, 578
epinephrine
    administration during transport, 503
    local, for circumcision, 311
epiphyseal plate, 367
epiphyses, ossification of, 367
epispadius, 579
    in bladder exstrophy, 260
    continent vs incontinent, 261, 265, 268, 271
    incidence of, 261
    isolated, 261
    surgical treatment of, 265, 267–268
epithalamus, 323
epithelial cells
    meconium, 177–179
    in wound healing, 461f, 462
epithelium, lower respiratory tract, embryology
        of, 59, 61, 63f
epoophoron duct, embryology of, 224f
equinovarus deformity, of foot, 382–391. See also
        talipes equinovarus
equinus deformity, of ankle, 382, 382f–383f, 385
equipment
    for circumcision, 310–311
    for fetal surgery, 542
    home care, 109, 516
Erb-Duchenne-Klumpke palsy, 400
Erb's palsy, 400
ERCP. See endoscopic retrograde
        cholangiopancreatography
erythema, abdominal, in necrotizing
        enterocolitis, 172
erythropoietin, kidneys activation of, 227
esophageal atresia (EA), 146–151
    associations of, 148–149, 177
    clinical presentation of, 148
    complications of, 150
    definition of, 146
    diagnosis of, 149–150
    differential diagnosis of, 149
    etiology of, 148
    with fistula, 147, 147f
    incidence of, 148
    outcomes of, 151
    pathophysiology of, 146–148
    proximal, 146, 147f
    surgical treatment of, 150
        postoperative nursing care, 150–151
    types of, 146, 147f
    without fistula, 147, 147f
esophageal diaphragmatic hernia, 87–88

esophageal pH study, for gastroesophageal
        reflux, 153
esophageal pressure, decreased proximal, 152
esophageal sphincter, lower, delayed maturation
        of, 152
esophageal variceal hemorrhage, 200
esophagoscopy, in vocal cord paralysis, 46
esophagus
    embryology of, 59, 61, 142
    gastric contents in, 151. See also
            gastroesophageal reflux (GER)
    malformations of, 146–151, 147f
essential fatty acid deficiency, 437
estradiol-17β, in reproductive physiology, 240
estrogen(s)
    maternal, in utero levels of, 303
    in reproductive physiology, 240
estrone, in reproductive physiology, 240
ethics, in neurosurgical disorders, 360–361, 361t
ethmoid bone, embryology of, 7, 7f
ethnicity
    DDH associated with, 393–394
    incidence related to. See inheritance patterns
Eustachian tube, 3, 32, 575
eutectic mixture of local anesthetic (EMLA)
        cream
    for painful procedures, 311, 444, 451
    for ventriculoperitoneal shunt management,
            334
evacuation, surgical, of brain hemorrhage, 354
evaporation, heat loss through, 107
    during infant transport, 492f, 494–495
EVD. See external ventricular drainage
eventration of diaphragm, 94–97
    associations of, 95
    clinical presentation of, 94–95
    congenital vs acquired, 94
    definition of, 94, 579
    diagnosis of, 95–96, 95f
    differential diagnosis of, 95
    etiology of, 94
    incidence of, 94
    nursing care for, 96
    outcomes of, 96–97
    pathophysiology of, 94
    treatment of
        conservative, 96
        postoperative nursing care, 96
        surgical, 96
evidence-based practice, for skin care, 457
ex utero intrapartum treatment (EXIT)
            procedure
    for congenital cystic adenomatoid
            malformation, 528
    for giant neck masses, 535–536
excision, surgical
    of arteriovenous malformation, 9
    of branchial apparatus remnants, 27–28
    of bronchogenic cyst, 70
    for bronchopulmonary sequestration, 82
    of choanal atresia, 30
    circumferential, for amniotic band syndrome,
            376, 376f
    of cystic hygroma, 14–15
    of neuroblastoma, 209–211
    of patent urachus, 259

of sacrococcygeal teratoma, 533
of spinal dimples/sinuses, 344–345
excision and drainage, of urachal cyst, 259–260
expectant management, 579
expert knowledge
in family-centered care, 509
for infant transport, 480t, 482
exploratory surgery, in testicular torsion, 253
contralateral, 253–254
exposure, heat loss related to, 107
exstrophy
of bladder, 260–271. *See also* bladder
exstrophy
cloacal, 271–279. *See also* cloacal exstrophy
splanchnic, 272
exstrophy-epispadius complex, defects of, 260,
271
extensor muscles, of extremities
defects of, 379
embryology of, 365, 366f
exteriorization techniques, in Kasai
portoenterostomy, 198
external auditory meatus, embryology of, 3, 6
external genitalia, embryology of, 225, 225f–
226f, 227
external manipulation and fixation, for testicular
torsion, 253
external ventricular drainage (EVD), for
hydrocephalus, 331–332, 331f
extracellular water, 579
composition of, 413–414
in hypernatremia, 419
in hyponatremia, 417–418, 419t
renal physiology of, 239, 414–416
extracorporeal membrane oxygenation (ECMO),
553–559, 579
cardiopulmonary bypass *vs*, 553
circuits for, 555–556
for congenital cystic adenomatoid
malformation, 75
for congenital diaphragmatic hernia, 90,
92–93
contraindications for, 554–555
criteria for use of, 553–554
indirect monitoring for, 556–557
initiation procedure for, 556
mechanical ventilation adjustments for, 556
nursing care for, 557–559
outcomes of, 559
parental support for, 559
for pulmonary hypertension, 553
team tasks for, 555
transport of candidates for, 491–492
weaning from, 559
extracranial hemorrhage, 351–356
associations of, 353
clinical presentation of, 353
complications of, 355
definition of, 351
diagnosis of, 353
differential diagnosis of, 353
etiology of, 352
incidence of, 352
nursing care for, 354–355
outcomes of, 356
pathophysiology of, 352

sites of, 350f, 351
treatment of, 354–356
immediate, 354
medical, 354
postoperative nursing care, 355–356
prior to transport, 354
surgical, 355
extradural hemorrhage, 350f, 351
extrahepatic bile ducts, obstruction of, 190–191,
191f, 203
extralobar sequestration (ELS),
bronchopulmonary, 77–79
outcomes of, 84
treatment of, 83
extrauterine circulation, intrauterine transition
to, 115
extrauterine gas exchange, 62, 554
extravaginal, 579
extravasation, intravenous, 467–468, 579
extravascular, 579
extravascular volume
changes in, 239, 414, 415f
in preterm *vs* full-term infants, 414
extremity(ies)
joint dimpling, in prune belly syndrome, 289
lower. *See* lower extremities
upper. *See* upper extremities
extrinsic, 579
exudate, 579
eye examinations
craniosynostosis and, 53
for retinopathy of prematurity, 21
eyelids, embryology of, 6
eyes
anomalies of, Robin sequence and, 38
choroid layer of, 576
embryology of, 5–8
neuroblastoma metastasis to, 205–206
retinopathy of, 16–25. *See also* retinopathy of
prematurity (ROP)

F

face
embryology of, 4–8
growth of with congenital defects. *See specific
anomaly*
Face, Legs, Activity, Cry and Consolability
(FLACC) pain scale, 463, 572f
facial activity, in pain response, 442t, 443–444
facial nerve (cranial nerve VII), pharyngeal arch
origin of, 2t, 3
failure to thrive
congenital diaphragmatic hernia and, 93
with gastrointestinal conditions, 151–153
laryngomalacia associated with, 40
falciform ligament, 143–144
fallopian tubes
in bladder exstrophy, 264
embryology of, 224, 224f
in inguinal hernia, 181, 182f
false passage, of tracheostomy, 549–550
familial associations. *See* genetics/genetic
disorders; inheritance patterns
family assessment, 511–514
family-centered care, 509–519

for biliary atresia, 197–198
communication in, 510–511
components of, 509–510
culturally competent, 510
definition of, 509, 579
family assessment in, 511–514
for grief and loss, 516–519, 519*t*
health care team relationship and, 515–516
for hydrocephalus, 330, 334
during infant transport, 498
parent involvement in infant care, 514–515
family education. *See* parent teaching
Fanconi's anemia, absent radius associated with, 379–380
fat(s)
brown, 107, 461
dermal. *See* subcutaneous fat
malabsorption of, common bile duct obstruction and, 191, 202
in renal physiology, 239
fat embolism, 437
fat emulsions, in parenteral nutrition, 436–437
fat necrosis, neuroblastoma *vs*, 206
fat-soluble vitamins
deficiency of, common bile duct obstruction and, 191, 195, 202
in parenteral nutrition solutions, 436
supplementation of, for intestinal malrotation/volvulus, 168
fatty acid deficiency, essential, 437
fecal diversion, indications for, 174, 179
feeding(s)
for cleft lip/palate, 32, 36
discontinuation for surgery, 432
enteral. *See* enteral nutrition
for gastroesophageal reflux, 153
gastrostomy tube. *See* gastrostomy tube (G-tube)
intragastric, for choanal atresia, 30
introduction of
in necrotizing enterocolitis, 175
in pyloric stenosis, 162
nasogastric, for laryngomalacia, 41
for ongoing pulmonary disorders, 109
oral. *See* oral feedings
transpyloric, 439
feeding problems
in cleft lip/palate, 32, 35–36
in esophageal atresia with fistula, 148, 151
vocal cord paralysis and, 45, 47
female gonads
in bladder exstrophy, 262, 264
in cloacal exstrophy, 273
embryologic differentiation of, 222–223, 223*f*
external, 225, 225*f*–226*f*, 227
internal, 224, 224*f*
preservation of, with ovarian cyst surgery, 307
femoral head
avascular necrosis of, 398–399
dysplasia of, 392–393
ossification of, 395
femur
dysplasia of, 391–399. *See also* developmental dysplasia of the hip
embryology of, 367
FENa. *See* fractional excretion of sodium

fentanyl citrate, 447
administration during transport, 403, 497–498
as anesthesia adjunct, 432
for bladder exstrophy repair, 270
ferritin, in neuroblastoma evaluation, 207
fetal circulation
development of, 114–117, 114*t*
transition to extrauterine, 115
fetal congenital cystic adenomatoid malformation, 528–530
definition of, 528
delivery of fetus with, 530
etiology of, 528
incidence of, 528
pathophysiology of, 528
postnatal care for, 530
prenatal assessment of, 528–529
surgical intervention for
indications, 529
procedures, 524*t*, 529–530
fetal congenital diaphragmatic hernia, 525–527
definition of, 525
delivery of fetus with, 527
etiology of, 525
incidence of, 525
pathophysiology of, 525
postnatal care for, 527
prenatal assessment of, 525
surgical intervention for, 524*t*, 527
fetal diagnosis and treatment center
additional resources required by, 542
essential services provided by, 541–542
function of, 541
fetal echocardiography, 117
in congenital heart disease, 117, 120, 129, 135
in fetal surgery, 523, 526, 529, 535, 538, 541
fetal hydrops. *See* hydrops fetalis
fetal movement
in amniotic band syndrome, 375
gestational evidence of, 367
fetal obstructive uropathy, 537–539
definition of, 537
delivery of fetus with, 539
etiology of, 538
fetal surgery for
indications, 538
interventions, 524*t*, 539
incidence of, 538
pathophysiology of, 537–538
postnatal care for, 539
prenatal assessment of, 538
fetal surgery, 523–543
for cleft lip/palate, 33
for congenital cystic adenomatoid malformation, 528–530
for congenital diaphragmatic hernia, 525–527
diagnosis and treatment center for, 541–542
equipment for, 542
fetal management for, 540–541
future directions for, 542–543
for giant neck masses, 535–537
maternal management for, 540–541
for myelomeningocele, 533–535
for obstructive uropathy, 537–539
for ovarian cysts, 307
patient candidates for, 523–524*t*

patient selection for, 523–525
perioperative care for, 540
postoperative care for, 541
preoperative care for, 540
for sacrococcygeal teratoma, 530–533
fetal ultrasound. *See* prenatal (fetal) ultrasound
fetus
    apoptosis in lungs of, 72
    development of. *See* embryology
    intrauterine surgery on. *See* fetal surgery
    viability of, 360
fever, ovarian cysts causing, 304
fiberoptic, 579
fiberoptic computed tomography, in choanal
        atresia, 30
fiberoptic laryngoscopy, flexible, in
        laryngomalacia, 40
fiberoptic nasopharyngoscopy, 30, 579
fibrin, 579
fibrinogen, 579
fibroblasts, 365
    in wound healing, 461–462, 461f
fibrocartilage, 368
fibrosis, in talipes equinovarus, 383
"fifth vital sign," 443. *See also* pain
fingerprints, 459
fingers
    defects of, in amniotic band syndrome,
        372f–373f, 373–378
    clubbing of, 125
    embryology of, 364f, 365, 366f
Finnegan scoring system, for opioid weaning,
        448f–449f, 450
FiO₂. *See* fraction of inspired oxygen
fissure(s)
    ileovesical, 272
    vesicointestinal, 272
fistula(s)
    anoperineal, 176f
    anorectal malformations associated with, 175,
        176f, 177
    branchial, 26–27
    cystic hygroma and, 15–16
    genitourinary, 175, 176f
    proximal esophageal atresia with, 146, 147f,
        150
    rectocloacal, 176f
    rectourethral, 176f, 180
    rectovaginal, 176f
    tracheoesophageal, 146–151, 147f
        tracheostomy risk for, 550–551
    urethrocutaneous, with circumcision, 313
    vesicointestinal, 272, 277
fixation
    external manipulation and, for testicular
        torsion, 253
    internal, for talipes equinovarus, 382, 387,
        389–391, 477
    for intestinal malrotation, 166, 167f
fixed wing aircraft (FWA), 489, 505, 579
FLACC. *See* Face, Legs, Activity, Cry and
        Consolability pain scale
flaccid, 579
flame-retardant clothing, for transport team,
        505–506, 505f
flap procedures

frontal-parietal, for brain hemorrhage, 355
    for laryngeal web, 44
    paraexstrophy, 582
    soft tissue, for cleft lip/palate repair, 34–35,
        34f, 35f
flexion-abduction brace, for DDH, 398
flexor muscle, of extremities, defects of, 379
flexures, of brain, 323
flights. *See* air transport; aircraft
fluid balance
    in congenital heart disease, 126, 128, 130, 137
    extracorporeal membrane oxygenation and,
        558
    in gastroschisis, 156
    kidney regulation of, 227, 229–230
    neonatal requirements for, 425–426
    in prune belly syndrome, 291
    in pyloric stenosis, 161
fluid overload, 426–427, 427t
fluid requirements, neonatal, 425–426
    abnormal factors, 426
    daily increase factors, 425
    initial factors, 425
    maintenance, 426
        in surgical infants, 430–431
    precise management of, 426
fluid restriction
    for arteriovenous malformation, 9
    for congenital heart disease, 137
    preoperative indications for, 430
    risks of, 426
    for SIADH, 419
fluid therapy/management, 413–439
    for biliary atresia, 201–202
    for cloacal exstrophy, 275
    in fetal surgery, 541
    general principles of, 413–426
    during infant transport, 493, 495–497, 503
    intraoperative, 432–433
    IV extravasation of, 467–468
    maintenance requirements for, 425–426
    nursing measures for, 431–432
    in nutritional support, 434–439
    postoperative, 433–434
    preoperative, 428–432
    for pulmonary disorders
        immediate stabilization, 107
        postoperative, 108
    for pyloric stenosis, 161
    rate of administration calculation, 495
    for specific conditions, 426–428, 427t
    for tetralogy of Fallot, 126, 128
    for D-transposition of the great arteries, 130
fluorescent *in situ* hybridization, for fetal
        chromosome karyotyping, 524
fluoroscopy
    airway, in tracheomalacia, 48
    in congenital lobar emphysema, 66
    in eventration of diaphragm, 96
    in patent urachus, 258
flush solutions, for IV lines, neonatal fluid
        requirements and, 426
foam dressings, 464, 579
focal, 579
Foley catheter
    in myelomeningocele management, 338, 340

for patent urachus, 260
for posterior urethral valves, 245–246
for rectourethral fistula, 180
folic acid supplements, for birth defects
reduction, 340, 369
folk treatments, 511
follicle-stimulating hormone (FSH)
in reproductive physiology, 239–240
in utero levels of, 303
Fontan procedure, for hypoplastic left heart
syndrome, 132
fontanels
in hydrocephalus, 328
ICP control and, 325
foot/feet
abduction of, in talipes equinovarus casting,
388
dorsiflexion of, in talipes equinovarus casting,
388
embryology of, 365, 366f, 367
equinovarus deformity of, 382–391. *See also*
talipes equinovarus
foot rays, 365, 366f
foramen of Monro, 579
foramen ovale
closure of, 115
embryology of, 115, 115f
in total anomalous pulmonary venous
connection, 134
in D-transposition of the great arteries, 129f,
130
force(s)
brain hemorrhage resulting from, 352
skull fractures resulting from, 348–349, 349f
in spinal cord injury, 356
forceps delivery
brain hemorrhage resulting from, 352
skull fractures resulting from, 348, 349f
spinal cord injury during, 356
forearm
absent radius in, 378–381
embryology of, 364f
forebrain, 2, 323, 364
forefoot, adduction of, 382, 382f–383f, 385
foregut, 2, 59, 579
embryology of, 142–144
in lung malformations, 68–69, 77
forehead, embryology of, 8
foreskin
in bladder exstrophy, 264
embryology of, 225, 225f–226f
inflammation of, 582
removal of. *See* circumcision
formula(s), specialized
chylothorax and, 99–100
elemental, 439
for intestinal malrotation/volvulus, 168
lactose-free, 439
for ongoing pulmonary disorders, 109
post-Kasai portoenterostomy, 203
fourth ventricle, of brain, 324, 324f
fovea, 579
fraction of inspired oxygen (FiO$_2$), 579
in extracorporeal membrane oxygenation,
554, 556
fractional excretion of sodium (FENa), 232, 233f

fractional reabsorption of chloride, 233
fractional reabsorption of potassium, 232
fracture(s)
skull, 348–351. *See also* skull fractures
of upper extremity, brachial plexus *vs,*
402–403
Fraser's syndrome, 535
Frejka pillow, for DDH, 397
French catheter, indwelling
infection control for, 109
for tension pneumothorax, 105
frenulum, embryology of, 6, 226f
fresh frozen plasma, 434
frontal bone, embryology of, 7, 7f
frontal bossing, 51f, 52, 576
frontal-parietal flap procedure, for brain
hemorrhage, 355
FSH. *See* follicle-stimulating hormone
full-term infants
body water composition in, 414
glucose production in, 435
functional assessment
in brachial plexus repair, 405–406
in myelomeningocele, 337, 340
in talipes equinovarus, during serial casting,
387–388, 391
fundal height, in fetal sacrococcygeal teratoma,
530
fundoplication
for gastroesophageal reflux, 152f, 153–154
complications of, 154
for gastrostomy tube placement, 564
funduscopic examination, in craniosynostosis,
53
fundus, retinopathy of prematurity and, 18
fungal rash, around stomas, 476
furosemide (Lasix), 123, 137, 421
fusion(s)
of cranial sutures, premature, 49–55
of joints, for brachial plexus injury, 405
of spine, for spinal cord injury, 358
FWA. *See* fixed wing aircraft

G

G-force. *See* gravitational force
G-tube. *See* gastrostomy tube
gait disturbances, 205, 399
galactosemia, biliary atresia *vs,* 194
Galeazzi sign, in DDH diagnosis, 395, 396f
gallbladder, 579
embryology of, 2, 59, 143, 579
fibrosis of, 197
surgical conditions of, 189–212
biliary atresia, 190–203
neuroblastoma, 203–212
overview of, 189
ganglia, sympathetic, malignancies arising
from, 203–204
ganglion cells, in colon, Hirschsprung's disease
and, 169–170
ganglioneuroblastoma, 204
ganglioneuroma, 204
gangrene, 174, 181
Gartner's duct, embryology of, 224f
gas dissolving in liquid, Henry's Law of, 488

gas exchange, extrauterine, 62, 554
gas expansion, in flight, infant transport and, 487–488
gastric decompression
 for biliary atresia, 201–202
 for bladder exstrophy closure, 270
 for cloacal exstrophy, 275
 for esophageal atresia with fistula, 150
 for gastroesophageal reflux, 154
 for Hirschsprung's disease, 170
 for intestinal atresia/stenosis, 163–164
 for malrotation/volvulus, 168
 for meconium ileus, 165
 for necrotizing enterocolitis, 173–175
 for omphalocele, 159
 for prune belly syndrome, 293
 for pulmonary disorders, 67, 90, 108–109
 for pyloric stenosis, 161
 for ureteropelvic junction obstruction, 301
gastric emptying time, 152–153
gastric motility, decreased, 152
gastrocnemius soleus muscle, in talipes equinovarus, 388–389
gastrocsoleus, in talipes equinovarus, 383
gastroesophageal reflux (GER), 151–154, 583
 associations of, 152
 clinical presentation of, 152
 complications of, 154
 congenital diaphragmatic hernia and, 93
 definition of, 151
 diagnosis of, 153
 differential diagnosis of, 152–153
 encephalocele associated with, 347
 etiology of, 151–152
 incidence of, 152
 laryngomalacia associated with, 40
 nursing care for, 153
 nutritional needs with, 109
 outcomes of, 154
 pathophysiology of, 151
 prevention of, 151
 pyloric stenosis associated with, 161
 tracheomalacia associated with, 49
 treatment of
  noninvasive, 153
  postoperative nursing care, 154
  surgical, 153–154
gastrointestinal bleeding, portal hypertension and, 200
gastrointestinal (GI) system/tract, 141–186
 air flight transport and, 487–488
 anomalies of, 141, 146–186. See also specific disorder
  prune belly syndrome associated with, 290
  ureteropelvic junction obstruction associated with, 297
 bronchopulmonary sequestration communication with, 79
 in cloacal exstrophy, 260, 272–274
 congenital diaphragmatic hernia involvement of, 91, 94
 embryology of, 141–146
 enteral nutrition considerations of, 438–439
 gastrostomy tube complications of, 569–570
 surgical conditions of, 146–186

anorectal malformations, 175–181, 176f
 male vs female, 178f, 179f
esophageal atresia, 146–151, 147f
fluid and electrolyte disturbances with, 427, 427t, 433, 436
gastroesophageal reflux, 151–154
gastroschisis, 155–158, 155f, 157f
Hirschsprung's disease, 169–171
inguinal hernia, 181–186, 182f
intestinal atresia and stenosis, 162–164
malrotation/volvulus, 166–169, 167f
meconium ileus, 164–166
necrotizing enterocolitis, 171–175, 172f, 173f
omphalocele, 158–160, 158f, 159f
overview of, 141
pyloric stenosis, 160–162
tracheoesophageal fistula, 146–151, 147f
gastroschisis, 155–158
 associations of, 155
 clinical presentation of, 155
 complications of, 157
 definition of, 155
 diagnosis of, 156
 differential diagnosis of, 155
 etiology of, 155
 incidence of, 155
 management during transport, 492f, 493–494
 outcomes of, 158
 pathophysiology of, 155, 155f
 treatment of, 156–158
  following delivery, 156
  obstetric management, 156
  postoperative nursing care, 157–158
  surgical, 157, 157f
gastrostomy, 579
gastrostomy button, 565
gastrostomy stoma, leaking, 568–569
gastrostomy tube (G-tube), 563–570
 complications of, 567–570
 components of, 563
 definition of, 563
 encephalocele indication for, 347
 for esophageal atresia with fistula, 150
 feedings guidelines, 567
 for gastroesophageal reflux, 154
  proper fit of, 154
 indications for, 439, 563
 location for, 564
 placement procedures
  alternate, 565
  radiologic, 564
  surgical vs percutaneous, 564, 579
 postoperative care, 565–567
 site care, 565–569
 stabilization of
  products used for, 566–566t
  techniques for, 566–567, 567f
gastrulation, 322, 579
gauze dressings, 463–464, 468
gel pillows, for positioning, in spinal cord injury, 359
gender assignment/reassignment
 in bladder exstrophy repair, 271
 in cloacal exstrophy repair, 278–279
gender identification, in cloacal exstrophy, 275–277

gene therapy, 542
general anesthesia, for inguinal hernia repair, 184
genetic consultation. *See also* karyotypic analysis
  for absent radius, 380
  for branchial apparatus anomalies, 27
  for cloacal exstrophy, 275–277
  for cystic fibrosis, 166
  for fetal anomalies, 524
  for Robin sequence, 38
genetics/genetic disorders. *See also* inheritance patterns
  absent radius associated with, 379–380
  in bladder exstrophy, 261
  chromosomal patterns in. *See* chromosome disorders
  congenital high airway obstruction associated with, 535
  encephalocele associated with, 345
  hydrocephalus as, 328–329
  of myelomeningocele, 335
  pyloric stenosis as, 160
  of sexual differentiation, 222, 223f
  talipes equinovarus as, 384–385
genital swellings, differentiation of, 225, 226f, 227
genital tubercle, embryology of, 225, 225f–226f
genitalia
  ambiguous, 178, 310
  in bladder exstrophy, 260, 262
  in cloacal exstrophy, 272–273
  embryology of, 222–227
    external structures, 225, 225f–226f, 227
    internal structures, 224, 224f
    male *vs* female differentiation, 222–223, 223f
    normal factors of, 240
  structural abnormalities of, circumcision and, 310
genitourinary (GU) tract, 217–313
  anorectal malformations and, 175, 176f, 177
    dermatitis risk with, 467
  embryology of, 217–227
  physiology of, 227–240
  surgical conditions of, 240–313
    bladder exstrophy, 260–271
    circumcision of newborn, 309–313
    cloacal exstrophy, 271–279
    fluid and electrolyte disturbances with, 427–428, 427t
    megaureter, 279–287
    ovarian cysts, 303–309
    patent urachus, 255–260
    posterior urethral valves, 240–252
    prune belly syndrome, 287–294
    testicular torsion, 252–255
    ureteropelvic junction obstruction, 294–302
gentamycin, 200, 497, 503
GER. *See* gastroesophageal reflux
germ cell tumors, neuroblastoma *vs*, 206
germ cells
  primitive, 530
  primordial, 222–223
germ plasm defect, primary, 384
gestational age

cerebral blood flow and, 324f, 325
  DDH associated with, 392–393
  neonatal fluid requirements and, 425
  pain expression related to, 444
  pain incidence correlated to, 441
  survival correlated to. *See* mortality; *specific diagnosis*
GFR. *See* glomerular filtration rate
glans
  clitoral, embryology of, 226f, 227
  penile
    in circumcision, 311–312
    embryology of, 225, 225f–226f
Glenn shunt, for hypoplastic left heart syndrome, 132
glioblasts, 323, 579
gliosis, 579
glomerular filtration, physiology of, 227–228
glomerular filtration rate (GFR)
  factors affecting, 230–231, 414, 433
  physiology of, 228–229, 238
  ureteropelvic junction obstruction impact on, 296
glomerulosclerosis, 579
glomerulus
  embryology of, 219–220, 219f
  physiology of, 227, 238
glossopexy, 38, 579
glossopharyngeal nerve (cranial nerve IX), pharyngeal arch origin of, 2t, 3
glossoptosis, 37–38
glottis, in laryngeal web, 43–44
glucagon, production of, 144, 237, 434
glucocorticoids, in reproductive physiology, 240
glucose
  cerebral metabolism of, 326
  endogenous production of, in pre- *vs* full-term infant, 435
  as major energy source, 434–435
  renal excretion of, 237
glucose infusion. *See* dextrose infusions
glucose level
  decreased, 424
  homeostasis physiology of, 424
  increased, 424–425
  management during transport, 496–497, 503
  postoperative management of
    congenital heart disease and, 138
    pulmonary disorders and, 108
  preoperative assessment of, 431
  in surgical stress response, 434
glucose load, daily, calculation of, 496
gluteal folds, in DDH, 394
glycogen, stores of, 107, 189
glycogenolysis, in surgical stress response, 434
glycoproteins, in reproductive physiology, 239
"goalpost" taping technique, for G-tube stabilization, 566–567f
Goldenhar syndrome, 26
Gomco clamp, 310–311
gonadotropin-releasing hormone (GnRH), 239
gonads. *See also specific anatomy*
  bladder exstrophy and, 262, 264, 266–267
    gender reassignment of, 271
  in cloacal exstrophy, 273, 278
  embryology of, 222–227

external structures, 225, 225f–226f, 227
internal structures, 224, 224f
male *vs* female differentiation, 222–223, 223f, 240
normal factors of, 240
in inguinal hernia, 181, 185
preservation of, with ovarian cyst surgery, 307
"goose bumps," 460
GORE-TEX tube graft, for tetralogy of Fallot, 127, 127f
Graf classification, of DDH, 396, 396f, 397t
grafts/grafting
bone, in cleft lip/palate repair, 36
chondral cartilage, in cleft lip/palate repair, 36
GORE-TEX tube, for tetralogy of Fallot, 127, 127f
nerve, for brachial plexus injury, 405
grandparents
reaction to neonatal death, 519
social support from, 512–513
granulation tissue, with gastrostomy tube, 568
gravitational force (G-force), 579
during infant transport, 487, 494, 504
gray matter, of CNS, 323
great arteries/vessels
embryology of, 114t, 116
transposition of, 114t, 128–130. *See also* D-transposition of the great arteries
greater omentum, 144
grief/grieving
anticipatory, 516–517, 575
birth crisis and
interventions for, 518–519, 519t
process of, 518
types of, 516–518
chronic, 516, 576
family-centered care for, 498, 516–519, 519t, 575
pinwheel model of, 518
groin swelling, in inguinal hernia, 183–184
ground vehicles, for infant transport, 505
Group C rotavirus, in biliary atresia, 191, 192t
growth abnormalities
congenital diaphragmatic hernia and, 94
fetal, 117, 384
growth and development, 578
delayed. *See* developmental delay
infant cues in, 514–515
measurements of, 438
skeletal defects and
interventions for promoting, 372, 380
surgery timing for, 363, 370–371
teaching to parents, 514
growth factors
hormonal
of ovarian follicles, 303
of pulmonary development, 61, 72
in wound healing, 461–462, 461f
GU. *See* genitourinary tract
gubernaculum, in inguinal hernia, 182f
guilt, as parental reaction, 517

H

"H" taping technique, for G-tube stabilization, 566–°567f
H-type fistula, tracheoesophageal, 146, 147f, 150
hair, embryology of, 460–461
hair buds, 460–461
hair bulbs, 460
hair follicles, 460–461
Hall classification, of amniotic band syndrome, 375–376
hamartoma, of lung. *See* congenital cystic adenomatoid malformation (CCAM)
hand plate, 365, 366f
hands
in absent radius, 379
movement of, in brachial plexus injury, 403, 403f
reduction defects of, 369–371
splinting of, for brachial plexus injury, 404–405
Hartmann's pouch, 579
hCG. *See* human chorionic gonadotropin
head and neck
congenital malformations of. *See* brain; cranium; neck
embryology of, 1–8
head circumference/size, 438
brain hemorrhage and, 355
enlarged, 327, 581
in hydrocephalus, 328, 329f, 339
headphones, for transport team, 505–505f
health care team, relationship with infant's family, 515–516
Healthcare Cost and Utilization Project Nationwide Inpatient Sample (NIS), 261
hearing loss/impairment
cleft lip/palate and, 36–37
conductive, middle ear surgery for, 28
Hirschsprung's disease and, 169
heart
embryology of, 2–3, 114–117, 114t
ischemic injury of, 9
malformations of. *See* congenital heart disease
heart failure. *See* congestive heart failure (CHF)
heart murmurs
in congenital heart disease, 118
in patent ductus arteriosus, 122
in tetralogy of Fallot, 125
heart rate
in congenital heart disease, 118, 120
in pain response, 442t, 443
heart rhythm, in congenital heart disease, 120
fetal, 117–118
heart shape/size, in congenital heart disease, 119
heart sounds
in congenital heart disease, 118
in tetralogy of Fallot, 125
in total anomalous pulmonary venous connection, 135
heart tube, 114, 114t
heart valves, embryology of, 114t, 115
heat loss. *See* body heat loss
heel, varus of, in clubfoot, 387

heel cord lengthening, for talipes equinovarus, 391
heelsticks
   pain expression during, 444
   pain management during, 445–446, 452t
Heimlich valve, 579
helmets, for transport team, 505–505f
hematocele, 579
hematocrit
   craniosynostosis repair and, 54
   extracorporeal membrane oxygenation and, 557
hematologic system, extracorporeal membrane oxygenation and, 557
hematopoiesis, 143
hematuria, 579
hemibladders, in cloacal exstrophy, 277
hemidiaphragm, paralysis of, brachial plexus vs, 402
hemodilution, in tetralogy of Fallot, 126, 128
hemodynamics
   arteriovenous malformation impact on, 9–10
   cerebral, 325
   in congenital heart disease, 118, 120, 131, 136
      shunting, 119, 125, 128–129, 131
      stabilization of, 136–137
   in congenital lobar emphysema, 67
   fetal
      in prenatal surgery, 540–541
      in sacrococcygeal teratoma, 532
   gastroschisis repair impact on, 157
   omphalocele impact on, 159–160
   ovarian cyst hemorrhage and, 307
   in pulmonary disorders, 84, 88
      postoperative management, 108
   renal, factors affecting, 230–231
hemoglobinopathies, cellular transplant for, 542
hemoptysis, 579
hemorrhage. See also bleeding
   cerebral, arteriovenous malformation associated with, 9, 11
   cystic hygroma and, 12
   extracranial, 351–356. See also extracranial hemorrhage
   intracranial, 351–356. See also intracranial hemorrhage
   intraventricular, 326–327
   neuroblastoma causing, 205, 210
   ovarian cysts and, 305, 307–308
   sacrococcygeal teratoma and, 532
   skull fractures causing, 349–351
   tetralogy of Fallot repair and, 127
   tracheostomy risk for, 550
hemostasis, 579
   for circumcision, 311
   in wound healing, 461–462, 461f
hemostat, for circumcision, 311
Henry's Law, of gas dissolving in liquid, 488
Hensen's node, 530
heparin, in nutrition solutions, 437
hepatic diverticulum, embryology of, 143
hepatic portoenterostomy, for biliary atresia, 197
hepatic veins, occlusion of, 160
hepatitis, neonatal, biliary atresia vs, 196
hepatobiliary iminodiacetic acid (HIDA) scan, 196

hepatobiliary scintigraphy, in biliary atresia, 196
hepatobiliary system
   embryology of, 2, 59, 143–145, 579
   surgical conditions of, 189–212
      biliary atresia, 190–203
      neuroblastoma, 203–212
      overview of, 189
hepatopulmonary syndrome, 200
hepatosplenomegaly, in biliary atresia, 193
hernia(s)
   of brain, 345, 347. See also encephalocele
   congenital diaphragmatic, 87–94. See also congenital diaphragmatic hernia (CDH)
   inguinal, 181–186. See also inguinal hernia
   of lung, 66, 66f
   umbilical, 145, 155, 158
herniorrhaphy, for inguinal hernia repair, 184
HIDA. See hepatobiliary iminodiacetic acid
high-frequency oscillatory ventilation (HFOV), 90
high-frequency ventilation (HFV)
   for congenital cystic adenomatoid malformation, 75
   for congenital diaphragmatic hernia, 90
   for congenital lobar emphysema, 67
high-output cardiac failure, 531
high output state, sacrococcygeal teratoma associated with, 532
high-risk pregnancy, maternal transport for, 524, 541
hindbrain, 2, 323, 364
hindfoot, varus deformity of, 382, 382f–383f, 385
hindgut
   in cloacal exstrophy, 277
   dilated end of. See cloaca
   embryology of, 146
hip
   anomalies of, prune belly syndrome associated with, 290–291
   dislocatable, 392, 578
   dislocated, 392, 578
   dysplasia of, 391–399. See also developmental dysplasia of the hip (DDH)
   evaluation of
      with myelomeningocele, 337
      in talipes equinovarus, 386
   subluxable/subluxation of, 392, 584
   teratologic dislocation of, 392, 584
Hirschsprung's disease, 169–171
   associations of, 169
   clinical presentation of, 169
   complications of, 170
   definition of, 169
   diagnosis of, 170
   differential diagnosis of, 170
   etiology of, 169
   incidence of, 169
   megaureter vs, 280
   outcomes of, 171
   pathophysiology of, 169
   surgical treatment of, 170
      postoperative nursing care, 170
histamine 2 (H$_2$) receptor antagonists, for gastroesophageal reflux, 153
histidine, in parenteral nutrition solutions, 436

histologic classifications, of congenital cystic
adenomatoid malformation, 71–72
histologic examination, 579
in congenital cystic adenomatoid
malformation, 73
in neuroblastoma, 204, 208
hoarseness, 43, 45
holoprosencephaly, 328, 579
Holt-Oram syndrome, 379–380
home care instruction, 516
for circumcision, 312
for congenital heart disease, 126, 138
for pulmonary disorders, 109
homecoming, preparing parents for, 516
homeobox-containing (Hox) genes, 365
homeostasis, renal physiology of
acid-base balance, 233–237
electrolyte, 227, 229–235
fluid, 227, 229–230
postnatal, 227–229
in utero, 227
Homer-Wright pseudorosettes, 579
homogenous, 580
homovanillic acid (HVA), in neuroblastoma, 207
hope, as parental reaction, 517
hormonal growth factors
of ovarian follicles, 303
of pulmonary development, 61, 72
hormone replacement therapy, for testicular
torsion, 255
Horner's syndrome, 15, 205–206
brachial plexus associated with, 400, 402, 405
Hox. See homeobox-containing genes
human chorionic gonadotropin (hCG), 240, 303
humerus
embryology of, 364f
fracture of, brachial plexus vs, 402
humidification, ventilator circuitry
for bronchogenic cyst, 70
for congenital cystic adenomatoid
malformation, 76
for congenital lobar emphysema, 67–68
inadequate, 425
Hutchinson syndrome, 206
HVA. See homovanillic acid
hyaline cartilage
bone models of, 367
distribution of, 367–368
hyaluronic acid, for retinopathy of prematurity,
23
hyaluronidase, for IV extravasation, 467
hydranencephaly, 328, 332, 580
hydration. See fluid therapy/management
hydration status
evaluation of, 428–429, 429t
in pulmonary disorders
immediate stabilization, 107
postoperative management, 108
hydrocele, 181, 182f
inguinal hernia vs, 183–184
hydrocephalus, 326–335
arteriovenous malformation associated with, 8
associations of, 329
clinical presentation of, 328, 329f
complications of, 333–334
definition of, 326

diagnosis of, 329
differential diagnosis of, 329
etiology of, 326–328
incidence of, 328
myelomeningocele associated with, 327, 332,
339
nursing care for, 329–330
outcomes of, 334–335
pathophysiology of, 326
transport of infant with, 329
treatment of, 329–335
delayed or palliative, 330
medical, 330
postoperative nursing care, 334
supportive, 330
surgical, 330–333, 331f, 333f
hydrocolloid dressings, 465–466, 580
hydrogel dressings, 464–465, 580
hydrogen ions, renal physiology of
in acid-base balance, 235–237, 416
in electrolyte balance, 228–230, 232–233
in immediate newborn period, 415
hydrolethalus syndrome, 329
hydronephrosis, 580
in bladder exstrophy, 265
in cloacal exstrophy, 274
in megaureter, 281
posterior urethral valves causing, 242, 244
in ureteropelvic junction obstruction, 295–
298, 300
grading system for, 298–299
hydrops fetalis, 580
bronchopulmonary sequestration and, 79–80,
82, 84
congenital cystic adenomatoid malformation
and, 73, 76, 528, 530
cystic hygroma and, 13
in fetal surgery, 540
with pleural effusion, 80
sacrococcygeal teratoma and, 531–532
hydrostatic pressure, in renal physiology, 230
hygromas, cystic, 11–16. See also cystic hygroma
hymen, embryology of, 226f, 227
hyoid bone, embryology of, 2t, 3, 7f
hyomandibulopexy, 38, 580
hyperalimentation. See parenteral
hyperalimentation
hypercalcemia, 422–423
in surgical infants, 427–458, 427t
hypercarbia/hypercapnia, "permissive," 90, 582
hyperextension, of head, spinal cord injury with,
357
hyperglycemia, 424–425
management during transport, 497–498
parenteral nutrition risk for, 435
hyperinflation, of lung tissue, 64, 66f–67f
hyperkalemia, 420–421
in surgical infants, 427–428, 427t
hypermagnesemia, 424
in surgical infants, 427–428, 427t
hypernatremia, 419
in surgical infants, 427–428, 427t
hyperoxia test, in congenital heart disease,
119–120
hyperphosphatemia, 423
in surgical infants, 427–428, 427t

hyperresonance, 580
hypertension
    neuroblastoma causing, 205, 210
    portal, 193, 200
    pulmonary. See pulmonary hypertension
hypertensive crisis
    pulmonary
        in D-transposition of the great arteries
            repair, 130
    in spinal cord injury, 359
hyperthermia, prevention of, in congenital heart
            disease, 126, 137
hypertonic dehydration, 429t, 430
hypertrichosis, 580
hypertriglyceridemia, 437
hypervolemia
    in fetal surgery, 541
    preoperative management of, 430
hypoblast, 321
hypocalcemia, 422
    in surgical infants, 427–428, 427t
hypodermis
    anatomy of, 457, 458f
    embryology of, 459f, 461
hypogenetic lung syndrome, 77
hypoglycemia, 424
    management during transport, 496–497
hypokalemia, 420
    in surgical infants, 427–428, 427t
hypomagnesemia, 423–424
    in surgical infants, 427–428, 427t
hyponatremia, 417–419, 419t
    dilutional, 417
    with normal extracellular volume, 418, 419t
    in surgical infants, 427–428, 427t
hyponatremic dehydration, 580
hypophosphatasia, 580
hypophosphatemia, 423
    in surgical infants, 427–428, 427t
hypoplasia
    distal radius, 378
    facial, craniosynostosis and, 52–54
    left ventricular, 131–133
    mandibular, 37
    prostate, in prune belly syndrome, 288
    pulmonary. See pulmonary hypoplasia
hypoplastic left heart syndrome, 131–133
    associations of, 132
    clinical presentation of, 132
    complications of, 132
    definition of, 131
    diagnosis of, 132
    differential diagnosis of, 132
    etiology of, 131
    incidence of, 131–132
    outcomes of, 133
    pathophysiology of, 131, 131f
    surgical treatment of, 132, 133f
        postoperative nursing care for, 136–138
hypoprothrombinemia, in biliary atresia,
            196–197
hypospadias, 267, 310, 580
hypothalamus, 323
hypothermia
    gastroschisis and, 156
    prevention of

    in congenital heart disease, 126, 137
    during infant transport, 484–485
hypotonic dehydration, 429t, 430
hypovolemia
    in craniosynostosis repair, 53–54, 54t
    in fetal surgery, 541
    intestinal malrotation/volvulus causing, 168
    postoperative correction of, 433
    preoperative management of, 429
hypovolemic shock, 429
hypoxemia, pulmonary hypertension and, 107
hypoxia
    altitude, during infant transport, 487–489, 505
    in congenital heart disease, 119, 138
    in tetralogy of Fallot, 125–126
hypoxic-ischemic encephalopathy, 357
hysterotomy, 580
    in fetal surgery, 532, 534, 536, 540

I

ICP. See intracranial pressure
idiopathic clubfoot, 384, 384f, 385
ileal atresia, 162–163
ileocecal exstrophy, 272
ileostomy, 470, 580
    for cloacal exstrophy, 277, 279
    for meconium ileus, 165
ileovesical fissure, 272
ileum
    defects of, 162–163
    embryology of, 145
ileus, meconium, 164–166. See also meconium
            ileus
illness, in infant, grief and loss reactions to, 517
ILS. See intralobar sequestration
iminodiacetic acid scan, hepatobiliary, in biliary
            atresia, 196
immobilization
    for circumcision, 310
    of lower limb anomalies, 278
    for painful procedures, 445
    for pelvic ring stability
        in bladder exstrophy closure, 269
        in cloacal exstrophy closure, 278
    postoperative
        for brachial plexus repair, 405
        for DDH, 398
    for spinal cord injury, 358–359
immune system, surgical risks for, 109
immunodeficiency
    chylothorax and, 97
    severe combined, cellular transplant for, 542
immunoglobulin(s)
    for chylothorax, 100
    sepsis risk and, 109
immunosuppression, neuroblastoma causing,
            210
imperforate anus, 176, 181, 272
    in cloacal exstrophy, 260, 272–273
implied consent, in emergencies, 501
in utero activity, of infant, 367, 375
in utero diagnosis. See prenatal diagnosis
in utero homeostasis, renal physiology of, 227
in utero surgery. See fetal surgery
incarcerated inguinal hernia, 181, 183–185

ovarian cysts and, 303, 308
incision and drainage, of cystic hygroma, 14
inclusion cysts, with circumcision, 313
incontinence
    myelomeningocele impact on, 337, 340
    in spinal cord injury, 359–360
    spinal dimples/sinuses and, 343–345
    of stool. *See* bowel incontinence
    tethered cord causing, 340–342
    of urine. *See* urinary incontinence
incubators
    for infant transport, 494, 501
    neonatal fluid requirements with, 425
incus, embryology of, 7*f*
indomethacin
    maternal, for fetal surgery, 527, 540–541
    for patent ductus arteriosus, 123, 427
induration, 580
infant development, 578. *See also* developmental
        entries
    teaching to parents, 514–515
infant transport, 479–507
    care of neonate during, 489–498
    disease-based protocol for, 483*t*, 484
    equipment for, 501–503
    evolution of, 479
    for extracranial hemorrhage, 354
    for hydrocephalus, 329
    impact on outcome, 479, 481
    medications for, 503
    for myelomeningocele, 338
    orientation programs for, 481
    physiologic stresses of, 484–489
    process-based protocol for, 484–484*t*
    quality assurance for, 481, 483, 489, 501,
        506–507
    safety issues of, 481, 504–506
    for skull fractures, 349
    standardized procedures for, 482*t*, 484
    system for, 516
    team communication for, 504
    team competency for, 480*t*, 482
    team composition for, 481
    team leadership for, 482–483
    team responsibilities for
        additional, 498–501
        infant-focused, 489–498
    team selection factors for, 481
infarction
    bowel, malrotation/volvulus causing, 168
    cerebral, 11, 352
infection(s)
    bronchopulmonary sequestration and, 77, 82
    with Broviac catheter, 561
    choanal atresia *vs*, 29
    with circumcision, 311, 313
    cystic hygroma and, 12, 14, 16
    extracorporeal membrane oxygenation and,
        558
    with gastrostomy tube, 567–568, 570
    genitourinary. *See* urinary tract infection
        (UTI)
    hydrocephalus and, 330, 333
    inner ear, cleft lip/palate and, 32
    limb reduction defects and, 370, 372

    maternal, congenital heart disease associated
        with, 116–117
    in megaureter, 282–284, 286–287
    in spinal dimples/sinuses, 344
    tetralogy of Fallot and, 126
    tracheostomy risk for, 550
    upper respiratory tract, in prune belly
        syndrome, 293–294
    in wounds, 468
infection control
    for invasive devices, 109, 210, 283
    postoperative
        for pulmonary disorders, 109
        for suprapubic catheters, 270
inflammation
    biliary atresia associated with, 191
    choanal atresia *vs*, 29
    of ears, 575
    of esophagus, 151. *See also* gastroesophageal
        reflux (GER)
    of foreskin, 582
inflammatory cells, in wound healing, 461, 461*f*
information sharing, in family-centered care,
        510–511, 515
    on grief process, 518–519
    during infant transport, 498
informed consent conference, for fetal surgery,
        524
inguinal canal, 225
inguinal hernia, 181–186
    associations of, 183
    in bladder exstrophy, 263, 266
    clinical presentation of, 183
    common types of, 181, 182*f*
    complications of, 185–186
    definition of, 181
    diagnosis of, 183–184
    differential diagnosis of, 183
    etiology of, 181–182
    hydrocele *vs*, 183–184
    incarcerated, 181, 183–185
        ovarian cysts and, 303, 308
    incidence of, 182–183
    nursing care for, 184
    outcomes of, 186
    pathophysiology of, 181
    recurrent, 186
    strangulated, 181, 185
    treatment of, 184–186
        manual reduction, 184
        postoperative nursing care, 186
        surgical, 185
inhalation anesthetics, 432
inheritance patterns
    of absent radius, 379–380
    of amniotic band syndrome, 375, 378
    of biliary atresia, 193–194
    of bladder exstrophy, 261
    of cloacal exstrophy, 272
    of inguinal hernia, 183
    of neuroblastoma, 205, 207
    of prune belly syndrome, 289
    of talipes equinovarus, 384–386
injury(ies). *See* trauma; *specific anatomy or
        mechanism*
inner ear infections, cleft lip/palate and, 32

innocent bands, 375
innominate artery, in tracheomalacia, 47–49
innominate osteotomy, anterior, for bladder
       exstrophy closure, 266f, 267
inotropic agents
    for arteriovenous malformation, 9
    for congenital heart disease, 120–121, 126
insensible water loss, 419, 425, 580
inservice education
    on fetal surgery, 542
    for transport team, 481, 485, 504
inspissated, 580
instability, 580
insulin
    administration during transport, 497
    for hyperkalemia, 421
    parenteral nutrition and, 435
insulin secretion, gestational, 144
intake and output
    gastroschisis and, 156
    postoperative assessment of
        in biliary atresia, 201
        in bladder exstrophy closure, 270
        in congenital heart disease, 137
        in pulmonary disorders, 108
    preoperative assessment of, 429, 432
interarytenoid region, laryngeal web in, 44
internal fixation, for talipes equinovarus, 382,
       387, 389–391, 477
internal genitalia, embryology of, 224, 224f
International Classification System, for
       retinopathy of prematurity, 18, 19f
International Staging System, for
       neuroblastoma, 208–209t
Internet, as information source, 515
interpreters, in family-centered care, 511
interstitial emphysema. See pulmonary
       interstitial emphysema (PIE)
interstitial tissue, 580
    pulmonary development of, 62
    in renal physiology, 239
interstitial volume, intravascular volume vs, 414
interventricular septal defects, cardiac, 114t,
       124, 124f
intestinal atresia, 162–164
    associations of, 163
    clinical presentation of, 162–163
    complications of, 164
    definition of, 162
    diagnosis of, 163
    differential diagnosis of, 163
    etiology of, 162
    incidence of, 162
    nursing care for, 163
    outcomes of, 164
    pathophysiology of, 162
    surgical treatment of, 163–164
        postoperative nursing care, 164
intestinal stenosis, 162–164
    associations of, 163
    clinical presentation of, 162–163
    complications of, 164
    definition of, 162
    diagnosis of, 163
    differential diagnosis of, 163
    etiology of, 162

incidence of, 162
    nursing care for, 163
    outcomes of, 164
    pathophysiology of, 162
    surgical treatment of, 163–164
        postoperative nursing care, 164
intestine(s)
    dysfunction of. See bowel incontinence
    ectopic, in bladder exstrophy, 265
    embryology of
        large, 144–146
        small, 144–145
    exstrophy of, 272
    herniation through umbilicus, 145, 155
    in inguinal hernia, 181, 182f
    large. See also colon
        ostomies of, 470–471, 470f
    obstruction of. See bowel obstruction
    perforation of
        in necrotizing enterocolitis, 173–174, 173f
        ovarian cysts associated with, 303
    small. See small intestine
intracellular water, 580
    composition of, 413
    renal physiology of, 239, 414–416
intracerebellar hemorrhage, 351
intracerebral hemorrhage, 351
intracranial hemorrhage, 351–356
    arteriovenous malformation associated with,
       9, 11
    associations of, 353
    clinical presentation of, 353
    complications of, 355
    definition of, 351
    diagnosis of, 353
    differential diagnosis of, 353
    etiology of, 352
    hyperkalemia associated with, 428
    incidence of, 352
    nursing care for, 354–355
    outcomes of, 356
    pathophysiology of, 352
    treatment of, 354–356
        immediate, 354
        medical, 354
        postoperative nursing care, 355–356
        prior to transport, 354
        surgical, 355
intracranial pressure (ICP)
    brain hemorrhage and, 356
    craniosynostosis and, 52–53
    CSF hemodynamics of, 325–326
    in hydrocephalus, 328
        medical management of, 330
        surgical management of, 330–335, 331f, 333f
    management during transport, 487, 494
    pain effects on, 442
intragastric feedings, for choanal atresia, 30
intrahepatic bile ducts, obstruction of, 190–191,
       191f
intralobar sequestration (ILS),
       bronchopulmonary, 77–79
    outcomes of, 84
    treatment of, 82–83
intramembranous bone, formation of, 367

intramuscular injections, pain management for, 452*t*

intraoperative care, fluid and electrolyte management in, 432–433

intrathoracic pressure
  chylothorax and, 97
  increased, gastroschisis repair and, 157

intratracheal pulmonary ventilation, for congenital diaphragmatic hernia, 91

intrauterine circulation
  fetal embryology of, 114–117, 114*t*
  transition to extrauterine, 115

intrauterine environment. *See also* prenatal conditions
  brachial plexus injury associated with, 405
  DDH associated with, 392–393

intrauterine surgery. *See* fetal surgery

intravascular, 580

intravascular volume
  changes in, 239, 414, 415*f*
  interstitial volume *vs*, 414
  postoperative maintenance of, 433
  postoperative stabilization of, 108
  preoperative maintenance of, 430–431

intravenous access. *See also* catheters/catheterization
  complications of, 210, 467, 579
  for pulmonary disorders, in postoperative management, 108–109
  site selection for, 467

intravenous extravasation, 467–468, 579

intravenous fluids. *See* fluid therapy/management

intraventricular, 580

intraventricular hemorrhage (IVH), 351
  grading of, 327
  hydrocephalus related to, 326–327
    outcomes of, 335

intravertebral foramina, neuroblastoma found in, 205

intrinsic, 580

intubation
  airway. *See* endotracheal intubation; *specific anatomy*
  intestinal. *See* gastrostomy tube (G-tube); nasogastric tube insertion

invasive devices, infection control for, 109, 210, 283

invasive monitoring
  management during transport, 491
  maternal, in fetal surgery, 540–542
  postoperative, for congenital heart disease, 136

invasive procedures
  aseptic technique for, 109, 210, 283
  pain expression during, 441–442, 444
  pain management during, 445, 451, 452*t*, 454

ion transport, in nephrons, 228, 231–233. *See also specific electrolyte*

ipsilateral, 580

iridotomy, 580

irrigation, ileal, for meconium ileus, 165

irritability, gastroesophageal reflux associated with, 152–153

ischemic injury

arteriovenous malformation associated with, 9, 11

of bowel, 171. *See also* necrotizing enterocolitis (NEC)
  in atresia and stenosis, 162
  in gastroschisis, 156–157

of brain, 9, 11
  cerebral circulation and, 326

of heart, 9

of penis, 269

of retinal capillaries, 17

of testes, 252–253

isotonic, 580

isotonic dehydration, 429, 429*t*, 580

isotope studies. *See also* radionuclide scanning
  in gastroesophageal reflux, 153
  hepatobiliary, in biliary atresia, 196
  in megaureter, 282
  in neuroblastoma, 208

isotretinoin (Accutane), Robin sequence association with, 37

IVH. *See* intraventricular hemorrhage

J

Jackson Pratt drain, for cystic hygroma, 16

jaundice, 195, 195*t*, 580

jaw, embryology of, 2*t*, 3, 5–6

jejunal atresia, 162–163

jejunostomy, 470, 580

jejunum
  defects of, 162–163
  embryology of, 145

joint(s). *See also specific joint*
  in amniotic band syndrome, 377, 377*f*
  dimpling of, in prune belly syndrome, 289
  embryology of, 365, 366*f*, 367
  fusion of, for brachial plexus injury, 405
  in limb reduction defects, 369
  releases of, for brachial plexus injury, 405
  in talipes equinovarus, 383

juxtamedullary cortex, embryology of, 219*f*, 220–221

K

Kabuki syndrome, 29

kallikrein-kinin system, in renal physiology, 231

kanamycin (Neomycin), for hepatic portoenterostomy, 197

kangaroo care, 514

karyotypic analysis
  in amniotic band syndrome, 378
  in cloacal exstrophy, 275–277
  in cystic hygroma, 13
  fetal surgery and, 524, 526, 529, 533

Kasai portoenterostomy
  for biliary atresia, 198–199
  complications of, 199–200
  outcomes of, 203
  postoperative nursing care, 201–203

Keel, 580
  for laryngeal web, 44

keratinocyte growth factor, 72, 462

keratinocytes, 580
  in epidermis, 458

in wound healing, 461f, 462
Kerley B lines, 86
Kerner-Morrison syndrome, 206
ketogenesis, 434
keyhole sign, 580
kidney transplant, for prune belly syndrome, 294
kidneys
    anomalies of
        in cloacal exstrophy, 274
        ureteropelvic junction obstruction
            associated with, 297
    cysts of, ovarian cysts vs, 305
    embryology of, 217–227
        excretory sets of, 217–220, 218f
        nephrons, 220–221
        permanent development, 219–220, 219f
        positional changes, 218, 218f
        primitive, 220
    physiology of, 227–240
    posterior urethral valves effect on, 241–242
    surgical conditions of. See genitourinary (GU)
        tract
Klumpke's palsy, 400, 406
knees, embryology of, 365, 366f
knowledge assessment, of family caretakers,
    511–512, 517
Kupffer cells, 143

L

labia, in bladder exstrophy, 262, 264
labia majora
    embryology of, 226f, 227
    in inguinal hernia, 181–182, 184
labia minora, embryology of, 226f, 227
labial commissure, embryology of, 226f, 227
labioscrotal swellings, differentiation of, 225,
    226f, 227
labor and delivery. See also specific delivery
        method
    brachial plexus associated with, 400, 402
    brain hemorrhage resulting from, 352–353
    delivery of fetus
        in fetal surgery
            with congenital cystic adenomatoid
                malformation, 530
            with congenital diaphragmatic hernia,
                527
            with giant neck masses, 536
            with myelomeningocele, 337, 534
            with obstructive uropathy, 539
        in gastroschisis, 156
    preterm. See also preterm infants
    skull fractures resulting from, 348–349, 349f
    spinal cord injury during, 356
laboratory tests
    in cloacal exstrophy, 275
    for fluid/electrolyte assessment
        postoperative, 433
        preoperative, 429
    for jaundice evaluation, 195, 195t, 197
    in necrotizing enterocolitis, 173–174
    in neuroblastoma, 207, 210
    for parenteral hyperalimentation monitoring,
        438
    post-Kasai portoenterostomy, 201

    for posterior urethral valves assessment,
        243–244
    in prune belly syndrome, 291
    in ureteropelvic junction obstruction, 298
lacrimal ducts, embryology of, 6
lactate dehydrogenase (LDH), in neuroblastoma
        evaluation, 207
lactose-free formula, 439
Ladd's bands, in intestinal malrotation/volvulus,
        168
lambdoidal synostosis, 51
    treatment of, 53–55
laminectomy, for spinal cord injury, 358
lancet, for heelsticks, 444
Langerhans cells, 458, 580
lanugo, 458, 460
laparoscopic surgery
    for anorectal malformations, 180
        male vs female, 178f, 179f
    for gastroesophageal reflux, fundoplication,
        154
    for Hirschsprung's disease, 170
    for ovarian cysts, 308
laparotomy
    for malrotation/volvulus, 168
    for meconium ileus, 165
large intestine. See also colon
    embryology of, 144–146
    ostomies of, 470–471, 470f
laryngeal nerve, in vocal cord paralysis, 45
laryngeal outlet, 61
laryngeal stridor, congenital, 39
laryngeal ventricles, 61
laryngeal web, 42–45
    associations of, 43
    clinical presentation of, 43
    complications of, 44
    definition of, 42
    diagnosis of, 43
    differential diagnosis of, 43
    etiology of, 42
    incidence of, 42–43
    nursing care for, 43
    outcomes of, 44–45
    pathophysiology of, 42
    surgical treatment of, 43–44
laryngomalacia, 39–42, 48
    associations of, 40
    clinical presentation of, 40
    definition of, 39
    diagnosis of, 40
    differential diagnosis of, 40
    etiology of, 39
    incidence of, 39–40
    nursing care for, 41
    outcomes of, 42
    pathophysiology of, 39
    surgical treatment of, 41
        postoperative nursing care, 41–42
laryngoscopy
    direct operative
        in laryngeal web, 43
        in vocal cord paralysis, 46
    flexible fiberoptic, in laryngomalacia, 40
    suspension, 584
laryngotomy, for laryngeal web, 44

laryngotracheal groove, 59, 61
laryngotracheal reconstruction, for laryngeal
    web, 44
laryngotracheal tube, 61
larynx
    congenital anomalies of, 39–42
    embryology of, 59, 60f, 61
laser therapy
    carbon dioxide. *See* CO$_2$ laser vaporization
    for choanal atresia, 30
    for cystic hygroma, 15
    freezing, for laryngeal web, 44–45
    for posterior urethral valves, 247
    for retinopathy of prematurity, 20t, 22, 24
lateral ventricles, of brain, 323–324, 324f
latex sensitization, prevention of, in
    myelomeningocele, 337–338, 360
LBW. *See* low birth weight
LDH. *See* lactate dehydrogenase
learning objectives, for infant transport team,
    481
learning style, parental, assessment of, 514
left ventricle, cardiac, hypoplasia of, 131–133
leg length discrepancy, in DDH, 399
legs. *See* lower extremities
lenses, embryology of, 5–6
leptomeningeal cyst, 350
leptomyelolipoma, 580
lesser omentum, 144
leukocytosis, ovarian cysts causing, 304
level of consciousness
    brain hemorrhage impact on, 354
    skull fractures impact on, 351
Leydig cells, ischemic elimination of, 252
LH. *See* luteinizing hormone
LHR. *See* lung-to-head ratio
licensure, for transport team, 481
life support, decision making for, 518
ligament(s)
    gastrointestinal, development of, 143–144
    head and neck, pharyngeal arch origin of, 2t, 3
    hip, laxity of, 392. *See also* developmental
        dysplasia of the hip (DDH)
    in talipes equinovarus, 387–388
    urogenital, embryology of, 221, 223, 256
limb(s)
    lower. *See* lower extremities
    upper. *See* upper extremities
limb-body wall complex, amniotic band
        syndrome *vs*, 375
limb buds, 364f, 365, 366f
limb reduction defects, 368–372
    associations of, 369
    clinical presentation of, 369
    complications of, 370–371
    definition of, 368
    diagnosis of, 370
    differential diagnosis of, 369
    etiology of, 368–369
    incidence of, 369
    intrinsic *vs* extrinsic, 368
    outcomes of, 372
    pathophysiology of, 368
    treatment of, 370–372

postoperative nursing care, 371–372
    surgical, 370
linear skull fractures, 348–351
lipolysis, 434
lipoma, 580
    lumbosacral, 580
lipomyelomeningocele, 580
lipoprotein lipase, 437
lips
    facial, 6
        cleft, 31–37. *See also* cleft lip
    genital. *See* labia
liquid adhesive agent, for arteriovenous
        malformation embolization, 10
liquid nitrogen. *See* cryotherapy
liquid ventilation, for congenital diaphragmatic
        hernia, 91
lithiasis, 580
liver
    congenital diaphragmatic hernia and, 525–526
    congenital heart disease and, 119
    embryology of, 2, 59, 143–144, 579
    functions of, 189
    herniation into umbilicus, 158
    neuroblastoma metastasis to, 206
    surgical conditions of, 189–212
        biliary atresia, 190–203
        neuroblastoma, 203–212
        overview of, 189
liver biopsy, in biliary atresia, 197, 201
liver function tests
    in jaundice evaluation, 195, 195t
    omphalocele impact on, 160
    in parenteral hyperalimentation monitoring,
        438
liver transplant
    for biliary atresia, 197–199, 203
    complications of, 200–201
lobar emphysema, congenital, 64–68
lobectomy
    for bronchopulmonary sequestration, 83
    thoracotomy with, for congenital lobar
        emphysema, 67–68
local anesthesia
    for circumcision, 311
    for inguinal hernia, 186
    for inguinal hernia repair, 184
    for ventriculoperitoneal shunt management,
        334
localized, 580
long bones, ossification of, 367
loop of Henle
    embryology of, 219–221, 219f
    physiology of, 229, 232–233, 236
loop stoma, 470–471f, 580
lorazepam, 503
loss, perinatal/neonatal
    family-centered care for, 516–519, 519t
    interventions for grieving, 518–519, 519t
    types of, 517–518
low birth weight (LBW), 580
    biliary atresia associated with, 193
    patent ductus arteriosus and, 122
    pulmonary air leak risk and, 101, 106
lower esophageal sphincter, delayed maturation
        of, 152

lower extremities
  anomalies of, in cloacal exstrophy, 273, 278
  developmental dysplasia of hip and, 391–399
  edema of, neuroblastoma causing, 206
  embryology of, 365, 366f, 367
  prostheses for, 380
  range of motion, myelomeningocele and, 337
  reduction defects of, 368–372
  talipes equinovarus and, 382–391
  tethered cord impact on, 340–342
lower respiratory tract, embryology of, 59–64
lower urinary tract obstruction (LUTO), fetal
      surgery for, 537–539
lucency, 580
  pulmonary air leak and, 103–104
lumbar puncture (LP)
  in brain hemorrhage, 353
  in hydrocephalus, 329–330
  pain management for, 452t
lumbosacral lipoma, 580
lung-to-head ratio (LHR), in congenital
      diaphragmatic hernia, 526
lung transplant
  for bronchopulmonary sequestration, 84
  for congenital diaphragmatic hernia, 91
  for pulmonary lymphangiectasia, 86
lungs
  acquired disorders of, 97–100
  congenital malformations of, 64–109
    associated disorders in, 97–100
    developmental impact of, 59
    diagnostic advances in, 59
    incidence of, 59
    specific disorders in, 64–97
  diaphragmatic disorders of, 87–97, 525
  echogenic mass of, 80
  embryology of, 59–64
    stages of, 60f, 61–63
  fetal, apoptosis in, 72
  nursing care for disorders of, 106–109
  obstructive uropathy impact on, 539
  parenchyma disorders, 64–87
  pulmonary air leak and, 101–106
  resection of, for congenital cystic
        adenomatoid malformation, 529–530
  stabilization maneuvers for
    immediate, 106–108
    postoperative, 108–109
  underlying disease of, pulmonary air leak risk
        and, 101
luteinizing hormone (LH), in reproductive
      physiology, 239–240
LUTO. See lower urinary tract obstruction
lymph nodes
  inferior mesenteric, 146
  inguinal, 146
  neuroblastoma metastasis to, 211
lymphangiectasia(s), pulmonary, 84–87
lymphatic system
  cerebral, CSF flow through, 325
  head and head
    cystic hygroma of, 11–16
    embryology of, 3
    pulmonary development of, 61–62

chylothorax and, 97–100
overgrowth of, 84–87
lymphocytes, in wound healing, 461f, 462
lymphoma, neuroblastoma vs, 206
lysis, laser technique for. See CO_2 laser
    vaporization

M

M-mode echocardiography, in congenital heart
      disease, 120
maceration, 469, 580
macrocephaly, 327, 581
macrocystic lesions, in congenital cystic
      adenomatoid malformation, 71, 76
macroglossia, in Robin sequence, 37–38
macrophages, 581
  in wound healing, 461f, 462
macula/macular region, 581
  retinopathy of prematurity and, 17f, 18, 23, 25
magnesium
  decreased level of, 423–424
  homeostasis physiology of, 422
  increased level of, 424
  physiologic functions of, 423
  renal regulation of, 234
magnetic resonance imaging (MRI)
  in anorectal malformations, 178
  in arteriovenous malformation, 9
  in bronchopulmonary sequestration, 81
  in cloacal exstrophy, 275
  in craniosynostosis, 53
  in cystic hygroma, 13
  in DDH diagnosis, 396
  in encephalocele, 346
  in eventration of diaphragm, 95
  fast-spin, in brachial plexus injury, 404
  in hydrocephalus, 329
  in myelomeningocele, 337
  in neuroblastoma, 208
  in spinal cord injury, 358, 358f
  in spinal dimples/sinuses, 344–345
  in talipes equinovarus, 386, 388
  in tethered cord, 341
  ultrafast, in fetal abnormality evaluation,
        523–524, 526, 529, 535, 538
malabsorption, of fats, common bile duct
      obstruction and, 191, 202
male gonads
  in bladder exstrophy, 262, 264, 266–267, 271
  in cloacal exstrophy, 273, 278
  embryologic differentiation of, 222–223, 223f
    external, 225, 225f–226f, 227
    internal, 224, 224f
Malecot tube, suprapubic, for bladder exstrophy
      closure, 266
malformation, congenital, 577, 581. See also
      congenital malformations
malignancy(ies). See also cancer(s)
  choanal atresia vs, 30
  neuroblastoma as, 203–212
  neuroblastoma vs, 206
Mallet classification system, of motor function,
      in brachial plexus injury, 404
malleus, embryology of, 7f
malnutrition

in biliary atresia, 194, 202
prevention of. *See* nutrition/nutritional
    support
malrotation
of gastrointestinal tract, 166–169
  associations of, 167
  clinical presentation of, 166
  complications of, 168
  definition of, 166, 167*f*
  diagnosis of, 167–168
  differential diagnosis of, 167
  etiology of, 166
  fixation of, 166, 167*f*
  incidence of, 166
  outcomes of, 169
  pathophysiology of, 166
  surgical treatment of, 168
    postoperative nursing care, 168
in talipes equinovarus, 383
Management of Myelomeningocele Study
    (MOMS), 533–535
mandible
branchial arch development and, 27
embryology of, 5, 7*f*, 8
hypoplasia of, 37
pharyngeal arch origin of, 2*t*, 3
manipulation, for talipes equinovarus correction
physical therapy in, 388
serial, 382, 387, 391
manipulation and fixation, external, for
    testicular torsion, 253
mantle zone, of brain, 323
manual muscle test, for myelomeningocele, 337,
    340
manual reduction, of inguinal hernia, 184
MAP. *See* mean arterial pressure
mass(es)
abdominal, 161, 304–305
cervical spine, neuroblastoma as, 205
cystic hygroma as, 12, 14
echogenic, 80, 306, 538
mediastinal, tracheomalacia and, 48
metanephric, 219*f*, 220
neck. *See* neck masses
sacrococcygeal teratoma as, 530–533
subcutaneous, neuroblastoma as, 205–206
mass effect, 78–79, 581
mastication muscles, embryology of, 2*t*, 3, 5
maternal-fetal intensive care unit (MFICU), 541
maternal-fetal problems, center for diagnosis
    and treatment of, 541–542
maternal history
gathering during transport, 498, 501
limb reduction defects associated with,
    368–370
in Robin sequence, 38
in talipes equinovarus, 384, 386
maternal infections, congenital heart disease
    associated with, 116–117
"maternal-mirror" syndrome, 528, 532, 581
maternal transport, for high-risk pregnancy,
    524, 541
maxilla(e)
in cleft lip/palate repair, 33
embryology of, 5–6, 7*f*, 8
McGovern nipple, for choanal atresia, 30

MCP. *See* medical control physician
MCT. *See* medium-chain triglycerides
mean arterial pressure (MAP), 554
in cerebral blood flow, 325–326
in renal physiology, 228
meatitis, with circumcision, 313
meatus, 581
mechanical factors, of DDH, 392
mechanical load/loading, in talipes equinovarus,
    388
mechanical ventilation
for bronchopulmonary sequestration, 82
for chylothorax, 99–100
for congenital cystic adenomatoid
    malformation, 75–76
for congenital diaphragmatic hernia, 90, 92
for congenital heart disease, 137
for congenital lobar emphysema, 66–67
for eventration of diaphragm, 96
for extracorporeal membrane oxygenation,
    556
for gastroschisis, 157
during infant transport, 501
for omphalocele, 160
pulmonary air leak and, 101, 104
for pulmonary disorders, pre- *vs*
    postoperative, 107–108
for pulmonary lymphangiectasia, 86–87
for spinal cord injury, 359
meconium
anorectal malformations and, 177–178, 180
Hirschsprung's disease and, 169–170
meconium epithelial cells, 177–179
meconium ileus, 164–166
associations of, 165
clinical presentation of, 165
complications of, 165
definition of, 164
diagnosis of, 165
differential diagnosis of, 165
etiology of, 164
incidence of, 164
outcomes of, 166
pathophysiology of, 164
treatment of
  noninvasive, 165
  postoperative nursing care, 166
  surgical, 165
meconium peritonitis, 165
median prosencephalic vein, 8, 581
median umbilical ligament, 221, 256
mediastinal shift
in congenital cystic adenomatoid
    malformation, 73
in congenital diaphragmatic hernia, 88, 91–92
in congenital lobar emphysema, 64, 67*f*
mediastinum, 581
air in, 101
masses in, tracheomalacia and, 48
medical control physician (MCP), 581
transport team responsibilities of, 482, 489,
    492, 501, 504
medical terminology, parents experience with,
    517
Medicare, infant transport requirements of, 481,
    501

medications. *See also* pharmacology; *specific agent or classification*
  congenital heart disease associated with, 116
medium-chain triglycerides (MCT), 99, 203
medulla, renal
  embryology of, 219f, 220–223
  urine concentration role, 238
medulla oblongata, 323
medullization, of vocal cords, for paralysis, 46
megaureter, 279–287
  associations of, 281
  classification of, 280, 280t
  clinical presentation of, 281
  complications of, 280–281, 285
  definition of, 279
  diagnosis of, 281–282
  differential diagnosis of, 281
  etiology of, 281
  incidence of, 281
  nursing care for, 282–284
  outcomes of, 286–287
  pathophysiology of, 279–281
  in prune belly syndrome, 287
  published series of, 283
  treatment of, 282–287
    medical, 282–283
    nephrostomy tube placement, 283–284
    postoperative nursing care, 285–286
    surgical, 284–285
melanocytes, 458, 581
membrane oxygenator, for extracorporeal membrane oxygenation, 555–56
meninges
  in encephalocele, 345
  protrusion of. *See* myelomeningocele (MMC)
meningitis, hydrocephalus related to, 328
meningocele
  cranial, 345
  management during transport, 492f, 493–494
mental retardation, Robin sequence association with, 38
Merkel cells, 458, 581
meromelia, 369, 581
mesencephalic flexure, of brain, 323
mesencephalon, 323–324, 581
mesenchymal chondrosarcoma, neuroblastoma *vs*, 206
mesenchymal plate, 28
mesenchymal tissue, 2–3, 5–6
  in bladder exstrophy, 261
  cavities of, 144
  in prune belly syndrome, 288, 290
  in skeletal development, 364f, 365, 367
    defects of, 378
  in skin, 460–461
  in spinal dimples, 342–343
  splanchnic, 61, 141–143, 221
mesenteric arteries
  inferior, 146
  occlusion during embryogenesis, 146
  superior, 145
mesentery(ies)
  embryology of, 144–145
  in intestinal malrotation/volvulus, 168
  ischemia of, 171. *See also* necrotizing enterocolitis (NEC)

large gaps of, 162
mesocolon, in intestinal malrotation/volvulus, 168
mesoderm, 1, 25, 581
  in nerve development, 322
  in pulmonary development, 61, 63
  in renal development, 217–218
  in skeletal development, 364–365
  in skin development, 460–461
mesogastrium, ventral, 143
mesonephric ducts, 221, 224, 224f, 242
mesonephros, 217–218, 218f, 219, 224f
metabolic acidosis
  in congenital diaphragmatic hernia, 90
  in congenital heart disease, 131–132, 135
  preoperative assessment of, 431
  treatment of, 421–422
metabolic alkalosis, 421, 431
metabolic screen, in jaundice evaluation, 195, 195t
metabolism
  cerebral, 326
  liver role in, 189
  surgery demands on, 434
metacarpals, embryology of, 364f
metal coils, for arteriovenous malformation embolization, 10
metanephric mass, 219f, 220
metanephros, 218–220
metastasis, 581
  of neuroblastoma, 205–206
    outcomes of, 211–212
metatarsus varus, developmental, 367
metencephalon, 581
methemoglobinemia, 451, 581
methyliodobenzylguanadine (MIBG) scintiscan, in neuroblastoma, 208
methylprednisolone, for cholangitis, 200
metoclopramide, for gastroesophageal reflux, 153
metopic synostosis, 51–52
  treatment of, 53–55
MFICU. *See* maternal-fetal intensive care unit
Michelow grading scale, for motor function, in brachial plexus injury, 403–404
microcephaly, 581
microcoils, 581
  for arteriovenous malformation embolization, 10
microcystic lesions, in congenital cystic adenomatoid malformation, 71, 76
β_2–microglobulins, urine, in obstructive uropathy, 538
micrognathia, 37–38, 581
  encephalocele associated with, 346–347
microscopy
  electron, of neuroblastoma, 204
  histologic. *See* histologic examination
microsurgical neurolysis, for brachial plexus injury, 405
midazolam, 270, 450
midbrain, 2, 323, 364
middle ear
  conductive hearing loss and, 28
  embryology of, 3
midgut

embryology of, 144–145
malrotation/volvulus of, 168
midgut loop
cranial *vs* caudal limb, 145
rotation of, 145
Millard forked flap procedure, for cleft lip/palate
repair, 34, 35*f*
mineralocorticoids, in renal physiology, 229–
230, 235
minerals. *See also specific mineral*
renal regulation of, 416
replacement of, during infant transport, 496,
503
MIS. *See* Müllerian-inhibiting substance
mitomycin-C, for choanal atresia, 30
MMC. *See* myelomeningocele
mobile phone, for transport team, 504
modified Blalock-Taussig shunt, for tetralogy of
Fallot, 126–127, 127*f*
modified Buck's traction, for bladder exstrophy
closure, 269
Mogen clamp, 310–311
molding, cranial, 52
molecular markers, of neuroblastoma, 207, 211
MOMS. *See* Management of Myelomeningocele
Study
monitors/monitoring
for infant transport, 501–503
invasive. *See* invasive monitoring
procedure indications for. *See specific
diagnosis or procedure*
monocytes, in wound healing, 461, 461*f*
monozygotic, 581
mons pubis
in bladder exstrophy, 263, 265, 267–269
in cloacal exstrophy, 274
embryology of, 226*f*, 227
morbidity
of arteriovenous malformation, 8, 11
of congenital diaphragmatic hernia, 92, 525
of congenital lobar emphysema, 68
of eventration of diaphragm, 96–97
during infant transport, 484
of meconium ileus, 166
Morgagni diaphragmatic hernia, 87–89
Moro response, in brachial plexus injury, 403
Morotti classification, of congenital cystic
adenomatoid malformation, 71
morphine sulfate, 447
administration during transport, 497, 503
as anesthesia adjunct, 432
for bladder exstrophy repair, 270
mortality, neonatal, 518
of arteriovenous malformation, 8, 10–11
of biliary atresia, 197, 203
of brain hemorrhage, 355
of cloacal exstrophy, 276
of congenital cystic adenomatoid
malformation, 528
of congenital diaphragmatic hernia, 92, 525
of congenital lobar emphysema, 68
of cystic hygroma, 16
of encephalocele, 347–348
of esophageal atresia, 151
of eventration of diaphragm, 96–97
of gastroschisis, 158

grief and loss reactions to, 518
of hydrocephalus, 330, 334–335
of hypoplastic left heart syndrome, 133
during infant transport, 484
of meconium ileus, 166
of necrotizing enterocolitis, 172–173, 175
of obstructive uropathy, 537
of omphalocele, 160
of posterior urethral valves, 251
of prune belly syndrome, 288
of pulmonary lymphangiectasia, 87
of Robin sequence, 38
of spinal cord injury, 360
of total anomalous pulmonary venous
connection, 136
motion sickness, during infant transport, 485
motor function. *See also* range of motion
myelomeningocele and, 337
spinal cord injury impact on, 358–360
tethered cord impact on, 340–342
mouth
cleft anomalies of, 31–37
embryology of, 141–142
Robin sequence and, 3, 37–39
movement
CNS developmental aspects of, 406
fetal
in amniotic band syndrome, 375
gestational evidence of, 367
movement assessment
in amniotic band syndrome, 377
in brachial plexus injury, 403
postoperative, 405–406
in limb reduction defects, 371–372
in talipes equinovarus, 383–384
during serial casting, 387–388, 391
MRI. *See* magnetic resonance imaging
mucoperiosteal flaps, vomer, in cleft lip/palate,
34
mucous glands, pulmonary development of, 61
Müllerian ducts, embryology of, 224, 224*f*
Müllerian-inhibiting substance (MIS), 224
multidisciplinary team
for cleft lip/palate management, 33
for fetal surgery, 523–524, 540–542
for myelomeningocele management, 338–340
for Robin sequence, 38
multiple births, neonatal death and, 518
multivitamin supplements, limb reduction
defects reduction with, 369
"mummy wrapping," for bladder exstrophy
closure, 269
murmurs, cardiac, 118, 122, 125
muscle(s)
abdominal, in prune belly syndrome, 287
absent radius impact on, 379
arrector, 460
in branchial arches, 24*t*, 25, 28
calf, in talipes equinovarus, 383, 388–389, 391
cremaster, 577
embryology of, 2, 365
extensor, of extremities, 365, 366*f*, 379
facial
embryology of, 5
pharyngeal arch origin of, 2*t*, 3
flexor, of extremities, 379

gastrointestinal
    development of, 142, 146
        incomplete development of, 158
head and neck
    pharyngeal arch origin of, 2t, 3
    shortening of, 52
mastication, embryology of, 2t, 3, 5
mouth, in Robin sequence, 37–38
palatal, in cleft lip/palate repair, 34
pelvic, in bladder exstrophy closure, 266
posterior tibial, in talipes equinovarus, 383,
    388
pulmonary, development of, 61–62
pyloric, inadequate relaxation of, 161
transfers of, for brachial plexus injury, 405
urogenital
    embryology of, 221
    in megaureter, 281, 287
    in prune belly syndrome, 281, 287–288
    in ureteropelvic junction obstruction, 295
muscle fiber defects, clubfoot associated with,
    384
muscle relaxants, for bladder exstrophy repair,
    270
muscle weakness
    myelomeningocele and, 337
    spinal cord injury causing, 357–359
    tethered cord impact on, 340–342
musculoskeletal examination, of talipes
    equinovarus, 386
musculoskeletal system, 363–406
    anomalies of
        in esophageal atresia with fistula, 148
        extremity defects and injuries, 368–408
        myelomeningocele associated with, 336–
            337
        prune belly syndrome associated with,
            290–291
        tethered cord causing, 340–342
        congenital diaphragmatic hernia impact on,
            94
    embryology of, 2, 365
        limb formation, 363–368, 364f, 366f
myelencephalon, 323, 581
myelodysplasia, 274, 581
myelomeningocele (MMC), 335–340, 581
    associations of, 336–337
    axial cross-section of, 338f
    clinical presentation of, 336
    in cloacal exstrophy, 275, 277
        postoperative nursing care, 278
    complications of, 339
    definition of, 335, 533
    delivery of fetus with, 337, 534
    diagnosis of, 337
    differential diagnosis of, 337
    embryology of, 335
    etiology of, 335, 533, 580
    fetal surgery for, 533–535
        indications, 533
        interventions, 524t, 534
    genetics factors of, 335
    hydrocephalus related to, 327, 332, 339
    incidence of, 335–336, 533
    neonatal surgery for, 533–534
    outcomes of, 340

pathophysiology of, 335, 533
postnatal care for, 534–535
prenatal assessment of, 533
recurrent, 336
treatment of, 337–340
    immediate protective, 337–338
    postoperative nursing care, 339–340
    surgical, 338–339, 338f
myelosuppression, neuroblastoma causing, 210
myoblasts, in pulmonary development, 63f, 64
myoclonic, 581
myoelastic, 581
myoelectric prosthetics, for absent radius, 381
myofibroblast-like cells, in talipes equinovarus,
    383–384
myogenic theory, of talipes equinovarus, 384
myopia, 581

N

N-myc, as neuroblastoma marker, 207, 211
NaCl (sodium chloride) infusion. See saline
    infusions
NANN. See National Association of Neonatal
    Nurses
nasal alae, 575, 581
nasal bone, embryology of, 7f
nasal cartilage, embryology of, 6
nasal cavity
    choanal atresia of, 28–31
    embryology of, 5–6, 8
nasal choanae, 576
    congenital obstruction of, 28–31
    narrowing of, 29
    primitive vs definitive, 5
nasal columella, 577
    lengthening of, in cleft lip/palate repair, 34
nasal continuous positive airway pressure
    (NCPAP), 38, 41
nasal pits, 5
nasal sacs, 5
nasal septum
    in cleft lip/palate repair, 34, 35f
    embryology of, 6
nasal suctioning
    choanal atresia and, 30–31
    cleft lip/palate repair and, 36
nasal trumpet, for Robin sequence, 38
nasogastric feedings, for laryngomalacia, 41. See
    also enteral nutrition
nasogastric tube insertions
    for abdominal decompression. See gastric
        decompression
    esophageal atresia with fistula and, 149
    for megaureter stenting, 284–285
    pain management for, 452t
nasopharyngeal airway, for Robin sequence, 38
nasopharyngoscopy, 581
    fiberoptic, in choanal atresia, 30
nasotracheal intubation, emergency, 547
National Association of Neonatal Nurses
    (NANN), 457
    transport team composition guidelines, 481
National Institutes of Child Health and Human
    Development, myelomeningocele
    study, 533–534

Index

National Safety Board, 506
navicular bone, in talipes equinovarus, 382
NBAS. *See* Neonatal Behavioral Assessment
 Scale
NCPAP. *See* nasal continuous positive airway
 pressure
NEC. *See* necrotizing enterocolitis
neck
 cystic hygroma of, 11–16
 embryology of, 1–8
 laryngeal web in, 42–45
 laryngomalacia of, 39–42
 pharyngeal (branchial) arch anomalies of,
  25–28
 Robin sequence and, 3, 37–39
 stabilization of, for spinal cord injury, 358–359
 tracheomalacia, 47–49
 vocal cord paralysis and, 45–47
neck masses, giant, 535–537
 definition of, 535
 delivery of fetus with, 536
 etiology of, 535
 fetal surgery for
  indications, 535–536
  interventions, 524t, 536
 incidence of, 535
 pathophysiology of, 535
 postnatal care for, 536–537
 prenatal assessment of, 535
necrosis
 avascular, in DDH, 398–399
 bowel. *See also* necrotizing enterocolitis
   (NEC)
  in gastroschisis, 156–157
  malrotation/volvulus causing, 166
 in inguinal hernia, 181
 of testes, 252–253
necrotizing enterocolitis (NEC), 171–175
 associations of, 172
 clinical presentation of, 172
 complications of, 174
 definition of, 171
 diagnosis of, 172f, 173
 differential diagnosis of, 173
 etiology of, 171
 gastroschisis repair and, 157
 incidence of, 171–172
 nursing care for, 173–174
 outcomes of, 175
 pathophysiology of, 171
 treatment of, 173–175
  immediate stabilization, 173–174
  postoperative nursing care, 175
  surgical, 174
needle aspiration
 of brain hemorrhage, 354
 of cystic hygroma, 14
 of ovarian cyst, 308
  ultrasound-guided, 309
 of rectal pouch, 178
 of tension pneumothorax, 105
negative sodium balance, 417–418
Neonatal Behavioral Assessment Scale (NBAS),
 514
neonatal death
 grief and loss reactions to, 518

 statistics on. *See* mortality
Neonatal Infant Pain Scale (NIPS), 442t, 443,
 571f
neonatal intensive care unit (NICU)
 parental orientation to, 511–512t
 parental visitation plan for, 515
neonatal nurse practitioner (NNP), transport
   team responsibilities of, 482–484
neonatal postoperative pain assessment score.
   See CRIES
neonatal pouch, for stomas, 471, 471f
Neonatal Resuscitation Program (NRP), 481–482
neonatal resuscitation room, for fetal surgery,
 542
"Neonatal Skin Care: Clinical Outcomes of the
   AWHONN/NANN Evidence-based
   Clinical Practice Guidelines," 457
neonatal wafer, for stomas, 471, 471f, 474f
Neonatal Withdrawal Score Sheet, 448f–449f,
 450
neoplasm(s). *See also* tumor(s)
 malignant. *See* cancer(s); malignancy(ies)
 ovarian cyst *vs*, 305–306
 urachal remnants developing into, 260
neostigmine, 503
neoumbilicus, 581
neovascularization, 581
 retinopathy of prematurity and, 17, 24
nephrons
 embryology of, 220–221
  excretory sets of, 217–220, 218f
  permanent development, 219–220, 219f
  positional changes, 218, 218f
 functions of, 221, 228
 physiology of, 227–240
nephrostomy tube
 for megaureter, 283
 percutaneous
  for posterior urethral valves, 247
  for ureteropelvic junction obstruction,
   300–301
nephroureterectomy, for posterior urethral
   valves, 249
nerve(s)
 abnormal, pyloric stenosis related to, 160
 absence of, limb reduction defects associated
   with, 369
 in brachial plexus, 400, 401f
  recovery potential of, 405–406
 in branchial arches, 24t, 25
 cranial
  in brachial plexus injury, 400–406
  embryology of, 2t, 3, 5
 dermal, 457–458, 460
 dorsal, in brachial plexus injury, 400–406
 laryngeal, in vocal cord paralysis, 45
 optic, retinopathy of prematurity and, 17, 17f
 peripheral
  in brachial plexus, 400, 401f
  Hirschsprung's disease and, 169
 phrenic
  damage to, brachial plexus *vs*, 402
  in eventration of diaphragm, 94
  pacing of, for spinal cord injury, 359

spinal
  in brachial plexus, 400, 401f
  in diaphragm development, 64
  embryology of, 2t, 3, 5
  urogenital, in megaureter, 280, 287
nerve block(s)
  dorsal penile, 311, 451
  with epidural anesthesia/analgesia, 454
  for megaureter repair, 286
  for talipes equinovarus, 388–389
nerve conduction studies, in brachial plexus
      injury, 404
nerve grafting, for brachial plexus injury, 405
nerve pathways, regeneration potential of, 406
nerve roots
  cervical, tears of, 400, 401f, 404
  CSF absorption in, 325
  spinal cord injury impact on, 358–359
net acid excretion, 235
neural crest/cells, 2, 6, 322
  in musculoskeletal development, 365
  in nerve development, 364
  tumors originating in, 189, 203
neural folds
  development of, 322–323
  in spinal dimples, 342–343
neural plate, 2, 322, 364
neural tube
  cytodifferentiation of, 323–324
  defects of, 335. See also myelomeningocele
      (MMC)
    reconstruction of, 338–339, 338f
  differentiation of, 322–323
  embryology of, 2, 322–323, 364–365
  flexure development in, 323
neuroblastoma, 203–212
  clinical presentation of, 205–206
  complications of, 210
  definition of, 189, 203
  diagnosis of, 206–208
  differential diagnosis of, 206
  etiology of, 204
  follow-up care for, 212
  histopathologic patterns of, 204
  incidence of, 204–205
  international staging system for, 208, 209t
  outcomes of, 211–212
  pathophysiology of, 204
  recurrent, 212
  surgical treatment of, 208–210
    postoperative nursing care, 211
neuroblasts, 323
  Homer-Wright, 579
neuroepithelium, of brain, 323
neurogenic theory, of talipes equinovarus, 384
neurologic impairment
  arteriovenous malformation and, 10–11
  brachial plexus injury associated with, 405
  brain hemorrhage causing, 354
  congenital diaphragmatic hernia and, 93
  cystic hygroma and, 15–16
  myelomeningocele and, 337
  in spinal cord injury, 358–360
  spinal dimples/sinuses and, 343–345
  in talipes equinovarus, 386
  tethered cord causing, 340–342

neurologic system
  embryology of, 2, 321–324, 364
  extracorporeal membrane oxygenation and,
      557–558
  management during transport, 494, 495t
  physiology of, 324f, 325–326
  surgical conditions of, 325–361. See also
      neurosurgical disorders
neurolysis, microsurgical, for brachial plexus
      injury, 405
neuromuscular examination, in talipes
      equinovarus, 386
neuron-specific enolase (NSE), in neuroblastoma
      evaluation, 207
neuropathy, peripheral
  in brachial plexus, 400, 401f
  Hirschsprung's disease and, 169
neurosurgical disorders, 321–361
  encephalocele, 345–348
  ethical considerations for, 360–361, 361t
  extracranial hemorrhage, 351–356
  fluid and electrolyte disturbances with, 427t,
      428
  hydrocephalus, 326–335
  intracranial hemorrhage, 351–356
  myelomeningocele, 335–340
  overview of, 321, 360
  posthemorrhagic hydrocephalus, 330, 332, 335
  skull fracture, 348–351
  spinal dimples, 336, 342–345
  spinal sinuses, 342–345
  tethered cord, 340–342
  traumatic spinal cord injury, 356–360
neurovascular lesion(s), arteriovenous
      malformation as, 8–11
neurulation, 322, 581
  secondary, 322
neutral thermal environment. See
      thermoregulation
neutrophils, in wound healing, 461–462, 461f
Newborn Individualized Developmental Care
      and Assessment Program (NIDCAP),
      514
newborn pouch, for stomas, 471, 472f
NICU. See neonatal intensive care unit
NIDCAP. See Newborn Individualized
      Developmental Care and Assessment
      Program
nipple(s)
  cleft lip/palate and, 32, 36
  large open, for choanal atresia, 30
NIPS. See Neonatal Infant Pain Scale
NIS. See Healthcare Cost and Utilization Project
      Nationwide Inpatient Sample
Nissen fundoplication, for gastroesophageal
      reflux, 152f, 153–154
nitric oxide (NO), 432, 581
  administration during transport, 491, 503
  for bronchopulmonary sequestration, 82
  for congenital cystic adenomatoid
      malformation, 75–76
  for congenital diaphragmatic hernia, 91
  in renal physiology, 231
Nitropaste 2%, for IV extravasation, 467
NNP. See neonatal nurse practitioner
NNS. See nonnutritive sucking

NO. *See* nitric oxide

nociception, 582

nodules, subcutaneous, neuroblastoma *vs*, 206

noise exposure, during infant transport, 485–486, 506

noninflammatory cells, in wound healing, 461, 461*f*

nonnutritive sucking (NNS), for pain management, 445

nonopioid analgesics, 445, 450

nonpharmacologic measures, for pain management, 443, 445–446

during infant transport, 498

nonverbal communication, in family-centered care, 511

Noonan's classification, of pulmonary lymphangiectasia, 85

norepinephrine, in neuroblastoma, 207

normal saline (NS). *See* saline infusions

normocephaly, 50*f*, 51

Norwood procedure, Stage 1, for hypoplastic left heart syndrome, 132, 133*f*

nose

choanal atresia of, 28–31

embryology of, 5–6, 8

reconstruction of, in cleft lip/palate repair, 35–36

trauma to, choanal atresia *vs*, 29

nostril, embryology of, 6

notochord, 7*f*, 322

notochordal process, 322, 365, 582

noxious stimuli, 444, 582

NRP. *See* Neonatal Resuscitation Program

NSE. *See* neuron-specific enolase

nuclear scanning

isotope. *See* radionuclide scanning

magnetic. *See* magnetic resonance imaging (MRI)

nursing care/measures

for fluid and electrolyte management, 431–432

during infant transport, 489–498

equipment for, 501–504

flow sheet for tracking, 499*f*–500*f*, 501

postoperative. *See specific diagnosis or procedure*

supportive. *See* supportive care

nutrition/nutritional support

absorption factors, 439

chylothorax and, 99

for cloacal exstrophy repair, 276, 278–279

for congenital heart disease, 137

enteral, 438–439. *See also* enteral nutrition

for esophageal atresia with fistula, 150

extracorporeal membrane oxygenation and, 558

for intestinal malrotation/volvulus, 168

parenteral, 434–438. *See also* parenteral hyperalimentation

for patent urachus repair, 260

post-Kasai portoenterostomy, 202

postoperative options for, 434–439

for pulmonary disorders, 96, 99–100, 109

O

observation, for ureteropelvic junction obstruction, 299–300

obstetric management. *See also* prenatal *entries*

of gastroschisis, 156

obstruction

airway. *See* airway obstruction

intestinal. *See* bowel obstruction

megaureter classification based on, 280–281, 280*t*

ureteropelvic junction, 294–302. *See also* ureteropelvic junction obstruction

urethral

with posterior urethral valves, 240–252

in prune belly syndrome, 287–288

urinary. *See* urinary tract obstruction

obturator, 582

occipital bone, embryology of, 7, 7*f*

occipitofrontal circumference (OFC), 438

brain hemorrhage and, 355

in hydrocephalus, 328, 329*f*, 339

occlusive dressings, for primary closure, 468

occupational therapy, for brachial plexus repair, 405

ocular torticollis, contralateral, 52

OEIS. *See* omphalocele-exstrophy-imperforate anus-spinal complex

OFC. *See* occipitofrontal circumference

OI. *See* oxygenation index

OK-432, for cystic hygroma, 14

olfactory bulbs, 5

olfactory groove, 5

olfactory nerve, embryology of, 5

olfactory receptor cells, 5

oligohydramnios, 582

in amniotic band syndrome, 373

DDH associated with, 392–393

in obstructive uropathy, 537–538

posterior urethral valves and, 243

in prune belly syndrome, 288, 290

omental bursa, embryology of, 144

omentum, embryology of, 144

omphalitis, 582

omphalocele, 158–160

associations of, 159

clinical presentation of, 158

in cloacal exstrophy, 260, 272–273, 275

closure technique for, 277

complications of, 159

definition of, 158

diagnosis of, 159

differential diagnosis of, 159

etiology of, 158

incidence of, 158

nursing care for, 159

outcomes of, 160

pathophysiology of, 158

surgical treatment of, 159

postoperative nursing care, 160

omphalocele-exstrophy-imperforate anus-spinal (OEIS) complex, 260, 272–273

one-stage posteromedial release, for talipes equinovarus, 382, 387, 389–391, 477

oogonia, 224

oophorectomy, for ovarian cysts, 307

opacity, 582
open lesions, external
    bladder exstrophy as, 264
    cloacal exstrophy as, 275
    encephalocele as, 346–347
    fluid and electrolyte losses through, 433
    gastroschisis, 155–158
    management during transport, 492f, 493–494,
        502–503
    myelomeningocele as, 337
    omphalocele as, 158–160
open reduction, surgical, of DDH, 398
open-sky vitrectomy, for retinopathy of
        prematurity, 20t, 23–24
operative stress, infants' response to, 434
opioid analgesics, 445–450, 582
    administration during transport, 497
    general principles of, 446–447
    indications for, 446
    intravenous, 447
    prolonged use of, 447
    types of, 446
    weaning from, 447, 450
    withdrawal score sheet for, 448f–449f, 450
opsoclonus myoclonus ataxia syndrome, 206
optic disc, embryology of, 5
optic nerve, retinopathy of prematurity and, 17,
        17f
ora serráta, 582
    retinopathy of prematurity and, 17, 17f, 18
oral cavity. See mouth
oral feedings
    postoperative, in myelomeningocele repair,
        339
    problems with
        in cleft lip/palate, 32, 35–36
        in esophageal atresia with fistula, 148, 151
        vocal cord paralysis and, 45, 47
orchidopexy, for prune belly syndrome, 293
orchiectomy, 253, 278
orchiopexy, 582
    for testicular torsion, 253–254
organic acids, renal excretion of, 229, 237–238
organogenesis. See embryology
orientation programs, for transport team, 481
orogastric tube insertions
    for gastroschisis, 156
    for omphalocele, 159
    pain management for, 452t
oronasal membrane, 5
oropharyngeal intubation
    for choanal atresia, 30
    emergency, 547
oropharynx, hygromas of, 12
orthodontics, in cleft lip/palate repair, 35–36
orthopedic consultation, for prune belly
        syndrome, 290–291
orthosis(es), for talipes equinovarus, 388, 391
Ortolani maneuver, for DDH diagnosis, 394, 394f
osmolarity, 582
    of IV infusions, 467
osmosis, in renal physiology, 230
osmotic pressure, in water regulation, 414
ossification
    of femoral head, 395
    of limb long bones, 367

of mesenchymal plate, 28
    in premaxillary and maxillary regions, 6
    of skull, 7, 7f, 367
osteoblasts, 365
osteopetrosis, 329
osteosarcoma, small cell, neuroblastoma vs, 206
osteotomy(ies)
    pelvic
        for bladder exstrophy closure, 266f, 267
        for cloacal exstrophy closure, 278
    sliding for brachial plexus injury, 405
ostomy(ies), 582. See also stoma(s)
    appliance bag for, 474f, 475–476
    appliances for, 471–476. See also appliances
    for cloacal exstrophy, 277–278
    effluent drainage from, 470, 473
    for Hirschsprung's disease, 170
    indications for, 469–470
    location determination for, 469
    for necrotizing enterocolitis, 174–175
    nursing care for, 471–476
    nutritional support and, 439
    stoma types for, 470, 470f
    types of, 470, 470f
otogenic theory, of talipes equinovarus, 384
ovarian cyst, 274, 303–309
    associations of, 305
    clinical presentation of, 304–305
    complex (complicated), 305–306
    complications of, 308
    definition of, 303
    diagnosis of, 305
    differential diagnosis of, 305
    etiology of, 303
    incidence of, 304
    outcomes of, 308–309
    pathophysiology of, 303
    simple (uncomplicated), 306
    treatment of, 306–309
        conservative, 306–307
        postoperative nursing care, 308
        surgical, 307–308
        in utero, 307
    "wandering," 306–307
ovarian follicles
    cysts developing from, 303. See also ovarian
        cyst
    in utero growth of, 303
ovarian ligaments, embryology of, 223
ovaries
    in bladder exstrophy, 264
    embryology of, 222, 223f
    in inguinal hernia, 181–182, 182f
    neonatal vs pubertal, 303
    torsion of, 303–309
overhydration, SIADH vs, 418, 419t
overriding aorta, 124, 124f, 126–127
oximetry
    in congenital heart disease, 120, 137
    in fetal surgery, 540
oxybutynin chloride (Ditropan), 270, 286
oxygen, partial pressure of, 554
    altitude impact on, 488
    in congenital diaphragmatic hernia, 90, 92
oxygen concentration/saturation
    in congenital heart disease, 119–120, 129, 137

in congenital lobar emphysema, 67
in extracorporeal membrane oxygenation, 556
during infant transport, 488–489
in pain response, 442t, 443
retinopathy of prematurity related to, 17–18
oxygen consumption, body heat loss and, 107
oxygen delivery, *in utero,* 227
oxygen therapy
    for bronchopulmonary sequestration, 82
    for congenital diaphragmatic hernia, 90–91
    for eventration of diaphragm, 96
    during infant transport, 490–491
        equipment for, 501–502
    for laryngomalacia, 41
    for pulmonary air leak, 104–105
    for pulmonary disorders, 107
    for pulmonary lymphangiectasia, 86–87
    with tracheostomy, 549
oxygenation index (OI), extracorporeal
        membrane oxygenation and, 554

P

"pacemaker" sites, in renal collecting system,
        295
pacifiers, for pain management, 445
pacing
    cardiac, for cardiopulmonary bypass, 127
    of phrenic nerve, for spinal cord injury, 359
pain, 582
    abdominal, neuroblastoma causing, 205
    expression of, contextual factors of, 444, 577
    incidence in NICU, 441
    ovarian cysts causing, 304
    parent education on, 454
    response to, factors of, 443
    sensitivity to, mechanisms increasing, 446
pain assessment, 443–445
    in bladder exstrophy closure, 270
    general principles of, 443
    during infant transport, 497
    in megaureter repair, 286
    scales for, 571f–573f
        multidimensional, 442t, 443
    standards of practice for, 442–443
pain management
    for circumcision, 310, 312–313
    for cleft lip/palate repair, 36
    clinical significance of, 441–442
    for congenital heart disease, 138
    for cystic hygroma, 16
    extracorporeal membrane oxygenation and,
        558–559
    for gastrostomy tube placement, 567
    during infant transport, 497, 503
    for inguinal hernia repair, 186
    for invasive procedures, 445, 451, 452t, 454
    for laryngomalacia, 42
    for limb reduction defects, 371–372
    maternal, in fetal surgery, 527, 540
    for megaureter repair, 286
    nonpharmacologic approaches to, 443,
        445–446
    pharmacologic approaches to, 443, 446–454
    for pulmonary disorders, 109
    for retinopathy of prematurity, 23–24

for skull fractures, 351
for spinal cord injury, 358
standards of practice for, 442–443
for tethered cord repair, 342
thoracotomy tubes and, 106
for ureteropelvic junction obstruction, 302
for ventriculoperitoneal shunt placement, 334
for wound care, 462–463
pain scales, 571f–573f
    multidimensional, 442t, 443
palate
    cleft, 6, 31–37. *See also* cleft palate
    embryology of, 6
    primary *vs* secondary, 6, 32f
palliative management
    of encephalocele, 347
    of hydrocephalus, 330
    of skull fractures, 349
palpation
    in congenital heart disease, 118–119
    of pyloric stenosis, 161
PALS. *See* Pediatric Advanced Life Support
        Course
palsy(ies), in brachial plexus injury, 400, 406
pancreas, embryology of, 144
pancreatic buds, 144
pancreatic ducts, embryology of, 144
pancreatic islets, embryology of, 144
pancuronium bromide, 270, 503
papillae, dermal, 460
papilloma, of choroid plexus, 328
paracentesis, 582
paradoxical, 582
paradoxical respiration, 94–97
paraexstrophy flaps, 582
    for bladder exstrophy closure, 266, 268
parafollicular cells, embryology of, 3
paralysis
    cystic hygroma and, 16
    spinal cord injury causing, 356, 359–360
paralytics, administration during transport, 503
paramesonephric ducts, embryology of, 224
paranasal sinus, embryology of, 6
paraphimosis, 309, 582
paraplegia, 205, 360, 582
paraspinal tumors, neuroblastoma as, 205, 210
parathyroid gland
    branchial arch development and, 27
    embryology of, 3, 6
parathyroid hormone (PTH), in renal physiology,
        233–235
paraxial mesoderm, 365
parenchyma, 582
    brain, hemorrhage in, 351
    lung disorders of, 64–87
        bronchogenic cyst, 68–70
        bronchopulmonary sequestration, 76–84
        congenital cystic adenomatoid
            malformation, 70–76
        congenital lobar emphysema, 64–68
        pulmonary lymphangiectasia, 84–87
    renal, echogenic mass of, 538
parent involvement, in infant care, 498, 514–515
parent support systems, 515–516
    for grief process, 518–519
    during infant transport, 498

social, assessment of, 512–514
therapeutic. *See* family-centered care
parent teaching
    on bladder exstrophy closure, 270–271
    on casting, for talipes equinovarus, 390
    on circumcision, 310
    on cleft lip/palate repair, 36
    on cloacal exstrophy, 275–276
    on congenital heart disease, 126, 138
    on craniosynostosis repair, 55
    culturally-competent, 510–511
    on extracorporeal membrane oxygenation, 559
    on fetal anomalies, 524, 539, 542
    on gastrostomy tube, 570
    on hydrocephalus, 330, 334
    on laryngomalacia, 41–42
    on limb reduction defects, 372
    on pain assessment/management, 454
    on pulmonary disorders, 109
    on stoma care, 476
    on tethered cord, 342
    on urinary diversion stomas, 250–251
parental consent
    for fetal surgery, 524
    for infant transport, 501
parental knowledge, assessment of, 511–512, 517
parental visitation, plan for, 515
parenteral hyperalimentation, 434–438
    for chylothorax, 99–100
    for cloacal exstrophy repair, 276, 278
    complications of, 438
        prolonged administration, 157
    for congenital heart disease, 137
    for gastroschisis, 157–158
    goals of, 437–438
    indications for, 434
    for intestinal atresia/stenosis, 164
    for intestinal malrotation/volvulus, 168
    laboratory tests for monitoring, 438
    for meconium ileus, 166
    nursing measures for, 438
    for omphalocele, 160
    post-Kasai portoenterostomy, 202
    solution composition, 434–437
        crystalline, 434–436
        fat emulsions, 436–437
parenteral solutions. *See* fluid therapy/management; *specific solution*
paresthesia, cystic hygroma and, 12
parietal bone, embryology of, 7, 7f
paroophoron duct, embryology of, 224f
partial pressures, of gases
    in alveolar/arterial oxygen gradient, 554
    in congenital diaphragmatic hernia, 90, 92
    Dalton's Law of, 487–488
passive range of motion
    for spinal cord injury, 358–359
    in tethered cord repair, 342
passive transport, in nephrons, 228
patent ductus arteriosus (PDA), 121–124
    associations of, 122
    clinical presentation of, 122
    complications of, 124
    definition of, 121
    diagnosis of, 123

differential diagnosis of, 122
    etiology of, 122
    fluid and electrolyte disturbances with, 426–427
    incidence of, 122
    management during transport, 493–494
    outcomes of, 124
    pathophysiology of, 122
    prostaglandin E_1 for, 120, 125, 130, 132, 135
    in D-transposition of the great arteries, 129–130
    treatment of
        pharmacologic, 123
        postoperative nursing care for, 136–138
        surgical, 123–124
        symptomatic, 123
patent urachus, 255–260
    associations of, 257–258
    in bladder exstrophy, 266
    clinical presentation of, 256–257, 257f
    complications of, 259
    definition of, 255
    diagnosis of, 258
    differential diagnosis of, 258
    embryology of, 255–256
    etiology of, 256
    incidence of, 256
    outcomes of, 260
    pathophysiology of, 255–256
    in prune belly syndrome, 290, 292
    treatment of
        patent *vs* sinus, 259
        postoperative nursing care, 260
        surgical, 259
Pavlik harness, for DDH, 397–399, 397f
PAX-3 gene, in myelomeningocele, 335
PDA. *See* patent ductus arteriosus
peak inspiratory pressure (PIP), 556, 582
Pediatric Advanced Life Support Course (PALS), 481–482
PEEP. *See* positive end expiratory pressure
PEG. *See* percutaneous gastrostomy tube
pelvic floor, in cloacal exstrophy, 274
pelvic muscles, in bladder exstrophy closure, 266
pelvic osteotomies
    for bladder exstrophy closure, 266f, 267
    for cloacal exstrophy closure, 278
pelvic ring, in bladder exstrophy closure, 265, 267
    postoperative nursing care, 269
pelvis
    in anorectal malformations, 176f
    in bladder exstrophy, 263, 265, 267
        osteotomy approaches, 266f, 267
    in cloacal exstrophy, 274, 277–278
penile nerve block, dorsal, 311, 451
penile raphe, embryology of, 226f
penis
    in bladder exstrophy, 263–264, 266–267
        ischemia of, 269
        multiple-stage reconstruction of, 271
    cancer of, circumcision and, 309
    in cloacal exstrophy, 273, 278
    embryology of, 225, 225f–226f
    foreskin removal from. *See* circumcision
Penrose drain

for megaureter repair, 285–286
for ureteropelvic junction obstruction, 301
Pepper syndrome, 206
peptides, in renal physiology, 237
percutaneous catheter insertion, pain
management for, 451, 452t
percutaneous gastrostomy tube (PEG), 564, 568
perfluorocarbons, for congenital diaphragmatic
hernia, 91
perforation
abdominal, in meconium ileus, 165
intestinal
in necrotizing enterocolitis, 173–174, 173f
ovarian cysts associated with, 303
performance improvement, in infant transport.
See quality assurance (QA)
perfusion
determinants of, 492–493
gastroschisis repair impact on, 157
management during transport, 492–494
peribronchial space, alveoli rupture into, 101
pericardial effusion, in pulmonary
lymphangiectasia, 86–87
pericardial patch, in bronchogenic cyst excision,
70
pericardium, air collection in, 101
periderm, in skin, 458, 459f
perineal anoplasty, for anorectal malformations,
180
male vs female, 178f, 179f
perineal fistula, in anorectal malformations,
176f, 177
perineal inspection, for anorectal
malformations, 177–178, 180
male vs female, 178f, 179f
perioperative care
for fetal surgery, 540
for neonatal surgery. See specific diagnosis or
procedure
periorbital hemorrhage, neuroblastoma causing,
205
periosteum, cerebral, hemorrhage in, 350f, 351
peripheral nerves
in brachial plexus, 400, 401f
Hirschsprung's disease and, 169
peripheral smear, in jaundice evaluation, 195,
195t
peripheral vascular resistance (PVR), in renal
physiology, 227
peristalsis
dysfunctional, in esophageal atresia with
fistula, 150
in Hirschsprung's disease, 169
ureteral
in megaureter, 280
in ureteropelvic junction obstruction, 295
peritoneal cavity
CSF shunting into, for hydrocephalus, 332–
333, 333f
embryology of, 144, 225
in inguinal hernia, 181, 183
peritoneal dialysis, inguinal hernia and, 183
peritoneal drain, percutaneous, for necrotizing
enterocolitis, 174
peritoneal sac, absence in utero, 155
peritoneum, embryology of, 144, 225

peritonitis
in Hirschsprung's disease, 169–170
meconium, 165
ovarian cysts and, 304, 308–309
perivascular space, alveoli rupture into, 101
permeability, 582
permissive hypercapnia, 90
permissive hypercarbia, 90, 582
persistent pulmonary hypertension of the
newborn (PPHN), 119
Pfeiffer syndrome, 31
PGE$_1$. See prostaglandin E$_1$
pH, of IV infusions, 467
pH probe study
in esophagus, 153
renal regulation of, 232, 235
in tracheomalacia, 49
phagocyte, 582
phagocytosis, 582
phalanges, embryology of, 364f
phallus. See penis
pharmacology
for infant transport, 490–491, 503
in pain management, 443, 446–454
pharyngeal arch
anomalies of, 25–28
associations of, 26
cleft lip and, 27, 27f
complications of, 28
definition of, 24t, 25
diagnosis of, 27
differential diagnosis of, 26–27
etiology of, 25–26
incidence of, 26
outcomes of, 28
pathophysiology of, 25
surgical treatment of, 27–28
embryology of, 3, 5, 24t, 61
structures derived from, 2t, 3
pharyngeal clefts, 3
pharyngeal flap/pharyngoplasty, for cleft lip/
palate, 35
pharyngeal grooves, 3, 6
pharyngeal pouches, 3, 6
pharynx
embryology of, 1–8, 142
Robin sequence and, 3, 37–39
phenobarbital, 494, 503
phenotype, 582
phentolamine mesylate (Regitine), for IV
extravasation, 467
phenytoin, 503
PHH. See posthemorrhagic hydrocephalus
phimosis, 309, 313, 582
phosphate
in immediate newborn period, 415
renal regulation of, 229, 231, 234–235
phosphate salts, 416
phosphorous
calcium ratio to, 422
homeostasis physiology of, 422
organic vs inorganic forms of, 234, 236
in parenteral nutrition solutions, 436
physiologic functions of, 423
renal reabsorption of, 235
skeletal development and, 367

photocoagulation, laser, 582
  for retinopathy of prematurity, 20*t*, 22, 24
phototherapy, fluid requirements with, 425, 495
phrenic nerve
  damage to, brachial plexus *vs*, 402
  in eventration of diaphragm, 94
  pacing of, for spinal cord injury, 359
physical deformity, 577, 581. *See also* congenital
      malformations
  grief and loss reactions to, 517
physical examination
  of bladder exstrophy, 263–264
  of brachial plexus injury, 402–404
  for circumcision, 310
  for congenital heart disease, 117–119
  of DDH
    after four months of age, 395, 396*f*
    newborn to four months of age, 394–395,
        394*f*–395*f*
  for hydration status, 429, 429*t*
  of limb reduction defects, 369–370
  of talipes equinovarus, 386
  of tethered cord, 341
physical therapy
  for brachial plexus injury, 404–405
  for pulmonary disorders sequelae, 109
  for spinal cord injury, 358–359
  for talipes equinovarus, 388–389
  for tethered cord repair, 342
physician consultation, during infant transport,
      482*t*, 484, 501, 504
physiologic parameters, in pain assessment,
      442*t*, 443–444, 571*f*–573*f*
physiologic shunting
  in congenital heart disease, 119, 125, 128–129,
      131
  in congenital lobar emphysema, 68
  extracorporeal membrane oxygenation and,
      554
physiologic stress, during infant transport,
      484–489
  management of, 489–498
PIE. *See* pulmonary interstitial emphysema
pilot, in transport team, 505
"Ping-Pong" depressed skull fractures, 348–349
pinwheel model, of grief process, 518
PIP. *See* peak inspiratory pressure
PIPP. *See* Premature Infant Pain Profile
piriform aperture stenosis, 582
pituitary gland, in reproductive physiology,
      239–240
placenta
  physiology of, 239
  in renal physiology, 227–228
placental bypass, for fetal surgery, 528
plagiocephaly, 582
  synostotic, 50*f*, 51–52
plantar flexion, of ankle, 390
Plastibell device, 310, 312
plastic surgery consultation, for IV
      extravasation, 467
plasticity, 582
platelets
  extracorporeal membrane oxygenation and,
      557
  necrotizing enterocolitis and, 174

in wound healing, 461, 461*f*
pleural cavity, embryology of, 62
pleural effusion
  bronchopulmonary sequestration and, 79–80,
      82
  chylothorax in, 97–100
  in pulmonary lymphangiectasia, 86–87
pleural space, air collection in, 101
pleurodesis, for chylothorax, 100
pleuroperitoneal folds, failure to close, 525
pleuroperitoneal shunt, for chylothorax, 100
PMR. *See* posteromedial release
pneumatic craniotome, 582
pneumatosis intestinalis, 173, 173*f*, 175
pneumomediastinum
  diagnosis of, 103, 104*f*
  pathophysiology of, 101
  treatment of, 105
pneumonectomy, indications for, 83, 105
pneumonia
  bronchopulmonary sequestration and, 78
  necrotizing enterocolitis *vs*, 173
  postoperative, in prune belly syndrome, 293
pneumopericardium
  diagnosis of, 103, 104*f*
  pathophysiology of, 101
  treatment of, 105
pneumoperitoneum, in necrotizing enterocolitis,
      173–174, 173*f*
pneumothorax
  diagnosis of, 103, 103*f*
  incidence of, 101–102
  outcomes of, 106
  pathophysiology of, 101
  posterior urethral valves and, 243
  simple *vs* tension, 104–105
  spontaneous *vs* acquired, 101
  treatment of, 104–105
    postoperative nursing care, 106
polyhydramnios, 582
  chylothorax associated with, 98
  congenital diaphragmatic hernia and, 88, 92
  ovarian cysts associated with, 303, 308
polymerization, 582
polyuria, 582
pons, 323, 582
Ponseti casting technique, for talipes
      equinovarus, 387–388, 391
pontine flexure, of brain, 323, 582
"pop-off" mechanism
  in patent urachus, 258
  in posterior urethral valves, 242, 244*f*
porta hepatis, 190, 198
portal hypertension, 193, 200
portal vein, occlusion of, 160
portal venous system, air in, 172*f*, 173
portoenterostomy
  hepatic, Kasai, for biliary atresia, 197–199
    complications of, 199–200
    outcomes of, 203
    postoperative nursing care, 201–203
positions/positioning
  in brachial plexus presentations, 401–402,
      403*f*
  for choanal atresia relief, 30
  for circumcision, 310

for cleft lip/palate repair, 35
for cloacal exstrophy, 275
for congenital diaphragmatic hernia, 90
for congenital heart disease, 126, 138
for esophageal atresia with fistula, 150–151
for eventration of diaphragm, 96
fetal, limb reduction defects and, 368–369
for gastroesophageal reflux, 153
for gastroschisis, 156
for hydrocephalus, 330, 334
during infant transport, 498
for inguinal hernia repair, 186
for laryngomalacia, 41–42
for myelomeningocele, 339
for ovarian cyst recovery, 308
for pulmonary air leak, 104
for pulmonary disorders, 107
for Robin sequence, 38
for spinal cord injury, 358–359
for talipes equinovarus casting, 390
teaching parents on, 514
for tethered cord repair, 342
positive end expiratory pressure (PEEP), 556, 582
positive pressure ventilation
for congenital cystic adenomatoid malformation, 75–76
for congenital diaphragmatic hernia, 90
posterior fossa subdural hemorrhage, 351–352
treatment of, 354–356
posterior sagittal anorectovaginourethroplasty, 180
posterior tibial muscle, in talipes equinovarus, 383, 388
posterior urethral valves (PUV), 240–252
associations of, 243
clinical presentation of, 242–243
complications of, 249
definition of, 240
diagnosis of, 243–244, 244f
differential diagnosis of, 243
etiology of, 242
incidence of, 242
obstructive anomalies of, 524t, 537–539
outcomes of, 251–252
pathophysiology of, 241–242
in prune belly syndrome, 288–290
treatment of, 244–251
algorithm for, 245, 245f
drainage methods, 245–247
postoperative nursing care, 250–251
priorities in, 244–245
supportive measures, 247
surgical, 247–249, 248f
types of, 241
in ureteropelvic junction obstruction, 299
urinary drainage for, 245–247
suprapubic catheter, 246–247
urethral catheter, 245–246
posterior vertical osteotomy, for bladder exstrophy closure, 266f, 267
posteromedial release (PMR), for talipes equinovarus, 382, 387, 389–391, 477
posthemorrhagic hydrocephalus (PHH), 330, 332, 335
posthitis, 582

postnatal care
for gastroschisis, 156
postoperative fetal surgery
for congenital cystic adenomatoid malformation, 530
for congenital diaphragmatic hernia, 527
for giant neck masses, 536–537
for myelomeningocele, 534–535
for obstructive uropathy, 539
for sacrococcygeal teratoma, 532–533
postoperative care
for fetal interventions, 541. See also postnatal care
fluid and electrolyte management in, 433–434
for neonatal surgery. See specific diagnosis or procedure
postoperative pain assessment score, neonatal, 572f
postpartum blues, 514
postures/posturing
in brachial plexus injury, 401–402, 403f
decerebrate vs decorticate, 577
postvoid residuals, in myelomeningocele repair, 340
potassium, body fluid content of, 430t, 431
potassium balance
ammonium role, 237
decreased, 420
factors affecting, 416
increased, 420–421
maintenance requirements for, 420
physiology of, 419–420
renal regulation of, 229, 232–233
potassium chloride, 420
potassium replacement
during infant transport, 496, 503
principles of, 420
pouch/pouching, for stomas
applications for, 473-476
neonatal, 471f
newborn, 472f
principles of, 471–472
powders, for stoma care, 475–476
PPHN. See persistent pulmonary hypertension of the newborn
preeclampsia, fetal malformations and, 528, 532
pregnancy
fetal abnormalities in
choices for, 523
diagnosis of. See prenatal diagnosis
genetic analysis of. See genetic consultation; karyotypic analysis
interventions for. See fetal surgery
high-risk, maternal transport for, 524, 541
parental expectations regarding, 516
pregnancy history
gathering during transport, 498, 501
in Robin sequence, 38
pregnenolone, in reproductive physiology, 240
Premature Infant Pain Profile (PIPP), 442t, 443, 463, 573f
premature newborns. See preterm infants
premaxilla, in cleft lip/palate repair, 34
prenatal conditions
brachial plexus associated with, 400–402

Neonatal Surgical Procedures: A Guide for Care and Management

congenital cystic adenomatoid malformation associated with, 73
interventions for. *See* fetal surgery
pulmonary lymphangiectasia associated with, 85
talipes equinovarus related to, 386
prenatal diagnosis
of amniotic band syndrome, 375
of bladder exstrophy, 263
of bronchopulmonary sequestration, 80
of congenital cystic adenomatoid malformation, 73, 74f, 528–529
of congenital diaphragmatic hernia, 89, 525
of congenital heart disease, 117
of esophageal atresia with fistula, 149
of eventration of diaphragm, 95
of giant neck masses, 535
of myelomeningocele, 533
of obstructive uropathy, 538
of sacrococcygeal teratoma, 531–532
prenatal referral, 479, 489, 583
prenatal (fetal) ultrasound
in absent radius, 379–380
in amniotic band syndrome, 375
in bladder exstrophy, 263
in bronchopulmonary sequestration, 80
in cloacal exstrophy, 272, 274
in congenital cystic adenomatoid malformation, 73, 74f
in congenital diaphragmatic hernia, 89, 525–526
in cystic hygroma, 13
in esophageal atresia with fistula, 149
in eventration of diaphragm, 95
in fetal surgery, 523, 528, 531, 535, 538, 540–542
in hydrocephalus, 329
in intestinal atresia/stenosis, 163
in limb reduction defects, 370
in meconium ileus, 165
in megaureter, 281
in ovarian cysts, 304
in posterior urethral valves, 243–244
in prune belly syndrome, 290
in ureteropelvic junction obstruction, 297–299
preoperative care
for fetal surgery, 540
fluid and electrolyte management in, 428–432, 429t, 430t
for neonatal surgery. *See specific diagnosis or procedure*
preparatory handling, for painful procedures, 445
prepuce, 226f, 311
preputial epithelium, in circumcision, 311
preputial ring, in circumcision, 311
pressurization, 582
preterm delivery, for gastroschisis, 156
preterm infants
body water composition in, 414
cloacal exstrophy of, 272
death trends of, 518
energy requirements of, 435
family-centered care for, 509–516
gastroesophageal reflux in, 152
glucose production in, 435
grief and loss reactions to, 517
inguinal hernia repair in, 185–186
necrotizing enterocolitis in, 171–172
pain expression in, 444
pain incidence in, 441
preterm labor, in fetal surgery, 541
prethreshold retinopathy of prematurity, 21
preventive measures
for hypothermia/hyperthermia, 126, 137
during infant transport, 484–485
in pain management, 445
prevesical space, 583
priapism, 583
primary acetabular dysplasia, 392
primary closure
of bladder exstrophy, 265, 267
of cloacal exstrophy, 277
of congenital diaphragmatic hernia, 91
dressings for, 468–469
of gastroschisis, 157
of omphalocele, 159
wound care/healing for, 468
primary germ plasm defect, 384
primary obstructive megaureter, 280–281, 280t
primary repair, complete, for bladder exstrophy closure, 267–268, 271
primitive brain, primary vesicles of, 322–323
primitive germ cells, 530
primitive kidneys, 220
primitive nasal choanae, 5
primitive streak, 322
primordial germ cells, in reproductive tract, 222–223, 225
primordial gut, embryology of, 141–142
primordial heart, 3
primordial phallus, 226f
procedures
invasive. *See* invasive procedures
nursing care. *See specific care*
for pain assessment/management, 443
surgical. *See specific procedure*
process-based protocols, for infant transport, 484–484t
processus vaginalis
failure to close, 181, 185
in inguinal hernia, 181–182, 182f, 185
proctodeum, 141, 146
progesterone, in reproductive physiology, 240
projectile vomiting, 161
prokinetic agents, for gastroesophageal reflux, 153
prolabium, 583
prolapse
rectal, in bladder exstrophy, 263, 267
stomal, 472f, 473
proliferation stage, in wound healing, 461f, 462
pronation, developmental, of foot, 367
pronephros, 217–218
propranolol, for tetralogy of Fallot, 126
proprioception, 406
prosencephalic tissue, 583
prosencephalic vein, median, 8, 581
prosencephalon, 323
prostaglandin E_1 (PGE$_1$), for congenital heart disease, 120, 125, 130, 132, 135
during infant transport, 493–494

prostaglandin inhibitors, for patent ductus
    arteriosus, 123
prostaglandins, in renal physiology, 231
prostate
    embryology of, 225, 226f
    hypoplasia of, in prune belly syndrome, 288
prostatic urethra, in prune belly syndrome, 288
prostatic utricle, 224f
prosthesis(es)
    for absent radius, 380–381
    cosmetic vs functional, 381
    dental, in cleft lip/palate repair, 35
    for lower vs upper extremities, 380
prosthetic patch, for congenital diaphragmatic
    hernia, 91, 94
proteases, 583
    in wound healing, 461f, 462
protective barrier, for stomas, 473, 474f, 475–476
protective function, of skin, 457, 459
protective gear, for transport team, 505–506,
    505f
protective mattresses, 359
proteins. See also amino acids
    in parenteral nutrition solutions, 436
    plasma, water regulation by, 414
    renal excretion of, 228–229, 237
    in skin, 460
prothrombin, 583
prothrombin time (PT), prolonged, biliary
    atresia and, 196–197
protocols, for infant transport, 482t, 484
    disease-based, 483t, 484
    emergencies, 504–505
    procedure, 482t, 484
    process-based, 484–484t
proximal convoluted tubule
    embryology of, 219–220, 219f
    physiology of, 228–229
proximal esophageal atresia, with fistula, 146,
    147f
prune belly syndrome, 287–294
    associations of, 290
    clinical presentation of, 289–290
    complications of, 293
    definition of, 287
    diagnosis of, 290–291
    differential diagnosis of, 290
    etiology of, 288–289
    incidence of, 289
    nursing care for, 291–292
    outcomes of, 294
    pathophysiology of, 287–288
    treatment of, 291–294
        immediate stabilization, 291–292
        postoperative nursing care, 293–294
        surgical, 292–293
pruritus, post-Kasai portoenterostomy, 201–202
pseudodiverticula, in prune belly syndrome,
    287–288
pseudoglandular stage, of lung development,
    60f, 62
pseudoparalysis, brachial plexus vs, 402
pseudorosettes, Homer-Wright, 579
PT. See prothrombin time
PTH. See parathyroid hormone

puberty, developmental changes during, 303,
    461
pubic bones
    in bladder exstrophy, 263, 265, 267–269
    in cloacal exstrophy, 274
    embryology of, 226f, 227
pubovesical cleft, 261
pulmonary air leak, 101–106
    associations of, 102
    clinical presentation of, 102
    complications of, 105
    definition of, 101
    diagnosis of, 103–104, 103f–105f
    differential diagnosis of, 102
    etiology of, 101
    incidence of, 101–102
    outcomes of, 106
    pathophysiology of, 101
    treatment of, 104–106
        postoperative nursing care, 106
        pulmonary compliance and, 104
        surgical, 105
        temporary measures in, 104–105
pulmonary artery
    embryology of, 61–62, 63f, 114t, 116
    shunts for obstruction of, 126–127, 127f
    transposition of, 128–129, 129f
        surgical switch procedure for, 130, 130f
pulmonary atresia, 114t
pulmonary capillaries, embryology of, 62, 63f
pulmonary disorders. See also specific disorder
    acquired, 97–100
    air leak in, 101–106
    diaphragmatic, 87–97
    nursing considerations for, 106–109
    outcomes of, 109
    parenchyma, 64–87
    stabilization maneuvers for
        immediate, 106–108
        postoperative, 108–109
pulmonary hypertension
    in congenital diaphragmatic hernia, 91–93
    crisis, in D-transposition of the great arteries
        repair, 130
    extracorporeal membrane oxygenation for,
        553
    hypoxemia and, 107
    persistent, of the newborn, 119
    in tetralogy of Fallot, 128
pulmonary hypoplasia
    congenital diaphragmatic hernia and, 92–93
    in eventration of diaphragm, 94
    ovarian cysts causing, 305, 309
    posterior urethral valves causing, 243, 251
pulmonary interstitial emphysema (PIE)
    complications of, 105
    diagnosis of, 103–104
    pathophysiology of, 101
    treatment of, 104–105
pulmonary lymphangiectasia, 84–87
    associations of, 85–86
    clinical presentation of, 85
    definition of, 84
    diagnosis of, 86, 86f
    differential diagnosis of, 86
    etiology of, 85

incidence of, 85
outcomes of, 87
pathophysiology of, 84–85
primary vs secondary, 85
treatment of
postoperative nursing care, 87
supportive, 86
surgical, 86–87
pulmonary stenosis, congenital, 114t, 124
surgical management of, 126–128, 127f
pulmonary system
air flight transport and, 487
altitude hypoxia of, 487–489
brain hemorrhage and, 354
in cloacal exstrophy, 273, 275–276
in congenital heart disease, 119
congenital malformations of, 64–109
associated disorders in, 97–100
developmental impact of, 59
diagnostic advances in, 59
incidence of, 59
specific disorders in, 64–97
embryology of, 59–64, 142
extracorporeal membrane oxygenation and, 557
posterior urethral valves effect on, 243, 251
prune belly syndrome impact on, 290–291, 293–294
pulmonary toilet
for cystic fibrosis, 166
suctioning for. See endotracheal intubation; nasal suctioning
for tracheostomy, 549
pulmonary veins
anomalous connections of, 114t
total, 134–136, 134f
embryology of, 61–62, 63f, 114t, 116
pulse(s)
carotid, in arteriovenous malformation, 8
in congenital heart disease, 118
in limb reduction defects, 372
in patent ductus arteriosus, 122
pulse oximetry
in congenital heart disease, 120, 137
in fetal surgery, 540
pump, for extracorporeal membrane oxygenation (ECMO), 555–556
pupillary reaction, in brain hemorrhage, 354
push-off strength, diminished, 390
PUV. See posterior urethral valves
PVR. See peripheral vascular resistance
pyeloplasty, for ureteropelvic junction obstruction, 300–302
pyelostomy, 248, 583
pyeloureteral junction, obstruction of, 294–302
pyeloureterostomy, temporary, for posterior urethral valves, 251
pyloric muscle, inadequate relaxation of, 161
pyloric stenosis, 160–162
associations of, 161
clinical presentation of, 161
complications of, 161
definition of, 160
diagnosis of, 161
differential diagnosis of, 161
etiology of, 160–161

incidence of, 161
nursing care for, 161
outcomes of, 162
pathophysiology of, 160
surgical treatment of, pyloromyotomy, 161
postoperative nursing care, 161–162

Q

quadriplegia, 360
quality assurance (QA), 583
for infant transport, 506–507
examples of, 481, 483, 489, 501
process of, 506–507, 506f
purpose of, 506
relevant topics for review, 506
quality of life, cloacal exstrophy and, 276

R

"raccoon eyes," 205
radial ray, 378
radiant warmers, neonatal fluid requirements with, 425, 495
radiation, heat loss through, 107, 484
radiation therapy. See radiotherapy
radiography
in anorectal malformations, 178
in cloacal exstrophy, 275
in DDH diagnosis, 395–396
in esophageal atresia with fistula, 149
in Hirschsprung's disease, 170
in inguinal hernia, 184
in intestinal atresia/stenosis, 163
in intestinal malrotation/volvulus, 167
in laryngeal web, 43
in laryngomalacia, 40
in meconium ileus, 165
in necrotizing enterocolitis, 172f, 173–173f
progressive, 174
in prune belly syndrome, 291
in spinal cord injury, 357
in talipes equinovarus, 386–387
in tethered cord, 341
in tracheomalacia, 48
radionuclide scanning
in bronchogenic cyst, 69
diuretic, in megaureter, 282–283
hepatobiliary, in biliary atresia, 196
in neuroblastoma, 208
in posterior urethral valves, 244
in prune belly syndrome, 291
in testicular torsion, 253
in ureteropelvic junction obstruction, 299, 302
radiosurgery, for arteriovenous malformation, 9
radiotherapy, 583
for cystic hygroma, 14
for neuroblastoma, 208–210
radius
absent, 378–381. See also absent radius
dysplasia of, 378–379
embryology of, 364f
function of, 378
reduction defects of, 370–371
range of motion
in brachial plexus injury, 403

assessment scales for, 403–404
  therapeutic, 404–405
in limb reduction defects, 371–372
lower body, myelomeningocele and, 337
in talipes equinovarus, 383–384
therapeutic. *See* passive range of motion
ranitidine, for gastroesophageal reflux, 153
rash(es)
  diaper dermatitis, 180, 466–467
  fungal, around stomas, 476
RBF. *See* renal blood flow
reanastomosis, primary, for esophageal atresia
  with fistula, 150
recanalization, of ureters, in ureteropelvic
  junction obstruction, 296
reconstructive surgery
  for bladder exstrophy
    of bladder neck, 265, 267
    complete primary, 267–268
  secondary, for brachial plexus injury, 405
  for spinal dimples/sinuses, 344–345
  staged, for prune belly syndrome, 293
rectal arteries, 146
rectal biopsy, in Hirschsprung's disease, 170
rectal examination, for anorectal malformations,
  177
rectal irrigation, for Hirschsprung's disease, 170
rectal pouch, needle aspiration of, 178
rectal prolapse, in bladder exstrophy, 263, 267
rectal veins, 146
rectocloacal fistula, 176f
rectourethral fistula, 176f, 180
rectovaginal fistula, 176f
rectum
  anomalies of. *See* anorectal malformations
  in bladder exstrophy, 263
  embryology of, 146
rectus abdominis muscle, in prune belly
  syndrome, 287
red blood cell transfusion, 174, 432–433
reduction
  closed, of DDH, 397–398
  manual, of inguinal hernia, 184
  open surgical
    of DDH, 398
    of inguinal hernia, 185–186
reduction defect, of limbs, 368–372. *See also*
  limb reduction defects
referral center, 479, 504, 583
reflux
  gastroesophageal, 583. *See also*
    gastroesophageal reflux (GER)
  megaureter and
    classification based on, 280, 280t
    pathophysiology of, 279–281
    postoperative, 285–286
  urinary, 537
  vesicoureteral, 242, 248–249, 271, 279
    circumcision for, 309
    in megaureter, 279–281, 280t, 286
    prune belly syndrome impact on, 292
    in ureteropelvic junction obstruction, 297
regional anesthesia, for pain management, 451
regurgitation, postprandial, 152
reimplantation, of ureters. *See* ureteral
  reimplantation

reliability, 443, 583
remodeling
  of bone, in talipes equinovarus, 390
  in wound healing, 461f, 462
renal arteries
  postnatal physiology of, 227–228
  in ureteropelvic junction obstruction, 295
  in utero physiology of, 227
renal blood flow (RBF)
  autoregulation of, 229
  determinants of, 227–228
  factors affecting, 230–231
  ureteropelvic junction obstruction impact on,
    296
renal capillaries, embryology of, 219f, 221
renal clearance, determinants of, 227–228
renal cortex, embryology of, 219f, 220–221, 223
renal dysplasia
  posterior urethral valves causing, 242, 251
  in prune belly syndrome, 288, 290
renal failure
  end-stage, posterior urethral valves and,
    251–252
  in prune belly syndrome, 294
renal function
  acid-base balance in, 235–237, 416–417
  assessment of, 416
  autoregulation of, 229
  body composition regulation, 239, 414–416
  in congenital heart disease, 137
  electrolyte regulation in, 231–235
  fluid regulation in, 229–230
  glomerular filtration rate in, 228
  hemodynamic factors of, 230–231
  megaureter impact on, 283
  neuroblastoma and, 207, 210
  in obstructive uropathy, 538–539
  organic components in, 229, 237–238
  posterior urethral valves effect on, 241–243
    outcomes of, 251–252
    urinary diversion indications for, 247–249,
      248f
  postnatal determinants of, 227–228
  prune belly syndrome impact on, 291–292, 294
  ureteropelvic junction obstruction impact on,
    295–296, 300
  urine output mechanisms, 238–239
  in utero, 227
renal medulla
  embryology of, 219f, 220–223
  urine concentration role, 238
renal parenchyma, echogenic mass of, 538
renal pelvis
  embryology of, 219f, 220
  in ureteropelvic junction obstruction, 295–296
    grading based on, 298–299
    surgical management of, 300–301
renal scan
  diuretic, in megaureter, 282–283
  in prune belly syndrome, 291
  in ureteropelvic junction obstruction, 299, 302
renal system
  anomalies of, in cloacal exstrophy, 274
  embryology of, 217–227

Neonatal Surgical Procedures: A Guide for Care and Management

excretory sets of, 217–220, 218f
  permanent development, 219–220, 219f
  positional changes, 218, 218f
physiology of, 227–240
surgical conditions of. *See* genitourinary (GU)
    tract
renal threshold, in acid-base balance, 415
renal tubules. *See* collecting tubules
renal ultrasound
  in bladder exstrophy, 264
  in cloacal exstrophy, 275
  in myelomeningocele management, 340
  in prune belly syndrome, 291
  in ureteropelvic junction obstruction, 302
renal vascular resistance (RVR), 227–228
renal veins
  postnatal physiology of, 227–228
  in utero physiology of, 227
renin, renal production, 230
reovirus Type 3, in biliary atresia, 191, 192t
reproductive system
  embryology of, 222–227
    external structures, 225, 225f–226f, 227
    gonad differentiation, 222–223, 223f
    internal structures, 224, 224f
  physiology of, 239–240
resection, surgical
  bowel
    for intestinal atresia/stenosis, 163
    for malrotation/volvulus, 168
    for necrotizing enterocolitis, 174
  for bronchopulmonary sequestration, 82
  for congenital cystic adenomatoid
        malformation
    complete *vs* partial, 75
  of fetal lungs, 529–530
  of neuroblastoma, 208–209
  for posterior urethral valves, 247
  for pulmonary interstitial emphysema, 105
  for pulmonary lymphangiectasia, 86
resectoscope, for posterior urethral valves
        ablation, 247
resonance, 583
respect, in family-centered care, 510
  mutual, 515–516
respiration
  opioids effects on, 447, 454
  paradoxical, 94–97
respiratory acidosis, 428, 431
respiratory alkalosis, 428, 431
respiratory distress
  in congenital heart disease, 137, 493
  gastroesophageal reflux associated with, 152
  laryngomalacia and, 39, 39f, 41
  management during transport, 490–491, 493
  mass effect causing, 78–79
  metabolic imbalance associated with, 428
  obstructive. *See* airway obstruction
  in patent ductus arteriosus, 122–123
  progressive, 64–65, 72–73
  Robin sequence and, 38
respiratory distress syndrome, 101
respiratory diverticulum, 59, 61
respiratory effort, in congenital heart disease,
        118, 122–123
respiratory failure

posterior urethral valves causing, 243, 251
  spinal cord injury causing, 358–359
respiratory rate, in congenital heart disease, 118
respiratory system. *See* pulmonary system;
    specific anatomy
respiratory tract
  lower, embryology of, 59–64, 142
  upper, embryology of, 1–8, 142
resting energy expenditure, 437
restraints
  during circumcision, 310
  during infant transport, 487, 504
  postoperative, for cleft lip/palate repair, 36
resuscitation medications, for infant transport,
        503
resuscitation room, neonatal, for fetal surgery,
        542
rete ridges, 460
retinal capillaries, injury mechanisms of, 17
retinal detachment, retinopathy of prematurity
        and, 19f, 23, 25
retinal reattachment, for retinopathy of
        prematurity, 23, 25
retinopathy of prematurity (ROP), 16–25
  associations of, 18
  cicatricial changes with, 20, 25
  clinical presentation of, 18
  complications of, 23
  definition of, 16–17
  diagnosis of, 18–20
  etiology of, 17
  extent of, 17f, 18, 20
  incidence of, 18
  international classification of, 18, 19f
  outcomes of, 24–25
  pathophysiology of, 17
  prethreshold, 21
  screening for, 21
  staging of, 18, 20
  threshold, 20t, 21
  treatment of, 21–24
    postoperative nursing care, 23–24
    surgical, 20t, 21–23
  zones of, 17–18, 17f
retracted stoma, 472f, 473
retrograde, 583
retrolental fibroplasia, 17
retrolental membrane, in vitrectomy, 23
return transport, of infant, 516
reversal agents, 503
rhabdomyosarcoma, 583
rhombencephalon, 323–324, 583
ribs, 149, 365
rickets, 580
right ventricular hypertrophy
  congenital, 124, 124f, 129
    surgical management of, 126–128
  in hypoplastic left heart syndrome, 132
ring block, subcutaneous, for pain management,
        451
Ringer's lactate, 108, 431–432
Robin sequence, 3, 37–39
  associations of, 38
  branchial apparatus anomalies and, 26
  cleft lip/palate and, 32, 37
  clinical presentation of, 38

definition of, 37
diagnosis of, 38
differential diagnosis of, 38
etiology of, 37
incidence of, 38
outcomes of, 37
pathophysiology of, 37
treatment of
postoperative nursing care, 38
symptomatic *vs* surgical, 38
Roe v Wade, 360
Ronald McDonald House, 534, 541–542
ROP. *See* retinopathy of prematurity
rotary wing aircraft (RWA), 505, 505f, 583
rotation(s)
of foot, 382, 382f, 385
of limbs, developmental, 365
pathologic
of gastrointestinal tract, 166–169. *See also*
malrotation
of testes, 252
rotavirus, Group C, in biliary atresia, 191, 192t
rudimentary heart, 2
rugae, 583
rupture, amnion, limb defects associated with,
372f–373f, 373–378
RVR. *See* renal vascular resistance
RWA. *See* rotary wing aircraft

S

saccular stage, of lung development, 62, 63f
sacral dimple, 343, 343f
sacrococcygeal teratoma (SCT), 530–533
AAP classification of, 530
definition of, 530
delivery of fetus with, 532
etiology of, 530–531
fetal surgery for
indications, 532
interventions, 524t, 532
incidence of, 531
pathophysiology of, 530
postnatal care for, 532–533
prenatal assessment of, 531–532
recurrent, 533
safety issues, of infant transport, 481, 504–506
safety officer, in transport team, 505
sagittal synostosis, 51–52
treatment of, 53–55
saline infusions
for dehydration, 429–430
for homeostasis maintenance, 108, 431
during infant transport, 496, 503
intraoperative indications for, 432
for negative sodium balance, 418
postoperative indications for, 433
principles of, 416–417
salivary glands, embryology of, 142
sarcomas, neuroblastoma *vs*, 206
SBS. *See* short-bowel syndrome
scaphocephaly, 583
synostotic, 50f, 51–52
treatment of, 53–55
scapula, embryology of, 364f
scars/scarring

cicatricial, 576
with circumcision, 313
Schweckendiek repair, of cleft lip/palate, 34, 34f
scimitar variant, of bronchopulmonary
sequestration, 77–78, 78f
differential diagnosis of, 80
treatment of, 82–84
scintigraphy. *See* radionuclide scanning
sclera, embryology of, 6
scleral buckle, for retinopathy of prematurity,
20t, 22, 24–25
scleral support ring, 583
sclerose, 583
sclerosing agents, for cystic hygroma, 14–15
screening
metabolic, in jaundice evaluation, 195, 195t
for neuroblastoma, 207
for retinopathy of prematurity, 21
scrotal sac, in inguinal hernia, 181
scrotum
in bladder exstrophy, 262, 264
edema of, neuroblastoma causing, 206
embryology of, 223, 223f, 224f, 226f
in inguinal hernia, 181, 182f, 183–185
testes descent into, 225, 252
in testicular torsion, 253–255
SCT. *See* sacrococcygeal teratoma
seatbelts, for infant transport, 487
sebaceous glands, 458, 460–461
"second look" surgery, for necrotizing
enterocolitis, 174
secondary intention, wound care/healing by, 469
secondary osteotomy, for brachial plexus injury,
405
secondary reconstructions, for brachial plexus
injury, 405
sedation/sedatives
administration during transport, 403, 490–
491
for congenital heart disease, 138
for gastroschisis, 157
for pain management, 450–451, 454
postoperative
for cleft lip/palate repair, 36
for laryngomalacia, 42
for retinopathy of prematurity, 24
segmentectomy, for bronchopulmonary
sequestration, 82
seizures
brain hemorrhage causing, 354–355
management during transport, 494, 495t
skull fractures causing, 350–351
self-blame, as parental reaction, 517
seminal vesicles, embryology of, 224, 224f
seminiferous tubule, 223f, 583
semipermeable membrane, in nephrons, 228
sensation assessment
in amniotic band syndrome, 377
in brachial plexus injury, 403
postoperative, 405–406
for limb reduction defects, 371–372
sensory function
in brachial plexus, 402
lower extremity, myelomeningocele and, 337
of skin, 457–458, 460
tethered cord impact on, 340–342

sepsis, 109
  anorectal malformations and, 179
  in necrotizing enterocolitis, 171–172
  posterior urethral valves causing, 244–245
septostomy, balloon
  for congenital heart disease, 121
  for total anomalous pulmonary venous
    connection, 135
  for D-transposition of the great arteries, 130
septum(s)
  cardiac
    congenital anomalies, 114t, 124, 124f
    embryology of, 114t, 115, 115f
  lower respiratory tract, 61, 63–64
  nasal
    in cleft lip/palate repair, 34, 35f
    embryology of, 6
  urorectal, 146, 272
septum primum, 115, 115f
septum secundum, 115, 115f
septum transversum, 143
sequence, 583
sequestration, bronchopulmonary, 76–84. See
    also bronchopulmonary sequestration
    (BPS)
serial casting, for talipes equinovarus, 387–388,
    391
serial manipulation, for talipes equinovarus
    correction, 382, 387, 391
serial stretching, for absent radius, 381
severe combined immunodeficiency, cellular
    transplant for, 542
sexual development. See reproductive system;
    specific anatomy
sexual differentiation, embryology of, 222–223,
    223f
sexually transmitted disease, circumcision and,
    309
SGA. See small for gestational age
shock
  brain hemorrhage and, 353–354
  cardiogenic, management during transport,
    494, 503
  hypovolemic, 429
  as parental reaction, 498, 517
  spinal, 357–358
shoes, straight-laced, for talipes equinovarus,
    388
short-bowel syndrome (SBS), 164, 168–169, 583
  in cloacal exstrophy, 274, 276–277, 279
short distal radius, 378
shoulder
  contractures of, in brachial plexus injury,
    405–406
  dystocia of, in brachial plexus injury, 405
  fracture, dislocation, or subluxation of, 402
shunt care teaching, for ventriculoperitoneal
    shunts, 334
shunts/shunting
  CSF
    ethical considerations of, 360
    for hydrocephalus, 332–333, 333f
    for myelomeningocele, 339
  fetal thoracoamniotic, for congenital cystic
    adenomatoid malformation, 530
  physiologic

    in congenital heart disease, 119, 125, 128–
      129, 131
    in congenital lobar emphysema, 68
    extracorporeal membrane oxygenation
      and, 554
  pleuroperitoneal, for chylothorax, 100
  systemic-to-pulmonary artery
    for hypoplastic left heart syndrome, 132,
      133f
    for tetralogy of Fallot, 126–127, 127f
  ventriculoperitoneal. See ventriculoperitoneal
    shunt
  ventriculosubgaleal, for hydrocephalus,
    333–334
  vesicoamniotic, for obstructive uropathy, 524t,
    537–539
SIADH. See syndrome of inappropriate
    antidiuretic hormone
siblings
  reaction to birth crisis, 513–514
  reaction to neonatal death, 519
sigmoid colon, embryology of, 146
silk sign, in inguinal hernia, 184
silo closure, silastic
  of gastroschisis, 157, 157f
  of omphalocele, 159, 159f
Simonart bands, 373
simple pneumothorax, treatment of, 104–105
single-stage closure, of cloacal exstrophy, 277
sinogram, in patent urachus, 258
sinus(es)
  branchial, anomalies of, 26
    surgical treatment of, 27–28
  cervical, embryology of, 4f, 5–6
  dermal, 578
  paranasal, embryology of, 6
  spinal, 342–345. See also spinal sinuses
  urachal. See urachal sinus
  urogenital. See urogenital sinus
69XXX syndrome, 535
skeletal tissue/structures. See also bone(s);
    cartilage
  defects and injuries of, 368–408
    absent radius, 378–381, 378f
    amniotic band syndrome, 373–378
    brachial plexus injury, 400–406
    developmental dysplasia of hip, 391–399
    limb reduction, 368–372, 372f
    myelomeningocele associated with, 336–
      337
    skull fractures resulting from, 348–349
    talipes equinovarus, 382–391
  embryology of, 2, 363–368, 364f, 366f
skin
  anatomy of, 457, 458f
  embryology of, 365, 458–461, 459f
  function of, 457
  healing of. See wound healing
  tearing or stripping of, 466
skin assessment/care
  for circumcision, 312–313, 468
  congenital heart disease and, 138
  evidence-based practice guidelines for, 457
  extracorporeal membrane oxygenation and,
    558
  for gastrostomy tube, 154, 567–569

general principles of, 463–466
goals of, 463
of injured skin, 466–468
in limb reduction defects, 371–372
for ostomy stomas, 469–476. *See also* stoma(s)
post-Kasai portoenterostomy, 202
in spinal cord injury, 358–359
for urinary diversion stomas, 250
skin barriers
for breakdown protection, 359
for stomas, 473, 474f, 475–476
skin breakdown
prevention of, 358, 467
risk factors for, 466–467
in spinal cord injury, 358–359
skin color
in congenital heart disease, 117–118
in limb reduction defects, 371
skin sealants, 467, 469
for stoma care, 472, 476
skin tears, nursing care for, 466
skull. *See also* cranium
in encephalocele, 345–348
ossification of, 7, 7f, 367
skull fractures, 348–351
associations of, 349
clinical presentation of, 349
complications of, 350
definition of, 348
diagnosis of, 349
differential diagnosis of, 349
etiology of, 348, 349f
"growing," 350
incidence of, 348
nursing care for, 349–350
outcomes of, 351
pathophysiology of, 348
treatment of, 349–351
delayed or palliative, 349
immediate, 349
postoperative nursing care, 351
surgical, 350
transport for, 349
types of, 348
sleep state, pain expression during, 444
slings, for brachial plexus injury, 405
"slit tape" taping technique, for G-tube
stabilization, 566–567f
small cell osteosarcoma, 206
small for gestational age (SGA), 272, 583
small intestine
embryology of, 144–145
obstruction of
anorectal malformations associated with,
177
atresia/stenosis associated with, 162–164
gastroesophageal reflux associated with,
152
in Hirschsprung's disease, 169
inguinal hernia causing, 183
malrotation/volvulus causing, 166–169
meconium causing, 164–165
pyloric stenosis associated with, 161
ostomies of, 470–471, 470f. *See also* stoma(s)
perforation of
in necrotizing enterocolitis, 173–174, 173f

ovarian cysts associated with, 303
smooth muscle
pulmonary development of, 61
urogenital, in prune belly syndrome, 281,
287–288
Sober-type diversion procedure, for posterior
urethral valves, 249
social support, parental, assessment of, 512–514
sociology, in family-centered care, 510
sodium
body fluid content of, 430t, 431
serum, renal regulation of, 228–230, 232, 233f
sodium balance, 416–419
decreased, 417–419, 419t
factors affecting, 416
increased, 419
maintenance requirements for, 417
negative, 417–418
physiology of, 416–417
sodium bicarbonate (NaHCO$_3$)
administration during transport, 503
intraoperative indications for, 432
for metabolic acidosis, 90, 422
renal production of, 236
sodium chloride (NaCl) infusion. *See* saline
infusions
soft tissue
contractures of, in absent radius, 381
deformities of, in talipes equinovarus,
382–384
in hip dysplasia, 391–399. *See also*
developmental dysplasia of the hip
(DDH)
soft tissue flap, for cleft lip/palate repair, 34–35,
34f, 35f
soft tissue procedures
for amniotic band syndrome, 377, 377f
for limb reduction defects, 370
for talipes equinovarus
outcomes of, 391
release techniques, 382, 387, 389, 391, 477
release timing, 389–390
solutes, kidneys reabsorption of, 227–229
somatic, 583
somites, 365
sonography. *See* ultrasound
Spasticity Study Group, 389
special care newborn, loss experienced with, 517
speech impairment, cleft lip/palate and, 36–37
spermatic artery, internal, 252
spermatic cord, twisting of, 252
spermatogenesis, ischemic loss of, 252
spermatogonia, 224
sphenoid bone, embryology of, 7, 7f
sphincters, 583
dysfunction of. *See* incontinence
spica cast
for bladder exstrophy closure, 269
hip, for DDH, 398–399
shoulder, for brachial plexus injury, 405
spina bifida occulta. *See also* myelomeningocele
(MMC)
clinical presentation of, 336
differential diagnosis of, 337
fetal surgery for, 524t, 533–535
multidisciplinary clinic for, 338

spinal anesthesia, for inguinal hernia repair, 184, 432
spinal column. *See* spine
spinal cord
    compression of, neuroblastoma causing, 205, 210
    embryology of, 2, 323
    fixed defect of, 340–342. *See also* tethered cord
    protrusion of. *See* myelomeningocele (MMC)
spinal cord injury
    complications of, 358–359
    nursing care for, 358
    outcomes of, 360
    traumatic, 356–360
        associations of, 357
        clinical presentation of, 357
        definition of, 356
        diagnosis of, 357–358, 358f
        differential diagnosis of, 357
        etiology of, 356–357
        incidence of, 357
        pathophysiology of, 356
    treatment of, 358–360
        immediate stabilization, 358
        postoperative nursing care, 359
        surgical, 358
spinal dimples, 342–345
    associations of, 343
    clinical presentation of, 343
    complications of, 344
    definition of, 342
    diagnosis of, 343–344
    differential diagnosis of, 343, 343f
    etiology of, 343
    incidence of, 343
    outcomes of, 345
    pathophysiology of, 343
    in spina bifida occulta, 336
    surgical treatment of, 344
        postoperative nursing care, 344–345
spinal dysraphism, occult, 341
spinal nerves
    in brachial plexus, 400, 401f
    cervical, in diaphragm development, 64
    cranial, embryology of, 2t, 3, 5
spinal shock, 357–358
spinal sinuses, 342–345
    associations of, 343
    clinical presentation of, 343
    complications of, 344
    definition of, 342
    diagnosis of, 343–344
    differential diagnosis of, 343, 343f
    etiology of, 343
    incidence of, 343
    outcomes of, 345
    pathophysiology of, 343
    in spina bifida occulta, 336
    surgical treatment of, 344
        postoperative nursing care, 344–345
spinal tract, abnormalities of, 344
spine
    anomalies of

    in cloacal exstrophy, 260, 272–273, 275, 279
        prune belly syndrome associated with, 290
        soft tissue, 342–345
    bony defect in, 533. *See also* myelomeningocele (MMC)
        reconstruction of, 338–339, 338f
    cervical, neuroblastoma in, 205
    embryology of, 365
    fusion of, for spinal cord injury, 358
    stabilization of, for spinal cord injury, 358–359
spirometry, 68, 583
splanchnic exstrophy, 272
splanchnic mesenchyme, 61, 141–143, 221
spleen assessment, in congenital heart disease, 119
splints/splinting
    for absent radius, 380–381
    for DDH, 397–398, 397f
    hand/wrist, for brachial plexus injury, 404–405
    of lower limb anomalies, 278
    for talipes equinovarus, 388, 389f
split heart sounds, 118, 135
spouses, social support from, 512, 514
stabilization maneuvers
    for brain hemorrhage, 354
    for congenital heart disease, 126, 136–137
    for DDH, 397
    for encephalocele, 346–347
    during infant transport, 479, 489–490
    for myelomeningocele, 337–338
    for pulmonary disorders
        bronchopulmonary sequestration, 82
        congenital cystic adenomatoid malformation, 74–75
        congenital diaphragmatic hernia, 90–91
        congenital lobar emphysema, 66–67
        immediate, 106–108
        postoperative, 108–109
    for skull fractures, 349
    for spinal cord injury, 358
Stage 1 Norwood procedure, for hypoplastic left heart syndrome, 132, 133f
staged closure
    of bladder exstrophy, 265–266
    of cloacal exstrophy, 277
    of gastroschisis, 157, 157f
    of omphalocele, 159
staged embolization, for arteriovenous malformation, 9–10, 11f
staged repair/reconstruction
    of amniotic band syndrome, 377, 377f
    of esophageal atresia with fistula, 150
    of urinary tract, for prune belly syndrome, 293
staging, of retinopathy of prematurity, 18, 20
standards of practice, for pain assessment/management, 442–443
stapes, embryology of, 7f
staples, for primary closure, 468
stasis, 583
state-of-the-art services, in fetal surgery, 541–542
static technique, in DDH diagnosis, 396, 396f, 397t
stenosis

anorectal, 175–181, 176f
aortic, 114t
of aqueduct of Sylvius, hydrocephalus related
     to, 327–328
intestinal, 162–164. *See also* intestinal stenosis
piriform aperture, 582
pulmonary, congenital, 114t, 124
     surgical management of, 126–128, 127f
pyloric, 160–162. *See also* pyloric stenosis
stents/stenting
external tracheal, for tracheomalacia, 49
for megaureter, 284–285
     postoperative nursing care, 285–286
nasal, for choanal atresia, 30–31
ureteral
     for bladder exstrophy closure, 266–267
          postoperative nursing care, 270
     for ureteropelvic junction obstruction, 301
stereotyping, in family-centered care, 510
Steri-Strips, for primary closure, 468
sternocleidomastoid muscle, branchial arch
          anomalies and, 24t, 25, 28
steroids
for cholangitis, 200
postoperative
     for cystic hygroma, 16
     for Kasai portoenterostomy, 201
     for laryngomalacia, 42
     for retinopathy of prematurity, 24
for spinal cord injury, 358
Stickler syndrome, 37
stillbirths, loss following, 517
Stocker classification, of congenital cystic
          adenomatoid malformation, 71–72, 528
stoma(s), 583
appliance bag for, 474f, 475–476
appliances for
     application of, 473–476, 473f–475f
     discharge teaching on, 476
     optional use of, 472–473
     principles of use, 471–472
     removal of, 472f, 473
     types of, 471–472f
double-barrel, 470, 471f, 578
end, 470, 470f, 578
gastrostomy, 564–565
     leaking through, 565–569
for Hirschsprung's disease, 170
for intestinal atresia/stenosis, 163
loop, 580
for meconium ileus, 165
for necrotizing enterocolitis, 174–175
nursing care for, 469–476
     for gastrostomy tube stoma, 565–569
for posterior urethral valves diversions,
          248–250
prolapsed, 472f, 473
retracted, 472f, 473
types, 470–471, 470f–471f
stoma measuring guide, 473, 473f
stoma paste, 475–476
stoma powder, 475
stoma size, template for, 474–475, 474f
stomach
decompression of. *See* gastric decompression
embryology of, 142–143

separation from wall, gastrostomy tube and,
          569
stomodeum, 3, 141
stool
acholic, 575
fetal. *See* meconium *entries*
strangulated inguinal hernia, 181, 185
stratum corneum, 458–459, 459f, 583
stratum germinativum, 459f, 460–461, 583
stratum granulosum, 459, 459f, 583
stratum lucidum, 459, 459f, 583
stratum spinosum, 583
Streeter dysplasia, 373
strengthening exercises, for brachial plexus
          injury, 404, 406
stress/stressors
fetal, echocardiogram for, 117
during infant transport, 484–489
     management of, 489–498
surgical, infants' response to, 434
stretching maneuvers
for DDH, 398
for talipes equinovarus, 387
stricture(s)
of anus, 180
of colon, in necrotizing enterocolitis, 174–175
of ureter
     in megaureter, 280t, 281
     in ureteropelvic junction obstruction, 295
stridor, 584
congenital laryngeal, 39–40
expiratory, tracheomalacia and, 48
laryngeal web and, 43
Robin sequence and, 38
vocal cord paralysis and, 45
stroke, brain hemorrhage resulting from,
          352–353
subarachnoid hemorrhage, 351–352
treatment of, 354–356
subarachnoid space, 325–326, 584
subcutaneous, 584
subcutaneous fat
anatomy of, 457, 458f
embryology of, 459f, 461
subcutaneous mass, neuroblastoma *vs,* 205–206
subcutaneous ring block, for pain management,
          451
subdural hemorrhage, 351–352
treatment of, 354–356
subdural space, 584
subdural taps, direct, for brain hemorrhage, 355
subgaleal area, 584
subgaleal hemorrhage, 350f, 351–352
treatment of, 354–356
subglottic region, laryngeal web in, 42–44
subluxable hip, 392, 584
subluxation
of hip, 392, 584
of shoulder, brachial plexus *vs,* 402
talonavicular, 385
submandibular gland, cystic hygroma and, 15
suboccipital craniectomies, for brain
          hemorrhage, 355
subsaccules, embryology of, 62, 63f
sucrose administration
oral, during circumcision, 310

for pain management, 445–446
suctioning
  of airway. *See also* endotracheal suctioning;
      nasal suctioning
    with tracheostomy, 549
  closed postoperative. *See* closed system
      drainage device(s)
  for esophageal atresia with fistula, 150–151
sump catheter, for esophageal atresia with
    fistula, 150
superior vena cava, chylothorax and, 98
support systems
  for parents, 515–516
  for urinary diversion patients, 251
supportive care
  for anorectal malformations, 178–179
  during birth crises, 512–519
  for brain hemorrhage, 355–356
  during circumcision, 310
  for congenital heart disease, 137
  during crises, 514
  for family. *See* family-centered care; parent
      teaching
  for grief facilitation, 518–519
  for hydrocephalus, 330
  for laryngomalacia, 41
  maternal, in fetal surgery, 525, 540, 542
  for necrotizing enterocolitis, 173–175
    surgery *vs*, 174
  nutritional. *See* nutrition/nutritional support
  positioning as. *See* positions/positioning
  for posterior urethral valves, 244–245, 245*f*
    postoperative referrals, 251
  for prune belly syndrome, 291
  for pulmonary lymphangiectasia, 86–87
  respiratory. *See* airway management;
      mechanical ventilation; oxygen
      therapy
  for spinal cord injury, 358–359
  thermal. *See* thermoregulation
  for vocal cord paralysis, 46
supraglottic airway, in laryngomalacia, 39, 39*f*
supraglottoplasty, for laryngomalacia, 41
suprahyoid, 584
suprapubic catheter
  percutaneous, for posterior urethral valves,
    246–247
  site care for, 247, 270
suprapubic cystostomy tube, for bladder
    exstrophy closure, 266, 268
  postoperative nursing care, 270–271
supratentorial hemorrhage, 355
surface area. *See* body surface area
surfactant, exogenous
  administration during transport, 490
  for congenital diaphragmatic hernia, 91
  pulmonary air leak risk and, 101
surfactant system, pulmonary development of,
    62
surgical instruments, for fetal surgery, 542
surgical procedures
  answering parent's questions about, 511, 513*t*
  indications for. *See specific diagnosis*
  techniques for. *See named procedure*
surgical repair
  open

of inguinal hernia, 185
of ovarian cysts, 308
reconstruction with. *See* reconstructive
    surgery
surgical stress, infants' response to, 434
survival training course, for transport team,
    485, 504
suspension laryngoscopy, 584
sutures/suturing
  cranial. *See* cranial sutures
  for primary closure, 468
swaddling
  DDH associated with, 393
  for pain management, 310, 445
swallow studies
  barium contrast
    in bronchopulmonary sequestration, 81
    in tracheomalacia, 48
  postoperative, for giant neck masses, 537
sweat chloride test, for cystic fibrosis, 166
sympathetic ganglia, malignancies arising from,
    203–204
sympathetic nervous system, neuroblastoma
    locations in, 205
symphysis pubis
  in bladder exstrophy, 263, 265, 267–269
  in cloacal exstrophy, 274
  embryology of, 226*f*, 227
syndactyly, 368, 374, 376–377
syndrome, 584
syndrome of inappropriate antidiuretic hormone
    (SIADH), 418–419
  overhydration *vs*, 418, 419*t*
  skull fracture repair and, 351
synergism, 584
synostosis, 584. *See also* craniosynostosis
systemic-to-pulmonary artery shunts
  for hypoplastic left heart syndrome, 132, 133*f*
  for tetralogy of Fallot, 126–127, 127*f*
systolic ejection murmur, in tetralogy of Fallot,
    125

T

tail closure, for stomas, 471, 472*f*
talipes equinovarus, 382–391
  associations of, 385
  classification of, 383–384
  clinical presentation of, 385
  complications of, 390
  congenital idiopathic, 384, 384*f*
  definition of, 382, 382*f*
  diagnosis of, 385, 385*f*–386*f*
  differential diagnosis of, 385
  etiology of, 384–385
  incidence of, 385
  outcomes of, 391
  pathophysiology of, 382–384, 383*f*
  treatment of, 386–391
    botulinum toxin type A injections, 388–389
    early, 386
    manipulation and casting, 382, 387–388
    postoperative nursing care, 390–391
    surgical, 389–390
talocalcaneal joint, in talipes equinovarus, 383
talocrural joint, in talipes equinovarus, 383

talonavicular joint, 383, 385
talus, in talipes equinovarus, 382–383
TAR syndrome, 379–380
tarsal bones, in talipes equinovarus, 382, 384, 390
taurine, in parenteral nutrition solutions, 436
tear(s)
    amnion, limb defects associated with, 372f–373f, 373–378
    of cervical nerve roots, 400, 401f
    skin, 466
TEARS. See early amnion rupture spectrum, the
technetium-99-IDM (TC-99) scan
    in gastroesophageal reflux, 153
    hepatobiliary, in biliary atresia, 196
    in neuroblastoma, 208
TEF. See tracheoesophageal fistula
telencephalon, 323, 584
telephone consultation
    facilitating, 511
    for fetal surgery, 525, 542
    during infant transport, 482t, 484, 501, 504
temporal bone, embryology of, 7, 7f
tendon(s)
    Achilles, in talipes equinovarus, 383, 388
    transfers of, for brachial plexus injury, 405
tenotomy, adductor, for DDH, 398
tension pneumothorax, treatment of, 104–105
teratogenic agents
    limb reduction defects associated with, 370
    neuroblastoma associated with, 204
    Robin sequence association with, 37
teratologic dislocation of hip, 392, 584
terminal conditions, hydrocephalus as, 330
termination, of pregnancy, 523–524
tertiary care centers, 479, 504
testes/testicles
    descent into scrotum, 225, 252
    embryology of, 222, 223f, 224
    in inguinal hernia, 181, 182f, 183
    torsion of, 183, 252–255. See also testicular torsions
testicular appendix, 224f
testicular torsions, 252–255
    associations of, 253
    clinical presentation of, 253
    complications of, 255
    contralateral management of, 254–255
    definition of, 252
    diagnosis of, 253
    differential diagnosis of, 253
    etiology of, 252
    extravaginal vs intravaginal, 252
    incidence of, 252
    outcomes of, 255
    pathophysiology of, 185, 252
    postnatal vs prenatal, 252–253
    treatment of, 254–255
        emergency, 254
        postoperative nursing care, 255
        surgical, 254
    unilateral vs bilateral, 252–254
    in utero, 252–253
testosterone
    gestational production of, 225
    in reproductive physiology, 240

sexual differentiation role, 222, 223f, 224–225
    in testicular torsion, 252, 255
"tet" spells, with tetralogy of Fallot, 125–126
tethered cord, 340–342
    associations of, 341
    clinical presentation of, 341
    complications of, 342
    definition of, 340
    diagnosis of, 341
    differential diagnosis of, 341
    etiology of, 340–341
    incidence of, 341
    outcomes of, 342
    pathophysiology of, 340
    in spinal dimples/sinuses, 343–344
    surgical treatment of, 342
        postoperative nursing care, 342
tethering, fetal
    in amniotic band syndrome, 375
    in talipes equinovarus, 385
tetralogic clubfoot, 383, 385
tetralogy of Fallot (TOF), 124–128
    associations of, 125
    clinical presentation of, 125
    complications of, 127–128
    definition of, 124, 124f
    diagnosis of, 125
    differential diagnosis of, 125
    ductal-dependent cyanotic, 125, 128
    etiology of, 124
    incidence of, 124
    nursing care for, 125–126
    outcomes of, 128
    pathophysiology of, 124
    "tet" or "blue" spells with, 125–126
    treatment of, 125–127
        immediate vs staged, 125
        postoperative nursing care for, 136–138
        preoperative stabilization, 126
        surgical, 126–127, 127f
Thal fundoplication, for gastroesophageal reflux, 153–154
thalamus, 323
THAM. See tromethamine
thecal sac, defects of, 335. See also myelomeningocele (MMC)
    reconstruction of, 338–339, 338f
thermogenesis, nonshivering, 461
thermoregulation
    for cloacal exstrophy, 275
    for congenital heart disease, 126, 137
    for gastroschisis, 156
    during infant transport, 484–485, 492f, 493–494, 502
    for pulmonary disorders
        immediate stabilization, 107
        postoperative, 109
    skin role in, 457, 459, 461
thighs, in bladder exstrophy, 263, 271
"third spacing," 108, 160
    fluid losses with, 430–431
        replacement guidelines for, 432–433
third ventricle, of brain, 324, 324f
third ventriculostomy, for hydrocephalus, 333
thoracentesis, 584
    for congenital lobar emphysema, 67–68

thoracic duct ligation, for chylothorax, 100
thoracoamniotic shunt, fetal, for congenital
    cystic adenomatoid malformation, 530
thoracostomy, 584
thoracostomy drainage
    for chylothorax, 99–100
    for congenital cystic adenomatoid
        malformation, 76
    for congenital diaphragmatic hernia, 91–92
    for congenital lobar emphysema, 67–68
    for tension pneumothorax, 105
thoracotomy, 584
    for bronchogenic cyst, 70
    for chylothorax, 98
    for congenital cystic adenomatoid
        malformation, 75
    left, for patent ductus arteriosus closure,
        123–124
    with lobectomy, for congenital lobar
        emphysema, 67–68
    nursing care for, 106
thoracotomy tube. See chest tube
thorax/thoracic cavity
    air collection in, 101
    embryology of, 62
    neuroblastoma found in, 205
    transillumination of, for air leak, 103
threshold altitude, for aircraft, 488
threshold retinopathy of prematurity, 20t, 21
threshold time, for transport dispatch, 507
throat. See also neck
    embryology of, 1–8
    Robin sequence and, 3, 37–39
thrombosis/thrombus, 584
    brain hemorrhage resulting from, 352
    in spinal cord injury, 357–358
through transmission, 584
thumbs
    in absent radius, 380
    embryology of, 365, 366f
    in limb reduction defects, 369
thymus gland
    branchial arch development and, 27
    embryology of, 3, 6
thyroglossal duct, 5
thyroid gland, embryology of, 5
tibial muscles, posterior, in talipes equinovarus,
    383, 388
tie-down devices, for infant transport, 487
tobacco, Robin sequence association with, 37
tocolysis, in fetal surgery, 541
toes
    in amniotic band syndrome, 373–378
    embryology of, 365, 366f, 367
TOF. See tetralogy of Fallot
tolerance, to drugs, 584
toll-free number, for fetal consultations, 542
tone
    in brachial plexus injury, 403
    general, in congenital heart disease, 118
tongue
    embryology of, 5, 61, 142
    in Robin sequence, 37–38
tonsils
    branchial arch development and, 27
    embryology of, 3, 142

topical agents, absorption factor of, 459
TORCH, in jaundice evaluation, 195, 195t
torsion
    of ovaries, cysts resulting from, 303–309
    of testicles, 252–255. See also testicular
        torsions
torticollis, contralateral ocular, 52
tortuous, 584
total anomalous pulmonary venous connection,
    134–136
    associations of, 134–135
    clinical presentation of, 134
    complications of, 135–136
    definition of, 134, 134f
    diagnosis of, 135
    differential diagnosis of, 135
    etiology of, 134
    incidence of, 134
    obstructed vs unobstructed, 134–135
    outcomes of, 136
    pathophysiology of, 114t, 134
    surgical treatment of, 135
        postoperative nursing care, 136–138
total bilirubin, in jaundice evaluation, 195, 195t
total body water
    changes in, 239, 414, 415f
    renal regulation of, 239
total parenteral nutrition (TPN). See parenteral
    hyperalimentation
totipotent cells, 530
toxins
    intestinal, necrotizing enterocolitis associated
        with, 171
    kidneys excretion of, 227
trabeculae, 584
trabeculation, 584
trace elements, in parenteral nutrition solutions,
    436
trachea
    embryology of, 59, 60f, 61
    hygromas of, 12
    malformations of, 146–151, 147f
    reconstruction of, with giant neck masses, 537
tracheal occlusion therapy, for fetal congenital
    diaphragmatic hernia, 527
tracheal stenting, external, for tracheomalacia,
    49
tracheoesophageal fistula (TEF)
    associations of, 148–149
    with atresia
        proximal, 147, 147f
        proximal and distal, 147f, 148
    clinical presentation of, 148
    complications of, 150
    definition of, 146
    diagnosis of, 149–150
    differential diagnosis of, 149
    etiology of, 148
    incidence of, 148
    outcomes of, 151
    surgical treatment of, 150
        postoperative nursing care, 150–151
    tracheomalacia associated with, 47, 49
    tracheostomy risk for, 550–551
    types of, 146–147, 147f
    without atresia, 147, 147f

tracheoinnominate fistula, 584
tracheomalacia, 47–49
  associations of, 48
  clinical presentation of, 48
  complications of, 49
  definition of, 47
  diagnosis of, 48
  differential diagnosis of, 48
  etiology of, 47
  incidence of, 47
  pathophysiology of, 47
  surgical treatment of, 48–49
    postoperative nursing care, 49
tracheostomy, 547–551, 584
  complications of, 548–549
  contraindications for, 547
  for giant neck masses, 537
  indications for, 547
  for laryngeal web, 44–45
  for laryngomalacia, 41
  materials needed for, 547
  postoperative nursing care, 549–551
  procedure for, 547–548
  for Robin sequence, 38
  for tracheomalacia, 49
  for vocal cord paralysis, 46
traction
  for bladder exstrophy closure, 269
  excessive during delivery, 400. See also
    brachial plexus injury
  preliminary, for DDH, 398
transalveolar pressure, air leak associated with,
    101–109
transarterial embolization, for arteriovenous
    malformation, 10, 11f
transcutaneous monitoring, in congenital heart
    disease, 120, 137
transillumination
  of cystic hygroma, 13
  of inguinal hernia, 183–184
  of thorax, for air leak, 103
transparent film dressings, 465, 584
transperitoneal incision, for ureteropelvic
    junction obstruction, 301
transplant(s), 584. See also specific anatomy
transport coordinator, responsibilities of, 483
transport equipment, 501–503
transport incubator, 494, 501
transport medications, 503
transport procedures, standardized, 482t, 484
transport record, 499f–500f, 501
transport system
  for infant. See infant transport
  maternal, for high-risk patients, 524, 541
transport team, 479–484
  additional responsibilities, 498–501
  care of neonate responsibilities, 489–498
  communication with, 492, 504–505
  competency of, 480t, 482
  composition guidelines for, 481
  disease-based protocol for, 483t, 484
  dispatch of, 489, 504
    delay analysis, 506f, 507
  equipment and medications used by, 501–503
  impact on infant outcome, 479, 481
  leadership of, 482–483

  orientation programs for, 481
  physiologic stresses on, 484–489
  process-based protocol for, 484–484t
  quality assurance for, 481, 483, 489, 501,
    506–507
  safety for, 481, 504–506
  selection factors for, 481
  standardized procedures for, 482t, 484
  survival training course for, 485
D-transposition of the great arteries, 128–130
  associations of, 129
  clinical presentation of, 129
  complications of, 130
  definition of, 128
  development of, 114t
  diagnosis of, 129
  differential diagnosis of, 129
  etiology of, 129
  incidence of, 129
  outcomes of, 130
  pathophysiology of, 128
  surgical treatment of, 130, 130f
    postoperative nursing care for, 136–138
transpyloric feedings, 439
transtorcular embolization, for arteriovenous
    malformation, 10, 11f
transvenous embolization, for arteriovenous
    malformation, 10, 11f
transverse abdominis muscle, in prune belly
    syndrome, 287
transverse colon, embryology of, 144–146
trauma
  birth. See labor and delivery
  chylothorax associated with, 98
  during infant transport, 504–505
  nasal, choanal atresia vs, 29
  skull fractures resulting from, 348–349, 349f
  spinal cord injury related to, 356–360
Treacher Collins syndrome, 3, 26
triad syndrome, 287
triceps surae muscle, in talipes equinovarus,
    388–389
trigeminal nerve (cranial nerve V)
  in brachial plexus injury, 400–406
  pharyngeal arch origin of, 2t, 3
triglycerides, serum, recommended ranges for,
    437
trigonocephaly, 584
  synostotic, 50f, 51–52
trilaminar embryo, development of, 322
triploidy syndrome, 329
trisomy(ies), in prune belly syndrome, 289–290
trisomy 18, in esophageal atresia with fistula, 149
trisomy 21, duodenal atresia associated with, 163
tromethamine (THAM), for metabolic acidosis,
    90, 422
TrophAmine solution, 436
"trumpet sign" posture, in brachial plexus, 403f
truncus arteriosus, embryology of, 114t, 115f, 116
trust, in family-centered care, 510, 517
  mutual, 515–516
tub baths, after circumcision, 312
tumor(s). See also neoplasm(s)
  choanal atresia vs, 29–30
  cystic hygroma excision cautions with, 14
  germ cell, neuroblastoma vs, 206

neuroblastoma as, 203–212
sacrococcygeal teratoma as, 530–533
spinal tract, 344
Turco procedure, for talipes equinovarus, 382, 387, 389–391, 477
Turner syndrome, 13
twinning accident, 531
twins
    cloacal exstrophy in, 272
    esophageal atresia in, 148
    prune belly syndrome in, 289
two-dimensional echocardiography, in congenital heart disease, 117, 120, 129
tympanic membrane, embryology of, 3
tyrosine, in parenteral nutrition solutions, 436

U

U-shaped cleft soft palate, 32, 37
ulna
    in absent radius, 379–381
    embryology of, 364f
    reduction defects of, 370–371
ultimobranchial body, embryology of, 3
ultrafast MRI, in fetal abnormality evaluation, 523–524, 526, 529, 535, 538
ultrasound
    in anorectal malformations, 178
    antenatal. See prenatal (fetal) ultrasound
    in biliary atresia, 196
    in brain hemorrhage, 353
    in bronchopulmonary sequestration, 80–81
    cranial, in arteriovenous malformation, 9
    in DDH diagnosis
        coronal view, 395–396, 396f
        transverse flexion view, 396
    Doppler
        color, indications for, 9, 81, 120
        in testicular torsion, 253
    in eventration of diaphragm, 95
    fetal. See prenatal (fetal) ultrasound
    in gastroschisis, 156
    in inguinal hernia, 184
    of kidneys. See renal ultrasound
    in megaureter, 282–283
    in neuroblastoma, 208
    in omphalocele, 159
    in patent urachus, 258
    in posterior urethral valves, 244
    in prune belly syndrome, 291
    in spinal cord injury, 358
    in spinal dimples/sinuses, 344–345
    in tethered cord, 341
    in ureteropelvic junction obstruction, 299
ultrasound-guided aspiration, of ovarian cysts, 309
umbilical catheter insertion
    during infant transport, 493, 495, 502
    pain management for, 451, 452t
umbilical cord. See umbilicus
umbilical hernia, 145, 155, 158
umbilical ligaments, median, 221, 256
umbilicus
    in bladder exstrophy, 263, 265–233
    drainage from, in patent urachus, 257f, 258
    embryology of, 220

in gastroschisis, 155, 155f
unconjugated bilirubin, 584
upper extremities
    absent radius in, 378–381, 378f
    brachial plexus injury of, 400–406
    embryology of, 364f, 365, 366f, 367
    prostheses for, 380
    reduction defects of, 368–372
upper gastrointestinal (GI) series
    in gastroesophageal reflux, 152–153
    for malrotation/volvulus, 168
    in tracheomalacia, 49
upper respiratory tract
    embryology of, 1–8
    infections of, in prune belly syndrome, 293–294
urachal cysts, 256, 257f
    diagnosis of, 258
    differential diagnosis of, 258
    treatment of, 259–260
urachal diverticulum, 256, 257f
urachal remnants, total removal of, 260
urachal sinus, 256, 257f
    diagnosis of, 258
    differential diagnosis of, 258
    treatment of, 259
urachus, 584
    anomalies of, 256
    embryology of, 221–222, 222f
    patent, 255–260. See also patent urachus
urea, physiology of, 229, 237
ureteral bud, 218
ureteral catheters, for bladder exstrophy closure, 266
ureteral orifices, in prune belly syndrome, 288
ureteral reimplantation, for megaureter
    complications of, 285
    extravesical approach, 285–287
    intravesical approach, 284–285
    postoperative nursing care, 285–286
ureteral stents
    for bladder exstrophy closure, 266–267
        postoperative nursing care, 270
    for ureteropelvic junction obstruction, 301
ureteral valves, in megaureter, 280t, 281
ureteric bud, 219–220
ureterocele, in megaureter, 280t, 281
ureteropelvic junction obstruction, 294–302
    associations of, 297
    clinical presentation of, 297
    complications of, 301
    conservative, 299–300
    definition of, 294
    diagnosis of, 298–299
    differential diagnosis of, 297
    etiology of, 296
    extraparietal (extraluminal), 295
    incidence of, 296
    intraparietal (intraluminal), 295
    outcomes of, 302
    parietal (luminal), 295–296
    pathophysiology of, 295–296
    in prune belly syndrome, 287
    treatment of, 299–302
        postoperative nursing care, 301–302
        surgical, 300–301
        temporary, 300

ureterostomy, 248, 284, 584
ureterovesical junction, 584
    obstruction of, 294–302
ureters
    in bladder exstrophy, 263, 271
    dilated or wide. *See* megaureter
    embryology of, 219, 219*f*, 221–222, 222*f*
    function of, 279
    in megaureter, 280
    in prune belly syndrome, 287–288
        reconstruction of, 293
    strictures of, 280*t*, 281, 295
    in ureteropelvic junction obstruction, 295–
        296, 298
        surgical management of, 301
urethra
    in bladder exstrophy, 263–264, 266–267
    embryology of, 146, 222, 222*f*, 225, 225*f*–226*f*
    obstruction of
        with posterior urethral valves, 240–252
        in prune belly syndrome, 287–288
urethral atresia, fetal surgery for, 524*t*, 537–539
urethral catheter
    for bladder exstrophy closure, 267
    for posterior urethral valves
        ablation therapy, 246*f*, 247, 249
        immediate drainage, 245–246
urethral groove, embryology of, 225, 225*f*–226*f*
urethral obstruction malformation complex, 287
urethral orifice, embryology of, 226*f*
urethral valve ablation, for posterior urethral
        valves, 246*f*, 247
    complications of, 249
    postoperative nursing care, 250–251
urethral valves, posterior, 240–252. *See also*
        posterior urethral valves (PUV)
urethrocutaneous fistula, with circumcision, 313
urethrotomy, for prune belly syndrome, 293
uric acid, renal excretion of, 238
urinalysis
    in anorectal malformations, 177–179
    during infant transport, 502
    in obstructive uropathy, 538
    in parenteral hyperalimentation monitoring,
        438
    in posterior urethral valves assessment, 244
urinary ascites
    posterior urethral valves and, 242–243
    in prune belly syndrome, 288
urinary bladder. *See* bladder *entries*
urinary calculi
    bladder exstrophy repair and, 268, 271
    megaureter and, 280*t*, 281, 284, 287
urinary diversion
    for anorectal malformations, 179
        male *vs* female, 178*f*, 179*f*
    for bladder exstrophy closure, 267
    for megaureter, 284
    for posterior urethral valves, 247–249, 248*f*
    for ureteropelvic junction obstruction, 300
urinary drainage
    for bladder exstrophy closure, 266, 268
    for patent urachus, 260
    for posterior urethral valves, 245–247
        nephrostomy, 247
        suprapubic catheter, 246–247

urethral catheter, 245–246
urinary incontinence
    in bladder exstrophy, 261, 265, 268, 271
    with cloaca repair, 181
    myelomeningocele and, 337, 340
    myelomeningocele impact on, 337, 340
    neuroblastoma causing, 205
    posterior urethral valves causing, 244, 251
    in spinal cord injury, 359–360
    spinal dimples/sinuses and, 343–345
    tethered cord causing, 340–342
urinary reflux, 537
urinary retention
    after circumcision, 312–313
    in myelomeningocele, 338
urinary system/tract. *See also* bladder *entries*
    anomalies of, in cloacal exstrophy, 274, 277, 279
    anorectal malformations and, 175, 176*f*, 177, 180
    dysfunction of. *See* urinary incontinence
    embryology of, 221–222, 222*f*
    fetal, obstructive anomalies of, 524*t*, 537–539
    obstruction of. *See* urinary tract obstruction
    staged reconstruction of, for prune belly
        syndrome, 293–294
urinary tract infection (UTI)
    in bladder exstrophy repair, 268, 271
    circumcision and, 309
    in megaureter repair, 285–286
    necrotizing enterocolitis *vs*, 173
    postoperative, prophylaxis for, 339
    in prune belly syndrome, 291–292, 294
    in ureteropelvic junction obstruction, 297–
        298, 300–302
    in urinary diversions, for PUV, 249–252
urinary tract obstruction
    bladder outlet, fetal surgery for, 524*t*, 537–539
    lower, fetal surgery for, 537–539. *See also* fetal
        obstructive uropathy
    ovarian cysts causing, 308
    with posterior urethral valves, 240–252
    in prune belly syndrome, 287–288
urine
    acidification of, importance of, 236
    concentration of
        physiology of, 229–230, 238
        post-vesicostomy, 251
    organic components of, 237–238
    renal buffers of, 235–237, 415
    in renal function assessment, 416
urine flow
    diversion of. *See* urinary diversion
    in megaureter, 280–282
        nephrostomy tube for, 283–284
    in prune belly syndrome, 288, 293
    in ureteropelvic junction obstruction, 295
urine output
    in congenital heart disease, 126, 137
    determinants of, 238–239
        developmental, 228
    fetal, 537
    postoperative
        adequate, 108
        maintenance of, 433
        in megaureter repair, 285–286
        in ureteropelvic junction obstruction, 301
    volume of, physiology of, 238–239

urine-reducing substances, in jaundice
    evaluation, 195, 195t
urine screening
    for jaundice evaluation, 195, 195t
    for neuroblastoma, 207
uriniferous tubule, embryology of, 219f, 220
urinoma, 584
urodilatin, in renal physiology, 231
urodynamic studies, of bladder, in posterior
    urethral valves, 244, 251
urogenital complex mobilization, for bladder
    exstrophy in females, 268
urogenital folds
    developmental abnormalities of, 242
    embryology of, 225, 226f
urogenital membrane, 146
    developmental abnormalities of, 242
    in external genitalia, 226f
urogenital sinus, 146, 220
    embryology of, 221–222, 222f, 224f, 227
    in patent urachus, 255–256
uropathy
    obstructive
        fetal surgery for, 524t, 537–539. See also
            fetal obstructive uropathy
        posterior urethral valves causing, 240–252
        sacrococcygeal teratoma associated with, 533
urorectal septum, 146, 272
ursodeoxycholic acid, for cholangitis, 200
uterine contractions, in fetal surgery, 540–541
uterus, 37
    in anorectal malformations, 176f
    in bladder exstrophy, 264
    embryology of, 224, 224f
    mechanical conditions in Robin sequence, 37
UTI. See urinary tract infection

V

VACTERL association
    absent radius associated with, 379–380
    anorectal malformations association with, 177
    in esophageal atresia with fistula, 149
    tetralogy of Fallot association with, 125
    ureteropelvic junction obstruction associated
        with, 297
vacuum delivery
    brain hemorrhage resulting from, 352–353
    skull fractures resulting from, 348, 349f
    spinal cord injury during, 356
VAD. See ventricular access device
vagina
    anorectal malformations and, 180
    in bladder exstrophy, 264
    embryology of, 224, 224f, 227
vaginal masculina, 224f
vaginal orifice
    in bladder exstrophy, 264
    embryology of, 226f
vagus nerve (cranial nerve X), pharyngeal arch
    origin of, 2t, 3
validity, 443, 584
values, cultural, 510
valve resection, for posterior urethral valves, 247
valve systems, for ventriculoperitoneal shunt,
    333–334, 333f

valves
    cardiac, embryology of, 114t, 115
    urethral, anomalies of posterior. See posterior
        urethral valves (PUV)
vanillylmandelic acid (VMA), in neuroblastoma,
    207
varus deformity, of hindfoot, 382, 382f–383f, 385
vas deferens, embryology of, 224, 224f
vasa recta, 219f, 221
vascular access. See also catheters/
        catheterization
    complications of, 210, 467, 579
    for pulmonary disorders, in postoperative
        management, 108–109
    site selection for, 467
vascular anomalies
    in bronchopulmonary sequestration, 80–81,
        84
    cerebral. See arteriovenous malformation
        (AVM)
    chylothorax associated with, 97
vascular compromise, fetal
    amniotic band syndrome associated with,
        373, 377
    limb reduction defects associated with, 368
    talipes equinovarus associated with, 384–385,
        390
vascular resistance
    cerebral, 325
    peripheral, in renal physiology, 227
    renal, 227–228
vascular ring, in tracheomalacia, 47–49
vascular sling, in tracheomalacia, 47–48
vasoactive medications. See vasodilators,
        vasopressors
vasoconstriction, retinopathy of prematurity
        and, 17
vasodilators
    for congenital heart disease, 120
    pulmonary. See nitric oxide (NO)
vasopressin, in renal physiology, 229–230, 238,
        415
vasopressors
    administration during transport, 494, 503
    brain hemorrhage resulting from, 352–353
    IV extravasation of, 467
    for postoperative pulmonary stabilization, 109
VATER association
    anorectal malformations association with, 177
    in esophageal atresia with fistula, 149
VCUG. See voiding cystourethrogram
VDRL, in jaundice evaluation, 195, 195t
vecuronium, 503
vehicle accidents, during infant transport,
        504–505
vein(s)
    cerebral, 584
        malformations of, 8, 328
    hepatic, occlusion of, 160
    median prosencephalic, 8, 581
    portal, occlusion of, 160
    pulmonary
        anomalous connections of, 114t, 134–136,
            134f
        embryology of, 114t, 116

rectal, 146
renal, physiologic role, 227–228
vein of Galen, 8, 328, 584
vein of Markowski, 8, 584
velocardiofacial syndrome, 43
velopharyngeal dysfunction (VPD), 36, 584
vena cava, embryology of, 114t, 116
venipuncture
    during infant transport, 502
    pain expression during, 444
    pain management for, 451
venous/arterial circuit, for extracorporeal
        membrane oxygenation, 555
venous embolization, for arteriovenous
        malformation, 9–10, 11f
venous engorgement, in patent ductus
        arteriosus, 122
venous reservoir, for extracorporeal membrane
        oxygenation, 555
venous/venous circuit, for extracorporeal
        membrane oxygenation, 555
ventilation-perfusion mismatch, 68, 437, 554
ventilation-perfusion scan, in congenital lobar
        emphysema, 66
ventilator circuitry, humidification of
    for bronchogenic cyst, 70
    for congenital cystic adenomatoid
        malformation, 76
    for congenital lobar emphysema, 67–68
    inadequate, 425
ventilators. See mechanical ventilation
ventral mesogastrium, 143
ventral rami, of spinal nerves, in brachial plexus,
        401f
ventricle(s)
    of brain. See cerebral ventricles
    of heart. See cardiac ventricles
ventricular access device (VAD), for
        hydrocephalus, 330–331
ventricular septal defect (VSD), 114t, 124, 124f
    surgical management of, 126–128
ventricular septum, cardiac, development of,
        114t, 116
ventricular tap, for hydrocephalus, 329
ventricular zone, of brain, 323
ventriculitis, 328, 585
ventriculoperitoneal shunt
    ethical considerations of, 360
    for hydrocephalus, 332–333, 333f
        complications of, 333–334
        diuretics vs, 330
        inguinal hernia and, 183
ventriculostomy, 585
    third, for hydrocephalus, 333
ventriculostomy catheter, for hydrocephalus,
        331–332, 331f
ventriculosubgaleal shunt, for hydrocephalus,
        333–334
vernix caseosa, 458
vertebrae/vertebral column. See also spine
    bony defect in, 533. See also
        myelomeningocele (MMC)
    embryology of, 365
    fusion of, for spinal cord injury, 358

vertebral arches, nonfusion of primordial halves
        of, 533. See also myelomeningocele
        (MMC)
vertical osteotomy, posterior, for bladder
        exstrophy closure, 266f, 267
verumontanum, 585
very low birth weight (VLBW) infants
    fluid therapy during transport, 495–496
    gastroesophageal reflux in, 152
vesicles, primary, of primitive brain, 322–323
vesicoamniotic shunts, for obstructive uropathy,
        524t, 537–539
vesicointestinal fissure, 272
vesicointestinal fistula, 272, 277
vesicostomy, 585
    for posterior urethral valves, 247, 248f, 249
        complications of, 249
        postoperative nursing care, 250–251
    for prune belly syndrome, 292
vesicoureteral, 585
vesicoureteral reflux, 242, 248–249, 271, 279
    circumcision for, 309
    in megaureter, 279–281, 280t, 286
    prune belly syndrome impact on, 292
    in ureteropelvic junction obstruction, 297
vesicourethral canal, 222
vestibule, embryology of, 226f
viability, of fetus, 360
vibration stress, during infant transport,
        484–485
    management of, 485–486, 506
vimentin, in talipes equinovarus, 383
viral infections
    in biliary atresia, 191, 192t, 193
    congenital heart disease associated with,
        116–117
visitation plan, parental, for NICU, 515
visual examination, rectal, for malformations,
        177
visual impairment, in retinopathy of
        prematurity, 16, 18, 20, 25
vitamin A deficiency, biliary atresia and, 195, 202
vitamin D
    deficiency of, biliary atresia and, 195, 202
    in renal physiology, 227, 235
vitamin E deficiency, biliary atresia and, 195, 202
vitamin K deficiency, common bile duct
        obstruction and, 191, 195–197, 202
vitamins
    deficiencies of
        biliary atresia and, 195, 202
        common bile duct obstruction and, 191,
            195–196, 202
        limb reduction defects associated with, 369
    in parenteral nutrition solutions, 436
vitrectomy, 585
    for retinopathy of prematurity, 20t, 22–24
vitreous humor, retinopathy of prematurity and,
        18
VLBW. See very low birth weight infants
VMA. See vanillylmandelic acid
vocal cord paralysis, 45–47
    associations of, 46
    clinical presentation of, 45–46
    complications of, 47
    definition of, 45

diagnosis of, 46
differential diagnosis of, 46
etiology of, 45
incidence of, 45
nursing care for, 4
pathophysiology of, 45
surgical treatment of, 46
unilateral vs bilateral, 45
vocal folds, laryngeal web of, 42–45
vocational therapy, for pulmonary disorders sequelae, 109
voice
    laryngeal web impact on, 43–44
    resonance of, 6
    vocal cord paralysis and, 45–47
voiding
    after circumcision, 312
    delayed, in newborns, 239, 243
    infant patterns of, 239
        abnormal, 242–243
voiding cystourethrogram (VCUG)
    in anorectal malformations, 178
    in megaureter, 282
    in myelomeningocele management, 39–340
    in patent urachus, 258
    in posterior urethral valves, 244, 244f
    in prune belly syndrome, 291
    in ureteropelvic junction obstruction, 299
volume expanders
    administration during transport, 493, 495–497, 503
    albumin as, 429, 434, 575
volvulus, of gastrointestinal tract, 166–169
    associations of, 167
    clinical presentation of, 166
    complications of, 168
    definition of, 166, 167f
    diagnosis of, 167–168
    differential diagnosis of, 167
    etiology of, 166
    fixation of, 166, 167f
    incidence of, 166
    outcomes of, 169
    pathophysiology of, 166
    surgical treatment of, 168
        postoperative nursing care, 168
vomer bone, 585
    in cleft lip/palate, 32f, 33f
vomer-plasty, in cleft lip/palate, 34, 585
vomiting. See emesis
Von Rosen splint, for DDH, 397
VPD. See velopharyngeal dysfunction
VSD. See ventricular septal defect

W

W-plasty repair, of amniotic band syndrome, 376
"waddling gait"
    in bladder exstrophy, 263, 271
    in cloacal exstrophy, 279
wafer, neonatal, for stomas, 471, 471f, 474f
"waiter's tip" posture, in brachial plexus, 403, 403f
Walker Warburg syndrome, 329
Wangensteen-Rice x-ray, in anorectal malformations, 178

warming procedures
    during infant transport, 484–485, 492f, 493–494, 502
    postoperative, in craniosynostosis repair, 54
water balance. See body water composition
water loss
    fluid and electrolyte disturbances with, 427, 427t
    hypernatremia associated with, 419
    insensible, 419, 425, 580
    skin role in, 457, 459
    in surgical infants, 429–431
        abdominal quadrants estimation of, 433
water overload, 426–427, 427t
water-soluble vitamins, in parenteral nutrition solutions, 436
WBC. See white blood cell
weaning
    from extracorporeal membrane oxygenation, 559
    from opioid analgesics, 447, 450
        withdrawal score sheet for, 448f–449f, 450
webs/webbing
    anal, 177
    digital, developmental, 364f, 365, 366f, 367
    intestinal atresia/stenosis associated with, 162
weight gain
    cloacal exstrophy repair and, 279
    poor, cleft lip/palate and, 32
weight loss
    in biliary atresia, 194
    immediate postnatal, 239, 414
Weinzwieg classification, of amniotic band syndrome, 376
wheeze, 585
white blood cell (WBC) count, in necrotizing enterocolitis, 173
white matter, of CNS, 323
withholding, of treatment, 360, 361t. See also delayed treatment
wolffian ducts, embryology of, 224f
work of breathing (WOB), in congenital heart disease, 118, 122–123
wound care/management
    documentation guidelines for, 468–469
    of gastrostomy tube, 565–569
    general principles of, 463–466
    during infant transport, 493
    of injured skin, 466–468
    in necrotizing enterocolitis, 174
    of ostomy stomas, 469–476. See also ostomy(ies); stoma(s)
    postoperative, 109
        for circumcision, 312
        for cleft lip/palate repair, 35–36
        for cystic hygroma, 16
        for inguinal hernia repair, 186
        for megaureter repair, 286
        for myelomeningocele repair, 340
    of surgical wounds
        by primary closure, 468–469
        by secondary intention, 469
    of ventriculoperitoneal shunt, 334
wound dehiscence, in bladder exstrophy repair, 268
wound healing

documentation guidelines for, 468–469
impaired, factors of, 462
schematic representation of, 460f
stages and components of, 461–462, 461f
in surgical wounds
    by primary closure, 468–469
    by secondary intention, 469
wrists
    in limb reduction defects, 369
    reduction defects of, 371
    splinting of, for brachial plexus injury,
        404–405

X

X chromosome, in sexual differentiation, 222–
    223, 223f

X-linked hydrocephalus, 328–329
XX chromosome, in sexual differentiation, 222
XY chromosome, in sexual differentiation, 223

Y

Y chromosome, in sexual differentiation, 222–
    223, 223f
yeast infections, topical, 467

Z

Z-plasty repair, of amniotic band syndrome, 376,
    376f
zinc, in parenteral nutrition solutions, 436
zones, of retinopathy of prematurity, 17–18, 17f

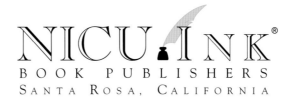

NICU Ink®
BOOK PUBLISHERS
SANTA ROSA, CALIFORNIA

Continuing Education Program

The examinations based on this text, that can be taken for continuing education credit are located at www.neonatalnetwork.com. Click on the link to NICU Ink and follow the link from there.

Tests are taken online and your certificate is immediately available if you pass the test by answering 80 percent of the questions correctly.

Cost for courses:
    Course 1: $75.00   25 contact hours
    Course 2: $50.00   15 contact hours

VISA and Mastercard are accepted for payment on our secure website.